Handbook of Social Development

A Lifespan Perspective

Perspectives in Developmental Psychology

Series Editor: Michael Lewis
Robert Wood Johnson Medical School
New Brunswick, New Jersey

ACTION IN SOCIAL CONTEXT
Perspectives on Early Development
Edited by Jeffrey J. Lockman and Nancy L. Hazen

ASSESSMENT OF YOUNG DEVELOPMENTALLY
DISABLED CHILDREN
Edited by Theodore D. Wachs and Robert Sheehan

COGNITIVE DEVELOPMENT AND CHILD
PSYCHOTHERAPY
Edited by Stephen R. Shirk

THE DIFFERENT FACES OF MOTHERHOOD
Edited by Beverly Birns and Dale F. Hay

FATHERING BEHAVIORS
The Dynamics of the Man–Child Bond
Wade C. Mackey

HANDBOOK OF SOCIAL DEVELOPMENT
A Lifespan Perspective
Edited by Vincent B. Van Hasselt and Michel Hersen

PSYCHOLOGY OF DEVELOPMENT AND HISTORY
Edited by Klaus F. Riegel

THE RISKS OF KNOWING
Developmental Impediments to School Learning
Karen Zelan

SOCIAL AND PERSONALITY DEVELOPMENT
An Evolutionary Synthesis
Kevin B. MacDonald

Handbook of Social Development

A Lifespan Perspective

Edited by

VINCENT B. VAN HASSELT

and

MICHEL HERSEN

Center for Psychological Studies
Nova University
Fort Lauderdale, Florida

PLENUM PRESS • NEW YORK AND LONDON

Library of Congress Cataloging-in-Publication Data

Handbook of social development : a lifespan perspective / edited by
  Vincent B. Van Hasselt and Michel Hersen.
      p.   cm. -- (Perspectives in developmental psychology)
    Includes bibliographical references and index.
    ISBN 0-306-44141-1
      1. Socialization. 2. Social intelligence. 3. Social skills.
  4. Developmental psychology.   I. Van Hasselt, Vincent B.
  II. Hersen, Michel. III. Series.
    [DNLM: 1. Human Development. 2. Interpersonal Relations.
  3. Socialization.   BF 7132 H2365]
  BF723.S62H36 1992
  303.3'2--dc20
  DNLM/DLC
  for Library of Congress   92-17058
                                                                  CIP

ISBN 0-306-44141-1

©1992 Plenum Press, New York
A Division of Plenum Publishing Corporation
233 Spring Street, New York, N.Y. 10013

Printed in the United States of America

Contributors

BROOKE A. BENSON, Department of Psychology, University of Mississippi, University, Mississippi 38677

GARY R. BIRCHLER, Veterans Affairs Medical Center, San Diego, California 92161 and University of California School of Medicine, San Diego, California 92093

INGE BRETHERTON, Department of Child and Family Studies, University of Wisconsin-Madison, Madison, Wisconsin 53706

EARNESTINE BROWN, Psychology Department, University of Pittsburgh, Pittsburgh, Pennsylvania 15260

CELIA A. BROWNELL, Psychology Department, University of Pittsburgh, Pittsburgh, Pennsylvania 15260

JEANETTE SMITH CHRISTOPHER, Department of Psychology, West Virginia University, Morgantown, West Virginia 26506-6040

JOSHUA EHRLICH, Department of Psychiatry, University of Michigan, Ann Arbor, Michigan 48104

RICHARD M. EISLER, Department of Psychology, Virginia Polytechnic Institute and State University, Blacksburg, Virginia 24061-0436

RAY FEROZ, Clarion University of Pennsylvania, Clarion, Pennsylvania 16214

ROBERT B. FIELDS, Allegheny Neuropsychiatric Institute, Oakdale, Pennsylvania 15071 and Department of Psychiatry, Medical College of Pennsylvania, Allegheny Campus, Pittsburgh, Pennsylvania 15212

CONSTANCE T. FISCHER, Department of Psychology, Duquesne University, Pittsburgh, Pennsylvania 15282-1705

ALAN FOGEL, Department of Psychology, University of Utah, Salt Lake City, Utah 84112

IGOR GRANT, Psychiatry and Research Services, Veterans Affairs Medical Center, San Diego, California 92161; Department of Psychiatry, University of California, San Diego, California 92093; and Department of Psychology, San Diego State University, San Diego, California 92182

ALAN M. GROSS, Department of Psychology, University of Mississippi, University, Mississippi 38677

DAVID J. HANSEN, Department of Psychology, University of Nebraska, Lincoln, Nebraska 68588

WILLARD W. HARTUP, Institute of Child Development, University of Minnesota, Minneapolis, Minnesota 55455

JEANNETTE M. HAVILAND, Department of Psychology, Rutgers University, New Brunswick, New Jersey 08903

THEODORE JACOB, Division of Family Studies, University of Arizona, Tucson, Arizona 85721

JEANNE KARNS, Department of Human Development and the Family, University of Nebraska, Lincoln, Nebraska 68588

LYNDA J. KATZ, University of Pittsburgh School of Medicine, Western Psychiatric Institute and Clinic, Pittsburgh, Pennsylvania 15213

HOWARD D. LERNER, Department of Psychiatry, University of Michigan, Ann Arbor, Michigan 48104

STEPHEN C. MESSER, University of Pittsburgh School of Medicine, Western Psychiatric Institute and Clinic, Pittsburgh, Pennsylvania 15213

DANIEL MESSINGER, Department of Psychology, University of Utah, Salt Lake City, Utah 84112

RICHARD K. MORYCZ, Western Psychiatric Institute and Clinic, Pittsburgh, Pennsylvania 15213

DOUGLAS W. NANGLE, Department of Psychology, West Virginia University, Morgantown, West Virginia 26506-6040

MARION O'BRIEN, Department of Human Development, University of Kansas, Lawrence, Kansas 66045

THOMAS L. PATTERSON, Psychiatry and Research Services, Veterans Affairs Medical Center, San Diego, California 92161; Department of Psychiatry, University of California, San Diego, California 92093; and Department of Psychology, San Diego State University, San Diego, California 92182

GREGORY S. PETTIT, Department of Family and Child Development, Auburn University, Auburn, Alabama 36849

KIM RAGSDALE, Department of Psychology, Virginia Polytechnic Institute and State University, Blacksburg, Virginia 24061-0436

LINDA ROSE-KRASNOR, Department of Psychology, Brock University, St. Catharines, Ontario L2S 3A1

KENNETH H. RUBIN, Department of Psychology, University of Waterloo, Waterloo, Ontario N2L 3G1

SUSAN B. SILVERBERG, Division of Family Studies, University of Arizona, Tucson, Arizona 85721

K. DANIELLE SMITH, Laboratory of Developmental Psychology, National Institute of Mental Health, Bethesda, Maryland 20891

LAWRENCE W. SMITH, Management Psychologists, 411 University Street, Seattle, Washington 98101

DANIEL L. TENNENBAUM, Department of Psychology, Kent State University, Kent, Ohio 44242

DOUGLAS M. TETI, Department of Psychology, University of Maryland Baltimore County, Baltimore, Maryland 21228

HEATHER WALKER, Department of Psychology, University of Utah, Salt Lake City, Utah 84112

ARLENE S. WALKER-ANDREWS, Department of Psychology, Rutgers University, New Brunswick, New Jersey 08903

CAROLYN ZAHN-WAXLER, Laboratory of Developmental Psychology, National Institute of Mental Health, Bethesda, Maryland 20891

Preface

Social development over one's lifetime is a complex area that has received considerable attention in the psychological, social-psychological, and sociological literature over the years. Surprisingly, however, since 1969, when Rand McNally published Goslin's *Handbook of Socialization*, no comprehensive statement of the field has appeared in book form. Given the impressive data in this area that have been adduced over the last two decades, we trust that our handbook will serve to fill that gap.

In this volume we have followed a lifespan perspective, starting with the social interactions that transpire in the earliest development stages and progressing through childhood, adolescence, adulthood, and, finally, one's senior years. In so doing we cover a variety of issues in depth.

The book contains 21 chapters and is divided into five parts: I, Theoretical Perspectives; II, Infants and Toddlers; III, Children and Adolescents; IV, Adults; and V, The Elderly. Each of the parts begins with introductory material that reviews the overall issues to be considered.

Many individuals have contributed to the final production of this handbook. Foremost are our eminent contributors, who graciously agreed to share with us their expertise. We also thank our administrative and technical staff for their assistance in carrying out the day-to-day tasks necessary to complete such a project. Finally, we thank Eliot Werner, Executive Editor at Plenum, for his willingness to publish and for his tolerance for the delays inevitable in the development of a large handbook.

Vincent B. Van Hasselt
Michel Hersen

Contents

I

Theoretical Perspectives

Whether one is concerned with normal development or psychopathology, a thorough understanding of social development over the lifespan is mandatory. From an empirical perspective, in the most ideal of worlds one would study individuals continuously over large blocks of time (i.e., decades) to precisely understand the development and changes in social interaction. Because this obviously is not highly feasible, the next best alternative is to study different, but yet similar, individuals at critical stages in their continuing development. However, to unite these sometimes disparate facts that emerge from such discontinuous study, a unifying theoretical perspective has proven to be a beneficial binding agent and a stimulus for new research.

In Part I, five overarching theoretical perspectives about a lifespan approach to social development are presented. Although each perspective is concerned with basically the same lifespan, vastly different theoretical views are presented. Gregory S. Pettit (Chapter 1) examines developmental theories. Central to his discussion of development is the concept of tension reduction or homeostasis as the desirable end state of interactions between the individual and the environment. When disequilibrium takes place, the individual's ability to cope is threatened, but such disequilibrium can also serve as an impetus to move to the next developmental stage. Jeannette M. Haviland and Arlene S. Walker-Andrews (Chapter 2) consider emotion socialization from the developmental and ethological viewpoints. In so doing, four primary components contributing to developmental change are examined in detail: structure, reflex, temperament, and knowledge. Howard D. Lerner and Joshua Ehrlich (Chapter 3) review psychodynamic models that recently have begun to look at the dimensions of development over the lifespan. Examples are the changes in narcissism in adulthood and separation–individuation, also in adulthood. Throughout the chapter the authors attempt to integrate the influence of intrapsychic processes across succeeding maturational stages. Brooke A. Benson, Stephen C. Messer, and Alan M. Gross (Chapter 4) describe learning theories as they relate to social development. Development is conceptualized as accumulated social interactions and accomplished via "organism action–environmental reactions." Most crucial to the behavioral position are the sequences of environmental events and subsequent effects or consequences.

1

Learning concepts included are classical and operant conditioning as well as cognitive and mediational factors. Although biological variables are given credence, learning is given prominence in this approach to the problem. Finally, Constance T. Fischer (Chapter 5) presents the humanistic approach to lifespan development, highlighting issues germane to development in women and the elderly. As a theoretical base and philosophical framework from which to operate, the phenomenological approach to research and understanding is promoted. However, the author does acknowledge that as a function of the major emphasis on the individual, longitudinal and comparative studies have received less attention from the humanists than they deserve.

Developmental Theories

GREGORY S. PETTIT

INTRODUCTION

The goal of this chapter is to present an overview of the major theoretical perspectives on social development, with particular emphasis on those theories that span the entire course of individual development. *Development* refers here to ontogenetic changes that are manifested in distinctive styles of relating to other individuals at different points in the lifecycle. These changes in interpersonal style represent reorganizations of behavior, cognition, and affect associated with certain developmental tasks or issues.

An integrative theme will be pursued, with the aim of bringing forth a greater understanding of the strengths and limitations of each perspective. Insofar as this chapter is primarily concerned with "strong" developmental theories (see Damon, 1983), it will necessarily exclude those perspectives that are explicitly or implicitly nondevelopmental. Most notably, social learning theory, discussed in a separate chapter of this volume, will be excluded. Standard textbook treatments of social-developmental theory typically focus on psychoanalytic theory and its derivatives and on cognitive-developmental theory. More recently, ethological-attachment theory has achieved sufficient status to be discussed in many texts alongside the more traditional intrapsychic and cognitive perspectives. Each of these perspectives continues to account for extensive research and theoretical commentary; consequently, these theories will serve as a guide for the discussion that follows.

Many of the theoretical positions to be discussed here have undergone significant transformation through the years. Important contributions of these perspectives are thus not limited to those made by the originators of the theories.

GREGORY S. PETTIT • Department of Family and Child Development, Auburn University, Auburn, Alabama 36849.

Handbook of Social Development: A Lifespan Perspective, edited by Vincent B. Van Hasselt and Michel Hersen. Plenum Press, New York, 1992.

Where possible, an effort will be made to trace existing positions to their earlier theoretical foundations and to outline the major conceptual developments responsible for these transformations. However, given space limitations, it is impossible to address the myriad offshoots of the major perspectives. Included in the discussion are positions judged to be fundamental to our understanding of social development and those providing a synthesis of social-developmental perspectives.

In the sections that follow, each theoretical perspective will be evaluated in terms of three developmental issues. The first issue concerns the *origins* of interpersonal exchange. How does the theory account for the initial development of social awareness, social skill, and more general social orientations? The second issue concerns the *mechanism for developmental change*: What factors are postulated to stimulate the continuing development of interpersonal style? The third issue, *transfer*, focuses on the processes governing interpersonal relationship coherence, that is, the manner in which interpersonal styles are carried over from one social situation or type of relationship to another (e.g., from child-with-parents to child-with-peers).

PSYCHOANALYTIC THEORY

Many of our current conceptions of social development are historically indebted to psychoanalytic theory, and more specifically to Freudian theory (e.g., Freud, 1940/1964). Although psychoanalysis has not served as a strong guide for scientific studies of human social development, its rich and insightful language—perhaps better viewed in metaphorical than empirical terms—has spurred a reappraisal of the processes governing interpersonal relations.

Psychoanalytic theory emphasizes the decisive role of the early childhood years in the development of personality and interpersonal style. This assertion stemmed from Freud's observation that his adult neurotic patients often dwelled on earlier, presumably traumatic, social experiences. The concomitant implications were that personality, once formed, is stable throughout life and that the general patterns of social behavior emerging from early childhood are largely irreversible (Hall, 1954).

Freud (1940/1964) argued that social development proceeds through a maturationally determined sequence of psychosexual stages. Each stage is associated with a particular bodily region serving as the focal point of sexual energy (*libido*). At each stage, the child faces a conflict of how to expend sexual energy in ways judged acceptable by society. Freud stressed that if too much energy was spent working through a conflict at a particular stage, the child might develop a "fixation" that would permanently scar personality development. The caregiving environment figures prominently in determining exactly what kind of impression each stage will leave on the developing child's personality.

The first psychosexual stage reflects Freud's observation that infants spend inordinate amounts of time in oral pursuits. Sexual pleasure in this *oral* stage emanates from stimulation of the lips and the oral cavity. At this time, brain structures associated with feeding activity are well developed, and oral skin receptors are sensitive to stimulation (McConnell, 1977). Here, the infant is faced with the challenge of seeking oral pleasure within the guidelines provided by the maternal caregiver, who provides the nourishment necessary for survival. If the infant's oral needs are thwarted, dependency needs may develop and carry forward into subsequent stages (e.g., as when a school-aged child behaves in a clingy, teacher-dependent manner).

In the second year of life, the libido shifts to the sphincter muscles, and matters of elimination and retention reign. Toilet training assumes great significance during this *anal* stage, as the caregiver attempts to combat the child's newfound pleasure in defecation with socially prescribed notions of appropriate toileting behavior. Lack of resolution of the conflict associated with this stage may result in retentive characteristics such as selfishness, occurring when caregivers overemphasize the importance of feces and the child comes to believe that he or she has lost something valuable.

The *phallic* stage, beginning around age 3, represents a libidinal shift toward the genitals. Owing to differences in genitalia, this stage differs somewhat for boys and girls. According to Freud, the boy has incestuous desires for his mother and sees his father as a rival (the well-known Oedipus complex). The boy fears that he will be discovered by the father and recognizes that he cannot compete with father for mother's affection. To alleviate the anxiety (fear of castration) created by this situation, he becomes overcompliant to the father's wishes, which is best accomplished by assuming characteristics of the father. Through this identification process, the boy adopts an appropriate sex-role identity and internalizes his father's (and presumably society's) moral values. The conflict associated with this stage and its resolution proceeds differently for girls. The girl, noting that she has no penis, seeks contact with the person having the desired organ—the father. She emulates the mother because of the close emotional bond she has shared with her mother and because this may be one way to attract her father. Through identification with her mother, she assumes the appropriate sex-role identity and internalizes suitable social mores. The theory suggests that because the process of identification for girls is based primarily on emotional attachment, girls may be less sex-typed and have a more poorly defined moral sense than boys, who operate according to the more powerful process of identification with the aggressor (Grusec & Lytton, 1988).

Following this intense period of sexual confusion is the *latency* stage (approximately ages 6 to 12), a time of relative calm in individual psychosexual development. During this period, sexual activity subsides as children channel their libinal energy into socially acceptable outlets, such as schoolwork and social play. This is an important time for the refinement of social skills and the acquisition of new roles and abilities.

The onset of adolescence signals the final psychosexual stage: the *genital* stage. Nascent sexual maturity, including increased hormonal activity, presumably underlies the renewed libinal focus on sexual matters. Unlike the earlier phallic period, sexual energy now is directed toward age-appropriate heterosexual relationships, with the instinctual aim of human reproduction. Love and tenderness begin to emerge, as does a fuller appreciation of friendships. This is the longest of the psychosexual stages, stretching from adolescence to old age.

Developmental Issues

ORIGINS

Freudian theory posits that social interests and skills originate because of instinctual, biological forces (libidinal energy) within the person. The libidinal energy eventually is distributed among the *id, ego,* and the *superego,* three personality components that interact to produce behavior (Hall & Lindzey, 1978). When libidinal energy is pentup, tension results. The id functions to relieve this tension (i.e., is pleasure seeking) but in social contexts is constrained by the contrary desires of others. The executive personality function (the ego) engages in reasoning and problem solving in an attempt to locate realistic sources of need gratification. Concomitant with the identification process occurring during the phallic stage, there emerges a "moral" and sometimes overcontrolling aspect of personality—the superego. It is the personality dimension that transcends individual needs and makes possible orderly, sociable society.

MECHANISM FOR DEVELOPMENTAL CHANGE

According to Freudian theory, individuals are propelled through the developmental stages because of perturbations (conflicts) in their intrapsychic systems (Miller, 1983). The sources of these conflicts include maturational shifts in the bodily focus of libidinal energy, external frustrations that interfere with the individual's efforts at discharging the buildup of this energy, and anxiety caused by anticipated physical and psychological pain. Developmental change takes place as individuals seek to reduce the tension associated with these conflicts (e.g., by employing more sophisticated coping strategies). Development does not, however, always proceed in a steady, incremental manner. A fixation, or halting, may occur at any stage to protect the individual from excessive anxiety surrounding progression to the next stage. For example, a child who is anxious about establishing relationships with peers may fixate at a stage marked by relative dependence on parents. In this particular case, fixation is considered more likely if the child has suffered parental rejection and is fearful of further rejection as he or she seeks to establish new and independent relationship (Hall, 1954).

TRANSFER

Interpersonal styles are generalized to new settings and new relationships by an instinctual process called *repetition compulsion.* This process refers to the tendency of the individual to repeat over and over a cycle of events beginning with bodily excitation (e.g., as when one is hungry or anxious) and ending in quiescence (e.g., as when one consumes food or displaces anxiety) (Hall, 1954). Within the social sphere, this process occurs as individuals strive to recreate experiences and types of relationships that are familiar to them. For example, an individual whose needs have been continually frustrated may seek out relationships that promise more of the same, even when the familiar experience is a painful one.

Continuity in interpersonal style across settings and relationships is also promoted by cognitive defenses and controls (Baldwin, 1980). Defense mechanisms (such as projection, reaction formation, and repression) interfere with rational thought and thereby constrain social perception, leading to traitlike behavior toward others. Cognitive controls also affect the ways in which information is processed. The social perceptions of the hysteric, for example, are diffuse and highly impressionistic, with little relevant contextual detail (Baldwin, 1980).

In summary, Freud's influential work spurred students of social development to consider intrapsychic aspects of human social behavior (e.g., anxiety, conflict, and tension reduction) and to examine childhood experiences for the origins of adult personality and social style. Likewise, his work provides direction for understanding some of the mechanisms underlying developmental change and coherence in personality and interpersonal style.

NEOPSYCHOANALYTIC PERSPECTIVES

The criticisms of Freudian theory are extensive and well known. Among the more commonly cited limitations are the theory's reliance on poorly defined terms (e.g., "penis envy") that are difficult to operationalize, the lack of objectivity and replicability in the way in which information is collected, and the absence of clear rules that would allow prediction of individual behavior (Hall & Lindzey, 1978). Although the theory continues to stimulate analytical writing and clinical work, its value to scientific psychology has declined through the years. Nonetheless, Freudian theory influenced many current research topics, including infant–mother attachment, moral development, sex typing, and aggression (Miller, 1983).

Freudian theory eventually spawned several revisionist theories, some of which have provided more testable—and hence more scientifically useful—propositions. The word of Erik Erikson is probably best known in this regard, although other theorists, particularly Harry Stack Sullivan, have also made lasting contributions to post-Freudian conceptualizations of social development. The key point of departure for these neopsychoanalytic theorists is that they place greater emphasis on the social environment, and less emphasis on biological drives, than does traditional Freudian theory. Moreover, both Erikson and Sullivan emphasize the importance of interpersonal relationships throughout life (although Sullivan does not describe postmaturity "stages"). Thus these theorists have extended the psychodynamic perspective by more explicitly addressing the social environment and by focusing more on the lifelong processes that govern the development of personality and interpersonal style.

Erik Erikson's Psychosocial Theory

Erikson's (1963, 1968) theory of *psychosocial* development parallels in many ways earlier Freudian theory: He acknowledges the role of instincts, stresses the importance of maturation, embraces the notion of conflicts associated with maturation, and describes social development in terms of successive stages. However, Erikson discounts the significance of sexuality as a motivating force in development and instead focuses on the role of interpersonal crises that emerge at different points in the life cycle.

Erikson describes eight stages of psychosocial development, each with a specific social conflict that results in a psychosocial crisis. The critical issue in the first stage is whether the infant experiences a reliable and responsive caregiving environment that is attuned to the infant's needs. Such a caregiving environment promotes a sense of trust, whereas an unreliable or unresponsive social environment engenders fear and uncertainty. Infants provided reliable care are more active and challenged by the environment, whereas infants experiencing unreliable caregiving may be passive and disinterested in a world they sense as unpredictable and uncontrollable. The second stage is marked by the crisis of autonomy, as the child seeks to exercise control over bodily functions and the external environment. During this toddlerhood period, parents attempt to socialize the child toward obedience and self-control. Parental disapproval and overcontrol result in shame; parental support and moderate amounts of control contribute to a sense of autonomy. In the third stage (ages 3 to 6), children expand on this autonomy by trying to act more "grown up" and by taking more initiative for their actions. Parental supportiveness contributes to a sense of initiative, whereas parental disapproval may interfere with initiative and produce guilt. It is also during this stage that attraction to the opposite-sex parent occurs, but according to Erikson, this is only an attempt to obtain that parent's affection. Feelings of guilt may arise, however, if the child's efforts are viewed by the same-sex parent as intrusive.

The fourth Eriksonian stage, occurring during middle childhood (and corresponding to Freud's latency stage), is characterized by the crisis of achieving social and academic competence in the extrafamilial learning environment. For the first time, the family is not the dominant social force determining how the conflict is resolved. Rather, teachers and peers provide an atmosphere where the child feels confident and acts industriously, or conversely, where the child feels (or is made to feel) inferior and behaves inadequately.

As the child enters adolescence, a conflict emerges between the demands for maturity associated with adulthood and the security (and immaturity) of the childhood years. This is a period marked by consolidation of varied self-perceptions and consideration of what role(s) one wants to play in society. Success in this endeavor results in a sense of identity; unsuccessful searching (or a lack of searching) may result in identity confusion (or diffusion). Social experience, particularly with peers, figures importantly in how the adolescent comes to view himself or herself in relation to others (i.e., the social-self component of personal identity). No other stage or concept in Erikson's theory has received as much research attention as "identity." In large measure this is because of the empirical work of Marcia (1966, 1976), who developed a typology of identity statuses based on the presence of conflict and the active searching for resolution. Even though there is some question as to whether Marcia's work actually represents an extension of, or break with, Erikson's theory (Coté & Levine, 1988), his operationalization of the identity construct provided a basis for numerous empirical studies.

The remainder of Erikson's stages pertain to conflicts in the adult years. Identity formation in adolescence paves the way for the establishment of intimate cross-sex relationships in early adulthood. Erikson contends that one must know oneself (i.e., have a coherent self-identity) before one can intimately know another. An inability to establish intimate relationships results in loneliness or isolation. Another way of thinking about the critical issue of this stage is that one's ego strength is dependent on a mutual partner with whom to share child-rearing responsibility and the productivity inherent in a shared and mutual relationship (Hall & Lindzey, 1978).

The next stage is represented by a concern with productivity and what is generated (children, ideas, etc.) and the setting forth of standards for future generations. These standards (or values) are determined by the particular culture in which one lives, but the root standard is one of caring, that is, concern for others and the sharing of material and emotional resources with others (termed generativity). Those who are unwilling or unable to accept these responsibilities will become stagnant or self-centered. This stage logically leads to the final of Erikson's stages, occurring during old age, which reflects the capacity of the individual to look back upon a fulfilled life. When products are left behind and a history of intimacy and caring is apparent, the individual moves into a stage of ego integrity. Conversely, individuals who look back on life with bitterness, resentment, and regret experience a sense of despair.

It should be noted that although a particular developmental crisis marks each of Erikson's stages, the crisis has "analogs" in both prior and subsequent stages. This feature of Erikson's theory is illustrated in Table 1 for the development of identity over the lifespan.

The diagonal lists the ascendant crisis marking each of the psychosocial stages. The search for identity may be traced along the vertical axis to its earlier and later forms. These analogs represent the nonascendant versions of the crisis, coexisting with the dominant crisis of each stage. The analogs provide the groundwork for resolution of the crisis during its period of ascendancy (Damon, 1983). Thus the analog of the search for identity during middle childhood is the issue of task identification versus futility. The horizontal dimension describes the components of the crisis at a particular stage of development. As can be seen in the table, crises have multiple components that are the by-product of earlier crisis resolution. As Damon (1983) notes,

> Adaptive psychosocial development means resolving each successive crisis as it arises during the stages of the life cycle [which] has implications both for the other aspects of psychosocial development that coexist with the crisis at that stage and for the resolution of all future crises as they appear in their own time. (p. 87)

Harry Stack Sullivan's Interpersonal Theory

Like Erikson, Sullivan (1953) proposed a stage theory in which the quality of interpersonal relationships, particularly with family members and peers, is critical in the development of personality and interpersonal style. Sullivan viewed maturational-biological forces as providing a substrate from which personality and social style emerge but argued that interpersonal experience accounts for variations in these styles, Individuals styles are characterized by *dynamisms*, or habitual patterns of interaction, which are modified as a result of maturation and life experience. An important dynamism is the self-system, which protects the individual from excessive anxiety associated with the conflicts and contradictions of human society. It serves a supervisory role by sanctioning behavior that minimizes interpersonal conflict. This protective mechanism often operates in an irrational manner, resulting in distorted perceptions of self and others. These rudimentary perceptions or images eventually lead to the development of *personifications*, which are complex summary descriptions of types of relationships (Hall & Lindzey, 1978).

Sullivan described six stages of development that roughly parallel those of Freud and Erikson. The first is *infancy*, when nursing provides the initial social experience, from which budding personifications of mother figures (e.g., good mother versus bad mother) emerge. The acquisition of language marks the beginning of *childhood*, when interpersonal experience may become more threatening because of the societal proscriptions for behavior imposed on the child. The *juvenile* stage (a latency-type stage) occurs when children are moving into extrafamilial social settings (e.g., school) and are beginning to develop their own set of social goals or orientations. *Preadolescence* follows and is the period in which intimate same-sex friendships are established and more mutual or reciprocal

TABLE 1. Erikson's Stages of Psychosocial Development

	1	2	3	4	5	6	7	8
VIII Mature age								Integrity vs. despair
VII Adulthood							Generativity vs. stagnation	
VI Young adults						Intimacy vs. isolation		
V Adolescence	Temporal perspective vs. time confusion	Self-certainty vs. self-consciousness	Role experimentation vs. role fixation	Apprenticeship vs. work paralysis	Identity vs. identity confusion	Sexual polarization vs. bisexual confusion	Leadership and fellowship vs. authority confusion	Ideological commitment vs. confusion of values
IV School age				Industry vs. inferiority	Task identification vs. sense of futility			
III Play age			Initiative vs. guilt		Anticipation of roles vs. role inhibition			
II Early childhood		Autonomy vs. shame doubt			Will to be oneself vs. self-doubt			
I Infancy	Trust vs. mistrust				Mutual recognition vs. autistic isolation			

Source: Erikson, 1968, p. 94.

conceptions of social rules develop (see Youniss, 1980). *Early adolescence* (similar to Freud's genital stage) emerges as biological changes trigger increasing interest in sexuality and heterosexual relations, and then *late adolescence* builds on these relations as individuals become more socially aware and socialized and begin the task of establishing families and contributing to the community.

Sullivan's theory departs significantly from Erikson's in its view on the developmental relation between identity and intimacy. For Erikson, intimacy follows from identity consolidation in adolescence, whereas Sullivan believed that intimate relations with others is a necessary step in the *subsequent* development of adolescent self-identity. According to Sullivan, the need for a close interpersonal relationship emerges in late childhood. This need cannot be fully met by parents because of inequities in power, authority, and nurturance in the parent–child relationship (Youniss, 1980). Thus, children turn to peer relationships—which are more symmetrical and reciprocal—to fulfill their intimacy needs. These intimate relationships with peers eventuate from same-sex "chumships" in late childhood to heterosexual longing (or "lust dynamism") during puberty, to more mature and respectful relationships with the opposite sex in late adolescence. These intimate relations then make possible the discovery of self because it is through intimate interactions with others that one acquires an image of oneself as worthy ("good me") or unworthy ("bad me") of intimacy.

Developmental Issues

Origins

For Erikson and Sullivan, social development originates in early biologically based needs requiring attention from significant others. The sequencing of the need states is maturationally determined, although considerable cultural and individual variation exists in both timing and amount of social attention required. These needs are more explicitly social than the sexually oriented needs described by Freud. Erikson's theory emphasizes the continuing search for identity through-out the lifespan as a key organizing construct, whereas Sullivan's theory stresses the individual's adaptation to society as the critical social–developmental function.

Mechanism for Developmental Change

Biological maturation triggers developmental change (i.e., stage progression) in both Erikson's and Sullivan's theories. However, social and cultural forces exert a strong moderating influence on the process of change. For Erikson, each stage brings forth a conflict of opposing forces that require resolution. The individual is seen as active in the pursuit of resolution and is guided by rational, ego-based motives.

For Sullivan, each developmental stage is marked by efforts to reduce anxiety arising from real or imagined threats to one's security. Interpersonal relations provide a context for the relief of tensions associated with this anxiety. Individuals naturally seek out these relations, and it is this interpersonal experience—not instincts or some epigenetic play—that provides the impetus for developmental change.

Neither Erikson's nor Sullivan's theory describes interpersonal style as "set" in early life. Due to the plasticity of the human organism, interpersonal style can undergo transformations at various points in development, given new and different types of social influence. However, both theories postulate powerful self-systems (or egos) that seek to organize social experience.

TRANSFER

Neither Erikson nor Sullivan explicitly address the transfer issue, but it would appear that for both, experiential "templates" are formed on the basis on the individual's interaction with significant others. These characteristic ways of interpreting and responding to social situations determine the cross-setting and intergenerational transfer of social style. For Erikson, the rudiments of conceptions of intimacy and trust in human relationships are established in infancy and influence the development of self-identity and how individuals perceive subsequent relationships with nonmaternal figures. For Sullivan, personifications of relationships emerge in response to social experience and serve to guide perceptions of self and others in later life (e.g., through processes of stereotyping and selective inattention).

COGNITIVE-DEVELOPMENTAL THEORY

Although cognitive-developmental theories have long had a pronounced impact on the conceptualization and study of knowledge and language acquisition, only in the past 20 years or so have these perspectives had a major influence on the study of social behavior. This recent shift is due in large measure to the efforts of several scholars to apply cognitive-developmental (especially Piagetian) concepts to social and emotional development (e.g., Cowan, 1978; Kohlberg, 1969; Turiel, 1983) and to integrate Piagetian theory with more psychodynamic and ethological principles (e.g., Breger, 1974; Youniss, 1980). A clear understanding of cognitive-developmental models requires grounding in the genetic epistemology of Jean Piaget (1983).

Piaget's Theory

Piaget was a prodigious contributor to the literature on normal aspects of children's cognitive development. His theory of genetic epistemology has generated innumerable research studies and theoretical critiques. Epistemology is that branch of philosophy concerned with knowing or understanding; genetic here refers to developmental origins. The theory thus concerns itself with how individuals come to understand their worlds and how these conceptions change over time.

Unlike the characterization of the passive infant and young child in psychoanalytic and traditional learning theories, Piagetian theory views the child as actively engaged with the environment and motivated not by inner biological drives nor external reinforcement but by curiosity and a "need" to engage and master the environment (Cowan, 1978). Like Freud, Piaget had an academic background in biology, and perhaps as a consequence of this training, adhered to a biologically oriented, organizational view of cognitive development. Most importantly, he viewed development as an organism's adaptation to its physical and social surroundings, represented by the continuous interplay of internally represented reality and externally based modifications of these representations. Development proceeds in qualitatively different, sequential stages as children acquire increasingly more complex mental structures (schemata). The impetus to cognitive (and social–cognitive) growth occurs when there is a mismatch between one's internal mental schemata and the external environment. Through assimilation (the processing of information from the environment) and accommodation (progressive cognitive reorganization as a result of environmental input), these schemata are elaborated so as to better represent veridical aspects of reality. These schemata influence social behavior by constraining social understanding. The preschool-aged child, for example, may have difficulty in playing games-with-rules, because the schema for "game" and an understanding of "fairness" are as yet poorly developed.

When the processes of assimilation and accommodation are out of balance, a dynamic tension (disequilibration) results. This tension is associated with cognitive conflict and confusion and often results in "compensatory" activities that push the organism toward the next stage of development. The motivation for this change is not externally produced but rather derives from the organism's biologically based need to actively engage the environment. For humans, this is particularly true for the processing of information because information about the environment is critical for survival (Breger, 1974). Nonetheless, there are instances in development in which disequilibrium predominates (see Cowan, 1978, pp. 26–29), particularly during pretend play, when assimilation overrides accommodation, and during "pure" imitation, when accommodation overrides assimilation.

Cognitive structures (schemata) undergo qualitative changes over the course of development and serve as the building blocks of information processing. At any given stage in development, all such schemata are assumed to be structurally coherent. Progression through the stages is governed by four principles: (a) each stage is qualitatively different from the other stages; (b) the stages are ordered in an invariant sequence; (c) each stage is viewed as a structural whole; and (d) the stages are hierarchically organized (Cowan, 1978). Cognitive reorganization across development reflects a stagelike graduation from dependence on immediate sensation in infancy to conceptual abstraction and independence in adolescence. Inherent in Piagetian thinking about social development is the notion of "cognitive primacy," namely that an individual's cognitions precede and are thus the primary determinants of social behavior.

Each Piagetian stage represents a complex reorganization of cognition and affect, characterized by numerous new interpersonally relevant attainments. The distinctiveness of the stages is best illustrated by describing salient social features of each stage. (More detailed descriptions of the cognitive and social–emotional characteristics of each stage are presented in Cowan [1978] and in Flavell [1963].) During the infancy period (the *sensorimotor* period), social behavior is reflexive and nonsymbolic. A key developmental outcome of this stage is the ability to mentally represent other people and to establish separate schemata for mother and non-mother figures (a prerequisite for attachment). Also during this period the infant acquires a sense of object permanency, whereby objects (including the mother) are recognized as continuing to exist even when they are no longer visibly present. From about ages 2 to 7 (the *preoperational* period) the child's social behavior is limited by appearance-based, primary-feature perceptions of social events. Children's behavior during this stage is guided by superficial understanding of social reality. For example, a preoperational child might describe peers in terms of external, observable qualities (e.g., how many toys they possess, physical appearance) rather than internal, dispositional qualities. Another hallmark of this stage is egocentrism, the inability to entertain perspectives other than one's own. During the early elementary-school years children pass into the stage of *concrete operations*, a period of logical analysis and preoccupation with rules and authority. Perspective taking emerges, and children are able to reason about social events in ways that go beyond a reliance on superficial features of these events. For example, attributions about the intent of a peer's action may involve judgments of covert characteristics (such as motives) as well as the obvious outcome of the event. Children are likely to disapprove of violations of normative social behavior during this stage. The final cognitive-developmental stage, *formal operations*, typically emerges in early adolescence. It is characterized by hypothetical-deductive thinking, the ability to mentally manipulate abstract concepts, and an awareness of the relativity of social rules and mores. Adolescent disagreements about moral standards and behavioral control (e.g., curfews) are typical of formal operational thinking. Also during this stage a form of earlier egocentric thinking reemerges. In this new form of egocentrism, possibilities seem endless, and adolescents fail to distinguish between their own (idealistic) conceptualizations and those of the rest of society (see Elkind, 1970).

Piaget's most enduring contributions to social-developmental theory are probably in the areas of peer relations and moral reasoning. More generally, however, the Piagetian notion that social development follows from cognitive development has brought the study of social cognition to the forefront of developmental research. Social-cognitive research is concerned with (a) how individuals come to understand the thoughts, feelings, intentions, and behaviors of themselves and others and (b) how this knowledge influences social behavior (Shaffer, 1988). The most significant early application of Piagetian concepts to social cognition was made by Kohlberg (1969).

Kohlberg's Cognitive-Developmental Theory

Kohlberg's extension of Piagetian theory rests on several assumptions. First, it is assumed that social-cognitive development proceeds through the same invariant sequence of stages as described by Piaget. Second, social-cognitive development is represented by changes that occur in the self-concept as children obtain more information about themselves in relation to others. Third, children's social cognitions are directly tied to their role-taking abilities. Finally, it is assumed that social development proceeds toward a state of *reciprocity* between the child's actions and the actions of others toward the child. This requires that others respond to the child in a predictable fashion, which requires in turn that the child acquire a stable individual identity (Kohlberg, 1969)

Kohlberg's theory is best illustrated in his views regarding moral development and sex-role identification. Kohlberg considered moral development to be part of a sequence that includes parallel advancements in logical thinking and perspective taking. Consistent with Piaget's primacy notion, Kohlberg viewed cognitive skill as having priority, in that acquisition of higher levels of moral judgment is not possible without the concomitant cognitive skills. Likewise, perspective taking follows from logical skill development and precedes moral judgment ability.

Kohlberg's position on identification differs significantly from neopsychoanalytic and social learning views (Damon, 1983). For Kohlberg (1969), *self-knowledge* precedes both modeling and the search for social rewards. That is, knowledge of certain defining characteristics of oneself allows the child to imitate those who exhibit similar characteristics and to seek rewards for doing so. Gender, a conspicuous (and hence cognitively accessible) characteristic, is established as a constant, unchanging attribute during early childhood. Same-sex identification occurs as children recognize the gender similarity between themselves and the same-sex parent, and development of sex-appropriate values and expectations follows. Thus, "Kohlberg's theory holds that judgments of similarity instigate the entire modeling process" (Damon, 1983, p. 176). Over time, extensive modeling results in the establishment of emotional attachments, which strengthen and extend the bases for identification.

Developmental Issues

ORIGINS

In cognitive-developmental theory, social behavior and the cognitive activity that precedes it are based on "innate" motivations to understand and control the social and physical environment (cf. White, 1959). Beginning at birth, the individual is endowed with rudimentary cognitive-reflexive structures that form a substrate for interpreting experience. These structures are increasingly elaborated as a by-product of continuing individual–environment interactions.

MECHANISM FOR DEVELOPMENTAL CHANGE

The interplay of internal constructions of reality, based on experience and maturation, and external (i.e., veridical) reality creates a tension that motivates the individual toward greater cognitive growth. Presumably this tension (disequilibrium) impels the individual toward greater structural differentiation and integration. Developmental progress is most likely (i.e., the cognitive structures undergirding the interpretation of social experience are most open to modification) when these social experiences are stimulating but familiar. This phenomenon has been documented most clearly in the social arena for the development of perspective taking (e.g., as when a late preoperational-stage child is repeatedly exposed to divergent points of view in interactions with familiar peers).

The mechanism responsible for these developmental transformations has not been well specified. It has been noted that disequilibrium and similar terms are descriptions rather than explanations because they fail to provide a precise account of the factors involved in the structural transitions (Langer, 1969) and the ways in which the structures themselves are manifested in actual social behavior (Cairns, 1979). It appears that Piaget (as well as Kohlberg) considered these processes to be enacted in a maturationally determined manner. However, the actual process whereby equilibrium is restored remains one of the central unanswered questions for cognitive-developmental theory.

GREGORY S. PETTIT

Cognitive-developmental theory has not explicitly addressed processes responsible for consistencies in social behavior across settings and relationships, primarily because it has focused on the normative sequence of social-cognitive development. It would seem likely, however, that structural representations (schemata) of self and others would account for coherence in individual style. In early childhood these schemata are characterized by egocentric conceptions of self, whereas in later development these conceptions broaden to include multiple social perspectives. These schemata function to organize social information and social experience throughout the lifespan.

Comment

Several writers have applied the cognitive-developmental concepts outlined by Piaget and Kohlberg to new arenas of inquiry. Most notable in this regard is the extensive theoretical and empirical work contributed by Turiel (1983) and Damon (1983). The reader interested in structural variations of cognitive-developmental theory as applied to morality and social understanding is encouraged to consult these authors. Of greater relevance in the present context are recent efforts aimed at merging structural concepts of normative development (from cognitive-developmental theory) with skills-based concepts of individual–environment interaction (from attribution theory). These hybrid models (e.g., Selman, 1980) provide a developmental context for interpreting variations in information-processing skills.

SOCIAL INFORMATION-PROCESSING APPROACHES

The roots of attribution theory lie in the early social-psychological writings of Baldwin (1902) and Mead (1934), who were concerned with individuals' efforts to understand themselves and their social worlds better. These theorists acknowledged the role of social interactions in learning who one is with respect to others. The basic premise guiding the attributional perspective is that individuals are active seekers of social information, intent on using this information to make sense of their own and others' behavior.

The social-psychological approach emphasizes judgments about the cause of behavior and the impact of these judgments on individual behavior. In contrast, cognitive-developmental theories stress psychological processes and underlying cognitive structures. In other words, "the social psychologist wants to know *why* people make judgments about others, whereas the cognitive developmental psychologist wants to know *how* they do it" (Grusec & Lytton, 1988, p. 257). Important early work by Heider (1958) demonstrated that explanations for behavior vary along an internal-external dimension (dispositional versus situational), depending on whether the one making the judgments is the actor or the observer. Subsequent work in this area has focused on judgment heuristics (e.g., Kahneman, Slovic, & Tversky, 1982), attitude–behavior relations (Bem, 1972), and information-processing biases and distortions (e.g., Dodge, 1980; Snyder, Tanke, & Berscheid, 1977). Increased interest in predicting individual behavior in social contexts led to the study of patterns of social information processing (e.g., social-cognitive problem solving) presumed to underlie socially skillful behavior (e.g., D'Zurilla & Goldfriend, 1971; McFall, 1982; Spivack, Platt, & Shure, 1976). These studies are important because they attempt to describe the sequence in which information from the social environment is processed (typically in terms of attending, considering, deciding, and enacting), and the types of social situations that are particularly problematic for children and adults.

Dodge's Social Information-Processing Model

Several models of social information-processing development have been advanced in the past decade (e.g, Huesmann, 1988; McFall & Dodge, 1982; Rubin & Krasnor, 1986), but the model receiving the greatest amount of empirical and theoretical attention was devised by Dodge (1980, 1986). In this five-step model, individuals process information about particular social situations in a sequential manner by encoding social cues, interpreting the cues, generating potential behavioral responses, deciding upon a response and evaluating the likely consequences of the response, and enacting the chosen response. This series of steps is thought to parallel brain functions of information processing and thus is dependent on various neurological structures for its development. Processing may be either automatic or conscious, depending on the characteristics of the individual (e.g., age, experiential history) and the nature of the social stimulus.

In a series of studies, Dodge (1980; Dodge & Frame, 1982; Dodge, Murphy, & Buchsbaum, 1984) has shown that variations in these processing steps predict individual social behavior. Moreover, comprehensive assessments of processing at each step provide impressive degrees of nonredundant prediction to behavior in specific social situations (Dodge, Pettit, McClaskey, & Brown, 1986). Dodge *et al.* (1986) maintain that the information-processing approach is more process oriented than structuralist approaches because it provides specific guidelines for predicting individual social behavior, whereas structuralist approaches mainly describe the *products* of social cognition.

Selman's Structuralist–Functionalist Synthesis

In an effort to link the structuralist interest in developmental progression with the functionalist concern with predicting individual social behavior, Selman (Selman, Beardsley, Schultz, Krupa, & Podorefsky, 1986; Selman & Demorest, 1984; Yeates & Selman, 1989) developed an integrated model of processes involved in social conflict resolution—the interpersonal negotiation strategy (INS) model. According to Yeates and Selman (1989), these strategies "serve to resolve the felt conflict, or intra- and interpersonal disequilibrium, that sometimes arises in interactions with other individuals" (p. 76). The strategies proceed through a series of four levels (impulsive/egocentric, unilateral, reciprocal, and mutual/collaborative), with each level describing a more sophisticated coordination of social perspectives (i.e., greater ability to place one's own social perspective in the context of multiple perspectives) (see Selman, 1980). Higher level strategies, reflecting a more balanced concern for others' perspectives, are more likely to result in satisfying outcomes for all participants. There is some research supporting the claim that higher level INS functioning is associated with more successful outcomes in peer relations (Selman & Demorest, 1984).

Of greatest relevance in the present context is the model's explication of those factors responsible for developmental variations in social conflict resolution. These variations are tied to specific steps in social information processing. Selman describes four such steps, which resemble steps identified by functionalist information-processing theorists. These steps are problem definition, generation of alternative solutions, selection and implementation of a specific strategy, and outcome evaluation. As can be seen in Table 2, the steps are integrated within the four levels of social perspective taking to create a four-by-four matrix of steps-within-levels.

As development proceeds, individuals presumably become more reflective in their problem solving (i.e., the four problem-solving steps become more under conscious control), although there are considerable fluctuations in reflectivity over time as individuals move into and out of periods of relative equilibrium or disequilibrium. Developmental transitions are more likely to occur during disequilibrium, when lower level strategies seem inadequate for resolving interpersonal conflict. During such times, gains in social perspective taking accrue as individuals reflect on the nature of the failure in terms of the specific problem-solving steps. During periods of equilibrium, these steps may become scripted so that they are no longer under conscious control. As the individual's interpersonal negotiation strategies mature, the within-level strategies grow more successful.

The hypothesized relations between developmental (structural) level and (functional) steps in information processing are interesting, but they remain for now just that—hypotheses. It is clear that the two approaches can be wed most

TABLE 2. Developmental Variations in the Four Functional Steps of Conflict Resolution

| Level | Functional Step | | | |
	Problem definition	Strategy generation	Strategy implementation	Outcome evaluation
0 (Impulsive)	Problem defined in physical terms, without reference to psychological states	Strategies are physical, with little differentiation of impulse and action	A strategy is selected to immediately gratify or protect the self	Outcomes are evaluated based on immediate needs of self
1 (Unilateral)	Problem is defined in terms of either the self's or the other's needs	Strategies emphasize assertion of power or appeasement, without balance	A strategy is chosen to please self or other in the short term	Outcomes evaluated based on personal satisfaction of either self or other
2 (Reciprocal)	Problem defined by contrasting both self and other's needs, at the same time	Strategies stress satisfying both participants in a "just" fashion	A strategy is selected to satisfy self and other and their relationship	Outcomes evaluated on basis of balance, with emphasis on fairness
4 (Collaborative)	Problem defined in terms of mutual goals and long-term relationship	Strategies reflect collaboration, with goals shared by self and other	A strategy is chosen to optimize sense of collaboration and to sustain relationship	Outcomes are evaluated in terms of long-term effects on relationship

Source: Yeates & Selman (1989).

profitably, but the legitimacy of the marriage will be judged on the basis of data generated in careful empirical study.

Developmental Issues

ORIGINS

For information-processing theorists, social understanding is closely tied to developing brain structures. Memory store, attentional capabilities, and behavioral enactment skill all affect how an individual will respond to a social cue. Information storage and retrieval are based on biologically determined storage capacity and retrieval efficiency, in interaction with individual learning history. Social information-processing skill, then, emerges from an interaction of prewired "hardware" and individual social experience. What emerges, however, is not a thought structure, such as might be described by Damon (1983), but a characteristic way of processing information.

MECHANISM FOR DEVELOPMENTAL CHANGE

What developmental mechanisms are postulated to account for the age-related changes in social information processing? Typically, the notion of development is merely implied (Gottman, 1986), with the "skills" associated with each step (e.g., attentional skills, memory store, accessibility of scripts) described as more sophisticated and refined with age. Unfortunately, this way of describing development does not distinguish between changes due to maturation from those due to experience. The information-processing model also fails to account for developmental improvements in basic processing capacity and strategy use that have been identified in the cognitive science literature (Dolgin, 1986). Finally, the model does not adequately address developmental changes in the social goals of children and the increasingly complicated social contexts in which children must learn what is expected of them (Gottman, 1986).

TRANSFER

Social information-processing patterns have been speculated to account for the transfer of individual social style across relationship contexts (Pettit, Dodge, & Brown, 1988). Children are presumed to develop characteristic patterns of processing social information (i.e., predictable ways of attending, interpreting, and responding to social stimuli) as a by-product of early family experience. These processing patterns may then be generalized to extrafamilial social settings. For example, a child whose parents repeatedly label ambiguous social provocations in a hostile fashion (e.g., as often happens in highway driving) may learn to assign hostile labels to similar ambiguous events and then may generalize these biases to other social contexts. When children are developmentally "ready" to acquire these kinds of biases and the exact sorts of experiences that trigger their acquisition are not yet clear. Moreover, it has not yet been demonstrated how closely stimuli must resemble one another for transfer to occur. Under what circumstances, for example, will the child who has learned to access aggressive strategies as a way of coping with parental intrusions display the same tendencies in interactions with others? Answers to these questions await future empirical scrutiny.

ETHOLOGICAL-ATTACHMENT THEORY

Having considered the intrapsychic and cognitive perspectives, we now turn to the third major perspective—ethological-attachment theory. The ethological perspective has had a pronounced impact on the conceptualization and study of many human social behaviors. Ethologists regard certain patterns of social behavior as the product of evolution. These patterns presumably assist the species in survival and continue throughout evolution because of natural selection. Many of the social behaviors of interest to ethologists are believed to have originated in "environments of evolutionary adaptedness," typically hunting and gathering ecological niches (Breger, 1974). These patterns continue to be passed down through the generations as inherited instincts. Because cultural evolution is far more rapid than biological evolution, many of these instinctual behavior patterns may no longer serve useful purposes (e.g., male sexual dominance). However, ethologists have provided extensive descriptive data on behavioral patterns that have historical as well as contemporary relevance. Best known in this regard are probably the ethological studies of aggression (e.g., Lorenz, 1966) and dominance (e.g., Blurton-Jones, 1972). More recently, however, ethological perspectives on infant–mother attachment have energized social-developmental research and have provided a rich groundwork for the cross-fertilization of ideas. The major theorists responsible for the emergence of ethological-attachment theory are Bowlby (1969, 1982, 1973) and Ainsworth (1973; Ainsworth, Blehar, Waters, & Wall, 1978).

Bowlby was originally trained in psychoanalysis and initially became interested in attachment because of concerns about disruptions in mother–infant relationships due to long-term separations (Bowlby, 1958). Bowlby integrated psychoanalytic concepts with control systems and ethological notions to formulate his theory of attachment. Bowlby's theory emphasizes the adaptive function of an infant–caregiver attachment, implying that infants reared in normal (i.e., predictable and nurturing) caregiving environments will become attached to one or more principal caregivers, usually the mother. Such attachments are critical for the survival of the species because they insure that the vulnerable infant stays in close proximity to mother and that the mother will be responsive to the infant in times of distress. Thus, infants are biologically "wired" to maintain close proximity to the mother and to be able to signal the mother in times of distress, whereas mothers are programmed to respond to infant social stimuli. Bowlby (1973) describes attachment in humans as the result of several interlocking behavioral systems. Signaling behavior (crying, smiling, babbling) brings the mother into proximity to the infant, whereas approach behavior (clinging, following, reaching) takes the baby to the mother. Attachment, for Bowlby, is represented by "control systems" that seek to minimize the discrepancy between the set goal (proximity) and the present state (physical separation from the mother). Subsequent theorists have expanded the physical proximity aspect of control systems to include a psychological dimension—termed *felt security* (see Sroufe & Waters, 1977). This felt security enables the infant to venture forth to explore the environment because of a sense that maternal protection will be available when needed. The extent to which early social experiences promote feelings of security hinges on the infant's internal representations (or working models) of pertinent attributes of the caregiver (e.g., the caregiver's responsive availability).

Interest in assessing mother–infant relationships characterized by "security" or "insecurity" led Ainsworth (Ainsworth & Wittig, 1969; Ainsworth *et al.*, 1978) to develop a typology of attachment quality and a procedure (the "strange situation") for evaluating this quality. These assessments are typically conducted between the ages of 8 and 18 months, when attachment behaviors are directed toward a single (usually) primary caregiver (almost always the mother).

In the "strange situation" procedure, infants are exposed to a series of increasingly stressful experiences with the mother and a stranger. The infant's reactions to brief separations from the mother and reunions with the mother provide a context for assessing attachment quality. Quality is reflected in a mixture of several attachment behaviors (e.g., proximity seeking, contact maintaining). Securely attached infants seek contact with the mother following separation (proximal contact if distressed, distal contact if not distressed), greet the mother, and quickly resume exploration of the play area. Insecurely attached infants either shun or avoid the mother upon her return (the avoidant group), or display a mixture of angry, resistant behavior and proximity-seeking behavior with mother (the resistant group). It is important to note that attachment behaviors are displayed by virtually all infants, but infants differ in the security of their attachment.

Individual differences in attachment security appear to have social-developmental antecedents in early patterns of infant–mother interaction (e.g., contingent responsiveness) (see Ainsworth *et al.*, 1978) and developmental sequelae in subsequent patterns of social adaptation (e.g., competence with peers) (see Bretherton, 1985). The underlying basis for such developmental continuity has been hotly debated. Some (e.g., Main, Kaplan, & Cassidy, 1985) maintain that internalized representations of the self and the attachment figure(s) mediate relations between early and later social development, but others argue that connections between attachment security and subsequent developmental outcomes are primarily due to infant temperament (Kagan, 1984) or consistency in caregiving (Lamb, 1987).

It should be noted that although attachment was originally introduced as an organizational construct to describe aspects of the mother–*infant* relationship, the term has more recently been applied to other close relationships (e.g., between older children, adolescents, and adults) (see Cassidy, 1988; Kobak & Sceery, 1988; Main *et al.*, 1985). These writers contend that later close interpersonal ties share many of the attributes of the primary attachment relationship, particularly proximity maintenance and felt security in times of distress, and that measures of attachment based on Q-sorts or clinical interviews can provide valid indexes of the quality of these attachment relationships.

Attachment as an Organizational Task

Sroufe (1979, 1983) has placed attachment within the broader framework of individual adaptation and has conceptualized continuity in social development in terms of key developmental tasks or issues. Rather than looking for simple continuities in behavioral development, Sroufe argues that we must specify the critical developmental tasks at different points in the life cycle and then evaluate the adequacy with which the individual meets the challenges associated with the tasks. Building on concepts of Erikson (1963) and his own empirical (e.g., Sroufe, 1983) and theoretical work (Sroufe, 1979; Sroufe & Waters, 1977), Sroufe specifies several organizational issues that characterize the early childhood period (e.g., physiological regulation, tension management, establishing an effective attachment, exploration and mastery, and so on). In keeping with the neopsychoanalytic views of Erikson and Sullivan, and the ethological-attachment perspective, Sroufe describes critical roles played by caregivers in promoting children's successful adaptation. Thus, for example, smooth routines assist in physiological regulation, sensitive interaction facilitates tension management, and responsive availability promotes the establishment of secure attachment. Each organizational issue lays the groundwork for succeeding issues, and the issues are not resolved and discarded but rather are continually reworked in subsequent development.

Developmental Issues

ORIGINS

Attachment to a primary caregiver, and later in life, to a significant other, originates in an inborn, environmentally stable propensity to seek physically and psychologically protective relationships. Although not labeled as a "drive" by the attachment theorists, such propensity nonetheless has been described as a motivational system rivaling the primary and secondary drives noted in psychoanalytic theory (Bretherton, 1985), and it appears to operate like a drive in that the tendency is strengthened when not gratified (e.g., an infant's efforts at maintaining proximity escalate—at least initially—when caregivers are unresponsive). The utility of this distinction has been questioned (Grusec & Lytton, 1988) because a drive is no more or less than a descriptive term for the initiation of a behavioral pattern, not why the behavior occurs.

MECHANISM FOR DEVELOPMENTAL CHANGE

Because ethologists focus on behaviors with evolutionary origins, their view of the process of development has a strong biological orientation. Maturation determines the timing and source of each developmental issue (Miller, 1983), but social experience and learning ultimately determine how each individual deals with the emerging developmental challenges. Evidence suggests that consistency in caregiving is necessary for stability in attachment security and presumably for coherence in social adaptation more generally. In contrast to the psychoanalytic view, which emphasizes the caregiver's role in helping the child to relieve tension, the ethological-attachment perspective stresses the supportive presence of the caregiver (or significant other) in helping the child (or adult) to maintain organized behavior when faced with novel or distressing situations (see Sroufe, 1979).

Behavioral adaptation is also a product of the individual's own history and active self-selection, or what Caspi and Elder (1988) refer to as cumulative and interactional continuity. Individual history plays a role because an individual may become "tracked" into a particular developmental path partly because of the cumulative effects of the types of experiences the individual has had. For example, an individual incapable of establishing a close emotional bond with another person early in life is unlikely to have friends or experience intimacy with the opposite sex as an adult. Related to this idea is the notion that the individual selects out life experiences that recreate the same types of relationships with which the individual is familiar (e.g., as when a child rejected by parents seeks out peer group experiences—indeed, fashions those experiences—that lead to rejection by those peers).

Transfer

Ethological-attachment theory has more to say about cross-setting and cross-relationship coherence in social behavior than any of the other perspectives that have been discussed. The postulated mechanism for this coherence is the internal working model. Although this model does not constitute "templates" of experience in social relationships (because it is more dynamic), it serves many of the same functions. Internal working models not only provide a guide for social behavior in new situations but also filter information from the social environment (Bretherton, 1985).

What exactly is internalized in these working models? In the original Bowlby (1969/1982, 1980) conceptualization, the models consist of complex cognitive-affective representations of the attributes of significant others and the self with respect to others. For example, when parents treat children with love and respect, children should internalize a view of parent figures as loving and of themselves as lovable. Sroufe and Fleeson (1986) have modified this view of working models somewhat by suggesting that individuals internalize *both sides* of relationships (e.g., an early experience of rejection may predispose an individual to reject others or to enact the role of victim of rejection, depending on the circumstance).

Some effort has been made to describe more precisely the defining attributes of internal working models (Crittenden, 1988; Main *et al.*, 1985) across the lifespan. Crittenden (1989) has gone one step further by offering comprehensive terminology to describe internal representational models of attachment relationships. The defining properties of such models consist of focus, memory system, content, cognitive function, metastructure, quality of and attitude toward attachment, and behavioral strategies. Memory systems and behavioral strategies would appear to have particular promise as guides for empirical study. Three memory systems are described and distinguished by the information encoded in each. Procedural memory consists of interactional patterns (e.g., scripts) elicited in specific situations. Episodic memory refers to more lengthy interactional episodes or vignettes that are encoded visually or linguistically. Semantic memory consists of generalizations of types of relationships. Each type of memory is subject to distortion. Encoding distortions may serve to systematically exclude certain information or to misrepresent information already stored. Retrieval distortions limit the availability of information for recall. Behavioral strategies are described in terms of patterns of behavioral responses to attachment figures. These strategies are context-specific and are displayed in accordance with expectations of self and attachment figure (i.e., judgments of the likely outcome of the behavior). Behavioral strategies displayed by infants in the Strange Situation include approach, resistance, and avoidance; those displayed by older children in play contexts include cooperation, difficultness, and passivity. Although each type of strategy may serve an adaptive function in a particular context (e.g., as when an infant avoids a mistreating mother), the same behavior may prove maladaptive in other contexts.

Crittenden's (1989) description of the properties of internal models suggests a conceptual compatibility between ethological-attachment theory and social information processing theory. Empirical support for the defining attributes is only now accumulating, but the concept of "working model" holds promise as a means of linking psychological experience to specific social–cognitive and behavioral skills.

Summary

Despite their varied histories and disparate disciplinary orientations, the theoretical perspectives described share several commonalities. Central to each is the notion of tension reduction, as homeostasis is the desired end state for individual–environment interactions. Disequilibrium occurs when the individual's capacity for coping has been exceeded. This applies to purely internal processes, such as proposed in the Freudian hydraulic model of tension reduction, or in more social or social-cognitive aspects of experience, such as described by Piaget, Erikson, Sullivan, and Bowlby. In its purest sense, disequilibrium refers to a mismatch between social-environmental input and internal representations of self and others. Active striving to reduce this unpleasant state is the impetus moving the individual through successive stages of development.

Each of the theoretical perspectives also emphasizes that individual patterns of apprehending the social environment (as well as oneself) are constructed from social experience and that these patterns serve to guide subsequent development. For the most part, the theorists discussed above describe this process in unidirectional terms (i.e., involving only the individual's construal of social experience). Dodge (1986) describes a process whereby each participant in an interaction contributes to the coherence in the other's behavior. In this reciprocal influence model of social interaction, each individual brings to a social interaction a distinct social history and characteristic way of processing social information. Social systems are normally conservative, and social interaction serves to maintain rather than to modify existing social organization. These maintaining functions are extremely important when individuals have deviant reputations (e.g., are viewed as aggressive) and respond to social situations in idiosyncratic ways (e.g., by making hostile judgments in ambiguous contexts). Others' processing of social information about the deviant individual will reflect these expectations (based on reputation), thus reinforcing the deviant child's negative reputation and biased judgments.

The theories differ substantially in the degree to which they describe the individual as actively pursuing social interaction. In Freudian theory, the individual is viewed as rather passive, preyed upon by conflicts associated with instinctual drives. Neopsychoanalytic theorists assign greater control over the course of development to the individual and view social development as more rational and ego based than did Freud. Cognitive-developmental theory describes a true interactionist position, with the individual actively seeking new environmental input, and then becoming transformed as a product of this input. Ethological-attachment theory posits active individual organization of experience, within the confines of a biologically derived blueprint of social-developmental functioning.

The theories vary widely in what they contribute to an understanding of social development across the life cycle. Although some theorists (e.g., Erikson) have made explicit efforts at describing developmental transitions throughout life, the majority of the perspectives either ascribe greater developmental significance to the childhood period, or simply fail to delineate how and why "postmaturity" stages may develop. At present, more attention has been paid to the notion of adult stages in the popular media (e.g., Sheehy, 1976) than in the scientific literature. Nonetheless, the theories described provide some strong clues as to how development may proceed across the lifespan. Conflicts are an inherent part of human social development, and adequacy in resolving these conflicts will always constitute a critical developmental adaptation. The source of conflict will vary in accordance with physical maturation, changes in social "roles" (e.g., from a young parent caring for offspring to an older parent being cared for by offspring), and cultural and historical evolution.

A critical issue in the study of lifespan social development concerns the notion of "carryover" effects; that is, coherence in interpersonal style across time and relationships. Underlying this issue are several key questions, such as those posed by Hartup (1989): "To what extent are the child's interactions specific to partner and place? Do the child's adaptations carry forward across developmental transformations? . . . Does the child carry forward holistic ideas and expectations about relationships, or bits and pieces of relationship information?" (p. 128). What do the theories reviewed in this chapter provide in the way of answers to these questions? What can be gained in our overall understanding of social-developmental processes by linking the theories around the "carryover" issue? One potentially valuable place to start is with the most obvious and observable sources of information—what an individual actually does in circumscribed social situations. We may then trace backwards in a concentric chain of increasingly hypothetical explanations. It would appear that the strongest predictions of behavior (requiring the least amount of inference) currently are provided by social information processing (SIP) assessments of interpersonal competence (see Dodge, 1986; McFall & Dodge, 1982). These patterns may then be viewed as partially determined by more general and abstract concepts such as internal working models, which are themselves comprised of mental representations (or structures). At an even more abstract level, the representational models may be based on unconscious conflicts and the affectively laden residue of significant early experiences. In a sense, then, the social information-processing constructs are the more proximal processes represented by underlying theoretical constructs, whether these be Freud's defense mechanisms, Erikson's ego states, Sullivan's personifications, Piaget's structures, or Bowlby's internal working models. Perhaps the theoretical constructs posited by structuralists may serve as a guiding developmental framework for functionalist approaches to understanding and predicting social developmental patterns. At present a key conceptual and empirical link remains only vaguely stated and tested: namely how the underlying (and possibly hypothetical) mental and emotional forces reveal themselves in behavior and social cognition.

ACKNOWLEDGMENTS   Preparation of this chapter was supported in part by Grant No. 42498 from the National Institute of Mental Health. Appreciation is expressed to Amanda Harrist, Sandra Twardosz, Ken Dodge, and Jan Allen for their helpful comments on earlier drafts of this chapter. A very special note of gratitude is extended to Joan Deer for her editorial assistance.

REFERENCES

Ainsworth, M. D. S., Blehar, M. C., Waters, E., & Wall, S. (1978). *Patterns of attachment: A psychological study of the Strange Situation*. Hillsdale, NJ: Erlbaum.

Ainsworth, M. D. S., & Wittig, B. A. (1969). Attachment and the exploratory behavior of one-year-olds in a strange situation. In B. M. Foss (Ed.), *Determinants of infant behavior* (Vol. 4, pp. 113–136). London: Methuen.

Baldwin, A. L. (1980). *Theories of child development* (2nd ed.). New York: Wiley.

Baldwin, J. M. (1902). *Social and ethical interpretations in mental development* (3rd ed.). New York: Macmillan.

Bem, D. J. (1972). Self-perception theory. *Advances in Experimental Social Psychology, 6*, 1–62.

Bowlby, J. (1958). The nature of the child's tie to his mother. *International Journal of Psychoanalysis, 35*, 350–373.

Bowlby, J. (1973). *Attachment and loss: Vol. 2. Separation*. New York: Basic.

Bowlby, J. (1980). *Attachment and loss: Vol. 3. Loss, sadness, and depression*. New York: Basic.

Bowlby, J. (1982). *Attachment and loss: Vol. 1. Attachment* (2nd ed.). New York: Basic. (Original work published 1969)

Blurton Jones, N. (1972). *Ethological studies of child behavior*. Cambridge: Cambridge University Press.

Breger, L. (1974). *From instinct to identity: The development of personality*. Englewood Cliffs, NJ: Prentice-Hall.

Bretherton, I. (1985). Attachment theory: Retrospect and prospect. In I. Bretherton & E. Waters (Eds.), Growing points of attachment theory and research. *Monographs of the Society for Research in Child Development* (Serial No. 209, Vol. 50).

Cairns, R. B. (1979). *Social development: The origins and plasticity of interchanges*. San Francisco: Freeman.

Caspi, A., & Elder, G. H. (1988). Childhood precursors of the life course: Early personality and life disorganization. In E. M. Hetherington, R. M. Lerner, & M. Perlmutter (Eds.), *Child development in life-span perspective* (115–142). Hillsdale, NJ: Erlbaum.

Cassidy, J. (1988). Child-mother attachment and the self in six-year-olds. *Child Development, 59*, 121–134.

Coté, J. E., & Levine, C. (1988). A critical examination of the ego identity status paradigm. *Developmental Review, 8*, 147–184.

Cowan, P. A. (1978). *Piaget with feeling: Cognitive, social, and emotional dimensions*. New York: Holt, Rinehart & Winston.

Crittenden, P. (1988). Distorted patterns of relationship in maltreating families: The role of internal representational models. *Journal of Reproductive and Infant Psychology, 6*, 183–189.

Crittenden, P. (1989, April). *Internal representational models of attachment relationships*. Paper presented at the biennial meeting of the Society for Research in Child Development, Kansas City.

Damon, W. (1983). *Social and personality development*. New York: Norton.

Dodge, K. A. (1980). Social cognition and children's aggressive behavior. *Child Development, 51*, 162–170.

Dodge, K. A. (1986). A social information processing model of social competence in children. In M. Perlmutter (Ed.), *Minnesota Symposia on Child Psychology* (Vol. 18, pp. 77–125). Hillsdale, NJ: Erlbaum.

Dodge, K. A., & Frame, C. M. (1982). Social cognitive biases and deficits in aggressive boys. *Child Development, 53*, 620–635.

Dodge, K. A., Murphy, R. M., & Buchsbaum, K. (1984). The assessment of intention-cue detection skills in children: Implications for developmental psychopathology. *Child Development, 55*, 163–173.

Dodge, K. A., Pettit, G. S., McClaskey, C. L., & Brown, K. A. (1986). Social competence in children. *Monographs of the Society for Research in Child Development, 51*, (1, Serial No. 213). Hillsdale, NJ: Erlbaum.

Dolgin, K. G. (1986). Needed steps for social competence: Strengths and present limitations of Dodge's model. In M. Perlmutter (Ed.), *Minnesota Symposia on Child Psychology* (Vol. 18, pp. 127–135). Hillsdale, NJ: Erlbaum.

D'Zurilla, T. J., & Goldfried, M. R. (1971). Problem solving and behavior modification. *Journal of Abnormal Psychology, 78*, 107–126.

Elkind, D. (1970). *Children and adolescents: Interpretive essays on Jean Piaget.* New York: Oxford University Press.

Erikson, E. H. (1963). *Childhood and society* (2nd ed.). New York: Norton.

Erikson, E. H. (1968). *Identity: Youth and crisis.* New York: Norton.

Flavell, J. (1963). *The developmental psychology of Jean Piaget.* Princeton, NJ: Van Nostrand.

Freud, S. (1964). An outline of psychoanalysis. In J. Strachey (Ed.), *The standard edition of the complete psychological works of Sigmund Freud* (Vol. 23). London: Hogarth Press. (Original work published 1940)

Gottman, J. (1986). Commentary on "Social Competence in Children." *Monographs of the Society for Research in Child Development, 51* (1, Serial No. 213).

Grusec, J. E., & Lytton, H. (1988). *Social development: History, theory, and research.* New York: Springer-Verlag.

Hall, C. S. (1954). *A primer of Freudian psychology.* New York: World.

Hall, C. S., & Lindzey, G. (1978). *Theories of personality* (3rd ed.). New York: Wiley.

Hartup, W. W. (1989). Social relationships and their developmental significance. *American Psychologist, 44,* 120–126.

Heider, F. (1958). *The psychology of interpersonal relations.* New York: Wiley.

Huesmann, L. R. (1988). An information processing model for the development of aggression. *Aggressive Behavior, 14,* 13–24.

Kagan, J. (1984). *The nature of the child.* New York: Basic.

Kahneman, D., Slovic, P., & Tversky, A. (1982). *Judgment under uncertainty: Heuristics and biases.* New York: Cambridge University Press.

Kobak, R. R., & Sceery, A. (1988). Attachment in late adolescence: Working models, affect regulation, and representations of self and others. *Child Development, 59,* 135–146.

Kohlberg, L. (1966). A cognitive-developmental analysis of children's sex-role concepts and attitudes. In E. E. Maccoby (Ed.), *The development of sex differences* (pp. 82–173). Stanford: Stanford University Press.

Kohlberg, L. (1969). Stage and sequence: The cognitive-developmental approach to socialization. In D. A. Goslin (Ed.), *Handbook of socialization theory and research* (pp. 347–480). Chicago: Rand McNally.

Kohlberg, L. (1976). Moral stages and moralization: The cognitive-developmental approach. In T. Lickona (Ed.), *Moral development and behavior* (pp. 31–53). New York: Holt, Rinehart & Winston.

Lamb, M. E. (1987). Predictive implications of individual differences in attachment. *Journal of Consulting and Clinical Psychology, 55,* 817–824.

Langer, J. (1969). *Theories of development.* New York: Holt, Rinehart & Winston.

Lorenz, K. (1966). *On aggression.* New York: Harcourt, Brace, & World.

Main, M., Kaplan, N., & Cassidy, J. (1985). Security in infancy, childhood, and adulthood: A move to the level of representation. In I. Bretherton & E. Waters (Eds.), Growing points in attachment theory and research. *Monographs of the Society for Research in Child Development* (Serial No. 209, Vol. 50).

Marcia, J. E. (1966). Development and validation of ego identity status. *Journal of Personality and Social Psychology, 3,* 551–558.

Marcia, J. E. (1976). Identity six years after: A follow-up study. *Journal of Youth and Adolescence, 5,* 145–160.

McConnell, J. V. (1977). *Understanding human behavior* (2nd ed.). New York: Holt, Rinehart & Winston.

McFall, R. M. (1982). A review and reformulation of the concept of social skills. *Behavioral Assessment, 4,* 1–35.

McFall, R. M., & Dodge, K. A. (1982). Self-management and interpersonal skills learning. In P. Karoly & F. Kanfer (Eds.), *Self-management and behavior change: From theory to practice* (pp. 353–392). New York: Pergamon Press.

Mead, G. H. (1934). *Mind, self, and society.* Chicago: University of Chicago Press.

Miller, P. (1983). *Theories of developmental psychology.* San Francisco: Freeman.

Pettit, G. S., Dodge, K. A., & Brown, M. (1988). Early family experience, social problem solving patterns, and children's social competence. *Child Development, 59,* 107–120.

Piaget, J. (1983). Piaget's theory. In W. Kessen (Ed.), *Handbook of child psychology, Vol. 1; History, theory, and methods* (pp. 103–128). New York: Wiley.

Rubin, K. H., & Krasnor, L. R. (1986). Social-cognitive and social behavioral perspectives on problem solving. In M. Perlmutter (Ed.), *Minnesota Symposia on Child Psychology* (Vol. 18, pp. 1–68). Hillsdale, NJ: Erlbaum.

Selman, R. L. (1980). *The growth of interpersonal understanding: Clinical and developmental analyses.* New York: Academic Press.

Selman, R. L., Beardslee, W., Schultz, L. Krupa, M., & Podorefsky, D. (1986). Assessing adolescent interpersonal negotiation strategies: Toward the integration of functional and structural models. *Developmental Psychology, 22,* 450–459.

Selman, R. L., & Demorest, A. (1984). Observing troubled children's interpersonal negotiation strategies: Implications of and for a developmental model. *Child Development, 55,* 288–304.

Shaffer, D. R. (1988). *Social and personality development* (2nd ed.). Pacific Grove, CA: Brooks/Cole.

Sheehy, G. (1976). *Passages: Predictable crises of adult life.* New York: E. P. Dutton.

Snyder, M., Tanke, E. D., & Bersheid, E. (1977). Social perception and interpersonal behavior: On the self-fulfilling nature of social stereotypes. *Journal of Personality and Social Psychology, 35,* 656–666.

Spivack, G., Platt, J. J., & Shure, M. B. (1976). *The problem-solving approach to adjustment.* San Francisco: Jossey-Bass.

Sroufe, L. A. (1979). The coherence of individual adaptation. *American Psychologist, 34,* 834–841.

Sroufe, L. A. (1983). Individual patterns of adaptation from infancy to preschool. In M. Perlmutter (Ed.), *Minnesota Symposia on Child Development* (Vol. 16, pp. 41–83). Hillsdale, NJ: Erlbaum.

Sroufe, L. A., & Fleeson, J. (1986). Attachment and the organization of relationships. In W. Hartup & Z. Rubin (Eds.), *Relationships and development* (pp. 51–71). New York: Cambridge University Press.

Sroufe, L. A., & Waters, E. (1977). Attachment as an organizational construct. *Child Development, 48,* 1184–1199.

Sullivan, H. S. (1953). *The interpersonal theory of psychiatry.* New York: Norton.

Turiel, E. (1983). *The development of social knowledge.* Cambridge: Cambridge University Press.

White, R. W. (1959). Motivation reconsidered: The concept of competence. *Psychological Review, 66,* 297–333.

Yeates, K. O., & Selman, R. L. (1989). Social competence in the schools: Toward an integrative developmental model for intervention. *Developmental Review, 9,* 64–100.

Youniss, J. (1980). *Parents and peers in social development: A Sullivan-Piaget perspective.* Chicago: University of Chicago Press.

2

Emotion Socialization

A View from Development and Ethology

JEANNETTE M. HAVILAND
AND ARLENE S. WALKER-ANDREWS

INTRODUCTION

In this chapter we are interested primarily in the social functions of emotion and how development may influence them. Our emphasis will be on the expressive, communicative aspects of emotion as they relate both to (a) interpersonal interactions and (b) the organization of one's own behavior. In our view, these two functions are inseparable facets in the expression of emotion. Throughout we take a developmental perspective because we are interested in the changes that occur in emotion and emotional expression. We also take an ecological perspective, as we assume that the emotional and perceptual systems interact, that affective perception is adaptive, and that there are developmental differences in the affective affordances of the environment.

SYSTEMS APPROACH

We will introduce a multicomponent systems approach to understanding the origins and development of affect extending from birth into adulthood. This approach begins to bring together the various approaches to emotion that have been the target of research in the past century. Past research on emotion has been

JEANNETTE M. HAVILAND AND ARLENE S. WALKER-ANDREWS • Department of Psychology, Rutgers University, New Brunswick, New Jersey 08903.

Handbook of Social Development: A Lifespan Perspective, edited by Vincent B. Van Hasselt and Michel Hersen. Plenum Press, New York, 1992.

JEANNETTE M.
HAVILAND and
ARLENE S.
WALKER-ANDREWS

confined to separate fields—social, physiological, developmental, cognitive, ethological—and has therefore atomized the emotion system. Reflexive theorists (e.g., Bekhterev, 1928; Watson, 1928) have been concerned with the biological, species-specific components. They have often come into conflict with social-cognitive and philosophical theorists (e.g., Harré, 1986), who analyze the influence of culture and learning on emotion. Not often in conflict but concerned with problems in different research fields, we find theories of temperament and of structure modifying our view of emotion socialization.

We propose that emotion development in an ecological system must be viewed as the outcome of development in several component systems or even modules (e.g., Leventhal, 1991). We propose that these components interact dynamically across developmental epochs (see Fogel & Thelen, 1987). Each one may be involved in the production of emotional behavior, but at any specific moment in time any one of them may be the controlling factor. In the summary section of this chapter we will discuss potential interaction patterns and their developmental significance. The probability that any one component is controlling or necessary will shift over time and shift within the demands of the ecological system; therefore, it is necessary to consider all components in an emotional system.

Our current knowledge of the components of emotion that should be included in the systems approach is uneven, and any discussion of emotion will reflect the gaps in that knowledge. However, we will emphasize the adaptive role of each component in promoting survival of an organism.

The first part of this chapter has four sections, each of which describes an overarching component of affect: structural affect, temperamental affect, reflexive affect, and affect knowledge. These four examples are not meant to identify the entire field of components that regulate emotion behaviors. However, at the moment each one reflects an important body of knowledge about emotion generated within a particular area.

We will consider each of the four components and then examine more fully the implications of our approach to the development of affect. Before progressing further, however, we will discuss how it is that the communicative and organizational functions of emotion are interrelated.

ECOLOGICAL PERSPECTIVE

Central to our approach to the development of emotion is the assumption that affective perception is direct and meaningful (Gibson, 1979). By this we mean that an organism detects information in its environment that specifies the affective "affordances" of that environment, what it provides to the adapting individual, for joy or sadness, and whether it is hostile, fearful, or disgusting. The ecological perspective emphasizes the action or response of an observer to affordances.

The ecological approach we are taking here is different from traditional accounts of the perception of socioemotional events in several respects. It focuses on the adaptive nature of perception and on the inherent connection between action and perception, with introduction of the affordance concept. This is not the first approach to suggest that one's goals or expectancies have an effect on perceptual attunement (e.g., Erdelyi, 1974), but the influence is perceptual rather than inferential. One of the most basic assumptions in the ecological approach is that perceivers can extract information from the environment before the development of conceptual structures or language. Neither is the ecological approach unique in its assumption that perception is selective, but the reasons for selectivity are different. We are most sensitive to adaptively relevant or useful information, and information that specifies the emotional state of other people is of critical importance to social interaction.

We allow adaptive emotional behavior to be considered part of the emotion system whether or not the individual expressing the behavior "knows" what the emotion is and can express in a nonemotion behavior system such as language that he "knows." This is akin to the Nisbett and Wilson's (1977) argument that consciousness of knowing is not necessarily a veridical component of behavior. We would argue that because we perceive emotion, we also experience emotion in the very act of perceiving. The percept does not depend upon the emotion, for an affordance is not a subjective value added to a neutral perception, but emotion accompanies perception because an affordance is a property of an object or event taken with reference to an observer. Likewise, perceiving other persons is no different from perceiving objects and events; we perceive the affordances of others for us by observing their expression, their actions, and their more permanent properties. As Gibson (1979) stated:

> The perceiving of these mutual affordances . . . is just as much based on stimulus information as is the simpler perception of the support that is offered by the ground under one's feet. For other persons can only give off information about themselves insofar as they are tangible, audible, tastable, or visible. (p. 135)

The ecological approach to perception is particularly amenable to a developmental perspective on emotion because an affordance is "inherently specific to a particular perceiver" (McArthur & Baron, 1983, p. 218). The stimulus information to which one is attuned varies as a function of one's perceptual system (phylogenetic variation), temperament (individual variation), perceptual learning, behavioral repertoire, goals, and ongoing actions. A human adult may detect information (for size, rigidity of substance, height) that specifies a surface of support on which a book may be placed; a crawling infant may detect information (for size, rigidity of substance, height in relation to the infant) that specifies an object to pull up on. Each observer is attuned to different affordances of the table, although the information that specifies the affordance may be the same objectively. So it is with emotional affordances. An adult and a child may detect the same information about affect, and yet the information may have different emotional affordances.

In summary, emphasis is on emotions as a guide to action rather than as purely phenomenological experience. Emotions are viewed as social affordances in the sense that they call forth various interpersonal behaviors. (See McArthur and Baron, 1983, for a more complete discussion of an ecological theory of social perception.)

FOUR COMPONENTS OF EMOTION: OVERVIEW

The rest of the chapter will describe four proposed components of emotion chosen to illustrate a multicomponent systems approach to emotional develop-

JEANNETTE M.
HAVILAND and
ARLENE S.
WALKER-ANDREWS

ment. Examples will be given as space allows. An underlying and very basic assumption of all that follows is that affect development is an organizational process involving many developmental elements. It does not assume that infant and child and adult emotions are the same; in fact, they are probably quite different. In spite of this, they seem to belong to a family of emotions. As Griffin (1981) reminds us, there has been resistance to the notion that infrahuman animals have subjective feelings. So, too, has there been difficulty for suggesting that human infants experience emotion, but "there is a serious danger of circular reasoning in basing a denial . . . on the mere assumption that this suggestion is anthropomorphic. The charge carries weight only if one assumes in advance that . . . [they] do *not* have such experiences" (Griffin, 1981, pp. 124–125). Affective experience and expression are likely to exist and to be ecologically appropriate at all developmental ages but in different forms, much as cognition exists in some form in humans at all ages.

AFFECT STRUCTURE

Definition and Background

Research pertaining to affect structure has largely resided in the area of ethology and has rarely been used in developmental theories. It is clear, however, to any biologist that the appearance, scent, and so forth, of an animal will influence the behavior of others to it. This is a design feature of the animal (an affordance to others of its species), just as the dot on a seagull is a design feature for involuntary behavior (Tinbergen, 1951). Changes in the perceptible qualities of an animal influence the behavior directed toward it and the range of responses allowed to it. Within the realm of affect development, more than in many other areas of development, these structural features are important, and their importance is likely to vary across developmental age and situation.

Affect structure refers primarily to static facial configuration without any identifiable affect pattern in the muscular movement in our description. Most studies of affect have focused on the information in the face with a very few concentrating on postures, communicative gestures (see Hall, 1969) or vocal information for affect (see Scherer, 1979; Wolff, 1969). Other aspects of appearance or of physiology could be considered under affect structure as well—aspects such as height or scent.

The study of static facial configuration and its effect on personality attribution has a long history, though it is studied little today. In the 1930s, Brunswick and Reiter (1937) demonstrated that adults made attributions about age, intelligence, and feelings, as well as personality, from facial cues such as the position of the features (see also Sternglanz, Gray, & Murakami, 1977). Similarly, the facial configuration and the round "babyish" characteristics will influence the judgment of state, as well as age of an infant. Such communication is incidental, but adults perceive age and expression and attribute an emotion to the infant (e.g., Haviland, 1976).

As several ethologists have commented, including Lorenz (1981), and as Gardner and Wallach (1965) have demonstrated, the infant face (relative to an adult face) is rounder, its eyes more widely spaced; it has a shorter chin, a pug nose, high forehead, fatty pads that obscure muscular markings, and thinly haired brows. Lorenz pointed out that some of these characteristics are displayed by the young of many species and also by species considered neotonized by humans, though he did not explain why these characteristics are so appealing. That they are is not just an intuitive observation. Brunswick and Reiter (1937) found that large eyes and a high brow were preferred features. Adult faces with childlike facial features are perceived as affording more warmth, more honesty, more naivete, but less physical strength and more submission (Berry & McArthur, 1986).

In the case of infants, facial structure imparts an appealing affective message (e.g., Darwin, 1872/1965). Specifically, the structural affect of an infant does not anger or threaten but elicits attention, care, and love from a caretaker (see Hoffman, 1978, 1982). This creates an adaptive environment for an infant that maximizes his or her likelihood of being interested and attentive. So the facial affect structure influences the caretaker and produces reciprocal motivational states in the infant.

Later, in the pubertal period, Steinberg (1981) found that the changing appearance of the preadolescent is the most likely causal factor in alterations in family social interaction including dominance behaviors. Cognitive development, age, and grade were unrelated to changes in adolescent dominance behaviors, whereas facial/bodily changes were related. Little is known about the potential for structural change in old age for altering affective communication, but it is also likely to be an important period of change in which structural components have a central controlling role to play. Further, there is some suggestion that gender differences in static facial structure also influence affective behaviors, in that women's faces are more like those of children than are men's faces.

What is an explanation for the function of structure? Darwin's explanation focused on the signal value of expressions. He suggested, for example, that threat signals were related to anger–rage configurations (gnashing teeth, roaring, biting, and tearing movements). More important to us here, Darwin also introduced the principle of *antithesis*, suggesting that movements that had no obvious original function but that produced an effect opposite to movements with clear functions would assume an opposite signal value. Using the same example, movements judged the opposite to those used to express anger might evolve to signal "antianger" or "antihostility." Thus, the static infant face portrays just the opposite of the angry face. The infant's face *affords* benevolent interest (Gibson, 1979). On the other hand, the adult male face is more flexible and may afford hostile information among other signals.

Stability and Change

Taking our hypothesis about the importance of facial affect structure still further, some individual differences in interaction may actually stem from or be related to the structure of the face. For example, developmental changes in the structure may signal or even trigger different responses from caretakers regardless of behavior (Maier, Holmes, Slaymaker, & Reich, 1984). Also, a mismatch between affect structure and affect behavior may elicit unusual or even hostile behavior from a caretaker (Field & Vega-Lahr, 1984; McCabe, 1984).

Finally, direction of the developmental change across the lifespan for overall face shape and placement of features has been outlined (Alley, 1983; Pittinger,

Shaw, & Mark, 1979) and contains the elements mentioned. The growth is best described as a cardiodal strain transformation that gradually alters the shape of the head and face. The specific changes occurring during the infant period have as yet to be documented, though these changes are discussed in the coding systems used by Oster and Ekman (1978).

Summary

Although we have emphasized the infant's facial structural affect in this section, a child or adult's "resting expression" has an impact on interactions with others as well, especially in the case where two individuals are not familiar with one another (Laser & Mathie, 1982). Extended observation of a face in motion will reveal which placements of features are truly expressive and which are static, but attributions may be made about an individual's personality merely on the basis of static characteristics. This is a component of emotion expression that deserves considerably more attention.

REFLEXIVE AFFECT

Definition and Background

A reflexive affect is an innately programmed affective response much like a fixed action pattern (Lorenz, 1965), as its name implies. As Thelen (1985) has written, they are

> conspicuous movements using large muscle groups. . . . [Like] rhythmical stereotypes, the different emotionally expressive behaviors have a characteristic age of onset, peak frequency, and decline. . . . [They are] quite adultlike in form but without the complex temporal and spatial sequencing of expressions in older children or adults. (p. 235)

According to Tomkins (1962), a reflexive affective response will vary according to the change-increasing or change-decreasing amplitude of any perceived event and to the frequency of the event. Considered are the objective qualities of a stimulus event such as the frequency and intensity of an auditory signal as well as the perceptual and sensing abilities of the individual. For example, if a feather were floating down from the ceiling toward one's eye, information about the event (magnification of contour and structure) would specify a slow approach. One's reaction would be to visually follow the event with mild interest. If, however, an object approaches very quickly and especially if it is accompanied by a whizzing noise, increasing its impact intermodally, the person will startle. One does not reflect on these reactions during the situation; at least initially they have "reflexive" qualities. It is on such responses that experiences of emotion are based.

As pointed out by Malatesta (1985) in support of Tomkins's (1962) gradient theory, several research studies suggest that early infant affect is elicited by gradients of physical stimuli:

> Certain types of tactile stimulation, depending on intensity, can produce smiles or laughter (Sroufe & Wunsch, 1972; Guillory, Self, Biscoe, & Cole, 1982; Washburn, 1929). Auditory stimuli, depending on their onset, intensity, and

pitch values, can elicit the startle response, smiling, and laughter (Guillory *et al.*, 1982; Cicchetti & Hesse, 1983). Various visual events such as looming stimuli and the gradients associated with depth . . . can elicit fear (Campos & Stenberg, 1981; Cicchetti & Hesse, 1983). . . . Distress crying is provoked by chronic unrelieved pain, hunger, and certain auditory events . . . (Sagi & Hoffman, 1976; Cicchetti & Hesse, 1983; Martin & Clark, 1982). Anger can be produced by sustained physical restraint (Wiesenfeld, Malatesta, & DeLoach, 1981; Stenberg, 1982) and by low-level distress that persists over a prolonged period of time (Malatesta & Haviland, 1982). (pp. 197–198)

Reflexive affect has a long history. Early in this century, Bekhterev (1928) defined a class of reflexes as the "emotion reflex" or the "somatomimetic" reflex. He did not specify the number of reflexive affects, but he could at least agree with Watson (1928) about joy (pleasure), fear, rage, and excitement and cites his own and coworkers' observations. He concluded that there are innate somatomimetic reflexes corresponding to qualitatively distinct affects and that these are controlled primarily in the "vegetative brain centers" or subcortically in the thalamic region (see also Cannon, 1928). It is not a new idea, but it is a neglected one in psychology because psychologists have had great difficulty incorporating reflexive affects into theories and descriptions of the adult experience of emotion. Our knowledge of reflexive affect has grown substantially since that time, emerging in cross-cultural studies (Ekman, 1972), in studies of the physiology of emotion (Ekman, Levenson, & Friesen, 1983; Schwartz, 1982), and is now coming to play a major role in dynamic theories of expressive behavior (Thelen, 1985).

In spite of its long history, considerable controversy continues (e.g., Ortony & Turner, 1990) about the existence or, given their existence, the number of basic emotions or reflexive affects that should be considered in any effort to discuss the development or socialization of emotion. Further, there are questions about the usefulness of considering some set of emotion signals as having an involuntary or possibly reflexive quality. For example, there are hundreds of words in English that connote various shades of emotion to adult speakers. Should all of these be considered indicative of basic emotions? Considered from a phylogenetic position or from knowledge of brain structure, there are very few basic emotions. Researchers give us from three to five (Panksepp, 1982). The approach adopted here lies in between the extremes and is based on the communication of emotion, as is appropriate for our task.

For the last 20 years or so (Ekman, 1972; Izard, 1971; Tomkins, 1962), it has been clear that there is an acceptable facial and/or postural symbol among all humans for joy, surprise, sadness, anger, disgust, and fear and probably for interest, shame, and contempt. The majority of these symbols seem to be related in fairly standardized ways to other aspects of emotion (to be noted later). We rely upon this body of research to argue that there is a set of basic, involuntary emotions that have independent signal value in human communication, both in the sense of communicating to others and to oneself.

Stability and Change

How might reflexive affects change developmentally? At least two sorts of change are possible—changes in the form and alteration in eliciting events for a reflexive affect.

JEANNETTE M.
HAVILAND and
ARLENE S.
WALKER-ANDREWS

One well-studied expression that occurs during infancy is the smile. It is a good example for us here because some researchers argue that the production of the smile alters during infancy and that the smile emerges in response to a sociocognitive timetable (e.g. Lewis & Michalson, 1983; Sroufe & Waters, 1976). Sroufe and Waters (1976) note that the smile of an infant is first detected during periods of low arousal, during REM sleep or in drowsy states. Subsequently, it is seen in periods of alertness in response to mild arousal. As a next step, it is detected in periods of cognitive effort in which successful comprehension occurs. Similarly, Oster (1978) has described the form of what is deemed a "social smile": It is typically preceded by a 3- to 20-second period of knit brows, accompanied by visual fixation of another's face; at the onset of the smile, the brows are relaxed. Oster interprets the knit brow to reflect an effort by the infant to comprehend, followed, when that cognitive effort is successful, by releasing of the brow and an ensuing smile. Such social smiles are not identical in form to the early, reflexlike REM smiles that Sroufe and Waters (1976) describe.

To explain how the eliciting events for a smile change, Sroufe and Waters posit a tension reduction system in which cognitive change leads to both tension production and reduction. The smile itself occurs at periods of tension reduction. The endogenous smiles of the neonate are said to reflect a "fluctuating level of moderate arousal. . . . It is not until about the third month, however, that *psychological processing of the stimulus content* (recognition) leads to the smile, which may be suggested to indicate *pleasure*" (Sroufe, 1979, p. 481). They also suggest that the form of the response itself changes during infancy, coming to include eye movements, becoming more intense, and finally including the laugh. This progression in the intensity of the expression of the joy response is confirmed in more detail by Oster and Ekman (1978). In all cases the smile follows a posited reduction in "tension" as predicted by Tomkins (1962).

The reflexive response can be inhibited; it can be linked to other affects that may serve to mask it; or it may receive its full display in one part of the face or body rather than in the whole. The display patterns may be transformed through socialization processes (Malatesta, Gugoryev, Lamb, Albin, & Culver, 1986; Malatesta & Haviland, 1982). For example, most adults and children learn to inhibit the vocal aspect of affect rather early in life (see Malatesta, 1981). Little children may roar with anger or cry with distress, but adults do so only under extreme circumstances. Many adults take their inhibition several steps farther by either inhibiting the facial display also, or by making part of the vocal inhibition a part of the display. For instance, the thin-lipped, closed-mouth anger facial expression results from the vocal inhibition of anger; otherwise the mouth would be open and teeth bared. One learns to respond also to some affects with other affects. Many people cry when they are angry, for example. In this case, the initial expressive anger response is quickly responded to by distress and thus is difficult to detect.

Summary

The importance of reflexive affect cannot be overemphasized theoretically, but it is equally important not to confuse reflexive affect with structural or temperament components, much less with the knowledge—conditioned, learned, or symbolic—component.

In conclusion of this section, reflexive affect is a primitive response to any kind of stimulus information. The infant responds to information, and part of that response is affective. He or she then also responds to the affect because that serves as information as well; there is a continuous chain of affective behavior in the infant.

Affect Temperament

Definition and Background

In some respects, the cry of every infant is the same; it has a message and a predictable behavior pattern. This is true of all reflexive affect and represents basic neurological commonalities. Infants also differ in their responses to specific events, and those responses differ in certain respects such as intensity, duration, onset. These individual differences in affective displays may be called "temperamental."

Affective temperament is a subset of what is commonly called *temperament*; it is the stereotypic response of a particular individual. It identifies an individual's affective response to particular events as well as the intensity and timing of the response. For example, affective temperament is the aspect of behavior that predicts whether one is interested or startled by a bell ringing. To one person it may be routinely interesting and to another of the same developmental age, routinely startling.

Affective temperament, thus, is similar to the definition of temperament provided by Goldsmith and Campos (1982):

> Temperament refers to individual differences in the intensive and temporal parameters of behavioral expressions of emotionality and arousal, especially as these differences influence the organization of intrapersonal and interpersonal processes. (p. 832)

Temperament is defined as individual differences in the expression of primary emotions and in generalized arousal.

Including temperament as a component in the emotion system allows us to consider aspects of emotion that have been addressed incompletely in previous theories. For example, discontinuous shifts in emotion behavior may be controlled at some times by temperamental differences, not by specific reflexive or knowledge-based components. Those aspects of behavior that may characterize an individual, but are not related to emotion, are not part of affective temperament; and affective temperament may be measured only with respect to each discrete emotion. These requirements separate affective temperament from other theories of temperament, but that separation is supported by close examination of available data.

In general, most theories of temperament include any aspect of behavior that is both stable and related to personality. Included in such approaches are actual affect categories as well as a number of other behaviors. For example, Buss and Plomin (1984) include emotionality (fear, anger, and upset), sociability (interest in people), activity level, and impulsivity as temperamental characteristics. Rothbart and Derryberry (1982) use the entire emotional system as one of the temperament systems. They apply temperament generally to constitutional differences in the workings of any system, including motoric, endocrine, and the like. Similarly, Thomas and Chess (1977; see also Thomas, Chess, Birch, Hertzig, & Korn, 1963)

JEANNETTE M.
HAVILAND and
ARLENE S.
WALKER-ANDREWS

originally defined temperament as content free, as a description of behavioral style that applied across situations and across behavior systems. However, they divided temperament into nine categories that permits one to separately examine the more affective aspects of their more global temperament.

Of the Thomas et al. (1963) nine categories of temperamental reactivity, four seem identified with affect: (a) "Activity level" embodies the excitement and interest of the affect *interest*. (2) "Approach/withdrawal" embodies both the *fear* and *interest* domains, depending upon the level of stimulation; it may often include *disgust* or *anger*, but one cannot differentiate these with descriptions provided. (3)"Quality of mood" is meant as an affect dimension but reflects the authors' initial hypothesis that affect is a linear positive/negative dimension. It probably includes any intense affect but is most likely to be used to differentiate enjoyment from distress and anger. (4) "Attention span/persistence" includes the interest affect but also would be related to cognitive processing; so it is more likely an amalgam.

The other categories used by Thomas et al. may include affective behaviors as well, but they are not quite so clear in the description—they are (a) rhythmicity of biological functions, (b) adaptability (changes in behavior with repeated exposure), (c) threshold (intensity of stimuli needed to achieve a response), (d) intensity (of the response to stimuli), and (e) distractibility (changes in behavior with distractors available). The components of these qualities appear to be either heavily physiological or cognitive without affective components playing a controlling role or even a major contributing role.

Stability and Change

In spite of the overlapping of affects and affect intensity and the lack of separation between affect and cognition across the temperament dimensions that most researchers propose, there is stability in certain aspects of temperament. In Thomas, Chess, and Birch (1969), four of nine temperament categories showed significant stability across several years for differentiating clinical groups from nonclinical groups. Activity, mood, attention, and persistence (the heavily affect-laden dimensions) were the best predictors; they loaded heavily on the principal factor that demonstrated stable differences. Those children who had symptoms requiring clinical intervention tended to continue to have negative moods and strongly exhibited affect; they were more likely to withdraw than to approach and were not adaptable to new situations. Two categories showed, not continuity, but developmental change: the threshold of response and intensity of response. In comparison with other children, those children with clinical symptoms did not "mature"; they tended to maintain uninhibited affect and to maintain low thresholds for affect display.

There were two major patterns of results in the Thomas et al. (1969) data. One pattern suggested that there are early, sustained differences that are moderately correlated with clinically distressing symptoms. The main difference is affective, called *negative mood*. The other pattern indicated that the clinical population increasingly demonstrates behaviors that intensify the negative affect response. Rather than decreasing the signal for negative affect, they maintained or possibly increased the intensity of the display. Because most infants began to restrain negative affect signals and to increase positive affect signals as early as 6 months, this suggests a problem in the socialization of affect displays (Haviland & Malatesta, 1981).

The difficult child is described as having

> irregularity in biological functions, a predominance of negative (withdrawal) responses to new stimuli, slowness in adapting to changes in environment, a high frequency of expression of negative mood and predominance of intense reactions. (Thomas, Chess, & Birch, 1969, p. 75)

In light of an affective perspective, we propose that the difficult child is very sensitive to perceived events. Instead of eliciting interest these stimulus events are more intense in the child's experience—the interesting being the surprising, the surprising becoming the fearful or startling. This child may have difficulty inhibiting, moderating, or attenuating fear reactions, which then seem immaturely uncontrolled from the parent's point of view (Kagan, Reznick, Snidman, Gibbons, & Johnson, 1988; See also Stiefel, Plunkett, & Meisels, 1987). This makes the child seem not only difficult, but as he or she gets older, to seem increasingly infantile. He or she has not "moderated" his or her surprise/fear affect display as other younger children have learned to do (beginning as early as 3 months; Malatesta & Haviland, 1982), but this may be because his or her threshold for phase shifts across the affects of interest, surprise, fear is lower.

Most theories of temperament propose that it is stable. Our definition, like that of Goldsmith and Campos (1982), does not require long-term stability. Certain temperamental characteristics may have long-term stability, but others may not. These latter characteristics may be stable only within certain developmental epochs. As noted, some of the most stable characteristics called temperament by Thomas and Chess are closely related to affect, but we are not claiming that affect temperament is necessarily consistent across the lifespan. Further, although differences in affective temperament may remain stable, they may provoke diverging coping strategies. These are important issues that must be dealt with empirically and that become bound up in assessing homotypic versus heterotypic continuity (see Kagan *et al.*, 1988).

Summary

The definition provided here for affective temperament requires that one examine the individual characteristics in the expression of each discrete emotion—joy, sadness, anger, disgust, fear, and the like. We would not predict a general "emotionality" across emotions or moods but specific affective temperament types. This approach is used in research on shyness, for example see Kagan *et al.*, 1988.

To some degree, researchers have moved toward separating affect and temperament or at least to looking more closely at their interactions (whether considered as the same construct or separate ones). Goldsmith and Campos (1982) tried to map selected dimensions of temperament from a variety of temperament scales (Buss & Plomin, 1986; Rothbart & Derryberry, 1982; Thomas, Chess, Birch, Hertzig, & Korn, 1963) onto affect dimensions as defined by Ekman (1972) and Izard (1977). This attempt clearly indicated that most systems describing temperament, affect categories, and social categories are intertwined, as noted earlier.

JEANNETTE M.
HAVILAND and
ARLENE S.
WALKER-ANDREWS

Definition and Background

Affect knowledge is that part of affect that is most related to social learning and cognitive development and eventually is symbolic. This component of affect is the aspect that includes what is learned or known to the self. It is that aspect that has been emphasized by those who believe that an awareness of self is necessary for the experience of emotion (e.g., Lewis & Michalson, 1983). It also comes to include our conscious understanding of our feelings and the conscious experience of emotion (Haviland, 1984; Haviland & Kramer, 1991). This component of affect is probably the most studied and best understood component, and therefore we will frequently refer to other reviews.

A description of the socialization of affect must include a child's developing knowledge of emotion. Cognitive changes can be controlling factors in any system including the affective system. The extensive investigation of cognitive development that emerged in the last 20 years has given this component the largest research literature. Accounts of children's developing knowledge of emotion have been made by Harter and Whitsell (1988), Lewis and Saarni (1985), and Harris (1989), among others. Different theoretical approaches to emotion knowledge vary in the interpretation they place on a cognitive component. At one extreme, social philosophers (see Harré, 1986) have long argued that emotions are only the values constructed by social groups about events, people or ideas that therefore cannot be experienced without acquired knowledge. They particularly wish to refer to "refined" emotions, such as "patriotism," but they also include the "baser" passions, such as fear or anger. Their concentration is on the socialization of ideas about emotion or emotional ideas about other types of events. Historical analyses (e.g., Stearns, 1986) of emotional writing support the thesis that emotional ideas change in concert with other cultural ideas. In this position, the entire emotion system is but an outgrowth of social knowledge. This extreme version, of course, does not include the research that has been reviewed previously in this chapter on other components of emotion. The social-cognitive component cannot always be considered the constraining component in emotion development.

Other social-cognitive theorists (e.g. Tomkins, 1989; Leventhal, 1991) retain some of the other components of emotion as building blocks in their theories. That is, they acknowledge that some type of reflexive or involuntary emotion behaviors may be available as tools to use in forming social-cognitive systems, especially early in development, but they assume that metacognitive functions are more important in predicting later behavior. In this way they retain the linear, goal-oriented systems approach in their theories. Emotion socialization is increasingly under the control of cognition, with the ultimate adult social-emotional system being composed in large part of functional or dysfunctional cognitive components. Although it is clear that affective knowledge increases with the differentiation of knowledge, it is not obvious that cognition outweighs all factors or that it is generally more important and perhaps it is not. If it were, then educational programs would have direct and obvious effects on affective disorders. Because they do not, treatment strategies vary from biochemical controls to desensitization behavior controls to psychotherapy, each of which may have a noticeable effect on one or more of the other components.

Changes in knowledge as an elicitor or as critical in the production of emotion can occur in a number of ways. We will begin with learning mechanisms that may be specialized for emotion and remind the reader of well-established learning mechanisms that appear to be more general. Emotion knowledge is influenced by contagion, modeling, association, and reinforcement. Most of these mechanisms are familiar ones and will not be reviewed in this chapter because they are learning modes that have fairly long research histories in psychology. The exception is contagion.

Emotional contagion is closely associated with the affordances of people. There is some evidence that an emotional expression is itself sufficient to produce the emotional expression in the perceiver. When this happens, and two or more people show the same emotion, we would say that the emotion had been contagious. Happy expressions are contagious, just as fear and angry expressions are. They produce the expression and probably the experience in others as other nonsocial stimuli may. Although Tomkins suggested this in 1962, evidence to support it is fairly recent (Field, Woodson, Greenberg, & Cohen, 1982; Haviland & Lelwica, 1987). There are several demonstrations that certain expressions that may be related to emotions can be contagious as early as 1 day of age (Sagi & Hoffman, 1976; Simner, 1971) and that emotion expressions of joy, sadness, and anger are contagious at 10 or 11 weeks of age (Haviland & Lelwica, 1987). The early occurrence of contagion suggests that it is not likely to have resulted from other associative learning.

One result stemming from the contagion of emotion as a mechanism for change in emotion is that the expression of particular emotions in one person may become routine in an intimate companion (child, spouse, etc.) just because they are routine for one of them. A well-cared-for infant may be distressed frequently if the caretaker expresses distress, for example. The limits of the contagion system have not been explored. It may be that certain expressions are not contagious until later in life (for example, see Lewis, 1992, for a discussion of shame). One should not, however, discount the possibility that even simple contagious emotion may constrain behavior.

Related research using adult subjects has shown that visual, auditory, or metacognitive stimulus materials may orient a broad spectrum of behaviors for at least a short time. For example, Teasdale and Fogarty (1979) have shown that people who listen to music characterized as "sad" will have a low range of activity with slow production rates. They also may have the experience of recruiting memories and producing other images related to sadness but do not always have these verbal associates. The associative processes in adulthood are appreciably different from those in infancy, but the example does suggest that contagious emotion mechanisms may influence emotion behavior in important ways.

When the potential of contagious aspects of emotion are considered along with various learning abilities of infants, then the mutability of the emotion system becomes clearer. Very young infants are capable of associative learning (e.g., Blass, Ganchrow, & Steiner, 1984) and have good memories (Rovee-Collier & Fagen, 1981). Even so, specificity of associations may limit the effect of such early learning because young infants are very sensitive to context or place and their ability to generalize on the basis of categories is very limited (Rovee-Collier & Hayne, 1987).

JEANNETTE M.
HAVILAND and
ARLENE S.
WALKER-ANDREWS

Not only are emotion functions influenced by contagion and association, but specific patterns of expression are reinforced, and infants quickly learn to change the mode and frequency of emotion expression during social interactions. The rate of facial expression of emotion slows during the early months of life, beginning to approach adult rates of conversational expression change. Familial and cultural preferences for using different muscles for the expression emerge in the infant. For example, if the caretaker uses the brow more frequently in expression, so will the infant (Halberstadt, 1984; Malatesta & Haviland, 1982). Though there are limitations on the simple knowledge mechanisms of young infants, it is not necessary to posit metacognition about emotion in order to understand how simple associative systems could be formed. Although the examples used here are from the infant research literature, similar processes may well pertain in later life—processes in which simple nonconscious cognitive mechanisms constrain emotion behavior.

With respect to later childhood, research moves away from contagion, social referencing, and perception of emotion signals. It begins to focus on coping and the growing awareness of the functions of emotion. For example, self-conscious emotions, such as shyness, begin to function as indicators that the child is aware of how he or she appears to others (Lewis, 1992); deception skills further testify to the child's growing awareness of others' perception of him or her and the possibility for manipulating that perception (Ekman, 1985; DePaulo, 1988); awareness of distinct possibilities for changing one's own feelings and expressions also begins to emerge later in childhood (Harris, 1989).

Research on the development in emotion knowledge later in childhood primarily offers cognitive explanations. The child learns to predict the emotional responses of others to situations, to understand that it is possible to experience more than one emotion at once, and how to hide and recognize that others mask their emotions. Success in meeting these goals can be explained in various ways. For example, the child could learn to predict another's emotional response by noting the typical association between an expression and a type of event (Borke, 1971; Trabasso, Stein, & Johnson, 1981) or by imagining how he himself would feel in that situation (Harris, 1989). On the other hand, children as young as 3 or 4 can conceal the expression of disappointment in the presence of a gift given long before they have any explicit understanding of display rules (Cole, 1986).

There is evidence from children's reports that they knowingly respond to the emotional behavior of others and devise explanatory systems for understanding emotion. (See Harris, 1989, for detailed review.) As an example, Cummings, Vogel, Cummings, and El-Sheikh (1989) have shown that children report that *they* are angry when they are shown films in which adults behave angrily toward each other. It is not necessary that the adults verbalize the emotion or that they physically demonstrate any hostility, only that they "silently" produce angry expressions. However, older children report less anger when the adults resolve the conflict, demonstrating that if an understanding of the situation occurs, it changes the affective response.

Not only are there changes in the healthy functions of emotion expression, but there are also changes in dysfunctions. For example, a considerable bank of research (see Cummings & Cummings, 1988, for a review) suggests that children and adolescents with conduct disorders and other forms of aggressive behaviors have "attractors" for organizing behavior in which anger functions centrally and is very difficult to mediate or to resolve. These children are themselves easily angered as well as excessively sensitive to anger cues in others. This suggests a continuing central organizing feature for emotion under certain circumstances. In this case, the emotion of anger is a common denominator in the child's behavioral problems in his or her social world, the families' problems with hostility, and the formation of dysfunctional social and personality systems. Whether this is directly constrained and centrally mediated by cognitive mechanisms as is often assumed is open to empirical questioning.

Summary

In summary, affect knowledge may be acquired and transformed through contagion, learning, and finally by metacognitive processes. Affect knowledge is an important component of an emotion system in that it can function as an elicitor of emotion expression and changes in knowledge can produce changes in emotion functioning.

THE DYNAMIC SYSTEM

Background

Throughout this chapter we have argued that emotion and its development should be considered as a dynamic system with several general components. We discussed a few choices for these components based upon major research arenas and balanced between exogenous and endogenous component types. Throughout the chapter we have illustrated the interaction of these components and the necessity for beginning to think of emotion as a dynamic system. We will conclude by considering directly the advantages of this new approach.

In our analysis we have been aided substantially by illustration of a dynamic system for crying and smiling proposed by Fogel and Thelen (1987), based on rhythmical stereotypes and motor development. In summary, with respect to crying, Fogel and Thelen noted that the initial production of crying shows that there are discontinuous phase shifts in types of cries (defined by respiratory and repetition behaviors) that are controlled by specific types of stimulation at differing levels of behavior activation. Later in the first year of life the cry becomes "more ritualized and perfunctory as it becomes incorporated into a demand/request function" (Fogel & Thelen, 1987, p. 755). Although there are continuing changes in the regulatory motor abilities (regulation of respiration, expulsion of air, control of articulation), as well as in temperament, there are also clear changes in the associative (knowledge) factors with the cry serving new social functions in communication. Fogel and Thelen argue that components other than cognition clearly effect the emergent cry (affective) behavior and that at different developmental periods a different component may control the type of cry. Although they did not directly acknowledge the temperamental component, only a structural component (and that in a different sense than the structural component as we discussed it), the usefulness of a component approach was demonstrated. At different points in time, changes in the cry are controlled by different facets of structure or of social knowledge.

Approaches to the impact of a multicomponent dynamic systems model are

JEANNETTE M.
HAVILAND and
ARLENE S.
WALKER-ANDREWS

not limited to molecular analysis. Similar approaches have been suggested by Cantwell (1990), in a discussion of the production of depression, and by Ashmore (1990), in reviewing the components of gender differences in personality/ social research. For example, depression components could include a biological/ temperament component, a cognitive component, a socialization component, and so forth. Any one or combination of these might be an elicitor of a depressive mood at a particular point in time.

It may seem confusing initially that in a dynamic system components may change, interact, serve different controlling functions, but that behavior may occur in a generally predictable manner; however, the principle is relatively simple. Although the elements in components and the components themselves have many degrees of freedom, the outcome behavior tends to have fewer degrees of freedom. The adaptive behaviors and the affordances of any physical or psychological event or setting tend to be limited. There may be many ways to feed oneself, and the controlling features will vary developmentally, but feeding oneself is a fairly discrete and predictable outcome with chronological markers that are interesting ontologically and culturally. Crying and smiling likewise are discrete and predictable outcomes, the occurrence of which at any specific time may be constrained by different combinations of variables, nevertheless resulting in similar outcomes.

Stranger Fear—A Classic Example

Because this is a relatively new approach to the development of emotion, we will illustrate it with an example that points to the interaction of large components (as opposed to Fogel & Thelen's, 1987, smaller components) in a series of social behaviors—the affective behavior to strangers. Stranger reactions have been studied at several ages (where they have not we will be speculative). Strangers have been characterized as the elicitors of a particular emotion—fear—with some authors claiming that fear itself, as a behavior, emerges at the end of the second year with cognitive advances leading to the "achievement" of stranger fear. This approach is not consonant with our position, however. We argue that stranger fear is not a goal of development but a phase. Further, within a phase it is further circumscribed by the conditions that afford stranger fear. Even at the designated time there are other reactions than fear that may be elicited by a stranger, and at other chronological times fear or other emotions may be elicited, also depending upon the affordances within a particular situation as well as the subject's "developmental stage."

Even in early infancy, a stranger may have the affordances that lead to fear responses. In the early months a stranger may influence the infant's affective state by behaving in a familiar and regulating manner thus affording alert, interested responses. Other stranger behaviors could produce a wide variety of infant behaviors. Dropping the infant or acting like a looming object could probably elicit a fearful behavior. One might argue that the fact that the person is a stranger in itself does not elicit fear. That does not mean that fear cannot be elicited, nor does it mean that the novel person is not recognized as novel. Quite early the stranger can probably modulate the infant's affective expression by modifying his or her own affective behavior. A persistent smiling stranger is likely to elicit joy in the baby; the distressed or fearful stranger may elicit avoidance behavior in the infant.

At the end of the first year of infancy, the typical stranger fear may certainly be elicited, but it is easier to elicit the fear under certain conditions. The child being approached at first attends the stranger with interest, often smiles. If the stranger smiles and maintains distance, the child's happy response can be maintained. If the stranger continues to approach and does not respond, as was typical in stranger-approach laboratory studies, the child will avert. If the stranger still does not respond to the infant's responses, the infant will probably shift into distressed, fearful behaviors. Characteristics of the stranger influence the probability of a phase shift from one emotion to another. Whether the stranger is a child or an adult, a male or a female, and so on, all tend to influence the probability of a phase shift, but there is not one, simple, absolute response. We speculate that an interesting shift might occur in adolescence when the sexual attraction of strangers may further influence "stranger fear." The structural qualities (age, gender, pubertal status) of the child will influence the behavior of a stranger, and the structural qualities of a particular stranger will influence the probability of different emotional responses by the child.

In contrast to linear or additive teleologic approaches, the dynamic approach allows new forms of behaviors to become apparent just because one component of the system becomes the controlling one. A shift may occur because of maturation of the structural (including motoric, hormonal, etc.) component, because of a change in the type of stimulation afforded by the environment (reflexive behavior elicited), because of a change in temperament affect, or because knowledge allows the detection of different categories of affordances. As in our example, when a child first shows that she or he is afraid of strangers, one does not need to assume that "fear" is a novel behavior; it is not necessarily a "big bang" affect. The child has probably shown similar motoric expressive fear behaviors in response to other stimuli such as looming objects. The empirical question concerns instead the discontinuous shift in behavior from interest to fear in a particular situation.

Many contemporary models of emotion socialization build toward a teleological desirable state; such models are limited in their ability to accommodate important ecological positions. Too often the presumption is that the desirable direction is one in which the individual learns to cope with or dampen emotion. The assumption is that primitive emotions exist as a result of phylogenetic history and that subsequent ontological development brings such primitive sets of behavior under social and cognitive constraints. The alternative is to consider that affective systems of behavior are usually adaptive within the affordances of a given setting. For example, affective expressions often are more vocal in infancy than they are later in life. This does not necessarily mean that the infant vocal expression is maladaptive or that some social force must work to force a rapid change. Various explanations could be offered for the importance of vocal affect expression in infancy, including restrictions on reaching across distances that nonambulatory infants encounter. The vocal mode may be essential for maintaining contact when major motoric systems are limiting factors (e.g., Bowlby, 1969). To cite an entirely different set of factors, it is often assumed that an important task of adolescence is learning to control hostile affects that may emerge in puberty. Once again, the potential adaptive aspects of hostile emotion are often ignored.

"In both real and developmental time, new states emerge when components are pushed past critical values or the relations among the components change, leading to discontinuous phase shifts" in behavior (Fogel & Thelen, 1987, p. 750). For emotion this principle has many implications. With respect to differential emotions within a single setting, a shift in any component may lead to a discontinuous shift in the emotion behavior. For example, simple repetition without contingent response to a happy expression by the mother in the mother–infant setting shifts a 10-week-old baby's expression from a matching one of joy, to watchful interest (Haviland & Lelwica, 1987). There is a discontinuous shift in behavioral expression that is apparently related to the context of repetition of a joy signal but without contingency. With contingency the behavior of the infant will shift back to joy. It is the patterning of the stimulus that leads to the shift change. This seems to function as we predicted reflexive affect would function.

Across the mix of components and across temperaments, there also are discontinuous phase shifts. The temperamentally shy child under stress will reveal his or her shyness at many developmental epochs, as though the shy behavior were an "attractor" pulling together scenes. Another child who does not have such an attractor is more variable in general, although even the temperamentally shy child can show flexibility if the child's parents provide training and support of alternate behavior (Kagan *et al.*, 1988).

Summary

The dynamic approach to emotional behavior is relatively new, as dynamic approaches to processes are emerging in many sciences (e.g., chaos theory). Much of what it has to offer needs to be explored. Theoretical impasses that lead to seemingly irresolvable conflict when linear explanations were tendered, however, can now be seen from a new position as empirically resolvable.

We have targeted four particular overarching components because each represents a research domain in emotion and because they represent both endogenous and exogenous factors. Dispute whether each plays a role in emotion expression at any real time or developmental time is open to empirical investigation. Individual differences in emotion can also be investigated, not as deviances from a norm or as distances from a goal, but as processes that are adaptive within particular ecological subsystems. From any static point there is heterochronicity in the path followed by the interaction of components that function to produce emotional behavior. Structure, reflex, temperament, and knowledge all must be considered.

References

Alley, T. R. (1983). Growth-produced changes in body shape and size as determinants of perceived age and adult caregiving. *Child Development, 54*, 241–248.

Ashmore, R. D. (1990). Sex, gender, and the individual. In L. A. Pervin (Ed.), *Handbook of personality theory and research* (pp. 486–526). New York: Guilford Publications.

Bekhterev, V. M. (1928). Emotions as somato-memetic reflexes. In M. L. Reymart (Ed.), *Feelings and emotions: The Wittenberg symposium*. Worcester, MA: Clark University Press.

Berry, D. S., & McArthur, L. Z. (1986). Perceiving character in faces: The impact of age-related craniofacial changes on social perception. *Psychological Bulletin, 100*, 3–18.

Blass, E. M., Ganchrow, J. R., & Steiner, J. E. (1984). Classical conditioning in newborn humans 2–48 hours of age. *Infant Behavior and Development, 7*, 223–235.

Borke, H. (1971). Interpersonal perception of young children: Egocentrism or empathy? *Developmental Psychology, 5*, 263–269.

Bowlby, J. (1969). *Attachment and loss, Vol. I, Attachment*. London: Hogarth.

Brazelton, T., Koslowski, B, & Main, M. (1974). The origins of reciprocity: The early mother-infant interaction. In M. Lewis & L. Rosenblum (Eds.), *The effect of the infant on its caregiver* (pp. 49–76). New York: Wiley.

Brunswick, E., & Reiter, L. (1937). Eindruckscharacktere schematiserter Gesichter. *Zeitschrift der Psychologische Bildung, 142*, 67–134.

Buss, A. H., & Plomin, R. (1984). *Temperament: Early developing personality traits.* Hillsdale, NJ: Erlbaum.

Buss, A. H., & Plomin, R. C. (1986). The EAS approach to temperament. In R. Plomin & J. Dunn (Eds.), *The study of temperament: Changes, continuities, and challenges* (pp. 67–79). Hillsdale, NJ: Erlbaum.

Campos, J. J., & Stenberg, C. R. (1981). Perception, appraisal and emotion: The onset of social referencing. In M. E. Lamb & L. Sherrod (Eds.), *Infant social cognition* (pp. 273–314). Hillsdale, NJ: Erlbaum.

Cannon, W. B. (1928). Neural organization for emotional expression. In M. L. Reymert (Ed.), *Feelings and emotions: The Wittenberg symposium* (pp. 257–283). Worcester, MA: Clark University Press.

Cantwell, D. P. (1990). Depression across the early life span. In M. Lewis & S. M. Miller (Ed.), *Handbook of developmental psychology* (pp. 293–309). New York: Plenum Press.

Cicchetti, D., & Hesse, P (1983). Affect and intellect: Piaget's contributions to the study of infant emotional development. In R. Plutchik & H. Kellerman (Eds.), *Emotion: Theory, research, and experience* (Vol. 2, pp. 115–169). Orlando, FL: Academic Press.

Cole, P. M. (1986). Children's spontaneous control of facial expression. *Child Development, 57*, 1309–1321.

Cummings, E. M., & Cummings, J. L (1988). A process-oriented approach to children's coping with adults' angry behavior. *Developmental Review, 8*, 296–321.

Cummings, E. M., Vogel, D., Cummings, J. S., & El-Sheikh, M. (1989). Children's responses to different forms of expression of anger between adults. *Child Development, 60*,1392–1404.

Darwin, C. (1965). *The expression of emotions in men and animals.* Chicago: University of Chicago Press. (Original work published 1872)

DePaulo, B. M. (1988). Nonverbal aspects of deception. *Journal of Nonverbal Behavior, 12*, 153–161.

Ekman, P. (1972). Universals and cultural differences in facial expressions of emotion. In J. K. Cole (Ed.) *Nebraska Symposium on Motivation*, Vol. 19. Lincoln: University of Nebraska Press.

Ekman, P. (1985). *Telling Lies.* New York: Norton.

Ekman, P., Levenson, R. W., & Friesen, W. V. (1983). Autonomic nervous system activity distinguishes among emotions. *Science, 221*, 1208–1210.

Erdelyi, M. (1974). A new look at the new look: Perceptual defense and vigilance. *Psychological Review, 81*, 1–25.

Field, T. M., & Vega-Lahr, N. (1984). Early interactions between infants with cranio-facial anomalies and their mothers. *Infant Behavior and Development, 7*, 527–530.

Field, T. M., Woodson, R., Greenberg, R., & Cohen, D. (1982). Discrimination and imitation of facial expressions by neonates. *Science, 218*, 179–181.

Fogel, A., & Thelen, E. (1987). Development of early expressive and communicative action: Reinterpreting the evidence from a dynamic systems perspective. *Developmental Psychology, 23*, 747–761.

Gardner, B., & Wallach, L. (1965). Shapes of figures identified as a baby's head. *Perceptual and Motor Skills, 20*, 135–142.

Gibson, J. J. (1979). *The ecological approach to visual perception.* Boston: Houghton Mifflin.

Goldsmith, H. H., & Campos, J. J. (1982). Toward a theory of infant temperament. In R. N. Emde & R. J. Harmon (Eds.), *The development of attachment and affiliative systems: Psychobiological aspects* (pp. 161–193). New York: Plenum Press.

Griffin, D. R. (1981). *The question of animal awareness: Evolutionary continuity of mental experiences.* New York: Rockefeller University Press.

Guillory, A. W., Self, P. A., Biscoe, B. M., & Cole, C. A. (1982). *The first four months: Development of affect, cognition, and synchrony.* Paper presented at the American Psychological Association meetings, Washington, DC.

Halberstadt, A. G. (1984). Family expression of emotion. In C. Z. Malatesta & C. E. Izard (Eds.), *Emotion in adult development* (pp. 235–252). Beverly Hills, CA: Sage.

Hall, E. T. (1969). *The hidden dimension.* New York: Doubleday.

Harré, R. (1986). *The social construction of emotions.* New York: Basil Blackwell.

Harris, P. L. (1989). *Children and emotion.* Oxford: Blackwell.

Harter, S., & Rumbaugh-Whitesell, N. (1988). Developmental changes in children's understanding of single, multiple, and blended emotion concepts. In C. Saarni & P. Harris (Eds.), *Children's understanding of emotion* (pp. 81–116). New York: Cambridge University Press.

48

JEANNETTE M.
HAVILAND and
ARLENE S.
WALKER-ANDREWS

Haviland, J. M. (1976). Looking smart: The relationship between affect and intelligence in infancy. In M. Lewis & L. Rosenblum (Eds.), *Origins of intelligence: Infancy and early childhood* (pp. 353–377). New York: Plenum Press.

Haviland, J. M. (1984). Thinking and feeling in Woolf's writing: From childhood to adulthood. In C. Izard, J. Kagan, & R. Zajonc (Eds.), *Emotions, cognition and behavior* (pp. 515–546). London: Oxford University Press.

Haviland, J. M., & Kramer, D. (1991). Affect-cognition relationships in adolescent diaries: The case of Anne Frank. *Human Development, 34,* 143–159.

Haviland, J. M., & Lelwica, M. (1987). The induced affect response: 10-week-old infants' responses to three emotion expressions. *Developmental Psychology, 23,* 97–104.

Haviland, J., & Malatesta, C. Z. (1981). Fantasies, fallacies and facts: The development of sex differences in non-verbal signals. In C. Mayo & N. Henley (Eds.), *Gender and non-verbal behavior* (pp. 183–208). New York: Springer-Verlag.

Hoffman, M. L. (1978). Empathy, its development and prosocial implications. In H. E. Howe, Jr. & C. B. Keasey (Eds.), *Nebraska Symposium on Motivation.* (Vol. 25). Lincoln: University of Nebraska Press.

Hoffman, M. L. (1982). The measurement of empathy. In C. E. Izard (Ed.), *Measuring emotions in infants and children* (pp. 279–296). Cambridge: Cambridge University Press.

Izard, C. E. (1971). *The face of emotion.* New York: Appleton.

Izard, C. E. (1977). *Human emotions.* New York: Plenum Press.

Kagan, J., Reznick, J. S., Snidman, N., Gibbons, J., & Johnson, M. O. (1988). Childhood derivatives of inhibition and lack of inhibition to the unfamiliar. *Child Development, 89,* 1580–1589.

Laser, P. S., & Mathie, V. A. (1982). Face facts: An unbidden role for features in communication. *Journal of Nonverbal Behavior, 7,* 3–19.

Leventhal, H. (1991). Emotion: Prospects for conceptual and empirical development. In N. J. Weingartner & R. J. Listner (Eds.), *Cognitive neuroscience* (pp. 325–348). Oxford: Oxford University Press.

Lewis, M. (1992). *Shame, the exposed self.* New York: Free Press.

Lewis, M., & Michalson, L. (1983). *Children's emotions and moods.* New York: Plenum Press.

Lewis, M., & Saarni, C. (Eds.). (1985). *The socialization of emotions.* New York: Plenum Press.

Lorenz, K. (1965). *Evolution and the modification of behavior.* Chicago: University of Chicago Press.

Lorenz, K. (1981). Die angeborenen formen moglicher erfahrung. *Zeitschrift der Tierpsychologie, 5* 1–23.

Maier, R. A., Holmes, D. L. Slaymaker, F. L., & Reich, J. N. (1984). The perceived attractiveness of preterm infants. *Infant Behavior and Development, 7,* 403–414.

Malatesta, C. Z. (1981). Infant emotion and the vocal affect lexicon. *Emotion and Motivation, 5,* 1–23.

Malatesta, C. Z. (1985). Developmental course of emotion expression in the human infant. In G. Zivin (Ed.), *The development of expressive behavior* (pp. 183–219). New York: Academic Press.

Malatesta, C. Z., Gugoryev, P., Lamb, C., Albin, M., & Culver, C. (1986). Emotion socialization and expressive development in preterm and full term infants. *Child Development, 57,* 316–330.

Malatesta, C. Z., & Haviland, J. M. (1982). Learning display rules: The socialization of emotion expression in infancy. *Child Development, 53,* 991–1003.

Martin, G., & Clarke, R. (1982). Distress crying in neonates: Species and peer specificity. *Developmental Psychology, 18,* 3–10.

McArthur, L. Z., & Baron, R. M. (1983). Toward an ecological theory of social perception. *Psychological Review, 90,* 215–238.

McCabe, V. (1984). Abstract perceptual information for age level: A risk factor for maltreatment? *Child Development, 55,* 267–276.

Nisbett, R. E., & Wilson, T. D. (1977). Telling more than we can know: Verbal reports on mental processes. *Psychological Review, 84,* 231–259.

Ortony, A., & Turner, T. J. (1990). What's basic about basic emotions? *Psychological Review, 97,* 315–331.

Oster, H. (1978). Facial expression and affect development. In M. Lewis & L. A. Rosenblum (Eds.), *The development of affect* (pp. 43–76). New York: Plenum Press.

Oster, H., & Ekman, P. (1978). Facial behavior in child development. In A. Collins (Ed.), *Minnesota Symposium on Child Psychology.* Vol. II. Hillsdale, NJ: Erlbaum.

Panksepp, J. (1982). Toward a general psychobiological theory of emotions. *Behavioral and Brain Sciences, 5,* 407–467.

Pittenger, J., Shaw, R. E., & Mark, L. S. (1979). Perceptual information for the age level of faces as a higher order invariant of growth. *Journal of Experimental Psychology: Human Perception and Performance, 5,* 478–493.

Rothbart, M. K., & Derryberry, D. (1982). Development of individual differences in temperament. In

M. E. Lamb & A. L. Brown (Eds.), *Advances in developmental psychology* (Vol. 1, pp. 37–86). Hillsdale, NJ: Erlbaum.

Rovee-Collier, C. K., & Fagen, J. W. (1981). The retrieval of memory in early infancy. In L. P. Lipsitt (Ed.), *Advances in infancy research* (Vol. 1, pp. 225–254). Norwood, NJ: Ablex.

Rovee-Collier, C., & Hayne, H. (1987). Reactivation of infant memory: Implications for cognitive development. In H. W. Reese (Ed.), *Advances in child development and behavior* (Vol. 30, pp. 185–238). San Diego: Academic Press.

Saarni, C., & Harris, P. L. (Eds.). (1989). *Children's understanding of emotion*. New York: Cambridge University Press.

Sagi, A., & Hoffman, M. (1976). Empathic distress in the newborn. *Developmental Psychology, 12,* 175–176.

Scherer, K. R. (1979). Nonlinguistic vocal indicators of emotion and psychopathology. In C. E. Izard (Ed.), *Emotions in personality and psychopathology* (pp. 495–529). New York: Plenum Press.

Schwartz, G. (1982). Psychophysiological patterning and emotion revisited. In C. E. Izard (Ed.), *Measuring emotions in infants and children* (pp. 67–93). New York: Cambridge University Press.

Simner, M. (1971). Newborn's response to the cry of another infant. *Developmental Psychology, 5,* 136–150.

Sroufe, L. A. (1979). Socioemotional development. In J. Osofsky (Ed.), *Handbook of infant development* (pp. 462–516). New York: Wiley.

Sroufe, L. A., & Waters, E. (1976). The ontogenesis of smiling and laughter: A perspective on the organization of development in infancy. *Psychological Review, 83,* 173–189.

Sroufe, L. A., & Wunsch, J. P. (1972). The development of laughter in the first year of life. *Child Development, 43,* 1326–1344.

Stearns, P. N. (1986). Historical analysis in the study of emotion. *Motivation and Emotion, 10,* 185–193.

Steinberg, L. (1981). Transformations in family relations at puberty. *Developmental Psychology, 6,* 833–840.

Stenberg, C. (1982). The development of anger facial expressions in infancy. Unpublished doctoral dissertation. University of Denver.

Sternglanz, S. H., Gray, J. L., & Murakami, M. (1977). Adult preferences for infantile facial features: An ethological approach. *Animal Behaviour, 25,* 108–115.

Stiefel, G. S., Plunkett, J. W., & Meisels, S. J. (1987). Affective expression among preterm infants of varying levels of biological risk. *Infant Behavior and Development, 10,* 151–164.

Teasdale, J. D., & Fogarty, S. J. (1979). Differential effects of induced mood on retrieval of pleasant and unpleasant events from episodic memory. *Journal of Abnormal Psychology, 88,* 248–257.

Thelen, E. (1985). Expression as action: A motor perspective on the transition from spontaneous to instrumental behaviors. In G. Zivin (Ed.), *The development of expressive behavior: Biology-environment interactions* (pp. 221–148). New York: Academic Press.

Thomas, A., & Chess, S. (1977). *Temperament and development*. New York: Brunner/Mazel.

Thomas, A., Chess, S., & Birch, H. G. (1969). *Temperament and behavior disorders*. New York: New York University Press.

Thomas, A., Chess, S., Birch, H., Hertzig, M., & Korn, S. (1963). *Behavioral individuality in early childhood*. New York: New York University Press.

Tinbergen, N. (1951). *The study of instinct*. Oxford: Oxford University Press.

Tomkins, S. (1962). *Affect, imagery, consciousness: Vol. I. The positive affects*. New York: Springer Publishers.

Tomkins, S. (1989). Script theory: Differential magnification of affects. In A. E. Howe, Jr. & R. A. Dienstbier (Eds.), *Nebraska Symposium on Motivation* (Vol. 26). Lincoln: University of Nebraska Press.

Trabasso, T., Stein, N. L., & Johnson, L. R. (1981). Children's knowledge of events: A causal analysis of story structure. In G. Bower (Ed.), *The psychology of learning and motivation* (Vol. 15, pp. 237–281). New York: Academic Press.

Washburn, R. W. (1929). A study of the smiling and laughing of infants in the first year of life. *Genetic Psychology Monographs, 6,* 397–537.

Watson, J. B. (1928). *Psychological care of infant and child*. New York: Norton.

Wiesenfeld, A., Malatesta, C., & DeLoach, L. (1981). Differential parental response to familiar and unfamiliar distress signals. *Infant Behavior & Development, 4,* 281–295.

Wolff, P. H. (1969). The natural history of crying and other vocalizations in early infancy. In M. Foss (Ed.), *Determinants of infant behavior* (Vol. 4, pp. 81–109). London: Metheun.

3

Psychodynamic Models

Howard D. Lerner and Joshua Ehrlich

Introduction

Psychoanalysis does not offer a single, coherent account of social development across the life cycle. This is so for two broad reasons. First, psychoanalysis does not represent one unified, tightly knit theory. Rather, as we explore in the first section of this chapter, it represents four internally consistent theoretical models, models that intersect and overlap but that cannot be readily melded into a single theory of psychoanalysis. Each model offers its own perspective on social development. Second, from the perspective of psychoanalytic theorists, social development is too complex and multiply determined to elaborate in terms of a single thread that extends through the lifespan. In this chapter, therefore, we examine social development in terms of eight "dimensions of development." These dimensions, as we will articulate, interdigitate with one another in complex ways. However, we will consider each separately in order to offer some idea of the rich tapestry that comprises social development from the perspective of psychoanalytic theory.

Psychoanalysis traditionally has focused little attention on social development throughout life. Its focus, as we explore in the second section of this chapter, has been on intrapsychic development during the first 5 or so years of life and the impact this early development exerts on all ensuing development. In recent decades, psychoanalytic theorists have paid attention to the vicissitudes of development at all stages of the life cycle and also to the ongoing influence that real-life experiences, such as trauma, aging, and close relationships exert on the individual's inner world. We seek throughout this chapter to integrate the central em-

Howard D. Lerner and Joshua Ehrlich • Department of Psychiatry, University of Michigan, Ann Arbor, Michigan 48104.

Handbook of Social Development: A Lifespan Perspective, edited by Vincent B. Van Hasselt and Michel Hersen. Plenum Press, New York, 1992.

phasis within psychoanalysis on intrapsychic experience (e.g., drives, internal representations) with its increased attention to the formative impact of ongoing processes of maturation and of life experience.

In the first section of this chapter, we examine briefly the four dominant conceptual paradigms of psychoanalysis both as a general introduction to contemporary psychoanalytic thought and to establish a general conceptual framework for the discussion that follows. We then examine issues in adult development in an effort to demonstrate how psychoanalysis has come to incorporate the role of ongoing life experience into a predominantly intrapsychic framework. In the third section, we examine eight "dimensions of development" in order to shed light on the question of *what*, in fact, develops in social development across the life cycle and what is the nature of this development. In the final section, to add specificity to our discussion, we examine four formative experiences of adulthood: the consolidation of the intimate sexual relationship, parenthood, aging, and mourning.

PSYCHOANALYTIC MODELS

In seeking to formulate a psychoanalytic approach to development across the life cycle, it is important to recognize that psychoanalysis is not one closed, totally coherent theory of personality. Rather, it consists of a loose-fitting composite of four complementary, internally consistent models. Each model furnishes concepts and formulations for observing and understanding crucial dimensions of personality development through the life cycle.

Freud, through the course of his writings, developed a wide range of formulations concerning psychological functioning and accordingly created various conceptualizations of the mind. He changed from one theory to another theory whenever prior concepts failed to explain newly observed phenomena. However, the transformation from one set of formulations to another did not indicate that one superceded the other. That is, Freud did not intend to dispense with older concepts as he proposed newer ones. He assumed that a given set of clinical phenomena might be understood most clearly by using one particular frame of reference, whereas another set of data demanded a different set of concepts for its understanding. This principle of several concurrent and valid avenues for organizing the data of observation has been termed *theoretical complementarity* (Gedo & Goldberg, 1973) and is consistent with Waelder's (1930) notion of the principle of multiple functioning of the psychic apparatus that acknowledges that the "final pathway" in behavior is a compromise that serves many masters or psychic agencies; no single motive or significant factor can ever be isolated.

Psychology of the Self

Kohut (1971, 1977), in a series of major publications, laid the theoretical foundation for a systematic psychoanalytic psychology of the self. In a paper with significant diagnostic implications, Tolpin and Kohut (1980) distinguished between more classical neurotic psychopathology and what they termed *pathology of the self*. Unlike the neurosis that is presumed to originate in later childhood and at a time where there is sufficient self–other differentiation and when the various agencies of the mind (id, ego, superego) have been firmly established, self-pathology is thought to begin in early childhood and at a point when psychic structures are still in formation. Stemming from the absence of a cohesive sense of self, in self-pathology symptoms occur when an insecurely established self is threatened by the dangers of psychological disintegration, fragmentation, and devitalization. Unlike the neurotic patient who develops a transference neurosis in which the therapist is experienced as a new addition of the parents as objects of libidinal and aggressive urges, patients with self-pathology develop a treatment relationship in which the therapist is used to correct or carry out a function that should have been managed intrapsychically; that is, as a "self-object." Kohut (1977) suggests that individuals need significant others who can assume self–object functions throughout the life cycle.

Object Relations Theory

A second major advance within psychoanalytic theory is modern object relations theory. Object relations theory, or "object-relational thinking" (Guntrip, 1974), does not constitute a singular organized set of concepts, principles, formulations, or a systematized theory. Instead, it represents a broad spectrum of thought that historically and collectively has taken the form of a movement within psychoanalysis. Within object relations theory, the concept of object representation has served as a superordinate construct. Defined broadly, object representation refers to the conscious and unconscious mental schemata, including cognitive, affective, and experiential dimensions of objects encountered in reality (Blatt, 1974). Beginning within an interpersonal matrix as vague and variable sensorimotor experience of pleasure and unpleasure, these schemata develop into increasingly differentiated, consistent, and relatively realistic representations of the self and the object world. Earlier forms of representation are based more on action sequences associated with the gratification of needs; intermediate forms are based on specific perceptual features; and higher forms are thought to be more symbolic and conceptual. Whereas these schemata evolve from and are intertwined with the developmental internalization of object relations and ego functions, the developing representations provide a new organization or template throughout for experiencing ongoing interpersonal relationships internally.

Modern Structural Theory

A third major advance in psychoanalysis has been what is termed *modern structural theory*. Taking as its starting point Freud's (1923/1957) tripartite model of id, ego, and superego and dispensing with concepts of psychic energy from the libido theory of his topographical model, modern structural theory remains as the "mainstream hypothesis of modern psychoanalysis" (Boesky, 1989).

Modern structural theory takes as its premise the ubiquitous nature of internal, intrapsychic conflict throughout the life cycle and the view that this conflict can be conceptualized through the interaction of the id, ego, and superego. Brenner has been one of the most articulate spokesmen for this point of view. According to this author, psychic conflict is at the heart of psychoanalytic theory and treatment, the components and interactions of which result in compromise formations. All thoughts, actions, plans, fantasies, and symptoms are compromise formations and are thought to be multidetermined by the components of conflict.

Specifically, all compromise formations represent a combination of a drive derivative (a specific personal and unique wish of an individual, originating in childhood, for gratification); of unpleasure in the form of anxiety or depressive affect and their ideational contents of object loss, loss of love, or castration associated with the drive derivative; of defense that functions to minimize unpleasure; and various manifestations of superego functioning such as guilt, self-punishment, remorse, and atonement.

According to Brenner, compromise formations are the observational bases for the study of all psychic functioning; that is, they are the data of observation when one applies the psychoanalytic method to observing all psychological phenomena. According to Brenner (1986):

> To say everything is a compromise formation, means everything. Not just symptoms, not just neurotic character traits, not just the slips and errors of daily living, but everything, the normal as well as the pathological. Just as nothing is ever just defense or only wish-fulfillment, so nothing is ever only "realistic" as opposed to "neurotic." One of the principal contributions of psychoanalysis to human psychology is precisely this. The various components of conflict over wishes of childhood origin play as important a part in normal psychic functioning as they do in pathological psychic functioning. (p. 41)

From this perspective, important questions asked for understanding all psychological phenomena are: What wishes of childhood are being gratified? What unpleasure (anxiety and depressive affect) are they arousing? What are the defensive and superego aspects? The answers to these questions, according to Brenner, provide a distinctive psychoanalytic understanding of all mental phenomena and in the treatment situation guide the timing and nature of interactions. From a lifespan perspective, conflict and compromise formation are as significant a part of normal psychological functioning and development as they are of psychopathology.

Developmental Theory

A fourth major model in psychoanalysis is a dynamically based, developmental theory. A host of contemporary authors have concluded independently that developmentally salient aspects of psychological structure and functioning are initiated in and stem from the early mother–child relationship. In terms of its application to an understanding of the vicissitudes of development throughout the life cycle, the developmental perspective provides an assimilative and unifying focus within which multiple approaches can be organized. The developmental perspective is rooted deeply in psychoanalysis and embraces all aspects of psychological functioning—specifically, the relationship between past experience and present functioning (temporal progression), between early trauma and present symptoms (phase-specific deficits), and between historical actualities and psychic realities. In addition, a developmental focus provides a framework for discerning the relative etiological weight of constitutional and experiential factors.

The developmental approach within psychoanalysis, especially as it has been built upon the systematic, naturalistic, and longitudinal study of infants and children, has provided a methodological link between psychoanalysis and the social sciences, as well as a bridge between clinical and research approaches to the individual. Mahler and her colleagues (Mahler, Pine, & Bergman, 1975) have carefully observed children and their caretakers and have described the steps in what they term the *separation–individuation process*. Beginning with the earliest signs of the infant's differentiation or "hatching" from a symbiotic fusion with the mother, the infant proceeds through the period of his or her absorption in his or her own autonomous functioning to the near exclusion of the mother (practicing subphase), then through the all-important period of rapprochement in which the child, precisely because of a more clearly perceived state of separateness from mother, is prompted to redirect attention back to the mother, often in provocative ways, and finally to a feeling of a primitive sense of individual identity and of object constancy. Several authors, including Behrens and Blatt (1985), have conceptualized the major task throughout the course of the life cycle as a continuation of the separation–individuation process, which is accomplished through progressive internalization of need-gratifying aspects of relationships with significant others.

The studies of Mahler and her colleagues combine many of the empirical values extant within the social sciences with the intensive, clinical study of single subjects favored by psychoanalysis. The developmental perspective and associated methodologies offer a corrective influence for both blind adherence to theoretical constructs and equally blind reliance on group data and inferential statistics. As such, this approach offers a flexible balance between ideographic and nomothetic methodologies, while providing a context from which to distill theoretical formulations as they emerge from and are rooted in human experience.

Adult Development: General Considerations

Psychoanalysts traditionally have viewed adulthood as the endpoint of psychological development. An epic of relative stagnation, adulthood has stood within psychoanalysis as a monument to the formative developmental experiences of the early years and the resurgence of developmental processes catalyzed by puberty that characterizes adolescence. In general, psychoanalytic theorists have conceptualized childhood in terms of its ongoing, age-specific developmental tasks; they have seen adulthood in terms of *already accomplished* (or, in more severe cases, not accomplished) developmental tasks.

In its inception, psychoanalysis focused its attention on the vicissitudes of infantile development, especially on the unfolding of the psychosexual drives during the first 5 years of life. Infantile development was viewed as decisive for all ensuing personality development. Emphasis was on the past and what was formative. Classical psychoanalytic thinkers stressed the repetitive nature of human behavior, emphasizing the individual's drive to reenact formative, unconscious early experience, conflict, and fantasy throughout life.

What has been termed the *genetic* point of view has been crucial to the psychoanalytic understanding of adult psychic life and reflects the psychoanalytic belief in the central role of infantile experience in adult psychic functioning. It is "limited to the past," especially in terms of how the past is retrospectively perceived, related to, and understood in the present (Shane, 1977). Within the genetic point of view, one seeks to elaborate adult experience in terms of its infantile antecedents. For example, one might examine a personality trait in adulthood in terms of the stage of infantile psychosexuality from which it is seen to derive or explore an adult relationship from the perspective of an early object relational paradigm.

Although the formative impact of infantile development remains a cornerstone of psychoanalytic theory and treatment, and the genetic point of view remains a critical vantage point, psychoanalysts increasingly have moved to explore the ways in which development proceeds across the life cycle. For many contemporary psychoanalytic thinkers, the close of the oedipal phase no longer represents the decisive endpoint of formative psychological development. Rather, many clinicians and theorists would suggest that infantile experience is worked and reworked in each developmental epic across the life cycle within the context of new achievements in functioning, maturational changes, new relationships, and changing environmental conditions.

A "developmental" orientation as opposed to the genetic, according to Shane (1977), "implies an ongoing process, not only with a past, but also with a present and a future" (p. 95). From this vantage point, each phase of life, not only early childhood, brings with it distinctive developmental challenges and possibilities. In addition, advances in psychic structuring are seen as accruing across all phases of the life cycle, so that each developmental experience incorporates all development that precedes it.

Recent contributions to adolescent development suggest that adolescence is not a simple recapitulation of early development. Rather, this stage brings with it distinctive developmental tasks involving object relations, moral, and cognitive development, the continued consolidation of gender identity, and other critical developmental tasks (Blos, 1979; Kaplan, 1986; Ritvo, 1971). Infantile experience is not repeated in adolescence but *reworked* in order to fulfill the specific developmental tasks that this epic requires.

One can find within psychoanalysis a rich thread of writings on adult development that is woven through the literature. Jung (1933) explored various dimensions of adult development, suggesting that previously suppressed thoughts, feelings, and aspects of the self could be further developed and integrated in midlife. He noted, for example, that men at midlife become significantly more introverted and better able to integrate the feminine side of their personalities, whereas women are better able to integrate the masculine.

Eric Erikson was the first psychoanalyst to advance an integrated psychosocial view of individual development through the course of the life cycle. Erikson has had an enormous influence in various fields throughout the social sciences and humanities. Through his numerous publications, he has highlighted the interaction between the individual's internal psychological state and external social events. Core to Erikson's perspective on development is the "epigenetic" principle, which assumes that anything that grows has an internal "game plan." Each stage of life, including those that comprise adulthood, brings with it new challenges that the individual must master. According to Erikson, individuals who are able to meet these challenges create the opportunity to confront life with renewed energy, creativity, and adaptive capabilities. Each of Erikson's eight stages centers on a crucial developmental task for the individual self in relation to the social world.

According to Erikson, in the sixth, or young adult stage (20s through 30s), the individual deals with issues of intimacy versus self-absorption. Issues of intimacy, sexuality, and empathy within the context of a cohesive sense of self in relationship to another person are paramount. In the seventh stage, or "midlife period," the conflict is between generativity and stagnation. Here generativity goes beyond the care of one's own children to guiding the next generation through teaching, creativity, and participation in society.

In light of a burgeoning interest in development across the life cycle, several recent psychoanalytic contributions have sought to clarify the particular features of psychological development in adulthood. Colarusso and Nemiroff (1981), as an important example, suggest that adult development is continuous with previous development in that the individual's exchanges with the external environment continue to affect evolving mental activity and functioning. However, where childhood development is concerned primarily with the formation of psychic structure, adult development is concerned with its continued evolution and its use.

As an example, the authors outline a developmental progression for identification. In childhood, identification is integral to such basic processes as the learning of speech and language and the acquisition of interests and ideals. In adulthood, these identifications are refined and reworked, for example, in the context of a mentor relationship. Adult identifications are not simply a repetition of early identifications, however: "The identification with the original objects deals with how the child builds psychological structure and becomes like the adult, whereas later identification provides specificity to the adult personality" (Colarusso & Nemiroff, p. 66).

In this context, adulthood is understood not simply in terms of infantile experience but as a developmental epic characterized by dynamic change. The adult's experience is affected not only by the childhood past, but by the adult past. As a developmental epic, adulthood brings with it its own developmental challenges—catalyzed by the specific life experiences and events of adulthood and confronted within the context of the adaptive capacities the individual has evolved to that point. Colarusso and Nemiroff illustrate the need for a developmental perspective on adulthood through the example of the male climacteric. Such an experience, they suggest, cannot reasonably be understood outside the context of the aging process and the man's ongoing and inevitable confrontation with bodily changes and mortality.

Settlage and his colleagues (Settlage *et al.*, 1988) contrast personality development in adulthood with the developmental processes of childhood and adolescence. Development, the authors suggest, is a

> process of growth, differentiation, and integration that progresses from lower and simpler to higher and more complex forms of organization and function. . . . The functions and structures resulting from development constitute additions to or advances in the self-regulatory and adaptive capacities. (p. 35)

As psychoanalysis traditionally has conceptualized it, personality development occurs at the interface between the individual's internal biological maturation and environmental pressures that he or she faces. More specifically, personality formation proceeds in the context of a predetermined unfolding of the oral, anal, phallic, and latency stages in childhood and the biologically driven resurgence of genital striving at puberty. Although biological maturation contributes to psychological development in adulthood, its impact is less dramatic and clear cut than in childhood and adolescence. No easily discerned, predetermined, generally uniform and invariant stages of maturation catalyze psychological development in the adult years. On this basis, Settlage *et al.* suggest, a stage theory of development is not useful for adulthood. Although adults may face similar developmental tasks, these are likely to be highly variable from one individual to the next.

In light of these considerations, Settlage *et al.* suggest that personality development in adulthood be conceptualized in terms of a "developmental process." In this framework, the stimulus for development is a disruption in the individual's previously adequate self-regulatory and adaptive functioning. Such a disruption can come in the form of biological maturation, environmental demand, a traumatic event such as a loss, or a self-initiated pursuit of better adaptation. As examples of the vast array of events or experiences that disturb the adult's psychic equilibrium, these authors cite potentially positive experiences such as marriage, parenthood, or a job promotion, and such threatening experiences as personal illness, the loss of a friend, or the loss of a function due to aging.

In response to developmental challenge that the event or experience poses, the individual experiences a developmental conflict in which he or she confronts the need to adapt and attempts to negotiate the anxiety and conflict that any change will entail. Resolution of developmental conflict potentially leads to structural change in self-regulatory and adaptive functioning. In turn, this can lead to a change in the individual's self and object representations, level of separation–individuation, sense of identity, and compromise formations.

MULTIPLE DIMENSIONS OF DEVELOPMENT: A LIFE CYCLE PERSPECTIVE

In formulating a psychoanalytic framework for development across the life cycle, it is essential to clarify *what*, in fact, develops. Anna Freud (1965) offered a significant conceptual framework in her discussion of "developmental lines." A. Freud described these developmental lines in terms of fundamental aspects of personality, which unfold in a regular sequence in the context of the child and adolescent's maturation. She described, as examples, one developmental line that leads from dependency to emotional self-reliance and another that leads from irresponsibility to responsibility in body management. Several past contributions (e.g., Greenspan, 1979, 1981; Sugarman, Bloom-Feshbach, & Bloom-Feshbach, 1980) offer perspectives on development that allow us to expand on A. Freud's valuable concept of developmental lines (what we will term *dimensions of development*) and to extend them across the life cycle.

The developmental–structural approach advocated by Greenspan (1981) is based on two fundamental assumptions. First, the organizational capacity of the individual progresses to higher levels as the individual matures; that is, phase-specific higher levels of development assume an ability to organize an increasingly broad and complex range of experience into stable patterns. The organizational level of experience can be delineated along a number of dimensions, including age or phase appropriateness, range and depth, stability, and personal uniqueness. Second, for each stage of development there are particular characteristic *tasks* that the individual must accomplish before advancing to the next stage of development. This suggests that certain *types* of experience must be organized by means of the structures available to the individual for development to proceed.

In keeping with this view, the major tasks of adult development will be seen as *synthesis*—specifically, the integration of the various dimensions of development (psychosocial, cognitive, moral, etc.). The dimensions may integrate and reintegrate at higher or lower levels of synthesis around nodal points or tasks in development such as adolescence, or, in adulthood, around marriage, parenthood, vocational achievement, or retirement—what Neugarten (1979) refers to as "the normal turning points, the punctuation marks along the life line" (p. 889). The dimensions of development may also be thought to integrate and reintegrate toward either higher or lower levels of adaptation around such crises as the decline in bodily function, serious illness, losses, and, ultimately, confronting death.

The eight dimensions of development that we examine next encompass salient aspects of psychological functioning that are transformed over time and are shaped by both maturation and experience. Although actual development is multifaceted and extremely complex, we will consider these dimensions of development separately for heuristic and conceptual reasons.

The Psychosexual Development: Drives and Bodily Experience

There is a consensus among most psychoanalytic theorists and clinicians that many of the major psychosexual passions and conflicts of the first 5 years of life are not only rekindled and reworked during adolescence but also at other nodal points of adulthood. Despite the continuum in sensual experience (G. Klein, 1976) suggested in Freud's theory of psychosexual development there are important qualitative differences between adult, adolescent, and prepubertal sexuality. At puberty an adult body combines with growing cognitive capacities intersecting with hormonal secretions, menstruation, or the discharge of semen (Lidz, Lidz, & Rubenstein, 1976) to impact on the adolescent in concrete bodily manifestations; that is, changing sexual status "feels" different. The metamorphosis of the body (Sugarman *et al.*, 1980) and with it clear sexual and gender distinctions is a defining characteristic of adolescent development. Integrating these changes, which are brought about according to an autonomous biological timetable, within the self, the family, and the peer group, can be problematic. Precocious or delayed puberty can pose a significant developmental interference (Nagera, 1970) that interacts with other developmental dimensions and can bear its stamp on one's identity. This is a period in which the adolescent makes the transition from self-love to love of another. A complicating factor is that sexual and affectional feelings must be distinguished and separated from those of the same sex while fused for those of the opposite sex. The adolescent is confronted with the need to reexperience the repressed sexual passions of the earlier years while maintaining the incest taboo.

As Colarusso and Nemiroff (1981) note, American society associates increasing age with a decrease in sexual interest and activity. This common view of diminished sexuality with age is certainly not biologically mandated. Far-reaching and deep social and cultural changes have brought about a loosening and flexibility in social norms regarding sex roles and increased external freedom. For many, however, this external freedom does not bring about a corresponding internal freedom from conflict. For example, the women's movement has brought new role conflicts for women who simultaneously pursue occupational success and motherhood and for men who seek new freedom and new combinations of roles as worker, parent, and homemaker. As Neugarten (1979) observes, for women there is a new freedom and increased energy available when children leave home, and freedom from unwanted pregnancy and, for many, new pleasures in sexual activity that

HOWARD D.
LERNER and
JOSHUA EHRLICH

accompanies menopause. Nevertheless, for both sexes through the life cycle, there is a realization that the body is increasingly less predictable than earlier, and there is increased attention to body monitoring. The psychological counterpart of the inevitable aging of the body are corresponding changes in the experience of time. Middle age is thought to bring with it a change in time perspective in that time becomes restructured in terms of time left to live rather than time since birth.

Harman (1978) and Martin (1977) have surveyed the literature on changes in sexual behavior with aging. The most important factor in determining the level of sexual activity with age appears to be health and survival of the spouse. Colarusso and Nemiroff (1981), after reviewing the biological literature on aging, conclude that some degree of declining sexual function and interest appears to be an inevitable consequence of aging, but health, social, and cultural factors rather than physiological changes *per se* seem to be responsible for most of the sexual changes seen with aging. These authors also noted that prevalent attitudes about brain functioning in middle and late adulthood are just as skewed as those about sexual functioning. They cite recent research indicating that mental functioning need not necessarily decline with age because of inevitable degenerative changes in the brain. Health, social factors, interpersonal relationships, and environmental stimulation appear to be the most important determinants of the course of mental development in middle and late adulthood rather than a decline in brain functioning and the central nervous system.

Attitudes toward the body change through development. During adolescence and early adulthood there is a casual acceptance of the body with concerns revolving around invincibility versus vulnerability as well as the development of physical abilities and care of the body. Through the 30s and 40s, there is a growing awareness of physical limitations, often heralded by baldness, gray hair, wrinkles, and changes in vision. These changes are reflected in fantasies having to do with the body of youth, a mourning process, and the emergence of a new body image, and with it an acceptance of physical limitations and an enjoyment of the body in new ways. Continued care or neglect of the body becomes an increasingly important issue. These issues continue in the 50s and 60s in a more intensified way and with them come increased efforts to compensate for diminished physical energy in terms of altering schedules, diets, and sleep patterns. These changes are also accompanied by increased fantasies of death, heart attacks, and for many women, widowhood. With increased time, the psychological focus becomes one of remaining active despite frequent physical infirmity and with it the acceptance of permanent physical impairment.

The Psychosocial Dimension: Strivings for Ego Identity

Whereas most classical psychoanalytic thinkers have conceptualized development from an intrapsychic perspective, Erikson (1964, 1968, 1978), in a series of influential papers and books, has stressed the importance of the broader social context. In concert with the task of integrating psychosexual and bodily changes, Erikson notes, the adolescent is also confronted with the difficult task of assessing society, assimilating those values that appear sensible, and finding a place within society. To do so, according to Erikson, is to develop a sense of identity, a sense of who one is as a unique individual across situations and through historical time, a sense of self-sameness. Erikson suggests that adolescence is a time of life when there is a simultaneous demand to achieve commitments to physical intimacy, to decisive occupational choice, and to psychosocial definition—all central to components of adult role identity.

Staples and Smarr (1980) assert that

the various identifications must be worked out and consolidated into forms that simultaneously satisfy certain internal and external needs. They must be internally consistent with each other and with the moral system that is chosen. Social roles must be adopted that are consistent with the predominant identifications and which provide a fulfilling life style for those identifications and value systems. Moreover, these social roles must also provide reality testing of those values and be compatible enough with them. (p. 485)

Adolescence is a stage of poignant encounters with adult role models outside the family that can potentially serve as important alternatives to or modulators of parental identifications. The process of identity formation facilitates the resolution of both pre-oedipal and oedipal conflicts through relatively conflict-free identifications with role models. Finding these role models may foster more positive identifications with the parent of the same sex. Identity formation may be viewed as combining the adolescent's sense of uniqueness, an unconscious striving for continuity of experience, and a solidarity with group ideals (Sugarman *et al.*, 1980). The formation of ego identity may be formulated intrapsychically as a process that results in the integration of self- and object representations with actual interpersonal behavior. Identity formation exerts a stabilizing effect on the personality.

The formation of identity, however, does not end with adolescence. The adult phases of the life cycle require a continuing although less rapid and dramatic evolution, refinement, and maturation of identity for the maintenance of optimal adaptation and functioning. Michels (1980) outlines four major themes of adult development that can be considered in terms of their impact on ego identity: work, sex, parenthood, and aging.

A major task of adult life involves the development and integration of a work identity, one that is integrated with other adult identities and, as Michels points out, incorporates its developmental precursors of play and school, yet tolerates the constraints of reality that require that work be different from each. During adolescence and young adulthood, the ability to make choices, to identify and develop work skills, to maintain a capacity for sustained work and derive pleasure from it, as well as success and failure in the workplace are pivotal determinants of an adult work identity. The role of a mentor relationship is often instrumental during this phase as well as during the 30s, in which there is a solidification of a work identity, the continued development of skills, increased attention to levels of achievement in terms of economic and social status, and increased internal and external pressures involving balancing of work and family life.

Through the fourth decade of life there is a transformation from student to mentor and with it an acceptance of limitations and a failure to reach certain goals. It is often at this point in development that one chooses a second or new career. Issues of facilitation versus competitiveness and jealousy as well as the use of power and position come into play. With age, the successful adult must also synthesize a work identity with the aging process and must be able to diminish the role of work in his or her life with a progressive diminution in capacity and yet still maintain self-esteem and a capacity for pleasure.

HOWARD D.
LERNER and
JOSHUA EHRLICH

In terms of sexuality, according to Michels (1980), the adult has two developmental tasks: to structure a pattern of sexual behavior that incorporates biological, psychological, and social reality, and to integrate that pattern with the rest of his or her personality and to achieve maximal satisfaction from it. Early adulthood involves the developmental tasks of finding appropriate heterosexual partners, cultivating the desire for both sexual and nonsexual closeness, the emergence of a capacity for heterosexual caring and tenderness, the ability to use the body comfortably as a sexual instrument, and the continued resolution of homosexual conflicts. Out of these trends comes during the 20s and 30s a greater capacity to invest in one person based on an ability to trust and tolerate imperfections in oneself and the partner. Included here are increased wishes for children as an expression of love and sexuality as well as a capacity to share children and child rearing with partners. With age comes increased pressure to redefine relationships to the partner, to care for the partner in the face of illness and aging, to develop capacities for sharing new activities, to continue an active sexual life, and eventually the capacity to tolerate loss and death.

According to Erikson (1978), aging begins at conception but has special characteristics at each phase of the life cycle. Jaques (1965) observes that the psychological meaning of death shifts in adult life from one of fear associated with traumatic experience and symbolically related to unconscious fantasies of punishment, characteristic of children and adolescents, to adulthood in which death begins to be more familiar and gradually accepted. The loss of one's parents, friends, and loved ones, as well as the inevitability of one's own death replace the child's unconscious fantasies as the symbolic equivalent of death. The social meanings of adulthood and of being elderly must be integrated into the adult identity. With development, the social significance of aging joins race, gender, and physical handicap as roles that must be redefined and reintegrated into the identity.

The Cognitive Dimension: The Emergence of Formal Operations

As with each dimension of adult development, the cognitive dimension underlies and interdigitates with other dimensions of adult development in important and complex ways. Nevertheless, for conceptual purposes, it will be considered here separately. Many attempts have been made to integrate formulations from cognitive psychology with drive theory (Wolff, 1960), ego psychology (Greenspan, 1979), and more recently with object relations theory (Lerner & Lerner, 1987).

An important cognitive transformation and development that is decisive for the remainder of the life cycle takes place during adolescence. In Piagetian theory (Inhelder & Piaget, 1958), this shift is from concrete to formal operations. As Piaget (1954) notes, the principle of formal operations involves the real versus the possible. According to Sugarman et al. (1980),

> During the stage of concrete operations, the child is increasingly able to think in terms of complex classes of things and to make linked statements about them. Formal operational thinking allows the adolescent to progress from combining the properties of objects into classes to combining classes into classes. The adolescent can, thereby, have access to a complete system of all possible combinations. This system can be used to solve problems, to generate hypotheses, and to integrate identifications. Reversibility of thinking develops. That is,

formal operations reverse the possible and the real. . . . Such reversibility frees adolescents from the constraints of concrete reality. With formal operations adolescents can act on representations of reality rather than on reality itself. (p. 483)

The transformation of thinking from concrete to formal operations enhances adaptation in a number of ways. In contrast to the concrete operational child, the adolescent and adult manifest increased freedom in dealing with wishes, affects, and interpersonal relationships—in that both the real and the possible can be considered. Fantasy can become an adaptive and creative modality. Affect-drenched issues, such as sex, death, and the meaning of life can be considered in the abstract, all possibilities and consequences can likewise be considered, and the internal world takes on the quality of a real place. New cognitive capacities permit increased freedom to experience a wider range of both internal and external issues.

Cognitive changes with development facilitate a quantum leap in self-awareness, particularly for the adolescent, but also for the adult, especially in psychoanalysis and psychoanalytic psychotherapy. The internal world can be considered in a propositional sense as not necessarily real—reality and fantasy can be distinguished, thought is freed from action. Beginning with adolescence and through adulthood, with the successful resolution of conflict and the negotiation of crises, the individual can experience his or her internal world in a more reflective and flexible manner because an enhanced appreciation of the possible significantly reduces the fearful aspects of internal stimuli. The shift from concrete to formal operations also facilitates identity formation by affording the individual the cognitive capacities to organize and integrate representations of the past with those of the present and the future.

The Object Relations Dimension: Separation–Individuation and Underlying Representations

In keeping with the hypothesis advanced by Colarusso and Nemiroff (1981) that the fundamental developmental issues of childhood continue as central aspects of adult development but in altered form, several authors have theoretically and clinically examined the basic process of separation–individuation through various phases of the life cycle, rather than only as a significant event of childhood. According to Mahler (1973):

> The entire life cycle constitutes a more or less successful process of distancing from an introjection of the lost symbiotic mother, an external longing for the actual or fantasized ideal state of self, with the latter standing for a symbiotic fusion with the all-good symbiotic mother who was at one time part of the self in a blissful state of well-being. (p. 138)

Colarusso and Nemiroff claim that the quest for clearer differentiation between self and other only ends with biological death. Formative adult experiences, such as shifting interpersonal relationships and investments, the recognition of interdependence on others, the experience of parenthood and grandparenthood as well as the relationship with the spouse, all involve enhanced separation–individuation secondary to the gradual acceptance of real over idealized aspects of relationships with significant others and the acceptance of the aging process in both self and others.

It has become a basic tenet of psychoanalytic theory that the mother–infant relationship is essential to subsequent psychological development and growth. The initial "dual unity" (Mahler, 1968) represents the first developmental prerequisite for internalization and, in fact, contains the chrysalis for all subsequent internalizations throughout the life cycle (Behrends & Blatt, 1985). Basch (1981) concludes that the essential function of the mother–infant unity is to provide order, harmony, and organization, using the language of self- and object representation. G. Klein (1976) suggested that the primary developmental objective is to maintain identity, unity, coherence, and overall integrity of the self-schema. These authors emphasize that the optimal stage that the developing child seeks to either maintain or restore is one of order, coherence, and integrity, and, as Behrends and Blatt (1985) observe, such optimal integration is only possible through continued relationships with others.

According to Behrends and Blatt (1985), psychological development occurs continuously through the life cycle through progressive internalizations of aspects of relationships with significant others. According to these authors, the underlying mechanism of the internalization process remains the same; that is, it involves first the establishment of a gratifying involvement with a significant other, followed by the experience of nontraumatic "incompatibilities" in the relationship, resulting in internalization, differentiation, and individuation. According to Behrends and Blatt (1985): "Psychic growth continues as these elemental steps occur in hierarchical spirality, over and over again throughout the course of the entire life cycle" (p. 35).

Nowhere are the dynamics and underlying processes of separation–individuation better seen than during adolescence. Blos (1979) formulates a "second individuation process" as essential to adolescent development in terms of providing an opportunity to finally resolve conflicts dating back to the first separation–individuation phase at the end of the third year of life. Both periods share a heightened vulnerability of the personality organization, an urgency for psychic restructuring in tandem with the maturational surge forward, and, if the process should miscarry, the development of psychopathology.

The Structural Dimension: Ego Development

The structural dimension of development refers especially to ego development; that is, a complex and multifaceted set of psychological functions based upon interactions among innate constitutional givens, maturational forces, and experiential and social influences. This dimension includes the innate and developmental strengths and weaknesses of cognitive and representational structures and of drive-and-affect modulating structures such as defense. Under optimal conditions, when these functions operate effectively, they facilitate adaptation and further development by freeing the individual for developmental tasks not related to conflict. When there is "ego weakness," regardless of etiology, there is either a diffusion or severe inhibition of drives and affects; there may be more pervasive regressions that impinge on personality structures, and the vulnerable individual confronted with such threats to structural integrity may decompensate. The integrity of overall personality function may be maintained at the high price of flexibility in the overall character structure. Inhibitions can include a limitation of experience, of feelings and/or thoughts, a restriction of the experience of pleasure, a tendency to externalize internal events, and a host of limitations of internalization necessary for the regulation of impulses, affects, and thought, as well as limitations in the maintenance of self-esteem.

Affect tolerance is an important aspect of the structural dimension. Although the intensity, depth, and range of affects can vary along both qualitative and quantitative dimensions both between individuals and across the lifespan, more pathological expressions of affect tend to be less differentiated and articulated. The level of development and structural integrity of the defensive organization represents an important aspect of affect tolerance and expression.

Vaillant's (1977) longitudinal study of adaptation focused on defensive organization. Core to Vaillant's study is the assumption that for individuals to master conflict adaptively and to utilize resources creatively, adaptive styles, that is, defense mechanisms, must mature throughout the life cycle. Ordering defenses into a theoretical hierarchy in terms of relative maturity, this author found in a group of normal men over time a decline in the less mature defense mechanisms of fantasy and action and a concomitant increase in the more mature defense mechanism of suppression. Whereas less mature defenses such as projection, hypochondriasis, and masochism were more common in adolescence, more developed processes such as sublimation and altruism increased in midlife. Such changes in defensive organization from adolescence to midlife provide evidence that internal structural change occurs throughout development.

The Moral Dimension: Superego and Ego Ideal

Psychoanalysis and developmental-cognitive psychology have both made important contributions to a theory of moral development that may lead to a synthesis of viewpoints (Greenspan, 1979). Although traditional psychoanalytic theory related moral development to psychosexual drive states, cognitive psychology is primarily concerned with moral judgment; hence, the scope of cognitive theory is narrower than formulations derived from psychoanalysis. Psychoanalytic inquiry has focused on moral development in terms of the socialization process and the progressive internalization of standards that modulate potentially disruptive drives and eventually take the form of an integrated value system. On the other hand, Piagetian theory has focused on the role of higher cognitive processes and role-taking ability in moral judgment.

Working within a Piagetian framework, Kohlberg and Gilligan's (1972) work on moral judgment indicates that adolescence marks a crucial transition from the conventional morality of preadolescence to the postconventional morality of adulthood. Conventional morality is defined by global conformity to a valued social order. Postconventional morality, according to these authors, involves the formation of autonomous moral principles that have validity separate from the groups that hold them and independent from the individual's identification with the group. Seen from this perspective, the attainment of postconventional morality is inextricably contingent upon the achievement of formal operations (Sugarman *et al.*, 1980).

Psychoanalytic theorists have approached moral development from the perspective of transformations and consolidation of the superego. According to psychoanalytic theory, during adolescence external changes in relationship to the parents are paralleled by internal changes in the superego in terms of a revival of oedipal and pre-oedipal conflict. It is thought that these changes exert a disruptive

HOWARD D.
LERNER and
JOSHUA EHRLICH

and destabilizing effect on self-regulation and self-esteem. Freud (1923/1957) described the superego as a precipitate of the ego, consisting of identifications with the parents and reactions against them. The function of the superego was seen as the repression of the Oedipus complex. According to Freud (1923/1957), functions involving judgment, prohibitions and injunctions, moral censorship, a sense of guilt, and social feelings and identifications are all subsumed under the superego. According to modern structural theory, all compromise formations include a superego or moral dimension, and the superego itself is a compromise formation. These formulations suggest that the moral dimension and superego functioning in particular is a dynamic process that develops through the life cycle.

Transitional Objects

In recent years the work of D. W. Winnicott has received increasing attention both within and outside of psychoanalytic thought. Winnicott's formulations, particularly concerning transitional objects, omnipotence, and self-development, all have important implications for understanding development through the life cycle. It is in describing the infant's experience of adapting to a shared reality through the transition from absolute to relative dependence that Winnicott's most original contributions reside.

The natural unfolding of the infant's growth potential, including developing cognitive and affective structures within a facilitating environment, make possible a dawning awareness of maternal care and the need for it. In turn, the "not me" gradually becomes separate from the "me," a capacity for objectivity is attained, and an active participation in a world where objects can be experienced as permanent in time and space is achieved. At this nodal point, gradual nontraumatic failures of maternal adaptation to the infant's needs become a crucial aspect of "good-enough mothering" and determinant of the growing infant's capacity to internalize the mother's caring functions, and in turn to regulate his or her own internal states and self-experience.

The transition from absolute to relative dependence (mature interdependence) and the acceptance of a "not-me" world corresponds to Freud's notions concerning the transition from the pleasure principle to the reality principle; that is, from a need-gratifying to an adaptive orientation. Winnicott (1951/1958) described the child's earliest experiences of decentering in efforts to bridge the gap between fantasy and reality. It was through his deceptively simple and direct clinical observations that Winnicott was led to the remarkable discovery of the child's first "not-me" possession; that is, the "transitional object." Winnicott traced the transitional object (e.g., a bundle of wool, the corner of a blanket, etc.) to very early forms of relating and playing. The relationship of the infant to the transitional object is marked by several qualities, including a decrease in omnipotence, a relationship in which the object is totally controlled by the infant, and in which the object becomes the target for love and hate. The transitional object takes on a reality of its own, combining the qualities of being paradoxically created and discovered:

> In the course of years it becomes not so much forgotten as relegated to limbo . . .
> it is not forgotten and it is not mourned. It loses meaning, and this is because the
> transitional phenomena have become diffused, have become spread out over the
> whole intermediate territory between 'inner psychic reality' and 'the external

world as perceived by two persons in common,' that is to say, over the whole cultural field. (p. 233)

Recently, Sugarman and Jaffe (1987) asserted that multiple developmental transitions occur throughout the life cycle and that transitional phenomena are psychologically called upon and used to "regain inner–outer equilibrium at each phase." In keeping with Winnicott's original formulations, transitional phenomena are conceptualized as adaptational mechanisms that are used throughout the lifespan. In this context, the transitional object is considered to be a type of transitional phenomenon that is specific to a particular developmental period. A core premise is that equilibrium between the individual and the environment is promoted through the internalization of key self-regulatory functions. Transitional phenomena are seen as central aspects of this process as they foster internalization. As a consequence, the "self-representation becomes increasingly differentiated and integrated through a series of internalizations" (p. 421). In essence, Sugarman and Jaffe (1987) demonstrate how the transitional object facilitates the modulation of tension created by internal and external stresses in development.

Although these authors focus on four nodal points of development— symbiosis, practicing and rapprochement, the oedipal phase, and adolescence— their formulations can be extended to include marriage, parenthood, and other developmental events. According to Sugarman and Jaffe (1987):

> The specific form of transitional phenomena will differ at each stage due to maturational and developmental shifts in cognitive functioning, libidinal focus, affect organization, and the demands of the environment. (p. 421)

The level of cognitive maturity as well as other dimensions of personality become particularly important in determining and delimiting the manifest forms of transitional phenomena. As other functions including self- and object representations become increasingly differentiated, transitional objects are thought to become increasingly less tangible and more abstract. For example, in contrast to the transitional objects of early childhood, the transitional phenomena of adolescence such as career aspirations, music, and literature are more abstract, ideational, depersonified, and less animistic. They are also increasingly coordinated with reality. Rather than the concrete fantasy representation, it is the ideas, the cause, or the symbolic value that becomes important. Regardless of manifest content of the transitional object, transitional phenomena are thought to promote the internalization of core self-regulatory functions that include narcissistic regulation in terms of sustaining self-esteem, drive regulation, superego integration, ego functioning, and interpersonal relationships. Through the use of increasingly abstract transitional phenomena, the individual is better able to synthesize discrepant events in his or her life experience. Representational capacities evolve in concert with and become more complex because more alternative solutions and choices can be conserved simultaneously. With increased development, the function of transitional phenomena may also change from one of self-soothing to one of enriching the quality of experience.

Narcissism

One of the most lively debates in contemporary psychoanalysis revolves around the concept and very nature of narcissism and its role in normal develop-

68

HOWARD D.
LERNER and
JOSHUA EHRLICH

ment. Freud's use of the term left many areas of ambiguity that subsequent investigators have attempted to clarify. The most widely used definition of narcissism was offered by Hartmann (1950): "the libidinal investment of the self." Hartmann's contributions and later elaborations by Jacobson (1964) distinguished the concept of self as a person, ego as structure, and self- and object representations as subsystems within the structural schema. Some recent attempts at definitional reformulation have involved a dispensing with the energy model and with it the concept of libido. Stolorow (1975) offers a functional definition of narcissism in terms of the "structural cohesiveness, temporal stability and positive affective coloring of the self-representation' (p. 174). Psychological functioning is seen as narcissistic to the degree that it serves to establish and maintain such cohesiveness, stability, and positive affective coloring of the self-representations.

Kohut (1971), in his earlier formulations, retained the energy metaphor but used it differently. According to Kohut (1971), narcissism is not defined as the "target of libido" (self vs. object), but rather the "quality" of libido that determines whether or not it is narcissistic. For Kohut, libido is narcissistic when it involves "idealizing" or "self-aggrandizing" features; that is, if an attachment, either of the self or to an object, serves idealization or self-aggrandizement, then that attachment is narcissistic. This formulation is in keeping with Kohut's clinical observation that patients with narcissistic disturbances, rather than withdrawing their interest from others, tend to relate to others in entirely inconsistent and intense ways. Such attachments can be understood in terms of the individual's needing the object to stabilize and bolster a threatened self as a result of a defect or developmental arrest in structural development.

Most authors implicate self-esteem in formulations of narcissism. Jacobson (1964), in particular, has drawn relationships among ego ideal formation, narcissism, and self-esteem. According to this author, self-representations are optimally and progressively based on accurate representations of the real and not the fantasized self as they gradually develop out of appropriately accurate perceptions of past and present experiences. By contrast, the ego ideal is based on the wished-for—potential self—idealized self as it would like to be in the future. The ego ideal serves the function of holding up to the ego an idealized addition of the self-representation to strive for. It is out of this developmental matrix that self-representations and ego ideal formation gradually evolve in tandem and that a cognitive-affective schema or attitude toward the self develops. It is the nature of the "ideal self" subsumed by the ego ideal that is thought to influence the level of self-esteem as well as the libidinal investment of the self; that is, narcissism.

Although little has been written systematically about the vicissitudes of narcissism throughout the life cycle, it is generally agreed that narcissism is either altered or transformed as development proceeds. According to this view, there are relatively immature and mature manifestations of narcissism, and healthy as well as pathological forms. Advances in the capacity to love another suggest advances in narcissism. According to Spruiell (1975), transformation of narcissism parallels transformations in object relations. In adolescence, this transformation is organized around the acquisition of an adult body image, is catalyzed by the first romantic love relationship, and massively reorganizes psychic equilibrium in terms of developmental advances in erotic self-love, a taming of omnipotence, and a more adaptive regulation of self-esteem. Colarusso and Nemiroff (1981) used the term *authentic self* to characterize the mature adult in that it describes the capacity to accept what is genuine within the self and the outer world regardless of narcissistic injury involved. According to these authors, significant influences in adulthood are narcissistic issues related to the aging body, significant relationship (spouse, children, parents), middle-age time sense, and the vicissitudes of work and creativity.

Normative narcissistic regressions can be expected to be precipitated by developmental tasks such as midlife, which lead to a reemergence of aspects of infantile narcissism. The reworking and eventual integration of aspects of infantile narcissism can be seen as an integral part of normal development throughout the life cycle. Fantasies of omnipotence, according to Tyson (1983), play an important role in the course of development as well as in pathological states. Mahler, Pine, and Bergman (1975) have traced the gradual decrease in age-appropriate feelings of grandiosity and omnipotence from about the fifteenth month of infancy: "[T]he repeated experience of relative helplessness punctures the toddler's inflated sense of omnipotence" (p. 213). The adaptive aspects of optimally implementing omnipotence in infancy and nontraumatically relinquishing it during development include recognition and tolerance of differentiation and separation from others; reassurance that expressions of aggression do not result in the loss of others, the recognition that idealized others are not omnipotent themselves, and finally, with these advances, a protection from a "basic depressive mood" (Mahler, 1968), a mood that can lead to intense, malignantly regressed yearnings to restore a state of infantile narcissistic well-being. According to Tyson (1983):

> If identification with the presumed omnipotence of the object has not taken place, then to the extent that feelings of omnipotence and power remain important in the person's narcissistic equilibrium and depend on the loved one for their persistence and potency, there exists a vulnerability to narcissistic injury in that area, by disappointment in or loss of the object. (p. 212)

Dimension of Adult Experience: Intimacy, Parenthood, Mourning and Aging

A consideration of the multiple dimensions of adult development leads us to an examination of the consolidation of the intimate, sexual relationship, parenthood as well as mourning and aging as nodal developmental milestones and challenges to both the adult man and woman.

INTIMATE SEXUAL RELATIONS

The consolidation of the intimate, sexual relationship poses a significant developmental challenge to both men and women in terms of initiating a reintegration of the developmental lines previously discussed. Each partner must continually adapt in the face of the powerful demands that a sexual relationship presents, developing new modes of relating, new skills, and attitudes in order to achieve and maintain a functional relationship. Psychoanalysts have long observed the regressive pull that sexual intimacy exerts. Infantile longings emerge in which primitive anxieties are awakened; patterns of relating to others, internalized in earliest development, infiltrate the experience and meaning of the interaction in the present.

The couple's capacity to negotiate these regressive forces is crucial to the success of the relationship. The partners must also counteract the intense wishes that each brings to the adult relationship to turn that relationship into a replica of a longed-for symbiotic relationship with the mother. Each partner must find new solutions to the current relationship as each unconsciously seeks to make the partner in the present conform to infantile prototypes. When the individual is insufficiently able to distinguish past relationships from love relations in the present, whether due to early trauma or to unresolved neurotic conflict, he or she is prone to reenact infantile patterns of relating, transferring onto the partner in the present wishes, demands, and perceptions that stem from childhood. This is to say that early formative experiences, such as disappointments, losses, and separations are regressively reexperienced in the present and can exert a disruptive impact on present relationships in the form of guilt, suspicion, or primitive rage reactions.

Although there is an extensive psychoanalytic literature that has examined the psychopathology of adult love relationships in great depth, it has offered relatively little insight into the nature of the mature love relationship, particularly in terms of the role it plays in psychological development across the life cycle. The paucity of psychoanalytic literature on sexual intimacy and its role in adult development reflects, in part, the lack until recently of a well-articulated framework for development in adulthood (Ehrlich, 1988). Although approaching the adult relationship from the perspective of its infantile precursors—a genetic perspective—has offered a powerful conceptual framework for clarifying the complex nature of adult relationships, it has also tended to frame the relationship exclusively as the end product of earlier development. In doing so, it has tended to neglect the role that the intimate relationship might play in the ongoing developmental process of adulthood. Past contributions (Kernberg, 1976; Person, 1988) have begun to broaden the psychoanalytic perspective on the adult love relationship in terms not only of its infantile precursors but as a vehicle for psychological growth.

From the perspective of the life cycle, it can be suggested that the adult enters into an intimate sexual relationship at a single point along the continuum of his or her development. This development, as described earlier, can be characterized in terms of complex interweaving developmental lines that are rooted in infantile development and are continually elaborated and reintegrated throughout the course of life. The intimate sexual relationship invariably influences development along these developmental lines, as significant relationships influence development from life's inception. Although the intimate relationship can promote stagnation or regression for the partners involved, it can also facilitate development.

For example, the developmental task of consolidating an identity, which comes to the fore in adolescence, represents a complex process of synthesis in which the individual gradually integrates the various identifications he or she has formed into a cohesive sense of self. Intrapsychically, the consolidation of identity represents a gradual process in which self- and object representations are integrated with actual interpersonal behavior. Kernberg (1980) suggests that even under optimal conditions, critical developmental tasks remain in the postadolescent years, especially in terms of integrating aspects of internalized self- and object relations into a consolidated identity. Adatto (1980) similarly stresses the central role of integrative tasks in early adulthood. Because ego functioning becomes more autonomous over the course of adolescence, the young adult is better able to integrate drives and to develop new adaptive capacities.

The intimate sexual relationship potentially plays a critical role in the integrative processes that contribute to the developing identity in early adulthood. Bergmann (1980) suggests that in the context of mature love relationships, the ego integrates sexual strivings, originally attached to many objects, into love for one person. Such a process, Bergmann emphasizes, occurs only in optimal circumstances in the relationship in which the partner is able to withstand the pressure to repeat early experiences and the wish to make the partner conform to patterns of infantile modes of relating. By finding new solutions to current relationships through withstanding the regressive pull that intimacy invariably elicits, the partners can achieve a restructuring of internal self- and object representations.

The intimate sexual relationship can facilitate the consolidation of identity through the mutual identifications in which lovers engage. Identification, according to Blum (1986), is a "process of internalization and structural transformation leading to a change in the self-representation based upon identification with features of an object" (p. 269). The concept of identification represents one important bridge between the intrapsychic and the interpersonal: It offers a conceptual framework for clarifying how an interaction between people can affect the intrapsychic processes within each.

Kernberg (1980) suggests that within the intimate sexual relationship, the lovers' mutual identifications facilitate a gradual integration of early pre-oedipal and oedipal identifications—a central task in the young adult's ongoing consolidation of an ego identity. This author focuses on the sexual interaction itself. Sexual intercourse, Kernberg suggests, activates both heterosexual and homosexual identifications from earlier development. Gratification derived from the partner's sexual pleasure represents a reconfirmation of and identification with the oedipal object of the opposite sex. Excitement at the partner's orgasm also represents an unconscious identification with the partner—a sublimated homosexual identification. Foreplay, as well, may represent a simultaneous identification with the complementary role of the partner and the reconfirmation of one's own sexual identity. The identification with the partner's complementary role in sexual intercourse allows for the integration of both heterosexual and homosexual identity components.

Binstock (1973) suggests that an ongoing, gratifying sexual relationship offers the couple the opportunity for resolving normative conflicts about sexual identity. By identifying with the partner of the opposite sex, the man variously satisfies his feminine wishes—a process that gradually facilitates his acceptance of his own masculinity. In a parallel fashion, the woman, in unconsciously identifying with the man, satisfies masculine strivings. In this way, Binstock suggests, the sexual relationship gradually facilitates an increasing differentiation for the partners into male and female identities. Such a process provides protection from the threat of regressive yearning that sexual interactions can potentially present, and, in turn, allows for increased sexual intimacy.

Barbour (1981), in a compelling study of women's development in late adolescence and early adulthood, found that intimate sexual relationships with men play the central role in women's development and maintenance of a stable feminine gender identity. She traced the development of a feminine gender identity through four phases. In Phase 1, the women were able to establish a sense of feminine attractiveness and to overcome a sense of adolescent inferiority in regard to their bodies through their partner's appreciation of them. In a second phase, in the context of a fully genital relationship with a man, the women made significant gains in self-acceptance and in claiming autonomy from and parity with their mothers. In the third and fourth phases, the women moved toward a greater sense of autonomy and mature femininity. Barbour highlights the critical role that the partner's consistent affirmation and appreciation of the woman's femininity plays in these developmental processes.

PARENTHOOD

Parenthood also poses a significant developmental challenge by calling upon the couple to adapt and evolve new ways of relating in order to fulfill the task that caring for an infant and then a developing child thrusts upon them. As with sexual intimacy, parenthood evokes powerful affects, fantasies, and memories, rooted in earlier developmentally formative experiences. Here too, the potential for regressively reexperiencing the present in terms of the past represents both a potential danger as well as new opportunity for enrichment and further development along the various developmental lines.

The reintegration of the developmental lines catalyzed by the experience of parenthood emerges before the birth of the child. For prospective fathers, the wife's pregnancy often elicits a range of powerful reactions—rooted both in the present reality of the experience and in its evocation of earlier, often conflict-ridden experiences (Osofsky, 1982). Especially during a first pregnancy, the man must negotiate shifts in his relationship with his pregnant mate who undergoes dramatic changes—physical, emotional, social. He must also begin to forge an identity as a father, which includes his gradually developing an attachment to the developing fetus.

Gurwitt (1986) suggests that prospective fatherhood represents a developmental crisis for the man. In addition to excited anticipation, many men might be confused and anxious during their wife's pregnancy, often manifesting psychosomatic symptoms and other indications of emotional distress (Osofsky, 1982). Though potentially painful and unsettling, the challenges with which the wife's pregnancy confronts the man also offer the opportunity for significant developmental shifts to occur. Osofsky found that the woman's pregnancy stimulates in the prospective father profound changes in his sense of responsibility, his feelings about his mate, and about himself. Gurwitt (1986) suggests that the expectant father reexamines and reworks his relationship with his own father as one aspect of the identity shift that occurs during his wife's pregnancy.

Bibring (1959) views pregnancy as a crisis for women, similar in many ways to puberty and menopause. In each of these experiences,

> new and increased libidinal and adjustive tasks confront the individual, leading to the revival and simultaneous emergence of unsettled conflicts from earlier developmental phases and to the loosening of partial and inadequate solutions of the past. (p. 116)

Bibring suggests that the psychic reorganization inherent in the experience of pregnancy has profound implications for the mother's ongoing psychological development. Pregnancy, like any major developmental task, prompts the reemergence of earlier conflicts that can potentially lead to either a regressive consolidation of neurotic solutions, or conversely, offer an opportunity to rework these conflicts and arrive at new, more creative solutions. Recent contributions (e.g.,

Notman & Lester, 1988; Novick, 1988) emphasize the influence of pregnancy on the woman's feminine gender identity and self-esteem. Notman and Lester (1988) suggest that pregnancy reevokes the early relationship with the mother, offering the pregnant woman the opportunity for reworking earlier identifications and conflicts that contribute to her sense of herself as a woman.

Each developmental stage through which the child progresses evokes strong emotional responses in the parents, which include memories, fantasies, and feelings from the corresponding developmental stage in the parents' own past. When the child evokes in the parent experiences that have been problematic in the parent's own development, the parent may be unable to respond appropriately to the child's needs. For example, an 8-year-old boy frightens the neighborhood children with angry, threatening outbursts, his parents seemingly unable to set appropriate limits. For the mother, the boy's anger evokes the chaos that ensued in her childhood home when she was the same age as her son. Deeply anxious about open confrontation, she wishes simply to smooth things over so as to avoid any confrontations reminiscent of that painful time. For the father, the boy's anger evokes his own, long-suppressed angry feelings. Frightened by these feelings, he tends to avoid his son's anger as he does his own. Such a circumstance may promote a serious stalemate in which the parents are unable to disengage from unresolved childhood conflicts of their own and respond realistically to the child in the present. Potentially, however, the parents may use such a crisis to develop in significant ways. The relationship with the child can catalyze new modes of adaptation and with it, shifts away from problematic modes of relating. In terms of the example, the father might come to recognize, in angry confrontation with his son, that he and others can tolerate the angry feelings that he long has fantasized would be overwhelming and destructive.

A common example of a developmental challenge that parenthood presents concerns how the early adolescent's sexual awakening can provoke in the parents powerful feelings about their own sexuality, including incestuous fantasies that lie dormant from their own adolescence. The parent may then reenact aspects of his or her own earlier conflicts with the adolescent child. Rangell (1985) describes how a father might project his own adolescent competitive strivings onto an adolescent son and, in identifying with an internal image of his own jealous father, engage the son in a fierce, rivalrous struggle.

Kernberg (1976) examines how middle-aged women, in interaction with their adolescent daughters, often reexperience the relationship they had with their own mothers when they were adolescents with all the intense feelings that such a relationship often entails: idealization, hatred, or hostile dependency. The failure to come to terms with such feelings can lead to depression and envy and even severe psychopathology. Conversely, Kernberg suggests, the activation of such a crisis offers the woman a rich opportunity for reconfirming her own self-worth and values. In doing so, the woman can come to find a new sense of freedom and creativity.

Mourning and Aging

Lerner and Lerner (1987) observed that Freud's original definition of mourning and its distinction from melancholia is still accepted by most psychoanalytic clinicians and theorists. According to Freud (1917/1951), the distinguishing mental

HOWARD D.
LERNER and
JOSHUA EHRLICH

features of mourning are profoundly painful dejection, loss of interest in the outside world, inability to love, and massive inhibition of all activity. Melancholia involves the identical features as well as "a lowering of the self-regarding feelings to a degree that finds utterances and self-reproaches and self-revelings and culminate in a delusional expectation of punishment" (p. 244). Freud goes on to note that whereas melancholia, like mourning, may be a reaction to the loss of a loved object, it differs in that "one cannot see clearly what it is that has been lost—[the person] knows whom he has lost but not what he has lost in him" (p. 245). These observations led Freud to conclude that "in mourning it is the world which has become poor and empty; in melancholia it is the ego itself" (p. 246).

The process of mourning involves a gradual relinquishment and severing of emotional ties to the lost object and a corresponding displacement of interest or attachment onto other objects. According to Freud,

> [E]ach single one of the memories and situations of expectancy which demonstrate the libido's attachment to the lost object is met by the verdict of reality that the object no longer exists; and the ego, confronted as it were with the question whether it shall share this state, is persuaded by the sum of the narcissistic satisfactions it derives from being alive to sever its attachment to the object that has been abolished. (1917/1951, p. 237)

Melancholia as well involved a withdrawal of interest or attachment from the lost object. However, rather than being displaced onto other objects, the libido, by means of regressive identification, is withdrawn back into the self. In this way the object loss is transformed into a loss of self, and the conflict between the self and the lost object is experienced as a "cleavage" within the self.

According to Lerner and Lerner (1987), the impact of loss on personality is dramatic, intense, exceedingly complex, and dependent on a multitude of internal and external factors, including levels of separation: individuation, drive development, level of defense, and most significantly, the developmental level of mental representations, as well as the availability of substitute objects and the degree to which inner psychological structures have become autonomous from supporting objects. According to these authors, the impact of object loss on object relations and narcissism can be viewed on a developmental continuum in relation to self–other differentiation, level of mental representation, and degree of self- and object constancy. When these particular lines of development are not fully structuralized nor autonomous from supporting objects, the response to object loss is more likely to be one of melancholia; that is, a loss of self, as opposed to mourning.

George Pollock, perhaps more than any other psychoanalyst, has studied the mourning process and has reported that this most poignant human experience potentially serves as an adaptation to various losses throughout the life cycle. According to this author, bereavement is only one dimension of mourning. Mourning can be set in motion not only after death, but also by loss, disappointment, or change, and is a normative part of development throughout life. Colarusso and Nemiroff (1981) quote Pollock (1979) who asserts:

> Mourning is a universal transformational process that allows us to accept the reality that exists, which may be different from our wishes and hopes, which recognizes loss and change, both externally and internally, and which . . . can result in a happier life, fulfilled and fulfilling for ourselves and for others. For the gifted the mourning process may be part of or the end-product that can result in creativity in art, music, literature, science, philosophy, religion. (p. 10)

Mourning, seen in this way, is an adaptive phenomenon that facilitates development. According to Shabad and Dietrich (1989), the death of the old gives way to the birth of the new in ways that are not always immediately apparent in the midst of grief. Loss, despite potentially pathogenic consequences, may also have other creative, more constructive, long-term consequences that are not always recognizable in the aftermath. The process of increased internalization of the representation of lost objects set the stage for what Pollock (1979) refers to as the mourning–liberation process. The pain of working through the process of mourning can be gradually replaced by the relative psychological freedom brought about by an acceptance that a loss is final. A person may then direct his or her creative capacities toward reconstituting a replacement for the lost object (Shabad & Dietrich, 1989). The relative balance between acceptance of or denial of the finality of loss and death significantly influences the individual's capacity to eventually work through and resolve the loss experience.

It is well documented in the extensive psychoanalytic literature on loss that the process of loss, mourning, and reorganization of the representational world brings about an active search for new, age-appropriate adaptations for obtaining gratification that can be contrasted to more pathological forms of mourning that include melancholia and the experience of loss as a loss of vital aspects of the self. As Colarusso and Nemiroff (1981) observe, in the psychological processes involved in these changes, the fantasized, idealized, or negatively distorted conceptions of life emanating from childhood and young adulthood are diminished in power and importance.

The lifelong experience of separation and loss is what links mourning and aging. Aging begins at conception but has unique characteristics at each phase of the life cycle (Erikson, 1978). According to Michels (1980), aging means for the first time a diminution of capacity and potential rather than the steady progressive growth associated with childhood. As Michels (1980) puts it,

> For the adult, death begins to be more familiar and gradually accepted. Friends and loved ones die; one's own death is no longer beyond the psychologically meaningful horizon of future time; and the inevitable diseases and disabilities of middle life begin to replace the child's unconscious fantasies as the symbolic equivalent of death. (p. 33)

Driven attempts in middle age to remain young, hypochondriacal preoccupations with health in the parents, the emergence of sexual promiscuity in order to prove oneself youthful and potent, and the lack of authentic enjoyment of life as well as the frequency of religious concern at middle age are familiar defensive patterns of coping with the inevitability of death (Jaques, 1980). The aging process, and with it the loss of physical and mental capacities, represents an adult life crisis. It intensifies narcissistic vulnerability, the recognition of mortality, and the inevitable approach of death, which demand adaptation to this most imminent threat and stress. Dealing with the issue of death itself, both for the individual approaching it as well as the survivors, involves a major shift in internal, interpersonal, and social factors and the need for psychological adaptation to these new circumstances. Mourning and the aging process require a continuing evolution and maturation for the maintenance of adaptation and functioning. Inevitably, the vicissitudes of life experience include separation, loss, and mourning—no one is immune to them. Positive adaptation to these vicissitudes is less significantly related to their existence than to the individual's capacity for conflict resolution and continued adaptation. These adaptations are the result of the multiple dimensions or lines of development considered in this chapter.

Summary

Recent contributions to psychoanalysis have begun to examine the elaboration and refinement of different dimensions of development as these extend across the life cycle. As noted, for example, Colarusso and Nemiroff (1981) have examined the vicissitudes of narcissism in the adult years. As another example, Sternschein (1973), Behrends and Blatt (1985), and others have offered initial conceptualizations of how individuals deal with the ongoing task of separation–individuation in the adult years. In line with the approach of such contributions, this chapter, in exploring development across the life cycle, has sought to integrate the formative, ongoing influence of intrapsychic processes with the continuous impact of maturation and life experience.

Many fascinating questions remain for the psychoanalytic theorist interested in social development across the lifespan. We know little, for example, about the evolution of the various dimensions of development during later life. One might ask, for instance, how internalized object relations develop when an individual is 60 or 70. The answer, in addition to its theoretical interest, has important implications for understanding individual adaptation throughout life and for developing interventions where necessary. Colarusso and Nemiroff (1981) have noted that a spur to study adult development recently has been that subjects involved in longitudinal studies since childhood have begun to enter adulthood. As these subjects are followed across the adult years, researchers will, in fact, have increasing opportunity to clarify the nature of development through senescence. Research, such as Vaillant's (1977) compelling study of the evolution of mechanisms of defense through to middle adulthood, highlights the rich potential for further study in this domain.

In addition, much work remains to be done on the impact that specific life experiences exert on adult development. Too often, researchers and theorists conceptualize significant experiences of adulthood—for example, close relationships, divorce, loss, illness—outside the context of an individual's ongoing development. This tendency has two results. First, it often means that we lose sight of the dimensions of development that set the stage for each adult experience. Second, we fail to consider the role that each new experience of adulthood potentially plays in the refinement and reorganization of previous dimensions of development. Individual experience thus becomes static and detached.

Research such as Barbour's (1981) study of women's elaboration of their feminine gender identities in the context of their intimate relationships with men exemplifies the power of a developmental perspective on adolescent and adult experience. By understanding the development of gender identity as an ongoing process, this research is able to fully capture the richness of its subjects' individual experiences. One understands how the subjects' ongoing development both *sets the stage* for a particular life event and then is *transformed* by it. Our understanding of critical life cycle experiences—such as divorce, illness, grandparenthood, retirement—can be greatly enriched by viewing such experiences in the context of multiple dimensions of development.

Adatto, C. P. (1980). Late adolescence to early adulthood. In S. Greenspan & G. Pollock (Eds.), *The course of the life cycle: Psychoanalytic contributions toward understanding personality development* (Vol. II, pp. 463–476). Washington, DC: National Institute of Mental Health.

Barbour, C. G. (1981). *Women in love: The development of feminine gender identity in the context of the heterosexual couple.* Unpublished doctoral dissertation. The University of Michigan.

Basch, M. (1981). Psychodynamic interpretation and cognitive transformation. *International Journal of Psycho-Analysis, 62,* 151–175.

Behrends, R. S., and Blatt, J. J. (1985). Internalization and psychological development throughout the life cycle. *Psychoanalytic Study of the Child, 40,* 11–40.

Bergmann, M. S. (1980). On the intrapsychic function of falling in love. *Psychoanalytic Quarterly, 49,* 56–76.

Bibring, G. L. (1959). Some considerations of the psychological processes in pregnancy. *Psychoanalytic Study of the Child, 14,* 113–121.

Binstock, W. A. (1973). On the two forms of intimacy. *Journal of the American Psychoanalytic Association, 21,* 93–107.

Blatt, S. (1974). Levels of object representation in anaclitic and introjective depression. *Psychoanalytic Study of the Child, 29,* 107–157.

Blos, P. (1979). *The adolescent passage.* New York: International Universities Press.

Blum, H. P. (1986). On identification and its vicissitudes. *International Journal of Psycho-Analysis, 67,* 267–276.

Boesky, D. (1989). A discussion of evidential criteria for therapeutic change. In A. Rothstein (Ed.), *How does treatment help: Modes of therapeutic action of psychoanalytic therapy.* Madison, CT: International Universities Press.

Brenner, C. (1986). Reflections. In A. Richards & M. S. Willock (Eds.), *Psychoanalysis: The science of mental conflict. Essays in honor of Charles Brenner.* Hillsdale, NJ: Analytic Press.

Colarusso, C. A., & Nemiroff, R. A. (1981). *Adult development.* New York: Plenum Press.

Ehrlich, J. (1988). *A perspective on men, intimacy, and developmental processes in the adult heterosexual relationship.* Unpublished Master's thesis. The University of Michigan.

Erikson, E. (1964). *Insight and responsibility.* New York: Norton.

Erikson, E. (1968). *Identity: Youth and crisis.* New York: Norton.

Erikson, E. (1978). *Life history and historical moment.* New York: Norton.

Freud, A. (1965). *Normality and pathology in childhood.* New York: International Universities Press.

Freud, S. (1951). Mourning and melancholia. In J. Strachey (Ed. and Trans.), *The standard edition of the complete psychological works of Sigmund Freud.* London: Hogarth Press. (Original work published 1917)

Freud, S. (1957). The ego and the id. In J. Strachey (Ed. and Trans.), *The standard edition of the complete psychological works of Sigmund Freud.* London: Hogarth Press. (Original work published 1923)

Gedo, J., & Goldberg, A. (1973). *Models of the mind.* Chicago: University of Chicago Press.

Greenspan, S. (1979). *Intelligence and adaptation.* New York: International Universities Press.

Greenspan, S. (1981). *Psychopathology and adaptation in infancy and early childhood.* New York: International Universities Press.

Guntrip, H. (1974). Psychoanalytic object relations theory: The Fairbairn-Guntrip approach. In S. Arieti (Ed.), *American handbook of psychiatry* (Vol. 1). New York: Basic Books.

Gurwitt, A. R. (1986). On becoming a family man. *Psychoanalytic Inquiry, 8,* 261–279.

Harman, S. W. (1978). Male menopause? The hormones flow but sex does slow. *Medical World, 20,* 11.

Hartmann, H. (1950). *Ego psychology and the problem of adaptation.* New York: International Universities Press.

Inhelder, B., & Piaget, J. (1958). *The growth of logical thinking from childhood to adolescence: An essay on the construction of formal operational structures.* New York: International Universities Press.

Jacobson, E. (1964). *The self and the object world.* New York: International Universities Press.

Jaques, E. (1965). Death and the midlife crisis. *International Journal of Psycho-Analysis, 46,* 502–514.

Jaques, E. (1980). The midlife crisis. In S. Greenspan & G. Pollock (Eds.), *The course of the life cycle: Psychoanalytic contributions toward understanding personality development,* Vol. III (pp. 1–24). Washington, DC: National Institute of Mental Health.

Jung, C. L. (1933). *Modern man in search of a soul.* New York: Harcourt-Brace.

Kaplan, L. J. (1986). *Adolescence: The farewell to childhood.* New York: Jason Aronson.

HOWARD D.
LERNER and
JOSHUA EHRLICH

Kernberg, O. (1976). *Borderline conditions and pathological narcissism.* New York: International Universities Press.

Kernberg, O. (1980). *Internal world and external reality.* New York: Jason Aronson.

Klein, G. (1976). *Psychoanalytic theory: An exploration of essentials.* New York: International Universities Press.

Kohlberg, L., & Gilligan, C. (1972). The adolescent as a philosopher: The discovery of the self in a post-conventional world. In J. Kagan & R. Coles (Eds.), *Twelve to sixteen: Early adolescence* (pp. 77–95). New York: Norton.

Kohut, H. (1971). *The analysis of the self.* New York: International Universities Press.

Kohut, H. (1977). *The restoration of the self.* New York: International Universities Press.

Lerner, H. (1987). Psychodynamic models of adolescence. In M. Hersen & V. Van Hasselt (Eds.), *Handbook of adolescent psychiatry* (pp. 53–76). New York: Pergamon Press.

Lerner, H., & Lerner, P. (1987). Separation, depression, and object loss: Implications for narcissism and object relations. In J. Bloom-Feshbach & S. Bloom-Feshbach (Eds.), *The psychology of separation and loss* (pp. 375–395). San Francisco: Jossey-Bass.

Lerner, P., & Lerner, H. (1985). Contributions of object relations theory toward a general psychoanalytic theory of thinking: A revised theory of thinking. *Psychoanalysis and Contemporary Thought, 3,* 3–30.

Lidz, R., Lidz, R., & Rubenstein, R. (1976). An anaclitic syndrome in adolescent amphetamine addicts. *The Psychoanalytic Study of the Child, 31,* 317–348.

Mahler, M. (1968). *On human symbiosis and the vicissitudes of individuation: Vol. 1. Infantile psychosis.* New York: International Universities Press.

Mahler, M. (1973). In M. Winestine (Reporter). The experience of separation-individuation in infancy and its reverberations through the course of life: Infancy and childhood (Panel Report). *Journal of the American Psychoanalytic Association, 21,* 135.

Mahler, M., Pine, F., & Bergman, A. (1975). *The psychological birth of the human infant.* New York: Basic Books.

Martin, C. E. (1977). Sexual activity in the aging male. In J. Morey & H. Musaph (Eds.), *Handbook of sexology.* Amsterdam: Elsevier/North Holland.

Michels, R. (1980). Adulthood. In S. Greenspan & G. Pollock (Eds.), *The course of the life cycle: Psychoanalytic contributions toward understanding personality development* (Vol. III, pp. 25–34). Washington, DC: National Institute of Mental Health.

Nagera, H. (1970). Children's reactions to the death of important objects: A developmental approach. *The Psychoanalytic Study of the Child, 25,* 360–400.

Neugarten, B. (1979). Time, age, and the life cycle. *American Journal of Psychiatry, 136,* 887–894.

Notman, M. T., & Lester, E. P. (1988). Pregnancy: Theoretical considerations. *Psychoanalytic Inquiry, 8,* 139–159.

Novick, K. K. (1988). Childbearing and child rearing. *Psychoanalytic Inquiry, 8,* 252–260.

Osofsky, H. (1982). Expectant and new fatherhood as a developmental crisis. *Bulletin of the Menninger Clinic, 46,* 209–230.

Person, E. S. (1988). *Dreams of love and fateful encounters.* New York: Norton.

Piaget, J. (1954). *The construction of reality.* New York: Basic Books.

Pollock, G. (1979). *Aging or aged: Development or pathology?* Unpublished manuscript.

Rangell, L. (1985). The role of the parent in the Oedipus complex. *Bulletin of the Menninger Clinic, 19,* 9–15.

Ritvo, S. (1971). Late adolescence: Developmental and clinical considerations. *The Psychoanalytic Study of the Child, 26,* 241–263.

Settlage, C. F., Curtis, J., Lozoff, M., Silberschatz, G., & Simburg, E. (1988). Conceptualizing adult development. *Journal of the American Psychoanalytic Association, 36,* 347–369.

Shabad, P., & Dietrich, D. (1989). Reflections on loss, mourning, and the unconscious process of regeneration. In D. Dietrich & P. Shabad (Eds.), *The problem of loss and mourning* (pp. 461–470). Madison, CT: International Universities Press.

Shane, M. (1977). A rationale for teaching analytic technique based on a developmental orientation and approach. *International Journal of Psycho-Analysis, 58,* 95–108.

Spruiell, V. (1975). Narcissistic transformation in adolescence. *International Journal of Psychoanalytic Psychotherapy, 4,* 518–535.

Staples, H., & Smarr, E. (1980). Bridge to adulthood: Years from eighteen to twenty-three. In S. Greenspan & G. Pollock (Eds.), *The course of the life cycle: Psychoanalytic contribution toward understanding personality development* (Vol. II, pp. 477–496). Washington, DC: National Institute of Mental Health.

Sternschein, I. (Reporter). (1973). The experience of separation-individuation in infancy and its reverberations through the course of life: Maturity, senescence, and sociological implications. *Journal of the American Psychoanalytic Association, 21,* 633–645.

Stolorow, R. (1975). Toward a functional definition of narcissism. *International Journal of Psycho-Analysis, 56,* 179–185.

Sugarman, A., Bloom-Feshbach, J., & Bloom-Feshbach, S. (1980). The psychological dimensions of borderline adolescents. In J. Kwawer, H. Lerner, P. Lerner, & A. Sugarman (Eds.), *Borderline phenomena and the Rorschach test* (pp. 469–494). New York: International Universities Press.

Sugarman, A., & Jaffe, L. (1987). Transitional phenomena and psychological separateness in schizophrenic, borderline, and bulimic patients. In J. Bloom-Feshbach & S. Bloom-Feshbach (Eds.), *The psychology of separation and love* (pp. 416–458). San Francisco: Jossey-Bass.

Tolpin, M., & Kohut, H. (1980). The disorders of the self: Psychopathology of the first year of life. In S. Greenspan & G. Pollock (Eds.), *The course of the life cycle: Psychoanalytic contribution toward understanding personality development* (Vol. 1, pp. 524–442). Washington, DC: National Institute of Mental Health.

Tyson, R. (1983). Some narcissistic consequences of object loss: A developmental view. *Psychoanalytic Quarterly, 51,* 205–224.

Vaillant, G. E. (1977). *Adaptation of life.* Boston: Little, Brown.

Waelder, R. (1930). The principle of multiple function. Observations on overdetermination. In S. Guttman (Ed.), *Psychoanalysis: Observation, theory, application* (pp. 68–83). New York: International Universities Press.

Winnicott, D. (1958). Transitional objects and transitional phenomena. In D. Winnicott (Ed.), *Collected papers: Through pediatrics to psychoanalysis* (pp. 229–242) New York: Basic Books. (Original work published 1951)

Wolff, P. (1960). The developmental psychologies of Jean Piaget and psychoanalysis. *Psychological Issues,* Monograph 5.

4

Learning Theories

BROOKE A. BENSON, STEPHEN C. MESSER,
AND ALAN M. GROSS

INTRODUCTION

To the developmental psychologist, social development is the process whereby children acquire their social roles, values, and behaviors (McGraw, 1987). The process of social development relies heavily upon the influence of the environment. Parents, peers, teachers, and others exert an undeniable impact upon the growing child. The outcome of this interactional process is the multifaceted behavioral repertoire referred to as personality.

In addition to the influence of significant others, however, children play a key role in their own social development. Children are not merely passive recipients of outside stimulation, but rather, actively participate in the social development process. Such reciprocal interplay of socioenvironmental forces and individual behavior results in the acquisition and expression of social behaviors in various contexts and at certain times.

With varying degrees of specificity and success, several models or general theoretical systems have attempted to explain the mechanisms by which social development (general or specific) emerges. Attachment, psychodynamic, maturational, social network, and cognitive-developmental theories are but some of the conceptual approaches utilized to understand the process of social development. The behavioral, or learning theory, perspective has provided a significant contribution to the developmental field. Typically invoked to help explain the acquisition of

BROOKE A. BENSON AND ALAN M. GROSS • Department of Psychology, University of Mississippi, University, Mississippi 38677.   STEPHEN C. MESSER • University of Pittsburgh School of Medicine, Western Psychiatric Institute and Clinic, Pittsburgh, Pennsylvania 15213.

Handbook of Social Development: A Lifespan Perspective, edited by Vincent B. Van Hasselt and Michel Hersen. Plenum Press, New York, 1992.

discrete behaviors or in the explication of individual differences, learning theories have generated substantial research and provided a clinically useful conceptual scheme of the socialization process.

From the behavioral view, one's social environment consists of stimuli presented by other individuals. Social behaviors are responses under the actual or potential control of social stimuli. Hence, the social learning of behavior defines a category and process of acquired adaptive behavior that involves the stimuli and contexts provided by people. This form of learning is indispensable given the cultural basis of human civilization (Gewirtz & Petrovich, 1983).

The purpose of this chapter is to present a general introduction to the basic assumptions and principles of learning theory, with a special emphasis on its relevance to the explication of social development. Our plan is to first review the historical development of the behavioral perspective; second, introduce the basic principles of learning; and third, apply learning theory to three basic areas encountered in social development research: temperament, infant attachment, and aggressive behavior.

HISTORICAL DEVELOPMENTS IN LEARNING THEORY: THE PARADIGM AND THE PRINCIPLES

The various theories of learning that have been proposed and studied over the years all share a high regard for the scientific method. These theories are designed to explain and predict events in terms of the lawfulness of behavior. They each search for an empirically demonstrated and parsimonious set of principles to account for these behavioral events. As with most theories, there are disagreements concerning the interpretation of both observable events and the methodologies most widely respected and utilized.

Depending on the theoretical orientation, the definition of learning is even somewhat disputed (Bachrach, 1985). Given certain environmental conditions, without reference to internal mechanisms, proponents of an experimental analysis of behavior (e.g., Skinner) emphasize the observable changes in the probability of a specific response's occurrence. In comparison, theorists with a neurophysiological orientation (e.g., Hebb) focus on learning as a change in neural processes in the central nervous system. Conversely, cognitive-behavioral theorists (e.g., Bandura) view learning as an intervening cognitive process that links organismic states together before and after a change in behavior occurs. Fortunately, most learning theorists can at least agree that learning is a more or less permanent change in behavior resulting from experience or practice, and is not a function of fatigue, maturation, illness, or drugs.

A central distinction for learning psychologists has been between the concepts of learning and performance (Bachrach, 1985). For those utilizing the intervening variable approach, learning is inferred from observed performance. Kimble (1989), for example, views learning as a change in behavior potentiality. The organism acquires capabilities to perform some act through learning, but the act itself may not occur. For Skinnerians, the performance of the response and the change in its probability of occurrence are considered isomorphic with learning. In this system, the proposal of mediating variables is unnecessary. There is even considerable disagreement regarding the importance of reinforcement in the learning process. Generally defined as a contingent relationship between an act and an environmental event that alters the future likelihood of the act, some theorists maintain that reinforcement is necessary for learning (e.g., Skinner). Others, however, propose that reinforcement is operative in performance but not necessarily in all learning (e.g., Bandura).

Though often regarded as comparable, learning theories display a good deal of variability. The purpose of this section is to provide an extremely brief review of learning theories affecting the domain of social development. Most important, the reader may come to better appreciate the evolution of learning theory as well as its past and potential contributions to social developmental phenomena.

WATSON

In 1912, John B. Watson was the first to formally state the assumptions and methodology of behaviorism. Behaviorism advocated the observation of overt behavior, rather than mental states, as the means by which psychology could become an objective science. Consistent with the tenets of behaviorism was an increasingly extreme perspective of environmentalism, which discounted innate contributions to behavioral development (Fantino & Logan, 1979). Watson's theory of environmentalism served to make the learning of observable responses fundamental to the field of psychology. Consequently, theories of learning become equivalent with theories of behavior (and development).

Watson's two most popular studies relating to social behavior involved the nature of emotional reactions in the infant and the acquisition of learned emotion (Watson & Rayner, 1920). These two studies provided the laboratory evidence for many of Watson's later positions on child development and child rearing.

Watson proposed that the human infant was endowed with only three emotions: fear, rage, and love. Consistent with his environmental emphasis, Watson believed that changes with age were solely produced by learning. In his famous "Little Albert" study, Watson attempted to demonstrate this phenomenon showing that the "innate" emotion of fear could be elicited by new objects through conditioning. He was, to a large extent, responsible for some of the stringent child-rearing practices advised (e.g., "hands-off" approach to infant crying to avoid reinforcement) before the permissiveness associated with the tenets of psychoanalysis. Watsonian behaviorism was fertile ground for the flourishing of the ideas and observations of Pavlov.

PAVLOV

Ivan Petrovich Pavlov, a Russian physiologist, explicated an important paradigm in learning theory currently known as classical conditioning, Pavlovian conditioning, or respondent conditioning. Studying the salivation reflex in dogs, Pavlov's prime interest focused on the physiological reflexes that occurred upon the presentation of food. As the dogs in this experiment were restrained for long periods of time, they were fed at regular feeding times. Over time, Pavlov noticed that as his assistant entered the room with food, the dogs would begin to salivate and secrete stomach acids. To study these anticipatory secretions, Pavlov isolated one animal from extraneous and influencing variables and presented the dog with food. Each presentation of food, however, was preceded by the tone of a tuning fork. After several pairings of the tone and food, Pavlov noticed that the dog began to salivate earlier and earlier in the procedure. Eventually the dog began to salivate prior to the presentation of food but subsequent to the sounding of the tone.

Unknown to Pavlov at the time, this basic paradigm became the model for classical conditioning and has become an important theory in the explanation of human behavior. This model provides an explanation of why certain reflexive behaviors are performed in response to stimuli which did not previously evoke the behavior. In general, there exists a natural relationship between various stimuli (called an unconditioned stimulus or US) and the reflexive or unconditioned response (UR) such stimuli evokes. In the case of Pavlov's experiment, the meat (US) reliably elicited the specific unconditioned response of salivation (UCR). In this experiment, the pairing of the neutral conditioned stimulus (CS) or the tone, with the unconditioned stimulus (US) of the food elicited the conditioned response (CR) of salivation. Pavlov coined the term *conditioning* to describe this new stimulus–response relationship. Because learning had taken place, the original neutral stimulus has become a *conditioned stimulus* (CS), and the response elicited is termed the *conditioned response* (CR).

The process of forming associations, however, can also be unraveled or disassembled. This weakening of associations, often referred to as extinction, occurs when an unconditioned stimulus is no longer presented with a conditioned stimulus. Over time and repeated unpaired CS presentations, the conditioned response will typically weaken and eventually will stop occurring in response to the presence of the CS.

The principles of classical conditioning have been used to account for a variety of developmental phenomena. In particular, the mechanisms of classical conditioning have been implicated in the development of fears and phobias. This association was first suggested by Watson and Rayner (1920) in the famous case of Little Albert and the white rat and was later expanded upon by Jones (1924). Today, many learning theorists believe that fears and phobias may develop through classical conditioning, and they utilize treatment strategies (such as systematic desensitization and flooding) based upon these conditioning principles (Davey, 1989; di Nardo, Guzy, Jenkins & Bak, 1988; Hygge & Ohman, 1978).

Generalized fears are common in a child's development. At some time or another, most children are fearful of such inanimate or animate objects as the dark, heights, flying, the doctor or dentist's office, large dogs, snakes, and so forth. It is suggested that repeated (or even single trial) pairings of these CSs with a UCS may elicit fear responses. To illustrate how this procedure can naturally occur in our environment, consider the development of a childhood fear about the doctor's office.

Small children frequently make visits to the pediatrician (the conditioned stimulus). On one such visit, the pediatrician prepares and gives the child a vaccination (UCS) resulting in a prick on the arm, a numbing or stinging sensation, facial expressions of pain, and crying behavior by the child (the unconditioned response). As a result of this interaction, the child has learned that certain salient stimuli at the pediatrician's office (the conditioned stimuli) are associated with receiving shots that produce painful sensations. Consequently, the child develops response dispositions toward the pediatrician that are consistent with a label of fear (conditioned response).

As indicated, this basic paradigm may be extended to account for many similar fears. These same principles also suggest why many childhood fears may disappear with time. With many fears, the unconditioned stimulus is not always followed by the conditioned stimulus. In our example, the doctor does not always given the child an injection. Consequently, with repeated, unpaired CS–US presentations, the conditioned fear response may gradually extinguish from the child's behavioral repertoire in this context.

Among the infant responses that have been successfully classically conditioned (see Davey, 1981, for studies) are sucking, the Babkin reflex, head turning, and eye movements. Classical conditioning has occurred with appetitive UCSs, including nipple-elicited sucking, vestibulation-elicited changes in respiration, heart rate, and motility, and adult-face-elicited head turning. Interestingly, the most potent CS for the early neonatal period appears to be time (Davey, 1981). Studies of temporal conditioning in human neonates suggest that conditioned responses of the autonomic nervous system are readily acquired through temporal conditioning but not motor responses (i.e., biologically constrained learning discussed later).

Finally, little evidence exists regarding the relationship between speed of conditioned response formation (i.e., learning capacity, Davey, 1981) and chronological age. However, Fitzgerald and Brackbill (1976) suggest that conditionability is a function of neurological maturation rather than chronological age.

THORNDIKE

Classical conditioning has been utilized to explain the acquisition of a variety of human behaviors, especially emotional- and motivational-based behavioral phenomena. This paradigm on its own, however, has been unable to explain many responses to our environment. The proposition that one learns by experiencing the consequences of one's behavior is an attempt to remedy the shortcomings of classical conditioning. Pioneered by Edward L. Thorndike, learning by consequences, or "trial and success" learning, was first systematically demonstrated in experiments with cats in a "problem box." In an attempt to understand whether animals solved problems by reasoning or by instinct, Thorndike placed food-deprived cats inside a box and placed a string capable of opening the door within reach of the cats paw. Once outside the door, the cats could feast on morsels of fish. Thorndike noticed that on successive tests in the cage, the animals took shorter and shorter periods to open the door. He concluded that this phenomenon was not due to an intelligent understanding of the problem but rather a "stamping in" of the stimulus–response connection between the door and the string. Thorndike further hypothesized that this "stamping in" process was mediated by the effects that followed the response. A response that was followed by a "satisfier" would be strengthened, but a response succeeded by an "annoyer" would be weakened.

Thorndike's theory that the "stamping in" of a stimulus–response connection was determined by its effects was termed the *law of effect*. It had a profound impact upon later theories of learning, including those addressing the process of social development.

BROOKE A.
BENSON *et al.*

The view that environmental consequences affected the probability of responding was enthusiastically embraced by Harvard psychologist B. F. Skinner. Skinner modified and furthered Thorndike's basic assumptions maintaining that most human behavior *operates* on the environment to secure particular consequences instead of simply *responding* to the environment. Skinner additionally changed the terms *satisfier* and *annoyer*. Although the concepts remained similar, Skinner espoused the notion of reinforcers in the shaping and maintenance of many human behaviors. According to Skinner, a positive reinforcer constitutes a reward given after a particular response. From this reasoning, an operant response that is followed by a reinforcer or reward will be more likely to occur again in that situation. Hence, the response was "reinforced," and the probability of the behavior occurring in the future is increased.

Jeremy Bentham's theory of psychological hedonism also plays an important role in Skinner's formulations. Essentially, Skinner's theory of instrumental conditioning "rests on the assumption of adaptive hedonism—we do what avoids pain and gets pleasure" (Zimbardo, 1988, p. 271). Instrumental responses that are positively reinforced are most likely to occur again. By the same token, it follows that negative reinforcers would decrease the probability of a behavior's occurrence. In reality, however, the reverse is true. Negative reinforcers are defined as aversive stimuli that the individual attempts to escape or avoid. The removal of a negative reinforcer will increase the probability of a response (referred to as escape–avoidance learning) just as the presentation of a positive reinforcer will increase response strength. Both positive and negative reinforcement increase the probability that the preceding response will occur again. It is important to note that reinforcement is operationally defined by its behavioral effects. The notion of what constitutes a reinforcer is usually empirically determined *after* its effects have been elicited.

The work of Skinner represents a significant and powerful divergence from the American tradition of learning theory (Fantino & Logan, 1979). Ironically, rather than formulating a specific theoretical position, Skinner is typically regarded as a self-proclaimed antitheorist. In fact, he rarely speaks of learning at all, instead referring to observable changes in behavior. For example, the concept of learning via "connections" in the nervous system is not given empirical consideration because it is an unobservable. Skinner's perceptive is characterized not by his position on the traditional theoretical issues but by his methodological emphasis that renders the issues irrelevant. He insists on the exclusive reliance of directly observable behavior. Skinner's approach does not include subjective mental constructs or hypothesized physiological constructs. In sum, behavior is not to be inferred but observed directly.

Skinner emphasized the principle of reinforcement in the shaping, differentiation, generalization, and extinction of behavior (see more about these principles later). Reinforcement is merely operationally defined as the presentation (or removal) of an event that alters the response (operant) rate. The theoretical question of why a reinforcer is reinforcing is considered a pseudoproblem. The operant is viewed as a group or class of responses that, by virtue of their similarity, are similarly affected by the consequences associated with any one class member. Though distinguishing between respondent (classical) and operant conditioning, the Skinnerian approach attributes more importance to operant conditioning among complex organisms.

Learning theorists have applied these reinforcement principles to a variety of social behaviors. Researchers have observed the impact that positive reinforcement has upon the development of altruistic and cooperative behavior (Aronfreed, 1968; Cialdini & Kenrick, 1976; Cook & Stingle, 1974; Darlington & Macker, 1966; Grusec & Redler, 1980; Kanfer, 1979; Midlarsky & Bryan, 1967, Midlarsky, Bryan, & Brickman, 1973; Miller, Brickman, & Bolen, 1975; Rosenhan & White, 1967; Weiss, Buchanan, Altstatt, & Lombardo, 1971) and sex-role behaviors and attitudes in children (Etaugh, Collins, & Gerson, 1975; Fagot & Patterson, 1969; Grusec & Brinker, 1972; Lamb, Easterbrooks, & Holden, 1980). The development of dominant or independent behaviors in children has also been linked to reinforcement contingencies. Social scientists have effectively demonstrated the ability of reinforcement to modify the development and maintenance of these behaviors (Barton, Baltes, & Orzech, 1980; Blum & Kennedy, 1967; Hilton, 1967; Serbin, Connor, & Citron, 1978). In addition, many learning theorists have argued for an S–R explanation in the development of attitudes and interpersonal attraction. A learning theory interpretation of interpersonal attitude and attraction formation has been postulated by Doob (1947), Staats (1968), Lott and Lott (1960, 1968, 1972), Byrne and Clore (1979), and Clore and Byrne (1974).

The principle of extinction is interwoven throughout our behavior patterns and is primarily responsible for which social behaviors we perform and which we do not. Extinction occurs when the reinforcer for a previously reinforced behavior is no longer presented contingently upon the response. As a result, the behavior decreases in frequency or magnitude. Unknown to many parents, maladaptive or annoying social behaviors, such as whining and temper tantrums, may be effectively reduced or eliminated simply through extinction. A parent who ignores a whining or tantrumming child eliminates reinforcement and extinguishes such attention-seeking behavior from the child's repertoire. Similarly, a teacher might praise and reward prosocial behaviors in the classroom with a star chart but ignore disruptive or aggressive actions. In some cases, the principle of extinction may accidently eliminate desirable behaviors. Parents who consistently attend to a child's normal fears or insecurities yet ignore more positive and adaptive verbalizations may mistakenly reinforce clinging and "dependent" behavior. Consequently, dependent behavior exhibited by the child increases.

A classic example of how extinction influences our behavior is evidenced in the case of a 5-year-old boy named Kraig (Rekers & Lovaas, 1974). Kraig exhibited many female-typed behaviors, including playing with cosmetics and dolls, dressing as a female, and engaging in traditional feminine role behaviors. To eliminate these behaviors and create appropriate male social behaviors, a treatment plan mixing positive reinforcement with extinction was implemented. Kraig was positively reinforced for social behavior, which was deemed appropriate (playing with trucks or guns), and ignored when engaging in feminine role behaviors. When consistently employed, the program led to a dramatic decrease in feminine activities and an increase in masculine social behaviors. Using extinction principles, the manipulation of Kraig's reinforcement contingencies enabled a dramatic change in his social and sex-role development.

From the preceding discussion, it is clear that positive and negative reinforcement and extinction are responsible for the maintenance and strengthening of many desirable and undesirable social behaviors. Although primarily utilized to reduce undesirable behaviors, punishment may also contribute to social development. Like positive reinforcement, punishment is empirically defined by the effect that it has upon the target behavior. By definition, punished behavior is always reduced in the frequency of its occurrence. Punishment may involve the presentation of an aversive event or the removal of a positive reinforcer following the occurrence of the targeted behavior. In either case, punishment requires a contingent consequence to occur, which results in the decrease in frequency of the behavior it follows.

Punishment can be effectively utilized to promote appropriate socialization skills in children (Doland & Adelberg, 1967; Lamb *et al.*, 1980). Consider a small child who does not share his toys or playthings with peers. This is a common occurrence faced by parents and is often dealt with by removing the child from the play area for a period of time. Often referred to as "time-out" (Drabman & Spitalnik, 1973), this punishment procedure may function to decrease the child's selfish behavior. Consequently, in a future, similar situation, the child will likely refrain from engaging in "selfish" responding and will share his toys with his peers.

Just as an individual can learn what response to make, he or she can learn to distinguish when that particular response will be reinforced and when it will not. This process is referred to as *discrimination* or *differential reinforcement* and is accomplished by recognizing stimulus cues that signal reinforcement. Stimulus discrimination trains the individual to recognize subtle differences among stimuli and to categorize stimuli into discrete categories. For example, an operant is produced in the presence of Stimulus A and Stimulus B. Reinforcement occurs only in the presence of Stimulus A but not in response to Stimulus B. The individual quickly learns to discriminate between these two situations; consequently, the tendency to respond when Stimulus B is present is gradually extinguished. For this individual, Stimulus A and Stimulus B have become reliable predictors of reinforcement. As this process continues and one's discrimination among stimuli becomes more sophisticated, responses to dissimilar items will weaken.

Discriminative stimuli can be categorized on the basis of their reinforcer potential. A positive discriminative stimulus, often abbreviated as SD or S+, indicates that responding will be reinforced. Similarly, a negative discriminative stimulus (SΔ) indicates that no reinforcer is available and responding will not be reinforced (Zimbardo, 1988). Skinner postulated that our behavior is controlled by discriminative stimuli, as we quickly learn to distinguish between and respond accordingly to positive and negative outcomes. When responses are controlled by antecedent discriminative stimuli, the individual's behavior is said to be under stimulus control.

Examples of stimulus control or discrimination pervade every developmental period. As early as infancy, children use environmental cues to discriminate and recognize their parents from other similar adults (McGraw, 1987). Similarly, newborns can imitate the components of facial expressions of surprise, fear, and sadness (Field, Woodson, Cohen, Garcia, & Greenberg, 1983; Ludemann & Nelson, 1988; Meltzoff & Moore, 1977), suggesting that infants can discriminate among basic facial expressions. The discrimination of facial cues enables infants to expect certain behavioral consequences and assists in the developmental progression of normal, social interaction.

Stimulus control is also evident in the classroom, when the teacher serves as a discriminative stimulus for quiet, nondisruptive behavior. As soon as the teacher leaves the classroom, however, chaos generally ensues. Using the teacher as a cue, children have made the discrimination concerning the appropriate types of behaviors in different situations (teacher is present or teacher is absent). Likewise, when interacting with their peers, children quickly learn to discriminate between accepted and shunned behaviors of their peer group (Fagot & Patterson 1969; Lamb *et al.*, 1980). This is especially evident in the adolescent years, when group membership and acceptance by one's peers become central issues. Consequently, stimulus discrimination fosters socialization skills, providing the ability to distinguish and interpret social cues.

In addition to other conditioning procedures, children also demonstrate stimulus discrimination when developing their sex-role identities. Capitalizing upon cues from parents, teachers, and other significant adults, young children quickly learn to distinguish between discriminative stimuli concerning traditional gender roles (Fagot, 1977; Fagot & Patterson, 1969; Lamb *et al.*, 1980; Maccoby, 1988). Through discrimination training, children learn to adopt traditional sex-role behavior. For example, in play situations, females are often reinforced for playing with dolls, wearing feminine clothing, and being interested in domestic activities; males, on the other hand, are typically reinforced when displaying rough-and-tumble behavior, playing with trucks or guns, and pursuing athletics. Consequently, the process of stimulus discrimination additionally contributes to the development of sex-role behavior in children.

Frequently, behavior that has been reinforced in a particular situation occurs in new environments. Considered to be a by-product of discrimination training, stimulus generalization involves the extension of a previously reinforced behavior to a novel stimulus. When a reinforced behavior in a particular setting also increases in another, similar setting, generalization is said to have occurred. As a rule of thumb, responses to novel stimuli that closely resemble the original SD are most likely to generalize to that setting. The phenomenon of generalization is especially important in the study of human behavior, as it illustrates how similar behavior can be elicited by different stimuli and helps account for across situational consistency of behavior.

The generalization of behavior to similar stimuli accounts for the development of many social behaviors. Stranger anxiety, often witnessed in infants and toddlers, occurs when the child is approached by an unfamiliar individual. In part, stranger anxiety may represent generalizations from prior interactions with individuals similar to the stranger (Greenberg & Marvin, 1982; Perry & Bussey, 1984). Prior unpleasant experiences with a stranger are likely extended and generalized to encompass all strangers resulting in fear-related behavior (Bronson, 1978). These generalizations dissipate as the child's ability to discriminate among social cues is enhanced.

In addition to stranger anxiety among infants, young children often generalize attachment behaviors to strangers. Despite an improvement in discriminative abilities, toddlers and preschoolers typically view strangers as resembling and embodying the attributes and behaviors of parental figures. As a result of this generalization, young children may be easily deceived by unfriendly adults and serve as gullible targets for manipulation.

As noted, the process of conditioning is profoundly affected by the concepts of stimulus generalization and stimulus discrimination. In essence, conditioning may be thought of as a virtual tug-of-war between these two processes. Stimulus generalization tends to be overresponsive to stimuli with similar properties; the task of stimulus discrimination, however, is to be selective in the choice of stimuli to which one responds. These two forces must be balanced in order for effective conditioning to occur.

The poser of reinforcement to influence new response patterns is unarguable. In some cases, however, a desired response may be so complex that reinforcement of the final behavior is not sufficient for its acquisition. In this situation, new behaviors may be shaped. The process of shaping involves the reinforcement of small approximations toward the final response. Behaviors that either resemble the desired response or are a component of the final response are reinforced. As each approximation of the desired behavior is performed, the criterion for success is altered to more closely resemble the final behavior. Through this process, the desired response is gradually learned.

The principle of shaping takes root at birth and contributes to the development of many of our everyday social actions. For example, in conjunction with neurological development, children must learn to roll over, sit up, crawl, and stand before they are able to walk. Without the preliminary motor behaviors and the experience gained through interacting with the environment, walking is an impossible task. Similarly, shaping is influential in the development of language in children (Rheingold, Gewirtz, & Ross, 1959). Although there are many current theories concerning language acquisition (Chomsky, 1980; Curtiss, 1977; Skinner, 1957), children may learn many of the fundamentals of any language system through the process of shaping. Fluent language is not automatically produced; successive approximations of correct speech in the form of sounds, syllables, and their combinations are progressively produced by the child. Appropriate speech steps are reinforced by parents, and inappropriate deviations (screaming, shrieking) are ignored and extinguished. The resultant, "shaped" behavior is a phonetically correct language system.

In addition to shaping, the concept of chaining is also an integral force in the development of new behaviors. Skinner suggested that both processes involve the use of reinforcement and focus upon a series of steps leading to a desired, terminal behavior. The steps involved in shaping a behavior are generally not evident when the process is completed. In chaining, however, the steps required to learn a new behavior are considered separate, discrete behaviors. Additionally, in a chaining sequence, each step is considered to be a discriminative stimulus (SD) or a predictor of reinforcement for the preceding step. When considered as a whole, the first step in the chain becomes an SD for the final, desired behavior. Consequently, the entire chain becomes reinforcing for the individual.

The idea that responses may be linked in a chain sequence helps explain the emergence of many social behaviors. Along with other conditioning concepts, children learn to feed and dress themselves through a chainlike sequence of behaviors. Responses elicited at the beginning of these chains (finger manipulation of food or of buttons and shoelaces) are necessary steps in the acquisition of appropriate feeding and self-care skills. Additionally, the behaviors at each step of the chain are discrete and independent responses.

Operant behavior chains are also evident in the process of toilet training (Azrin & Foxx, 1974). Considered a minor milestone in the development of a toddler, toilet training is often used as a criterion for school admittance and is an important determinant of future social behavior (McGraw, 1987). As parents eventually learn, efficient toilet training requires a series of sequential responses. Behaviors in the chain include walking to the bathroom, closing the door, removing one's garment, sitting on the toilet, and so forth. Again, each behavior in the chain serves as a discriminative stimulus for the preceding response and, by itself, may be considered a discrete behavior.

In many situations, behavior is not immediately followed by reinforcement or punishment. The rate at which behavior is followed by a functional consequence may vary according to several patterns. These patterns or schedules of reinforcement determine the timing and spacing of behavioral consequences and significantly influence the effectiveness of the reinforcer. In their book, *Schedules of Reinforcement*, Ferster and Skinner (1957) discussed six basic patterns of reinforcement: continuous intermittent, fixed ratio, variable ratio, fixed interval, and variable interval.

The simplest schedule, known as continuous reinforcement, reinforces each emitted response. This schedule of reinforcement is usually implemented when an individual is being trained to produce a specific behavior. Parents utilize this type of reinforcement schedule when teaching their child new behaviors. Once the behavior has been learned, however, reinforcement is typically shifted to an intermittent schedule, during which only some behaviors are reinforced. Intermittent schedules are capable of maintaining conditioned behaviors provided the shift in reinforcement schedules is gradual and systematic.

In a ratio schedule, the frequency with which reinforcers are presented depends upon the rate at which responses are emitted. With interval schedules (often referred to as time-dependent schedules), the frequency of reinforcement depends upon the passage of time. These two types of schedules may be further differentiated by a constant, fixed pattern of reinforcement or an irregular, variable rate of reinforcement.

On a fixed ratio schedule, reinforcement is delivered after the completion of a set number of responses. After each reinforcement, a postreinforcement pause will be evidenced before the behavior resumes. Typically, the length of the pause is related to the size of the ratio. High reinforcement ratios generally yield rapid responding but involve a longer pause after each reinforcement; the converse is true for low reinforcement ratios. This type of continuous reinforcement schedule is the most efficient for the rapid acquisition of a new response.

Although fixed ratio schedules are readily seen in the scientific laboratory or in factories, its occurrence in our everyday environment is much less noticeable. A fixed ratio schedule is in place when schoolchildren are reinforced with recess after completing a set number of assignments. In contrast, a variable ratio schedule involves reinforcing the individual's behavior after a variable number of responses have been emitted. Initially, an individual may be reinforced after four responses but may be required to emit eight responses on the next reinforcement trial. This type of schedule makes discrimination of reinforcement difficult and consequently generates the highest level of responding. A pause in responding after reinforcement is not observed in variable ratio schedules. Additionally, because each new response is likely to yield reinforcement, variable ratio schedules are extremely resistant to extinction.

Variable ratio schedules of reinforcement are usually associated with gambling or fishing. In both activities, reinforcement occurs after a variable number of responses. This type of schedule may additionally be utilized by children to control parental behavior. Many children learn that they may receive reinforcement (cookies, toys) through consistent nagging and whining. On some occasions, reinforcement may occur after the first response; other times, reinforcement may require more episodes of nagging and whining. In any case, reinforcement is received from the parent after a variable number of whining responses are made.

On a fixed interval schedule, reinforcement is delivered after a fixed period of time has elapsed. Once this interval has elapsed, the first response will be reinforced. Individuals under this type of schedule have nothing to gain from rapid responding during the interval. Consequently, a pause in responding is seen after reinforcement with a gradual increase in the rate of responding before the next reinforcer. This effect is known as scalloping, due to its appearance when the rate of responding is graphed against cumulative time.

Fixed interval schedules of reinforcement are apparent in any situation in which a deadline is imposed. In the developing child, fixed interval schedules are most commonly imposed upon entering school. Exams, class projects, term papers, and report cards illustrate school requirements that are reinforced after a period of time has elapsed. As is characteristic of most children (and adults), assignments are often postponed until the imposing deadline approaches. It is only in anticipation of the deadline that one's behavior drastically changes and takes the shape of the fixed interval scallop. Reinforcement is delivered only after meeting the assignment deadline.

With a variable interval schedule, varying lengths of time must pass before reinforcement occurs. As with the variable ratio schedule of reinforcement, it is possible to obtain a reinforcer at a different time on each trial. Reinforcement only becomes available, however, if the individual makes the appropriate and timely response. Consequently, a continuous but low response rate is characteristic of this schedule. The extinction of behavior controlled by this schedule, however, is gradual and much slower than behavior controlled by fixed interval schedules.

Behavior that is controlled by variable interval schedules of reinforcement are often overlooked in the environment. Parents who are inconsistent or sporadic in reinforcing good behavior place children on variable interval schedules of reinforcement. Components of interpersonal relationships may involve the passage of variable amounts of time before reinforcement is delivered.

As noted, these four schedules differ in the patterns of responding that they produce. Ratio schedules typically produce higher rates of responding than do interval schedules. This phenomenon is not unexpected, as quick responses from the individual in a ratio schedule will yield more reinforcement than in an interval schedule. Similarly, higher response rates are evidenced on most kinds of intermittent schedules than on continuous schedules. Resistance to extinction is also greater after being exposed to an intermittent schedule of reinforcement than a continuous schedule as discrimination of reinforcement potential is more difficult.

Regarding the empirical human evidence for schedules of reinforcement, the behavior of human subjects (including children) exhibits enormous intra- and intersubject variability. Although human responding is comparable to animal behavior on some schedules, there is little correspondence on the fixed interval schedule (Davey, 1981). The major factor in explaining these differences in responding appears to be the linguistic abilities and verbal cues that come to control behavior through the development of expectations and motivation.

Last, in our brief review of operant conditioning principles, it is important to note that Skinner introduced a number of methodological advances that have radically changed the study of learning. Among these are the in-depth analysis of the behavior of individual subjects observed under various, manipulable, conditions, a reluctance to make reference to any unobservable factors in the explanation of behavioral development, and the assessment of behavior as a continuous process rather than an isolated event (Fantino & Logan, 1979).

The Skinnerian approach has had a tremendous impact on the study and control of behavior. His influence is especially notable in the child development research during the 1950s and 1960s by Bijou and Baer.

BIJOU AND BAER

Our historical review concerning major developments in the field of learning leads us to two learning theorists who explicitly addressed the issue and nature of child development. According to Sidney Bijou (1976), and consistent with his colleague Donald Baer, the major task of the child psychologist is "to relate the well-known facts of early development to probable observable conditions" (p. xi). Their behavioral analysis of child development (Bijou, 1976; Bijou & Baer, 1961, 1965) interprets behavior according to the empirical concepts and laws of Skinner's radical behaviorism. Hypothetical mental events, such as cognitive structures, superegos, and physiological correlates of the mind, are not considered appropriate for a scientific functional analysis of behavior. Similarly, stage theories are rejected if based upon hypothetical constructs. Their justification of this approach is to simplify the complex analysis of development.

The authors have explicitly addressed two early periods of development, descriptively referred to as the universal stage (prenatal to second year of life) and the basic stage (second to fifth year of life). The universal stage is characterized by the acquisition of body management, locomotion, manual dexterity, initial socialization, and verbal behavior; the basic stage includes exploratory, cognitive, intellectual, play, and moral development. Throughout their work, social development is continually addressed reflecting their belief that social variables are intertwined with every aspect of the child's behavior. Social interaction leads to the development of personality defined as the total organization of all the child's behavioral repertoires.

Bijou and Baer (1961) provide several guiding assumptions in their behavioral approach to development. First, they propose that psychological development consists of progressive changes in interactions between a biologically maturing child and the successive changes in the environment. Second, the child is conceptualized as a unique biological structure in continuous interaction with environmental stimuli and containing a wide variety of species-typical characteristics. This unique biological makeup is itself the product of genetic and individual history. Third, the environment is functionally understood as the stimuli that interact with the child. According to Bijou and Baer (1961), stimuli may originate in the child's external environment (physical and social stimuli), through his or her own behavior (self-generated stimuli), or from biological functioning (organismic stimuli). Fourth, stimuli are assessed according to their physical dimensions and their functional meanings for an individual child (reinforcement and discriminative functions and setting factors). Last, classes of behavior are influenced by the mechanisms of respondent and operant conditioning and their interactions (i.e., reinforcers are also potential respondent unconditioned stimuli: Davey, 1981).

To illustrate these assumptions, consider the development of social abilities. According to Bijou (1976), social abilities refer to a child's knowledge of appropriate responding to adults and peers. Children act on certain occasions (discriminative stimuli), and the form their actions take are a function of environmental contingencies provided by family members, peers, teachers, and so on. These daily interactions are additionally influenced through societal social practices, standards, and values. In relation to adults, important social abilities displayed by young children include socially acceptable requesting behavior (behaving in ways to obtain reinforcers through the behavior of others) and following instructions. In relation to peers, social abilities are a function of the child's history with family members, interactions with peers, and the practices of supervising adults. An important acquisition in peer relations is the transition from responding to the peer-as-an-object to the peer-as-a-person. Requiring considerable adult supervision, the child must be assisted in the learning of acceptable ways to manage the emotional behavior generated by chain breaking or the frustration inherent in sharing and taking turns.

There is little doubt that operant and respondent conditioning and their interactions are responsible for much of what we are, including basic aspects of personality. The contingencies of reinforcement and punishment mold our most intimate interactions, even those with ourselves. Lewis (1976) suggested that operant conditioning plays a significant role in the formation of "self-esteem," which includes private events such as self-observations and self-verbalizations.

Regardless of the contributions of Skinnerian approaches to learning and development, discontent with the dismissal, neglect, and avoidance of cognitive constructs led to a new era in learning theory (i.e., the "cognitive revolution"). Among the most notable cognitive-behavioral approaches is the work of Albert Bandura and his colleagues.

BANDURA AND WALTERS

The idea that we can learn different forms of behaviors through imitation is not a new concept. Both Plato and Aristotle noted the importance of observational learning in the acquisition of new behavior patterns. Nevertheless, learning theorists gave little notice to this concept until the publication of Miller and Dollard's (1941) classic text, *Social Learning and Imitation*. Despite their text and the general acceptance of imitation as a form of learning, systematic analysis of the concept was virtually neglected until the work of Albert Bandura. With publication of *Social Learning and Personality* (Bandura & Walters, 1963) and *Principles of Behavior Modification* (Bandura, 1969), Bandura established social learning theory as a viable means for acquiring and explaining human behavior.

Bandura's theory of observational learning has evolved in contemporary psychological thought as an additional means of acquiring new behaviors. Until this point, applied behavior analysis had concentrated solely upon observable, overt behavior and environmental contingencies. Bandura extended the idea of conditioning to include cognitive mediational processes. These cognitive processes are based upon prior experiences and determine which operants are attended to, how they are perceived by the observer, whether they will be remembered, and how they will affect future actions. Consequently, Bandura proposed a social learning theory based upon the reciprocal interaction among three factors: behavior, cognitive or personal factors, and environmental influences (Bandura, 1969).

Bandura (1969) asserted that much learning occurs in situations where learning would not be predicted by traditional conditioning theory. In such cases, the learner has not made an active response and has received no tangible or observable reinforcer. What learning does occur, however, is referred to as *modeling* or *imitation*. Through the process of modeling, Bandura claims that behavioral dispositions may be acquired simply from watching and cognitively processing the actions of another individual. Essentially, modeling is learning by observation and vicarious experience (hence, the term *observational or vicarious learning and conditioning*).

As a passive form of learning, modeling provides us with information so that we may rapidly acquire new behaviors. This process does not require that the individual perform the behavior; consequently, our behavior does not have to be shaped in a trial-and-error fashion. Simply put, modeling involves observing

> what the model does, note[ing] what the consequences to the model are, remember[ing] what he has learned, mak[ing] various inferences from it, and either then or later tak[ing] account of it in his own behavior. What is learned is not responses in the connectionist sense, but knowledge about responses and their consequences. (Hill, 1986, p. 154)

Though Bandura proposes that exposure to a model is sufficient to promote learning, the performance of modeled behavior is influenced by the mechanisms of reinforcement. When we observe a model whose behavior is rewarded, we are more likely to imitate that behavior. A model whose behavior is punished, however, decreases the probability that the observer will adopt that behavior (Walters & Parke, 1964). In essence, the consequences of the modeled behavior significantly influence whether or not the observer will choose to imitate the model. This manner of learning, often termed *vicarious reinforcement*, determines whether or not the modeled behavior will be performed.

As a learning mechanism, modeling is effective in both increasing and decreasing behaviors. Behaviors may be increased in frequency through the process of acquisition, disinhibition, or facilitation. Similarly, behaviors may be reduced in frequency through inhibitory effects or incompatible behavior effects. It is through these modeling processes, discussed later, that many social behaviors emerge.

New behaviors may be acquired as a result of viewing a model. The process of behavior acquisition is a primary source for many of our socialization skills. In conjunction with other conditioning mechanisms, modeling often provides a first look for children at socialization skills, such as speech (Lovaas & Newsom, 1976), interpersonal behaviors (Perry & Bussey, 1984; Walters & Parke, 1964), gender role behaviors (Bandura, 1969; Perry & Bussey, 1979), prosocial and altruistic behaviors (Bandura, 1977; Coates, Pusser, & Goodman, 1976; Elliott & Vasta, 1970; Grusec,

Kuczynski, Rushton, & Simutis, 1978; Midlarsky & Bryan, 1967; Presbie & Coiteux, 1971; Rosenhan & White, 1967; Rushton, 1975; White & Burnam, 1975; White, 1972), and aggression (Bandura, Ross, & Ross, 1963; Collins, Berndt, & Hess, 1974; Hicks, 1965).

Models have additionally been effective in promoting the development of morality and self-control (Bandura, 1977; Bandura & McDonald, 1963; Brody & Henderson, 1977; Cowan, Langer, Heavenrich, & Nathanson, 1969). Modeling allows children to observe relevant factors when considering the morality of an act. According to Bandura (1977), "the nature of the act, its motivating conditions, its consequences, characteristics of the actor, the situation in which the act occurs, the remorse of the transgressor, and the number and type of people victimized" are critical features in morality development and may be readily observed through the process of modeling (Perry & Bussey, 1984, p. 180).

Modeling may also increase the occurrence of a previously learned behavior through disinhibition. Disinhibition occurs when the rate of an observer's inhibited behavior increases after viewing a model display the behavior. This process is only effective, however, when the model is reinforced for the targeted behavior and suffers no adverse consequences. The role of disinhibition in the modeling process has been documented extensively and is often utilized in the treatment of behavioral disorders.

The disinhibitory effect in modeling has been effectively utilized to promote the development of numerous social behaviors in children. By viewing a model perform an unpunished behavior, social scientists have increased social interaction among withdrawn children (Evers & Schwartz, 1973; Keller & Carlson, 1974; O'Connor, 1969), have decreased phobic reactions to feared objects (Bandura, Blanchard, & Ritter, 1969; Rachman & Lopatka, 1988; Ritter, 1968), have encouraged the development of assertive behaviors (Hersen, Eisler, & Miller, 1974), and have taught interpersonal social skills (Goldsmith & McFall, 1975; Ladd, 1981; Twenty-man & McFall, 1975). Clearly, disinhibition in modeling is a valuable means of increasing social behaviors.

Facilitation effects in modeling may additionally increase or promote the occurrence of social behaviors in children. Facilitation occurs when an already learned behavior increases solely from observing another individual perform the behavior. In contrast to the acquisition and disinhibitory effects of modeling, a novel behavior is not performed. Watching another individual perform the behavior serves to encourage the observer to do the same. A common example of the facilitation effect may involve altruistic behaviors such as volunteering for or donating money to a charitable cause after viewing a model perform the behavior. This form of modeling has been employed most effectively in the development of cooperative behavior in children (Liebert & Poulos, 1975).

Observing a model perform a targeted behavior may also serve to decrease occurrences of the behavior by the individual. Often, the behavior of an individual becomes "inhibited" as the observer watches a model engage in a behavior that is not reinforced. More often, however, decreases in behavior result from viewing a model perform an action that is incompatible with a targeted behavior. Referred to as the *incompatible behavior effect*, this form of modeling is most commonly employed in the reduction of fear-related behaviors. Observations of the coping model tend to reduce fear behaviors and teach effective coping skills.

Modeling of incompatible behavior has been effectively employed by researchers in the reduction of many common childhood fears. In particular, fear behaviors in children concerning painful stimuli (Vernon, 1973, 1974), the dark (Klingman, 1988), snakes (Meichenbaum, 1971), dental procedures (Melamed, Weinstein, Hawes, & Katin-Borland, 1975; Melamed, Hawes, Heiby, & Glick, 1975), and surgery and anesthesia (Melamed & Sieel, 1975; Vernon & Bailey, 1974) have been successfully reduced through the use of incompatible behavior modeling.

As indicated, modeling processes may have a dramatic influence upon the acquisition or reduction of behavior patterns. There are several factors, however, that significantly contribute to the effectiveness of modeling. Characteristics pertaining to the model are particularly relevant as models identical in age, sex, and ethnicity to the subjects are most likely to be imitated (Kornhaber & Schroeder, 1975; Perry & Perry, 1975). In addition, a model who is perceived positively, is of high status, and is well liked by the observer will be most effective. In general, modeling is most effective when the observer perceives similarities between features and traits of the model and himself or herself.

The effectiveness of modeling is also dependent upon characteristics of the observer. Simple exposure to a model is not sufficient for the development or decrease of a behavior. The observer must be able to attend to, comprehend, and retain in memory the information presented. In addition, the observer must have the necessary motoric skills required in the production of the behavior. Without these necessary components, imitation of a model is unlikely.

Provided the prerequisites for modeling are present, the effects of modeling are most likely to take place under certain conditions. The observer is most likely to perform the behavior when environmental context cues are similar to those present in the original learning situation, when reinforcement for the performing the behavior is imminent, and when the observer is highly motivated to achieve a certain goal.

Despite the voluminous research data involving modeling processes, few of the early social learning theorists explicitly addressed the issue of developmental factors and their influence on social learning processes (Foster, Kendall, & Guevremont, 1988). Currently, recent investigations have addressed age-related differences in life situations and mastery tasks (Mize & Ladd, 1991), changes in selective attention and memory of environmental stimuli (Mize & Ladd, 1991), increases in symbolic activity, problem-solving skills, and planning (Bierman, 1983), the development of outcome and self-efficacy expectations, and the differential effects of rewards and punishers for various ages (Robinson, 1985). Further analysis of the interactions among developmental factors and learning will undoubtedly contribute to our understanding of social development.

LEARNING THEORY AND SOCIAL DEVELOPMENT: APPLICATIONS

Children's Contribution to Their Own Development

Although the behavioral perspective has often been criticized for its exclusive emphasis on environmental contingencies, recent theorists have investigated the role of biological constraints upon learning (Davey, 1981). Current behavioral thought includes the role of organismic factors in learning and asserts that behavior is both a function of phylogenetic natural selection and ontogenetic environmental selection (Skinner, 1989). Therefore, learning theories do not reject the notion that organisms are endowed with physical structures and processes shaped by evolutionary pressures. Some of the infant's behaviors are a product of genetic propensities (e.g., temperamental attributes), and some of their earliest social responses (e.g., sucking, crying, smiling, and looking) appear to function as unconditioned reflexes (or fixed action patterns, to borrow an ethological term).

Rather than concentrating on these innate characteristics or predispositions, behaviorists are concerned with how organisms acquire and maintain responses. More specifically, behaviorists are primarily interested in the manner in which organisms act upon and react to the environment while being constrained within a range of biologically limited possibilities (e.g., *preparedness*: Seligman, 1970). This position means that researchers must not take an environmental-extremist approach. For example, some researchers suggest that infants are biologically prepared to learn certain stimulus–response associations, such as sucking at the sight of a breast, crying when the caregiver exits, and calming at the sight and sound of the caregiver's return (Sameroff & Cavanaugh, 1979). As we are first and foremost social organisms, an appreciation of genotypical factors in learning and perception is essential to the study of social development.

Despite the disapproval of radical behaviorists, current behavioral thought incorporates the role of organismic variables in learning. In examining the child's contribution to his or her own development, behaviorists consider temperament to be an important organismic construct. Kagan (1989) described temperament as "those psychological qualities that display considerable variation among infants and, in addition, have a relatively, but not indefinitely, stable biological basis in the organism's genotype, even though the inherited physiological processes mediate different phenotypic displays as the child grows" (p. 668). Temperamental qualities, such as motor activity, smiling, adaptability to new situations, irritability, and inhibition have generated considerable theory and research (Kagan, 1989).

As a behavioral characteristic and stimulus complex, infant temperament can contribute to attachment, for example, through the mechanisms of learning. One well-known pattern of temperament-based responding are those behaviors described as *difficult* temperament. Difficult infants are often characterized as irritable, irregular, slow to adapt, and moody. Because of their patterns of responding, difficult infants may inhibit maternal sensitivity and affection (Crockenberg, 1981), which potentially may impede the attachment process (Waters, Vaughn, & Egeland, 1980).

The behaviors comprising difficult temperament can influence parental behavior through learning mechanisms. One can speculate that the difficult infant (for some caregivers in certain contexts) provides an abundance of aversive stimulation to the caregiver. Such stimulation may be in the form of negative affectivity, as well as the sporadic presentation of positive reinforcers (i.e., a net aversive effect). Consequently, the difficult infant likely elicits irritable reactions from the parents. Parents may come to avoid interacting with their infant or interact in an inconsistent and hesitant manner. Unpredictable or relatively few positively reinforcing exchanges with the infant could shape unresponsive parental behavior. As a result, the infant has influenced his or her own social development by indirectly shaping caregiver behaviors.

To illustrate how the infant may influence parental behaviors, consider a hypothetical situation involving two mother–infant pairs. One infant may produce intensely loud, lengthy cries. The mother may slowly respond to the infant's crying, finding it difficult to ignore the crying when it reaches a certain intensity level or duration. Conversely, a second infant may respond with short, low-intensity cries requiring more prompt and decisive responding from the mother. Through the behavior of crying, both infants have shaped caregiving responses and have significantly influenced the manner and style of interaction between parent and child.

Social interactions, however, are a two-way process. Caregivers may exacerbate their infants' "difficultness" through the inadvertent reinforcement and elicitation of temperamental attributes. For example, a caregiver may become anxious, changing her fussy infant's diapers, responding with uncertainty, and handling the baby in a rough manner. Such interaction elicits more infant and adult distress that may result in an extended period of attention and vocalizing. Consequently, this sequence of behaviors may reinforce the infant's utilization of fussy behaviors in similar situations.

Observations of playful interactions between mother and child demonstrate the mutually reinforcing and discriminative functions of both participants' behavior (Stern, 1974). For example, adults reinforce infant smiling and vocalizing by tickling or vocalizing (Millar, 1976). Conversely, the mother's behavior (e.g., speech, facial expressions) varies as a function of her infant's behavior (e.g., gaze). Other studies have found that newborns and infants contribute to caregiver interactions with vocalizations (Rosenthal, 1982), head turning (Peery, 1980), and facial expressions (DeBoer & Boxer, 1979).

As illustrated, the organismic factor of temperament may play a significant role in social development. Behaviorists acknowledge the role of organismic variables in learning and recognize the importance of the child's contribution to his or her social development. Essentially, organismic factors such as temperament set the stage for certain interactional or response patterns. These emitted responses, however, are not immutable. Although influenced by biological variables, exchanges between the child and the environment are reciprocal.

Infant Attachment

Attachment behaviors are proximity-seeking responses that serve the role of gaining or maintaining contact with an attachment figure. In most situations, this is usually the mother (McGraw, 1987). Attachment behaviors evidenced by human infants can include tracking the mother with the eyes, crawling to her, smiling at her, and crying when she is not present. Separation "protest" is characteristic of human infants somewhere in the period of 6 months to 3 years, peaking at 8 to 18 months (McGraw, 1987). The separation reaction is apparently universal, occurring in infants among all cultures studied. Most protest is mild, consisting of some crying and attempts to cling to the mother as she departs from the vicinity. Protests, however, may be more severe. The severity of protest appears to be a function of the "unusualness" of the separation (Spelke, Zelazo, Kagan, & Kotelchuck, 1973). Prolonged separations may result in expressions of "despair," whereby the active physical movements diminish, crying becomes monotonous or intermittent, and the infant appears withdrawn and inactive (Bowlby, 1951).

From the preceding observations regarding attachment behaviors, we can utilize learning theory to explain the emergence of these behaviors. Behaviorists might first define attachment behavior as a complex set of response dispositions characteristic of infants whose function is to maintain proximity to the caregiver. Next, learning theory might propose that the mother's (or primary caregiver's) most essential function is to provide positive reinforcers to the infant and remove negative ones (Bijou & Baer, 1965). Thus she feeds her infant several times a day, moderates skin temperature, caresses and strokes the child, rescues him or her from aversive situations, plays with the child, and moves him or her about in a stimulating world. Interacting with the infant in these and other ways sets the occasion for the mother to become a discriminative stimulus. Certain features of her behavior are perceived by the infant and come to predict certain outcomes. In this manner, the mother acquires reinforcing properties and provides a foundation for the infant's further social development.

The majority of reinforcing events presented by the mother occurs in a close physical relationship with the baby (Bijou & Baer, 1965). Of course, the mother cannot feed, warm, or protect the infant easily from a distance. Consequently, the proximity of the mother becomes an important social discriminative stimulus. Infant behaviors that produce closeness to the mother will generally be strengthened. Therefore, behaviors such as crying, cooing, babbling, and smiling will promote proximity to the mother and be reinforced. When the toddler becomes mobile, proximity seeking of "tagging along" can be understood as a set of discriminated operants maintained by the proximity function acting as a positive reinforcer.

The mother also provides discriminative cues signaling reinforcement through her attentive and affectionate behaviors toward the child. The physical components of attention include looking, orienting the body, vocal stimuli, facial changes, and cessation of other activity (Bijou & Baer, 1965). These responses are emitted by the caregiver and serve as cues for the infant. These cues become discriminative stimuli as the mother attends to the child during various reinforcement occasions.

The variability in style of attending to the child evidenced by different mothers may correlate with the various kinds of attention that prove reinforcing to their children in later life (Bijou & Baer, 1965). For example, some children may be more reinforced by highly talkative persons and others by more quiet interactions. This process may help account for individual differences in response to attention observed among children.

A mother's affectionate behavior may consist of smiles, kisses, hugs, vocal and verbal stimuli, tickling, and others (Bijou & Baer, 1965). A major component of affectionate behavior is "contact comfort" (Harlow & Zimmerman, 1959). Compared to attention and proximity, affectionate behavior may display more variation among mothers. The child's reinforcement history will influence whether subtle or dramatic displays of affection are most rewarding. Regarding undesirable behaviors emitted by the child, attending and approaching the child may be difficult to control, and inadvertent reinforcement may occur. However, the ease of providing affection for good behavior and the tendency not to present it when confronted with bad behavior result in an effective set of stimuli for strengthening desirable infant responses. Children who are responsive to affection as a positive reinforcer may be more readily influenced by the mother's goals and prompts, and therefore, more amenable to socialization practices.

In sum, a conditioning account of attachment behavior rests on three basic assumptions. First, the caregiver must acquire conditioned or secondary reinforcer value following the provision of primary reinforcers (e.g., tactual stimulation, distress reduction, vocal and auditory stimulation). Second, the caregiver acquires discriminative stimulus properties for the infant. Finally, the infant's individual pattern of attachment behaviors will be shaped by the schedule of reinforcers and punishers applied and removed by the caregiver in their mutually regulated interactions.

Regarding attachment security, Ainsworth and her colleagues (1978) identified three basic patterns: (1) secure (Group B)—babies exhibit both contact seeking and positive interaction (i.e., smiling, eye contact, vocalizing) upon reunion with the mother and protest further separation; (2) avoidant (Group A)—the infant avoids the mother upon reunion, moves past her, averts her gaze, and generally does engage in contact-promoting behavior; and (3) ambivalent (Group C)—the infant vacillates between acts of seeking contact and then resisting it, often angrily. Secure and insecure infants also differ in their responses to "strangers." Secure infants behave "warily" around strangers, whereas avoidant infants do not exhibit distress and if so are as easily comforted by the stranger as by their own mother. Finally, ambivalently attached infants display "resistance" to the stranger.

From a behavioral perspective, one would expect that contingencies of reinforcement have shaped infant behaviors characterizing different types of attachments. It might be predicted that secure infants have discriminated the mother clearly as a generalized positive reinforcer. Consequently, proximity-seeking and separation-protest behaviors are evidenced. The mother has successfully acquired her proximity, attention, and affection functions through her interactions with her infant. Conversely, insecurely attached infants manifest behavior that is consistent with less successful discrimination of the mother's caregiving functions. The avoidant infants emit less approach behavior upon reunion. This might be due to a history of positive reinforcement for doing so, or more likely, the infant may be responding to the mother or situation as a negative reinforcer (aversive stimulus), and thus, avoid her. The ambivalent infants appear to respond to the mother and the reunion situation as if the interaction was loaded equally with positive and negative reinforcers. Consequently, interactions result in contradictory approach avoidance behavior.

Some evidence supporting environmental correlates of secure attachment does exist. During early infancy, Ainsworth and her colleagues (1978) discovered that mothers of securely attached infants held their infants more carefully and tenderly and for longer periods of time than did mothers of insecurely attached babies. With infants classified as securely attached, mothers appear to respond more reliably and quickly to their infants' distress signals (Bell & Ainsworth, 1972) and engage in more smiling and verbalizations (Clarke-Stewart, 1973). Conversely, mothers of 3-month-old avoidant infants appear to display an aversion to physical contact. Mothers of these infants often withdraw from their approaching infants, appear impatient while holding their babies, and hold their infant in an unusual manner. In a similar vein, investigations of abused and neglected children demonstrated a higher probability of insecure attachment (e.g., Schneider-Rosen & Cicchetti, 1984). Insecurely attached infants are less cooperative with their mothers as well as with other adults (Londerville & Main, 1981), suggesting stimulus generalization. Inconsistency of parental responding to children's cues for attention is associated with exaggerated, intense proximity seeking in children of various ages (Maccoby, 1980).

In sum, it is likely that mothers of secure babies provide less aversive stimulation and more contingent and consistent reinforcement (including distress relief) of their infants' behavior. The mother establishes high reinforcement value, elicits positive affect in the infant, and thereby, successfully shapes the child's behavior.

Child Aggression and Antisocial Behavior

Learning theory regards aggression as an environmentally shaped behavior. An operant conditioning conception of aggression views external factors as crucial in strengthening the probability of aggressive behavior in certain situations. Consequently, contingencies of reinforcement and punishment represent basic mechanisms for aggressive responding.

Initial aggressive behavior may occur by chance or be elicited by aversive stimulation (Perry & Bussey, 1984). Numerous studies have demonstrated that frustration and other noxious stimulation (e.g., verbal assault, deprivation of reinforcers, physical attack) do increase the probability of aggression in both children and adults (Barker, Dembo, & Lewin, 1941; Mallick & McCandless, 1966; Rocha & Rogers, 1976). If the aggressive response is successful in reducing or alleviating the aversive condition, the response may be strengthened, and its probability of future occurrences is heightened. To illustrate this point, imagine that a child's toy is taken by a peer. The child responds by yelling, pushing, and hitting the peer, which results in reobtaining the toy. In this situation, the aggressive behavior is likely strengthened.

As with any other behavior, discrimination and generalization principles apply in controlling aggressive behavior. Classical conditioning is relevant insofar as conditioned stimuli elicit emotional responding that interact with the operant learning of aggressive behavior. For example, a gun may function as both a discriminative stimulus and a conditioned stimulus by setting the occasion for a potentially reinforced aggressive response and by eliciting emotional arousal labeled as *anger* (Berkowitz, 1974).

Gerald Patterson and his colleagues (Patterson, 1976; Patterson & Cobb, 1971; Patterson & Reid, 1970) have utilized direct observations of aggressive and delinquent boys in their home environments to assist in the derivation of a comprehensive social interactional theory of child and adolescent aggression. Patterson begins by hypothesizing that many aggressive behaviors function as coping behaviors in the child's attempt to reduce aversive stimulation presented by siblings and parents. These aversive events include commands and instructions, expressions of disapproval and contempt, teasing and laughing, and the absence of desired attention in an environment with minimal positive interactions. Aggression serves as behavior directed at reducing or removing the aversive stimuli produced by the family environment.

As expected, observations demonstrate that highly aggressive children are likely to live in homes where aversive stimuli represent a large percentage of the social stimuli present. Family members are reluctant to initiate conversation, tend to ignore each other, and often disapprove and criticize. These high-frequency, aversive events may provoke angry and aggressive responding that is negatively reinforced. In addition, the aggressive child is positively reinforced on occasion by family members for acting in an aggressive manner. Therefore, Patterson posits that aggressive actions are elicited by aversive stimuli presented by a family member and reinforced by the family member's removal of the aversive stimulus.

A complicating aspect of the family's interactions is the rapid escalation of the child's aggressive behavior when the initial responses are not successful in alleviating the aversive stimulation. Patterson refers to the child's behavior as coercive, because the effect of these aggressive interactions is an aggressive manipulation of the behavior of others to meet the child's goals. Family members find themselves confronted by a whining or threatening child; they have fallen into a "negative reinforcement trap," and by discontinuing their commands or insults, have reinforced their child's aggressive behavior. Parents of aggressive children often react to their misbehavior inconsistently, sometimes giving in and at times resisting (Katz, 1971). As a result, the child learns to be aggressive on a partial reinforcement schedule (making this behavior very persistent). Also, parental threats of punishment acquire cue properties for escalating their aggression. Paradoxically, threats of punishment or control may increase rather than suppress aggression (Peterson, 1971). Aggressive interchanges may also be the most effective means for the child to obtain attention or simply escape a boring or noxious environment (Perry & Bussey, 1984).

Patterson suggests that aggression in settings other than the home is largely maintained by positive reinforcement (Patterson, Littman, & Bricker, 1967). Victims who provide the child aggressor with positive consequences are likely to be aggressed upon again in a similar manner. When the victim presents a negative consequence, the aggressor often alters the form of attack, the victim, or both. Nonaggressive children learn aggressive habits as a result of the positive consequences they sometimes experience by interacting with aggressive children. More specifically, (1) nonaggressive children who have been frequently victimized by aggressive children, and (2) who defend themselves by counterattacking, and (3) were reinforced by these defensive aggressions, are likely to initiate aggressive acts in the future (Patterson, DeBaryshe, & Ramsey, 1989).

Supportive evidence for peer-related learning of aggression comes from various sources. For example, members of delinquent gangs often reinforce each other for aggressive behaviors and may even make membership contingent upon violent acts (Bandura, 1973). Parents of aggressive children have been reported to reinforce their children for peer-directed aggression (Bandura & Walters, 1959), while harshly punishing parent-directed aggression, setting the occasion for discriminated aggression. In addition, response generalization has been demonstrated in laboratory studies of childhood aggression (Lovaas, 1961).

Recently, Patterson and colleagues have elaborated a more complex developmental model of antisocial behavior, with learning mechanisms proposed as mediating the process (Patterson, DeBaryshe, & Ramsey, 1989). Patterson begins with the consistently reported observation that families of antisocial children are characterized by harsh and inconsistent discipline, little positive parental involvement, and poor adult monitoring and supervision. As described, Patterson provides empirical support that parents train aggressive and antisocial behaviors. The parents typically are noncontingent in their utilization of positive reinforcers for prosocial behavior and punishment for misconduct. The escalating, coercive family process develops and is largely controlled by escape-conditioning contingencies.

Patterson further develops his model by hypothesizing (with empirical support) that coercive child behaviors produce two sets of reactions from the social environment: rejection by normal peers and academic failure. Furthermore, lax parental supervision, antisocial behavior, and peer group rejection often lead to deviant peer group membership. This peer group provides much reinforcement for deviant behavior and punishment of socially conforming acts. Patterson also emphasizes that a number of variables, referred to as "disruptors," contribute to child aggression by their negative effects on parenting skills (e.g., family history of antisocial behavior, disadvantaged socioeconomic status, and stressors). In sum, dysfunctional family processes directly and indirectly influence antisocial behavior through training and later involvement in a deviant peer group.

Other factors influential in the development of aggression are addressed by the Bandurian social learning perspective, stressing the importance of observational learning and cognition (Bandura, 1973). Bandura accepts the importance of direct contingencies of reinforcement but emphasizes the power of observation in shaping aggressive behavior. He asserts that aggressive models teach children potential responses, especially if reinforced in the process, and observing their behavior may disinhibit previously learned aggressive behaviors in the observers. More important, children are not likely to behave aggressively unless expectancies of reinforcement or nonpunishment are present. A distinguishing feature of the social learning approach is the proposition that aggression also comes under the control of internal self-evaluative processes (Perry & Bussey, 1984). Children learn rules and standards concerning the appropriateness of certain behaviors that guide future behavior. Direct instruction and modeling contribute to the formation of the rule that contribute to self-regulation.

Classic research by Bandura and his colleagues (Bandura *et al.*, 1963) provided support for the modeling of aggression hypothesis. Children who observed an adult model attacking a Bobo doll subsequently responded more aggressively to the Bobo doll themselves. Similarly, children observing an aggressive cartoon were more likely to later destroy a toy (Mussen & Rutherford, 1961). Bandura (1979) proposed that aggressive models have several effects. First, aggressive models teach children both new responses and the consequences of aggressive behavior via observational learning. Second, disinhibition of aggression results when a child observes another performing aggressively and not encountering aversive consequences, thereby increasing the likelihood of the observers on aggression. Third, stimulus-enhancing functions occur when aggressive models teach observers how to use objects (e.g., sticks, knives, guns) in harmful ways. And last, observing aggressive models may serve an emotional arousal function, increasing the tendency to respond impulsively. It is now widely accepted that aggressive behavior is, at least in part, shaped by the mechanisms of observational learning.

Summary

The purpose of this final section is to address the characteristics, potential contributions, and compatibility of a behavioral model in the understanding of the developmental process. Development is defined empirically as "progressive changes in the way an organism's behavior interacts with the environment" (Bijou & Baer, 1961, p. 1). The major operational mechanism in development is assumed to be learning. As a developmental mechanism, learning involves short-term changes in behaviors. These short-term changes are combined and are "hierarchically organized" (Staats, 1971), resulting in what is generally referred to as psychological development.

Social development is, therefore, the result of accumulated social (and non-social) interactions linked together over time. It is assumed that such apparent linking and evolving of behaviors is accomplished by the "organism action–environmental reaction" chains that shape and mold the child's behavior. The child progresses from the acquisition of basic repertoires of social skill to the learning of more advanced competencies based upon earlier learning (Staats, 1971). This more or less observable process represents social development. In this sense, development reflects "the cumulative effects of learning" (Gagne, 1968). However, modern social learning theory takes a more complex conceptual approach. Consequently, with cognitive-mediational processes, it is capable of addressing in more detail the organizational aspect of these cumulative experiences which define development.

Consistent with this view, behaviorists generally deemphasize biological age or stages of development. Age is used as a convenient means of noting change along some continuum but is considered a poor explanation of developmental change. The crucial factor in development is the sequencing of events in the environment and their subsequent effects. Nevertheless, though behaviorists do not adhere strictly to a stage theory, they do not dismiss the potential influence of evolutionary history predisposing the organism to behavioral patterns and sequences. Therefore, it is not totally inconsistent that many contemporary behaviorists endorse a basic interactionist position, viewing the organism as both active and reactive, and possessing mediational or cognitive properties.

Compared with other theoretical perspectives or models of human behavior and development, learning theories can be distinguished by their assumptions, level of analysis, concepts, measures, methods, and proposed mechanisms. First, learning theories give greatest weight to environmental influences and conditions, both present and past. Second, typical investigations are conducted at the micro-social (molecular or face-to-face) level, directly observing interactions between the person and the effective environment. Third, learning concepts include those associated with the established principles of learning (e.g., UCS, discrimination) as well as the more contemporary cognitive or mediational constructs tied to overt behavior (e.g., self-efficacy and outcome expectancies). Fourth, behavioral measures are directly observable with the necessity of minimal inference (though more inference is allowed in the social learning approach). Measures include response rate, probability, magnitude, duration, latency, and intensity. Fifth, the preferred research methods are the experimental or single-subject designs. Lastly, the crucial mechanisms of behavioral development are proposed to be the basic learning processes and operations: habituation, sensitization, respondent and operant conditioning, observational learning, and for the social learning theorists, a concern with information processing. Of course, these learning mechanisms could have developmental parameters such as neurological maturation, but data are lacking.

Modern learning conceptions and approaches have tempered the extreme environmentalism characterized by Watson's behaviorism. Increasing recognition is directed to organismic factors by some theorists (e.g., Patterson, *et al.*, 1989, with temperament and self-esteem) and their interactions over time with the social environment. Similarly, in an attempt to address behavior in its natural context, some contemporary learning theorists (e.g., Patterson, *et al.*, 1989) are increasingly utilizing multiple designs (single-subject, prospective, cross-sectional) and multiple indicators (molar and molecular) and are searching for linkages between molecular and molar levels of observation.

These contemporary developments bode well for the field of social development research and practice. As learning theory expands and grows, so does our knowledge base and skills at prevention and intervention. The traditional polarity of learned versus innate aspects of behavior is allowed its place in the early history of psychology. Interdisciplinary research and methodologies are necessary precursors for a mature learning theory and developmental psychology. Similarly, longstanding intellectual conflicts, such as that between the nomothetic and idiographic approaches to investigation, are potentially resolvable when viewed in an integrative context. As Kimble (1989) noted:

> Every individual is a unique expression of the joint influence of a host of variables. Such uniqueness results from the specific [idiographic] effects on individuals of general [nomothetic] laws. . . . People are the same in that they represent the outcome of the same laws operating on the same variables. They differ in degree not kind. People are unique in that the details of those operations differ from person to person. (p. 495)

REFERENCES

Ainsworth, M. D. S., Blehar, M. C., Waters, E., & Wall, S. (1978). *Patterns of attachment: A psychological study of the strange situation*. Hillsdale, NJ: Erlbaum.

Aronfreed, J. (1968). *Conduct and conscience: The socialization of internalized control over behavior*. New York: Academic Press.

Azrin, N. H., & Foxx, R. M. (1974). *Toilet training in less than a day*. New York: Simon & Schuster.

Bachrach, A. J. (1985). Learning theory. In H. I. Kaplan & B. J. Sadock (Eds.), *Comprehensive textbook of psychiatry* (4th ed.). Baltimore: Williams & Wilkins.

Bandura, A. (1969). Social learning theory of identificatory processes. In D. A. Goslin (Ed.), *Handbook of socialization theory and research*. Chicago: Rand McNally.

Bandura, A. (1973). *Aggression: A social learning analysis*. Englewood Cliffs, NJ: Prentice-Hall.

Bandura, A. (1977). *Social learning theory*. Englewood Cliffs, NJ: Prentice-Hall.

Bandura, A. (1979). Psychological mechanisms of aggression. In M. von Cranach, K. Foppa, W. Lepenies, & D. Ploog (Eds.), *Human ethology: Claims and limits of a new discipline*. Cambridge: Cambridge University Press.

Bandura, A., Blanchard, E. B., & Ritter, B. (1969). The relative efficacy of desensitization and modeling approaches for inducing behavioral, affective, and cognitive changes. *Journal of Personality and Social Psychology, 13*, 173–199.

Bandura, A., & McDonald, F. J. (1963). The influence of social reinforcement and the behavior of models in shaping children's moral judgments. *Journal of Abnormal and Social Psychology, 67*, 274–281.

Bandura, A., Ross, D., & Ross, S. A. (1963). Imitation of film mediated aggressive models. *Journal of Abnormal and Social Psychology, 66*, 3–11.

Bandura, A., & Walters, R. H. (1959). *Adolescent aggression*. New York: Ronald Press.

Bandura, A., & Walters, R. H. (1963). *Social learning and personality development*. New York: Holt, Rinehart & Winston.

Barker, R. G., Dembo, T., & Lewin, K. (1941). Frustration and regression: An experiment with young children. *University of Iowa Studies in Child Welfare, 18*, 1–314.

Barton, E. M., Baltes, M. M., & Orzech, M. J. (1980). Etiology of dependence in older nursing home residents during morning care; the role of staff behavior. *Journal of Personality and Social Psychology, 38*, 423–431.

Bell, S. M., & Ainsworth, M. D. S. (1972). Infant crying and maternal responsiveness. *Child Development*, *43*, 1171–1190.

Berkowitz, L. (1974). Some determinants of impulsive aggression: Role of mediated associations with reinforcement for aggression. *Psychological Review*, *81*, 165–176.

Bierman, K. L. (1983). Cognitive development and clinical interviews with children. In B. B. Lahey & A. E. Kazdin (Ed.), *Advances in clinical child psychology* (Vol. 6). New York: Plenum Press.

Bijou, S. W. (1976). *Child development: The basic stage of early childhood*. Englewood Cliffs, NJ: Prentice-Hall.

Bijou, S. W., & Baer, D. M. (1961). *Child development: A systematic and empirical theory* (Vol. 1). Englewood Cliffs, NJ: Prentice-Hall.

Bijou, S. W., & Baer, D. M. (1965). *Child development: Universal stage of infancy* (Vol. 2). New York: Appleton-Century-Crofts.

Blum, E. R., & Kennedy, W. A. (1967). Modifications of dominant behavior in school children. *Journal of Personality and Social Psychology*, *7*, 275–281.

Bowlby, J. (1951). *Maternal care and mental health*. Geneva: World Health Organization.

Brody, G. H., & Henderson, R. W. (1977). Effects of multiple modal variations and rational provision on the moral judgments and explanation of young children. *Child Development*, *48*, 1117–1120.

Bronson, G. (1978). Aversive reactions to strangers: A dual process interpretation. *Child Development*, *49*, 495–499.

Byrne, D., & Clore, G. L. (1970). A reinforcement model of evaluative responses. *Personality International Journal*, *1*, 103–128.

Chomsky, N. A. (1980). *Rules and representations*. New York: Columbia University Press.

Cialdini, R. B., & Kenrick, D. T. (1976). Altruism as hedonism: A social developmental perspective on the relationship of negative mood state and helping. *Journal of Personality and Social Psychology*, *34*, 907–914.

Clarke-Stewart, K. A. (1973). Interactions between mothers and their young children. *Monographs of the Society of Research in Child Development*, *38* (Whole No. 153).

Clore, G. L., & Byrne, D. (1974). A reinforcement affect model of attraction. In T. L. Huston (Ed.), *Foundations of interpersonal attraction*. New York: Academic Press.

Coates, B., Pusser, H. E., & Goodman, I. (1976). The influence of "Sesame Street" and "Mister Rogers' neighborhood" on children's social behavior in the preschool. *Child Development*, *47*, 138–144.

Collins, W. A., Berndt, T. J., & Hess, V. L. (1974). Observational learning of motives and consequences for television aggression: A developmental study. *Child Development*, *45*, 799–802.

Cook, H., & Stingle, S. (1974). Cooperative behavior in children. *Psychological Bulletin*, *81*, 918–933.

Cowan, P. A., Langer, J., Heavenrich, J., & Nathanson, M. (1969). Social learning and Piaget's cognitive theory of moral development. *Journal of Personality and Social Psychology*, *11*, 261–274.

Crockenberg, S. B. (1981). Infant irritability, mother responsiveness, and social support influences on the security of infant-mother attachment. *Child Development*, *52*, 857–865.

Curtiss, S. (1977). *Genie: A psycholinguistic study of a modern day "wild" child*. New York: Academic Press.

Darlington, R. B., & Macker, C. E. (1966). Displacement of guilt produced altruistic behavior. *Journal of Personality and Social Psychology*, *4*, 442–443.

Davey, G. (1981). *Animal learning and conditioning*. Baltimore: University Park Press.

Davey, G. C. (1989). Dental phobias and anxieties: Evidence for conditioning processes in the acquisition and modulation of a learned fear. *Behaviour Research and Therapy*, *27*, 51–58.

DeBoer, M. M., & Boxer, A. M. (1979). Signal functions of infant facial expression and gaze direction during mother-infant face-to-face play. *Child Development*, *50*, 1215–1218.

di Nardo, P. A., Guzy, L. T., Jenkins, J. A., & Bak, R. M. (1988). Etiology and maintenance of dog fears. *Behaviour Research and Therapy*, *26*, 241–244.

Doland, D. J., & Adelberg, K. (1967). The learning of sharing behavior. *Child Development*, *38*, 695–700.

Doob, L. W. (1947). The behavior of attitudes. *Psychological Review*, *54*, 135–156.

Drabman, R., & Spitalnik, R. (1973). Social isolation as a punishment procedure: A controlled study. *Journal of Experimental Child Psychology*, *16*, 236–249.

Elliott, R., & Vasta, R. (1970). The modeling of sharing: Effects associated with vicarious reinforcement, symbolization, age, and generalization. *Journal of Experimental Child Psychology*, *10*, 8–15.

Etaugh, C., Collins, G., & Gerson, A. (1975). Reinforcement of sex-typed behaviors of two year old children in a nursery school setting. *Developmental Psychology*, *11*, 255.

Evers, W. L., & Schwartz, J. C. (1973). Modifying social withdraw in preschoolers: The effects of filmed modeling and teacher praise. *Journal of Abnormal Child Psychology*, *1*, 248–256.

Fagot, B. I. (1977). Consequences of moderate cross gender behavior in preschool children. *Child Development, 48,* 902–907.

Fagot, B. I., & Patterson, G. R. (1969). An in vivo analysis of reinforcing contingencies for sex role behaviors in the preschool child. *Developmental Psychology, 1,* 563–568.

Fantino, E., & Logan, C. A. (1979). *The experimental analysis of behavior: A biological perspective.* San Francisco: W. H. Freeman.

Ferster, C., & Skinner, B. F. (1957). *Schedules of reinforcement.* New York: Appleton-Century-Crofts.

Field, T., Woodson, R., Cohen, D., Garcia, & Greenberg, R. (1983). Discrimination and imitation of facial expressions by term and pre-term neonates. *Infant Behavior and Development, 6,* 485–490.

Fitzgerald, H. E., & Brackbill, Y. (1976). Classical conditioning in infancy: Development and constraints. *Psychological Bulletin, 83,* 353–376.

Foster, S. L., Kendall, P. C., & Guevremont, D. C. (1988). Cognitive and social learning theories. In J. L. Matson (Ed.), *Handbook of treatment approaches in childhood psychopathology.* New York: Plenum Press.

Gagne, R. (1968). Contributions of learning to human development. *Psychological Review, 75,* 177–191.

Gewirtz, J. L., & Petrovich, S. B. (1983). Early social and attachment learning in the frame of organic and cultural evolution. In T. M. Field, A. Huston, H. C. Quay, L. Troll, & G. E. Finley (Eds.), *Review of human development.* New York: Wiley.

Glavin, J. P., & Moyer, L. S. (1975). Facilitating extinction of infant crying by changing reinforcement schedules. *Journal of Behavior Therapy and Experimental Psychiatry, 6,* 357–358.

Goldsmith, J. B., & McFall, R. M. (1975). Development and evaluation of an interpersonal skill training program for psychiatric inpatients. *Journal of Abnormal Psychology, 84,* 51–58.

Greenberg, M. T., & Marvin, R. S. (1982). Reactions of preschool children to an adult stranger: A behavioral systems approach. *Child Development, 53,* 481–490.

Grusec, J. E., & Brinkler, D. B. (1972). Reinforcement for imitation as a social learning determinant with implications for sex-role development. *Journal of Personality and Social Psychology, 21,* 149–158.

Grusec, J. E., Kuczynski, L., Rushton, J. P., & Simutis, Z. (1978). Modeling, direct instruction, and attributions: Effects on altruism. *Developmental Psychology, 14,* 51–57.

Grusec, J. E., & Redler, E. (1980). Attribution, reinforcement and altruism: A developmental analysis. *Developmental Psychology, 16,* 525–534.

Hall, R. V., Axelrod, S., Tyler, L., Grief, E., Jones, F. C., & Robertson, R. (1972). Modification of behavior in the home with a parent as observer and experimenter. *Journal of Applied Behavior Analysis, 5,* 53–64.

Harlow, H. F., & Zimmerman, R. R. (1959) Affectional responses in the infant monkey. *Science, 130,* 421–432.

Hersen, M., Eisler, R. M., & Miller, P. M. (1974). An experimental analysis of generalization in assertive training. *Behaviour Research and Therapy, 12,* 295–310.

Hicks, D. J. (1965). Imitation and retention of film mediated aggressive peer and adult models. *Journal of Personality and Social Psychology, 2,* 97–100.

Hill, W. F. (1985). *Learning: A survey of psychological interpretations.* Cambridge: Harper & Row Publishers.

Hilton, I. (1967). Differences in the behavior of mothers toward first- and later-born children. *Journal of Personality and Social Psychology, 7,* 282–290.

Hygge, S., & Ohman, A. (1978). Modeling processes in the acquisition of fears: Vicarious electrodermal conditioning to fear relevant stimuli. *Journal of Personality and Social Psychology, 36,* 271–279.

Jones, M. C. (1924). The elimination of children's fears. *Journal of Experimental Psychology, 1,* 383–390.

Kagan, J. (1989). Temperamental contributions to social behavior. *American Psychologist, 44,* 668–674.

Kanfer, F. H. (1979). Personal control, social control, and altruism: Can society survive the age of individualism. *American Psychologist, 34,* 231–239.

Katz, R. C. (1971). Interactions between the facilitative and inhibitory effects of a punishing stimulus in the control of children's hitting behavior. *Child Development, 42,* 1433–1446.

Keller, M. F., & Carlson, P. M. (1974). The use of symbolic modeling to promote social skills in preschool children with low levels of social responsiveness. *Child Development, 45,* 912–919.

Kimble, G. A. (1989). Psychology from the stand-point of a generalist. *American Psychologist, 44,* 491–499.

Klingman, A. (1988). Biblioguidance with kindergartners: Evaluation of a primary prevention program to reduce fear of the dark. *Journal of Clinical Child Psychology, 17,* 237–241.

Kornhaber, R. C., & Schroeder, H. E. (1975). Importance of model similarity on extinction of avoidance behavior in children. *Journal of Consulting and Clinical Psychology, 43,* 601–607.

Ladd, G. W. (1981). Effectiveness of a social learning method for enhancing children's social interaction and peer acceptance. *Child Development, 52,* 171–178.

Lamb, M. E., Easterbrooks, M. A., & Holden, G. W. (1980). Reinforcement and punishment among preschoolers: Characteristics, effects, and correlates. *Child Development, 51,* 1230–1236.

Lee, C. L. & Bates, J. E. (1985). Mother-child interaction at two-years and perceived difficult temperament. *Child Development, 56,* 1314–1325.

Lewis, M. (1976, November). *The origins of social competence.* Paper presented at the NIMH conference on mood development, Washington, DC.

Liebert, R. M., & Poulos, R. W. (1975). Television and personality development: The socializing effect of an entertainment medium. In A. Davids (Ed.), *Child personality and psychopathology: Current topics* (Vol. 2). New York: Wiley.

Londerville, S., & Main, M. (1981). Security of attachment, compliance, and maternal training methods in the second year of life. *Developmental Psychology, 17,* 289–299.

Lott, A. J., & Lott, B. E. (1968). A learning theory approach to interpersonal attitudes. In A. G. Greenwald, T. C. Brock, & T. M. Ostrom (Eds.), *Psychological foundations of attitudes.* New York: Academic Press.

Lott, A. J., & Lott, B. E. (1972). The power of liking: Consequences of interpersonal attitudes derived from a liberalized view of secondary reinforcement. In L. Berkowitz (Ed.), *Advances in experimental social psychology* (Vol. 6). New York: Academic Press.

Lott, B. E., & Lott, A. J. (1960). The formation of positive attitudes toward group members. *Journal of Abnormal Social Psychology, 61,* 297–300.

Lovaas, O. I. (1961). Interaction between verbal and nonverbal behavior. *Child Development, 32,* 329–336.

Lovaas, O. I., & Newsom, C. D. (1976). Behavior modification with psychotic children. In H. Leitenberg (Ed.), *Handbook of behavior modification and behavior therapy.* Englewood Cliffs, NJ: Prentice-Hall.

Ludemann, P. M., & Nelson, C. A. (1988). Categorical representation of facial expression by 7 month old infants. *Developmental Psychology, 24,* 492–501.

Maccoby, E. E. (1980). *Social development: Psychological growth and the parent-child relationship.* New York: Harcourt Brace Jovanovich.

Maccoby, E. E. (1988). Gender as a social category. *Developmental Psychology, 24,* 755–765.

Mallick, S. K., & McCandless, B. R. (1966). A study of catharsis of aggression. *Journal of Personality and Social Psychology, 4,* 591–596.

McGraw, K. (1987). *Developmental Psychology.* New York: Harcourt Brace Jovanovich.

Meichenbaum, D. H. (1971). Examination of model characteristics in reducing avoidance behavior. *Journal of Personality and Social Psychology, 17,* 298–307.

Melamed, B. G., & Siegel, L. J. (1975). Reduction of anxiety in children facing hospitalization and surgery by use of filmed modeling. *Journal of Consulting and Clinical Psychology, 43,* 511–521.

Melamed, B. G., Weinstein, D., Hawes, R., & Katin-Borland, M. (1975). Reduction of fear related dental management problems with use of filmed modeling. *Journal of the American Dental Association, 90,* 822–826.

Melamed, B. G., Hawes, R. R., Heiby, E., & Glick, J. (1975). Use of filmed modeling to reduce uncooperative behavior of children during dental treatment. *Journal of Dental Research, 54,* 797–801.

Meltzoff, A. D., & Moore, M. K. (1977). Imitation of facial and manual gestures by human neonates. *Science, 198,* 75–78.

Midlarsky, E., & Bryan, J. H. (1967). Training charity in children. *Journal of Personality and Social Psychology, 5,* 408–415.

Midlarsky, E., Bryan, J. H., & Brickman, P. (1973). Aversive approval: Interactive effects of modeling and reinforcement on altruistic behavior. *Child Development, 44,* 321–328.

Millar, W. S. (1976). Operant acquisition of social behaviors in infancy: Basic problems and constraints. In H. W. Reese (Ed.), *Advances in child development and behavior* (Vol. 11). New York: Academic Press.

Miller, R. L., Brickman, P., & Bolen, D. (1975). Attribution versus persuasion as a means for modifying behavior. *Journal of Personality and Social Psychology, 31,* 430–441.

Miller, N., & Dollard, J. (1941). *Social learning and imitation.* New Haven: Yale University.

Mize, J., & Ladd, G. W. (1991). Developmental issues in social skill training. In S. R. Asher & J. D. Cole (Eds.), *Children's status in the peer group.* New York: Cambridge University Press.

Murray, A. (1979). Infant crying as an elicitor of parental behavior: An examination of two models. *Psychological Bulletin, 86,* 191–215.

Mussen, P. H., & Rutherford, E. (1961). Effects of aggressive cartoons on children's aggressive play. *Journal of Abnormal and Social Psychology, 2,* 461–464.

O'Connor, R. D. (1969). Modification of social withdrawal through symbolic modeling. *Journal of Applied Behavior Analysis, 2,* 15–22.

Patterson, G. R. (1976). The aggressive child: Victim and architect of a coercive system. In L. A. Hamerlynck, L. C. Handy, & E. J. Mash (Eds.), *Behavior modification and families. I. Theory and research*. New York: Brunner/Mazel.

Patterson, G. R. (1982). *Coercive family process*. Eugene, OR: Castalia.

Patterson, G. R., & Cobb, J. A. (1971). A dyadic analysis of "aggressive" behaviors. In J. P. Hill (Ed.), *Minnesota Symposium on Child Psychology* (Vol. 5). Minneapolis: University of Minnesota Press.

Patterson, G. R., DeBaryshe, B. D., & Ramsey, E. (1989). A developmental perspective on antisocial behavior. *American Psychologist, 44*, 329–335.

Patterson, G. R., Littman, R. A., & Bricker, W. (1967). Assertive behavior in children: A step toward a theory of aggression. *Monographs of the Society for Research in Child Development, 32* (5, Whole No. 113).

Patterson, G. R., & Reid, J. B. (1970). Reciprocity and coercion: Two facets of social systems. In C. Neuringer & J. L. Michael (Eds.), *Behavior modification in clinical psychology*. New York: Appleton-Century-Crofts.

Peery, J. C. (1980). Neonate-adult head movement: No and yes revisited. *Developmental Psychology, 16*, 245–250.

Perry, D. G., & Bussey, K. (1979). The social learning theory of sex differences: Imitation is alive and well. *Journal of Personality and Social Psychology, 37*, 1699–1712.

Perry, D. G., & Bussey, K. (1984). *Social development*. Englewood Cliffs, NJ: Prentice-Hall.

Perry, D. G., & Perry, L. C. (1975). Observational learning in children: Effects of sex of model and subject's sex role behavior. *Journal of Personality and Social Psychology, 31*, 1083–1088.

Peterson, R. A. (1971). Aggression as a function of expected retaliation and aggression level of target and aggressor. *Developmental Psychology, 5*, 161–166.

Presbie, R. J., & Coiteux, P. F. (1971). Learning to be generous or stingy: Imitation of sharing behavior as a function of model generosity and vicarious reinforcement. *Child Development, 42*, 1033–1038.

Rachman, S., & Lopatka, C. (1988). Return of fear: Underlearning and overlearning. *Behaviour Research and Therapy, 26*, 99–104.

Rekers, G. A., & Lovaas, O. I. (1974). Behavioral treatment of deviant sex role behaviors in a male child. *Journal of Applied Behavioral Analysis, 7*, 173–190.

Rheingold, H. L. Gewitz, J. L., & Ross, H. W. (1959). Social conditioning of vocalizations in the infant. *Journal of Comparative and Psychological Psychology, 52*, 68–73.

Ritter, B. (1968). The group treatment of children's snake phobias, using vicarious and contact desensitization procedures. *Behavior Research and Therapy, 6*, 1–6.

Robinson, E. A. (1985). Coercion theory revisited: Toward a new theoretical perspective on the etiology of conduct disorders. *Clinical Psychology Review, 5*, 597–626.

Rocha, R. F., & Rogers, R. W. (1976). Ares and Babbitt in the classroom: Effects of competition and reward on children's aggression. *Journal of Personality and Social Psychology, 33*, 588–593.

Rosenhan, D., & White, G. M. (1967). Observation and rehearsal as determinants of prosocial behavior. *Journal of Personality and Social Psychology, 5*, 424–431.

Rosenthal, M. K. (1982). Vocal dialogues in the neonatal period. *Developmental Psychology, 18*, 17–21.

Rushton, J. P. (1975). Generosity in children: Immediate and long term effects of modeling, preaching, and moral judgment. *Journal of Personality and Social Psychology, 31*, 459–466.

Sameroff, A. J., & Cavanaugh, P. (1979). Learning in infancy: A developmental perspective. In J. D. Osofsky (Ed.), *Handbook of infant development*. New York: Wiley.

Sameroff, A. J., & Seifer, R. (1983). *Sources of continuity in parent-child relations*. Paper presented at the meeting of the Society for Research in Child Development, Detroit.

Schneider-Rosen, K., & Cicchetti, D. (1984). The relationship between affect and cognition in maltreated infants: Quality of attachment and the development of self-recognition. *Child Development, 55*, 648–658.

Seligman, M. E. P. (1970). On the generality of the laws of learning. *Psychological Review, 77*, 406–418.

Serbin, L.A., Connor, J. M., & Citron, C. C. (1978). Environmental control of independent and dependent behaviors in preschool girls and boys: A model for early independence training. *Sex Roles, 4*, 867–875.

Skinner, B. F. (1957). *Verbal behavior*. New York: Appleton-Century-Crofts.

Skinner, B. F. (1989). The origins of cognitive thought. *American Psychologist, 44*, 13–18.

Spelke, E., Zelazo, P., Kagan, J., & Kotelchuck, M. (1973). Father interaction and separation protest. *Developmental Psychology, 9*, 83–90.

Staats, A. W. (1968). Social behaviorism and human motivation: Principles of the attitude-reinforcer-discriminative system. In A. G. Greenwald, T. C. Brock, and T. M. Ostrom (Eds.), *Psychological foundations of attitudes*. New York: Academic Press.

Staats, A. W. (1971). *Child learning, intelligence, and personality: Principles of a behavioral interaction approach*. New York: Harper & Row.

Stern, D. N. (1974). The goal and structure of mother-infant play. *Journal of the American Academy of Child Psychiatry, 13*, 403–421.

Twentyman, C. T., & McFall, R. M. (1975). Behavioral training of social skills in shy males. *Journal of Consulting and Clinical Psychology, 43*, 384–395.

Vernon, D. T. (1973). Use of modeling to modify children's responses to a natural, potentially stressful situation. *Journal of Applied Psychology, 58*, 351–356.

Vernon, D. T. (1974). Modeling and birth order in responses to painful stimuli. *Journal of Personality and Social Psychology, 29*, 794–799.

Vernon, D. T., & Bailey, W. C. (1974). The use of motion pictures in the psychological preparation of children for induction of anesthesia. *Anasthesiology, 40*, 68–72.

Walters, R. H., & Parke, R. D. (1964). Influence of response consequences to a social model on resistance to deviation. *Journal of Experimental Child Psychology, 1*, 269–280.

Waters, E., Vaughn, B. E., & Egeland, R. R. (1980). Individual differences in infant-mother attachment relationships at age one: Antecedents in neonatal behavior in an urban, economically disadvantaged sample. *Child Development, 51*, 208–216.

Watson, J. B. (1912). Psychology as the behaviorist views it. *Psychological Review, 20*, 158–177.

Watson, J. B., & Rayner, R. (1920). Conditioned emotional reactions. *Journal of Consulting and Clinical Psychology, 33*, 448–457.

Weiss, R. F., Buchanan, W., Altstatt, L., & Lombardo, J. P. (1971). Altruism is rewarding. *Science, 171*, 1262–1263.

Werner, E., & Smith, R. (1977). *Kauai's children come of age*. Honolulu: University of Hawaii Press.

West, D., & Farrington, D. P. (1977). *The delinquent way of life*. London: Heinemann Educational Books.

White, G. M. (1972). Immediate and deferred effects on model observation and guided and unguided rehearsal on donating and stealing. *Journal of Personality and Social Psychology, 21*, 139–148.

White, G. M., & Burnam, M. A. (1975). Socially cued altruism: Effects of modeling, instructions, and age on public donations. *Child Development, 46*, 559–563.

Zimbardo, P. G. (1988). *Psychology and life*. 12th ed. Boston: Scott, Foresman & Co.

5

A Humanistic Approach to Lifespan Development

Constance T. Fischer

Introduction

Shifts in metaphors and methods afford fresh visions of human diversity, richness, and possibility. When we look beyond measured variables, our vision can include individuals shaping their lives even as they are influenced by societal context and dominant theories. This chapter encourages all of us who study human development to incorporate into our work postmodern humanistic psychology's perspectives and qualitative methods. In that way we can self-consciously choose the influence that our academic conceptions may have on human development. Perhaps we can also encourage positive societal and personal growth.

Humanistic psychology has always been concerned with the themes that all Western disciplines are now addressing as we enter a postmodern era. The modern era was ushered in by the Enlightenment that inspired belief that rationality, technology, and hard science were the routes to truth and advancement. Like other social sciences, psychology is undergoing what we may metaphorically name a midlife crisis: one that is related to disillusionment with the Enlightenment's promise.

This chapter will introduce psychology's developmental crisis, describe the approaches of humanistic and human-science psychology, and overview the themes of postmodernity pertinent to psychology. Rather than collate numerous

Constance T. Fischer • Department of Psychology, Duquesne University, Pittsburgh, Pennsylvania 15282–1705.

Handbook of Social Development: A Lifespan Perspective, edited by Vincent B. Van Hasselt and Michel Hersen. Plenum Press, New York, 1992.

sundry human-science studies, the chapter will review just two areas that reflect and encourage the directions postmodern humanistic lifespan developmental research is taking. These two areas are women's development and old age. The language of these reviews will be grounded in the metaphors of story telling, family, weaving, journeying, and authoring one's life.

Psychology's Developmental Crisis

Psychology (initially the study of psyche—mind, spirit) struggled for about 150 years to be accepted among the empirical sciences. Minority voices throughout psychology's development have argued that not all of human "nature" lends itself to what came to be known as logical positivism. Nevertheless, at this stage in the story of psychology, we are well-established as a social science, accepted within the united natural sciences as the "study of behavior." Beyond that, we are imbued with status as an autonomous discipline. We have systematically built a body of knowledge independent of philosophy, pedagogy, sociology, and psychiatry. Other fields borrow our tools and methods, rely on our data, and use our theories as frameworks for their own endeavors. We have earned our position as a mature science. Within this stage of maturity, however, we now find ourselves in a midlife crisis, even while glimpsing foreshadows of wisdom akin to Erikson's eighth stage of individual development.

In addition to the midlife crisis metaphor, I will also tell this part of the story through an analogy to our having grown into an expanded but divided family. The critical issue in either instance is the same. Through our maturity, and through awareness of the increasing philosophical emphasis on interpretation (hermeneutics) in all disciplines, we now can acknowledge that although the methods that grew out of positivism have served us well, these methods, their data, and their related conceptions of reality are social constructions. Our notions of truth are necessarily perspectival, historical, contextual; there is no absolute, external reality-in-itself knowable to humans except through language, culture, and values. We coauthor our knowledge. Hence there is no external guarantor of validity; we must turn instead to one another to seek validation, correction, and refinement of our accounts of human phenomena. We must rely on consensual criteria that are now acknowledged as contingent on historical moment and on implicit as well as known values. We find ourselves more circumspect about where we have been, and we question our direction. We have entered the postmodern era, subdued by this second enlightenment.

We are rightly proud of psychology's steadfast accomplishment, but from midlife we look around and know, with a sigh, that our accomplishment has been at a certain cost. Perhaps it is time to pay heed to the dimensions of human life that have not lent themselves to quantification, manipulation, and deduction. Dare we attend seriously and openly to such dimensions as spirituality and mutuality? Dare we fully acknowledge both the ambiguity of existence and our responsibility for the sense making we do? Dare we look beyond interactionism for ways to characterize the participation of the psychological and the material within one another? Would these moves mean losing our identity as an independent discipline? Does continued development mean leaving behind our earlier certainties?

Could it mean moving toward the eighth stage, where wisdom is not accumulation of data or guaranteed truth but a sense of community with all humankind across differences?

Within its midlife crisis, psychology is also contending with family tensions. The once unifying creed of behaviorism/positivism is now a frequent source of dissension. Some members of our expanding family argue with the patriarchs and traditionalists that their dogmatic empiricism is dead, passé; other members have simply gone their own way, convinced that psychology will be more meaningful in a postpositivist mode. Among the family factions that have gone their own way, more or less, are cognitive psychologists, who increasingly are welcoming not only strict cognition but affect and existential meaning under their roofs. The most numerous and diverse faction (the practicing clinicians), while maintaining a spoken allegiance to psychology's research base, persists in ignoring logical positivism when it fails to help clients in their daily lives.

The smallest, but rapidly growing, faction is devoted to developing foundations and methods suited specifically to the more-than-object character of being human. These folks see their subject matter as human science in contrast to natural science and have looked to the philosophies of phenomenology and existentialism, and to philosophical anthropology's studies of human structures and of how linguistics preforms human knowing and possibility. They are making contact with the clans within sociology, education, human development, and nursing, who, setting out in a similar fashion, are also working with qualitative research methods and data. The best known faction, humanistic psychology, has persistently promoted values, holism, and personal growth. These developments are not just a matter of broadening the family tree or of accommodating offshoots. In some quarters they have contributed to a radical rift. As the American Psychological Association has become increasingly responsive to and even guided by the divergent family factions, some traditionalists have disowned the parent organization and have formed a competing home base, the American Psychological Society.

Where will we go from here? How will the story of the postmodern era be told by later generations?

POSTMODERN HUMANISTIC PSYCHOLOGY

Humanistic and Human-Science Psychology

Humanistic psychology came of age in the 1960s in protest of partitive, deductive, reductive behaviorist psychology and of deterministic and pathology-oriented psychoanalytic theory. Its founders and followers emphasized that adult growth continues throughout one's life, that we ought to optimize each person's potential for such positive states as joy, creativity, love, self-affirmation, and expression of affect and belief. "With a little help from one's friends," one could take advantage of opportunities for self-direction. Positive values, such as respect for personhood, were to be a mainstay of psychology rather than being eschewed as unscientific. Finally, the unit of study or of counseling was to be the whole person—the feeling, thinking, valuing, emotional, embodied, behaving person.

The Journal of Humanistic Psychology continues to publish contributions to personal growth, psychotherapy, and transpersonal study, and *The Humanistic Psychologist* promotes philosophical reflection and qualitative research methods.

Kindred scholars sought to broaden psychology's scientific base to address human characteristics that go beyond those suitable to natural science methods. Giorgi's (1970) *Psychology as a Human Science: A Phenomenological Approach* served as one of the reference points for scholars who wanted to put aside academic preconceptions and to look freshly at the world as humans comprehend it—both to understand more about that structured/structuring process and to describe human phenomena in themselves, without reducing them to reactions, parts, and numbers. Husserl, Heidegger, and Merleau-Ponty provided philosophical starting points. Existential themes from Camus, Kierkegaard, and Sartre were elaborated in the North American context (e.g., May, 1958). In particular, we took seriously the ordinary and the disturbed ways in which people are responsible for what they make of their lives—for how they take up limits and givens as well as options and possibilities. Research-minded psychologists worked within a phenomenological framework to build empirical content, by asking subjects to describe an experience (e.g., of learning, being anxious, being victimized), and then by systematically describing the interrelated themes invariant across the subjects' experience. The themes were not necessarily explicit for the subject at the time but in transcribed form are readily evident as that person's living of the situation (cf. *The Journal of Phenomenological Psychology; Methods*; Aanstoos, 1987; Fischer & Wertz, 1979; Wertz, 1985).

Sociologists and educators developed related qualitative research methods geared to exploring the worlds of groups and of individuals and to then reflecting on social implications. Well-established approaches include ethnomethodology, symbolic interactionism, ethnography, grounded theory, phenomenography, and action theory (cf. Tesch, 1990). The journal *Phenomenology & Pedagogy* and *Qualitative Studies in Education* contain representative studies and applications in education.

Berger and Luckmann's (1967) *The Social Construction of Reality* was influential for sociology and social psychology, as is Gergen's (1985) contemporary work. North American psychology and pedagogy have been influenced by Riegel's (1976) dialectical psychology, Luria's (1973) research on social mediation of brain structure and function, and Vygotsky's (1962) emphasis on the "zone of proximal development," wherein we assess not native ability but readiness to take the next step by learning with peers. Together, such efforts at systematically exploring the structure, detail, and process of life worlds variously have been called humanistic, third force, and human-science (cf. Aanstoos, 1990a,b). For purposes of this chapter, I sometimes use *humanistic* as an umbrella term, in that it is most familiar to readers.

Although humanistic psychology did not evolve from Greek and Renaissance humanism, their respective themes resonate with each other and with our postmodern situation. In particular, the early humanism held that human nature includes goodness and that moral conduct arises out of knowing other lives. The good life was to come not through prescriptive socialization and authority, but through reflection, consultation, and discussion. Indeed, humanistic psychology has moved from its early celebration of self to an increased interest in community and to an acknowledgment of contingencies. Likewise, human-science psychology has matured to the point of looking beyond philosophy and qualitative research methodology to address how this knowledge might shape our communities. So, too, as we enter postmodernity, psychology in general asks how we ought to use our technical and scientific power in moral ways. Indeed, we are coming to accept that we are responsible for asking what we mean by *moral* and by the *good life*.

Themes of Postmodernity

The modern era is said to have begun in the eighteenth century, with the Age of Enlightenment. That era is seen as a shift toward believing that humans (then called *man*) could apply rationality and worldly (empirical) methods to discover the laws according to which the universe had been put in motion by Higher Powers. Biology, physics, and physiology, with the assistance of the formal science of mathematics, steadily demonstrated their reliability, independence from theology, and their utility for daily affairs. Indeed, the Age of Enlightenment was to be one in which rationality and application of empirical research would result in a new world of reason and progress through control of nature.

At today's juncture, practitioners across disciplines, from literature and architecture to physics and psychology, are using an increasingly popularized term, *postmodernity*, to evoke our point in history. Our place is similar to that of the minister who comes to see that although his or her church has thrived on denominational belief and ritual, no particular denomination is the only way to be spiritual, moral, united, and so on. Religion and science are in large part devised by humans, who are necessarily bound to their culture. Religionists and scientists, by choice or by inculcation, can follow their credentialed leaders and the accepted texts and belief systems, but increasingly leaders and practitioners know that there is no external, absolute, universal truth-in-itself. Human sense making, construing, philosophizing, theory building, and so on are of course contoured by human ways of knowing, asking, and hoping, which are always within particular historical, cultural, political, and motivational contexts. Some commentators on postmodernity's emergence are disheartened or cynical—what are we to do if religion and science are not independent authorities for us to rely on and appeal to?

Others, however, regard this stage in the Western world's development as an opportunity to more knowingly and responsibly shape our knowledge base, our relations to one another, and the earth's future. The modern era's grand project of precise knowledge and control becomes a postmodern circumspect effort to understand contextually and to influence responsibly. The social sciences, of course, should continue to use our measurement instruments, experimental and statistical methods, and theory building but with recognition that these are human constructions whose use in turn shapes our ways of knowing as well as our knowledge base. A new criterion for rigor is respect for uncertainty, for ambiguity, and for data's relativity to myriad contexts.

Validity, then, becomes radically contextualized. To study old age, for example, we would ask *old* according to whom, what are the possible social consequences of focusing on particular "variables," in what physical and economic circumstances are our subjects living, what oppressions and invitations face them, and what are the backgrounds, assumptions, life circumstances, and personal motives of the researchers? Yes, evermore life-world contexts become apparent; exploration and understanding are always unfinished. Validity is no longer demonstrated by hypothetical-deductive procedures alone but through hermeneutic spirals—continual relooking in light of different perspectives, and of revised understanding of parts.

Paying heed to social context and construction also requires going beyond numbers and beyond searches for underlying determinants to describing layered situations as they are lived and as they viewed from different perspectives. Researchers can now describe narratively; we become reporters and storytellers. Validity now is determined not just through the persuasion of deductive proof but through the interpersonal persuasion of lifeworld evidence, of personal descriptions that reverberate with the listener's or reader's life. Scientific knowledge is now developed through hermeneutic consensus, through a rhetoric of description. Conversation, discussion, sharing of illustrations, joint modification of understandings are at once means of demonstrating, testing, and revising knowledge. In these efforts we become more aware of the power of language to evoke one's own experience, to preform inquiry, and to break up old assumptions. We use and form language more advisedly, just as we come to respect local differences and are not so quick to categorize, judge, or ignore.

This presentation of emerging postmodern themes in the social sciences is a variation of what have been minority voices—those of humanistic and human-science psychology. As Toulmin (1990) points out, postmodernity can be taken up as a revitalizing form of Renaissance humanism. We can move from the so-called enlightened quest for logical certitude and universal truth and return to a respect for inherent ambiguity, diversity, and complexity, as we address the particular, the evolving, and the local through conversation, the arts, and storytelling. However, because of media and other technology, contemporary humanism is also global. What difference does this make, and how might we guide a twenty-first century humanist humanistic/human-science developmental psychology?

A Postmodern Developmental Psychology Approach

Much of the research and thinking presented in these two sections, on women's development and on older age, appears in other chapters of this handbook. It is presented here to highlight what can be done when we take seriously the co-authoring of lives and visions, the social construction of theory, and the importance of language in shaping knowledge. This work points to the promise of intermittently putting aside theoretical assumptions, of looking freshly at human situations, and of finding ways to narrate the rich and complex scenes we witness.

Women's Development*

Listening for the Female Voice

Sometimes, in family arguments or discussions, the voice of a child or a heretofore silent spouse is heard clearly for the first time. Similarly, the feminine voice now emerges in arguments and discussions about human development. This voice speaks of familiar themes—emotional, moral, cognitive, and spiritual devel-

---

*Kathleen Mulrenin is first coauthor of this section.

opment, yet it speaks differently. A metaphor increasingly invoked to speak of feminine experience is that of weaving (e.g., Aptheker's *Tapestries of Life*, 1989). Historically, women gathered in the evening to weave fabric from communally grown crops or to quilt. They wove blankets and rugs from remnants. Through daily practice, women often continue to be adaptive caretakers. Through their activity, they are attuned to texture, to layers, to the between, to context and relatedness, and, in weaving terminology, to the warp and woof of internal and external authorities, of intuition and reason, and of connectedness and separateness. Their voices tell a different story; they weave a different tapestry.

This emerging voice speaks from studies of women's narration of their experience, either through stories told in clinical settings (Eichenbaum & Orbach, 1982; Miller, 1976; Stiver, 1986; Surrey, 1984) or through formal qualitative research (Belenky, Clinchy, Goldberger, & Tarule, 1986; Gilligan, 1982, 1990; Gleason, 1985; Lyons, 1990; Randour, 1987). These direct approaches to women's development tell the stories not only of "statistically significant" women but of those who may not be counted by quantitative research methods.

FINDING A VOICE IN RELATION TO OTHERS

In the tradition of Freud, Erikson, Kohlberg, and Piaget, development follows a male norm. Maturation has been said to occur in terms of separation and individuation, without regard for how intimacy, care, empathy, and connectedness develop. These latter phenomena become visible when emotional development is looked at freshly by women such as Nancy Chodorow, and the scholars affiliated with the Stone Center (Jean Baker Miller, Irene Stiver, Janet Surrey, and others). These observers have unraveled traditional psychoanalytic theory and insights and reworked them to depict the story of women in human development.

In their writings on infancy, neither Freud nor Erikson attended to gender differences nor to the reciprocity of the parent–infant relationship. In contrast, Chodorow (1978) and Stiver (1986) carefully describe differences in boys' and girls' relationship to the mothering one (usually the woman). Citing research by Stoller (1968), Stiver (1986) tells us how girls and boys develop a "core gender identity" as early as 18 months. Later the young girl knows she is like mother, and the young boy knows he is not like mother. Does the young girl learn that to be like mother is to care for others and to attend to their feelings? It appears so. Chodorow (1978) and Surrey (1983), among others, take this thread of "connectedness" as experienced by young girls and draw out its positive character. Rather than pathologizing it as a failure of female development, a tendency toward fusion and dependency, we can see it as the warp—the foundational yarns—of empathy and as a vibrant emotional attending to others. We can also see how women's valuing of closeness can render them hesitant to risk asserting autonomy and authority (Gilligan, 1982; Miller, 1976).

Conversely, this perspective allows us to understand the difficulties that men often experience with intimacy as being grounded in the early disconnecting from and disidentifying with their mothers that Freud described (Gilligan, 1982; Miller, 1976). Furthermore, Chodorow's sociological analysis suggests that attending to different models of parenting infants and encouraging fathers to "mother" more may significantly influence psychological development of both boys and girls, particularly in the areas of intimacy, assertiveness, and empathic presence to others. As this shift occurs, society as a whole ought to consider the socioeconomic and cultural ramifications of fathers "mothering." Parenting takes place within the larger context of finances, emotions, family, and community.

Stages beyond infancy, from Erikson's "autonomy vs. shame and doubt," to Freud's "oedipal," through adolescent, can be reunderstood by listening to the feminine voice. Miller (1984) and others observe that even in the traditional "autonomy vs. shame and doubt" phase, as described by Erikson (1950), the child does not so much move away from the caregiver as that the environment presents more invitations to the developing boy and girl. As the complex pattern of relationships with a widening world grows, anchoring threads are *not* severed. Similarly in regard to the next, the so-called oedipal stage of development (characterized by Freud and others in terms of castration anxiety and its corollary, penis envy), Miller has remarked that for girls "there is no big crisis of cutting off anything, and especially relationships" (1976, p. 7). Stiver (1986), concurring with Horney (1926/1967) and others, echoes that there is little evidence for the notion of castration anxiety and its counterparts for girls. Unlike the traditional psychoanalytic view of girls at the oedipal stage angrily separating from mothers and turning to fathers, Chodorow and Stiver see the young girl remaining in an intense, although often conflicted, relationship with the mother.

New interpretations of oedipal "penis envy" regard the phallus as a symbol of the privileged position of men in the social world, with envy being of social status rather than of the penis. Envy of anatomical differences includes male envy of motherhood, pregnancy, breasts, and so on (Horney, 1926/1967). Moreover, studies suggest that both boys and girls desire to have babies and that the wish for babies precedes the understanding of anatomical differences (Parens, Pollack, Stern, & Kramer, 1977). Stiver provides an extensive analysis of the oedipal period, including reflections on the "sexual component of the father–daughter relationship," "competence and mastery," and "the birth of a sibling." When we put traditional psychoanalytic theory aside and observe girls' lives directly, we cannot help but see and hear that there is no evidence for, nor need for, traditional oedipal concepts.

As Gilligan (1982) points out, for most girls the primacy of relationships continues through preadolescence. While boys busily compete physically and argue about rules, in general girls talk with each other about personal appearance, family conflicts, and other intimate concerns. Girls learn to gossip and to weave intricate understandings of their social lives.

Although girls in late adolescence talk about sex, many struggle consciously about whether to express their sexual desire (Gleason, 1985). This struggle may suggest an acceptance of social codes that teach women not to assert themselves sexually (Eichenbaum & Orbach, 1982; Irigaray, 1985; Miller, 1976). Miller (1984) likewise emphasizes that girls' reluctance to assert themselves typically is in response to a perceived risk of becoming disconnected from others. Sassen (1980) reinterprets Horner's (1968) work on women's fear of success as their concern that achievement may be accompanied by disconnection from and harm to an other.

This shift within a psychoanalytic theory from a phallocentric to a gynocentric perspective has bypassed the dictums of evolutionary and biological theory and taken as its starting point direct observation of, and discussion with, females. So, too, in moral development: New truth becomes apparent when male norms are set aside long enough to listen to female voices in their own right.

Gilligan's *In a Different Voice* (1982) follows the threads of girls' and women's moral reasoning as they intertwine with cognitive and emotional development. Gilligan begins with studies involving preadolescent and adolescent children, noting differences between the genders (although the differences do not always fall strictly along gender lines). She continues with studies of the moral reasoning of women who are faced with the dilemma of whether to have an abortion. In general, Gilligan's females focused on interpersonal responsibility and care, for which the appropriate mode of thinking is contextual and narrative rather than formal and abstract. Males typically responded in terms of rights and rules. Lyons (1990) found that girls used one or both styles of thinking about their lives and sees these modes of reasoning as complementary.

Gilligan's description of females' moral reasoning reveals traditional biases in the prevailing stage theory of moral development (Kohlberg, 1981). That system consistently rates as higher the typical male criteria of rules, contracts, and logical deduction, in contrast to the more typical female criteria of interpersonal care and responsibility.

Gilligan, Lyons, and Hanmer (1990) are careful not to rank these different approaches to moral dilemmas. To set one manner of reasoning as more advanced or on a higher plane than another would repeat previous hierarchical and norm-setting biases. They attentively affirm both orientations, consistently following a contextual and perspectival approach to theory building rather than assuming linear progressive stages.

Listening and Speaking: Silence and Other Ways of Knowing

Belenky *et al.* (1986) interviewed women in different contexts (prestigious colleges, rural social service agencies, and community colleges) to gain a fresh understanding of, as their title says, *Women's Ways of Knowing: The Development of Self, Voice, and Mind*. These authors describe five positions through which women view, understand, and interact. The first of these they named *silence*. Silent women were found in "the most socially, economically, and educationally deprived" circumstances of all the women in their study (pp. 23–24). In this context, women are selfless and voiceless, their lives structured and dictated by powerful others; they have little appreciation for their individual intellectual and emotional resources. As one woman said, "I don't like talking to my husband. If I were to say no, he might hit me" (p. 24).

The relational context of the women in the second position is described as *hierarchical* and as conforming to sex-role stereotypes, with fathers and husbands as speakers and mothers and wives as listeners. The women in these contexts they named *received knowers*, for whom learning is based exclusively on the authority of others. Life is viewed through rigid categories, such as "should and ought," "right and wrong." What is right involves doing for others. Within these relational contexts, girls and women do not question.

In contrast to received knowers, women who hear their inner voice and actively search for a self grew up in family contexts of rebellion and self-assertion. Their histories frequently are highlighted with "strong-minded mothers" or "supermoms." Women from this position questioned the conventional view of women as selfless, dependent, and silent. However, they, too, may experience difficulty finding ways to speak publicly of their subjective understandings.

The relational contexts of women in the forth and fifth positions are similar. Perhaps key to their histories are personal, intimate, empathic connectedness to and dialogues with intellectually gifted mothers and an appreciation of their fathers' reasoning and emotional capacities.

Women identified as being in the fourth position, *procedural knowers*, for the most part attended prestigious colleges and universities. In this context, women learned how to defend their subjectivist positions by using [the procedures of] both logical reasoning and empathic feeling. For procedural knowers, however, priority is given to defending one's stance with the anticipated external authorities of 'objective truth.' Such skill serves one well in law, corporate business, and academia, where logic and argumentation are valued.

The fifth position integrates knowledge gleaned from external authorities with what is felt intuitively. Belenky *et al.* consider this as an integration of voices and a reclaiming of the self. *Constructivist knowers* see the relativity of truth, its construction within particular contexts. These women compassionately apply their intuitive and procedural skills to improve the quality of life for others. Belenky *et al.* emphasize the importance of the contexts in which each of the five epistemological positions develops. "The eventual path a woman takes is, in large measure, a function of the familial and educational environments in which she is struggling with these problems" (p. 79).

RELATING WITHIN A SPIRITUAL CONTEXT

Concomitant with the growth of feminist psychology and the ordination of women in some denominations, women's spiritual development has become open to qualitative study. Randour's (1987) work, *Women's Psyche, Women's Spirit*, highlights spirituality in terms of ways of relating and how a woman perceives herself in relation to others, including God. Randour delineates four groups of women in her qualitative study of 94 women: selves-in-conflict, emerging women, resolute women, and mystical women. She notes, consistent with the theory of knowing described above, that

> many of these women grew up equating self-assertion and self-definition with egocentricity and selfishness; they were given both spoken and unspoken messages to conform and to be directed by outside forces. As adults they could not trust their own inner sense of who they were and what they wanted, yet they also deeply yearned to find that self. . . . Much of the psychological work of these women was to shift from an external to an internal authority. (p. 22)

"Selves-in-conflict," all under the age of 21, described struggling with God, trying to balance self-assertion and the traditional understanding of sin. "Emerging" women described their spiritual experiences as part of self-development, of discovering themselves, their beauty and power. Not one of these emerging women referred to God in masculine terms, such as "God, the Father." They located authority within themselves and comfortably asserted themselves in a balanced manner while relating with others. Resolute women were older women, of whom Randour writes:

> Talking in the tones of traditional religious voice, they strive for submission to a higher authority, not self-enhancement. Accepting the traditional Christian

conception of sin for them means that self-assertion endangers their relationship to God and that acquiescence enhances it. (p. 48)

Finally, for "mystical" women, a relationship to or experience of God is that of experiencing oneself as one with God. This experience differed from that of resolute women in that mystical women did not experience themselves as handing over their power or authority but experienced God within themselves, or in Belenky *et al.*'s terms, as an integration of voices. Looking freshly and listening respectfully has yielded promising understandings of spiritual as well as emotional, moral, and cognitive development.

COMMENT

The tapestry of human development as woven by feminist theorists contains several strong and persistent strands, the first of which is the centrality of relationships throughout one's lifespan. Second, differentiation is seen not as a separating from significant others but as developing a whole and authentic self who maintains connectedness with others. From their various particular situations, women can speak with their own authority, empathy, and care, which inform their moral and epistemological interactions.

Research from this contextual and relational perspective has only begun. The focus thus far has been on grown daughters and their mothers. Nevertheless, this work *is* corrective in that it addresses women's development in its own right, through direct observation, interviews, and qualitative description. The relational fields of men and women, fathers and sons, fathers and daughters, preadolescent boys and girls, and so on, await research and restorying. In the meantime, feminist research also is the beginning of a new way of conceptualizing, researching, and speaking of development, while maintaining a dialogue with traditionally named categories and stages. The spinning and weaving of research and theory will grow in richness and texture to the extent to which we continue to attend to individuals in their family and sociocultural contexts.

Elders' Development*

The lives of older-age persons, like those of women, are a recent topic of study, similarly open to postmodern approaches. Researchers are finding that older age is directly accessible through conversation and through subjects' descriptions, including diaries. Just as the language of weaving and relating facilitates openness to new truths about women's development, so a language of continuity, biography, meaning making, and journeying–journaling affords new visions of growing older.

FROM CHAPTERS TO CONTINUITY

Psychology's story of human development has been written within a framework of quantification and explanation. In the past we have characterized the flow of life as a linear sequence of chapters each, in part, a preface for the next. We have regarded the individual much as we do a book, as separate and self-contained. We have read that book as though it were organized by two principles. The first is

*Jeffrey D. Freedman is first coauthor of this section.

Freud's emphasis on the early years of psychological development and the importance of these first few chapters to the ongoing story. The second principle is stage theory, such as Erikson's, which, although still emphasizing childhood, highlights one's ordered ascension through developmental stages. With the aging of America, we have begun to realize that these principles fall short of describing the experiences and meanings of living the later years of life.

Emphasis on formative years and stages to explain human development have perpetuated "gerontophobic" myths and stereotypes (Dychtwald, 1989; Neugarten, 1979). Among these myths are: People over 65 are old; older people are in poor health; older minds are not as bright as young minds; older people are unproductive; older people are unattractive and sexless; and all older people are the same (Dychtwald, 1989). With the increasing number of active elderly people participating in our communities, these long-standing myths are becoming increasingly difficult to accept. According to the Census Bureau, in 1890 only 4% of the U.S. population was over 65. Today, there are more than 30 million U.S. citizens over the age of 65, which is about 12% of the population. These 12% defy the expected roles, activities, needs, and experiences set by stage theories. Indeed, Americans of all ages are participating in our communities, in our workplaces, and in our families differently than the dated characterizations predict. Today we hear of "the 35-year-old grandmother, the 50-year-old retiree, the 65-year-old father of a preschooler, the 70-year-old student, and even the 85-year-old mother caring for 65-year-old son" (Neugarten, 1979). It is time to adopt alternative perspectives from which we can reexamine and restory the meanings, experiences, and life worlds of our elder citizens.

Only in the last 10 to 15 years have we attended to the inaccuracies of traditional stories of the later years of life. Slowly but concertedly we are revising the dated versions. Alternative words, phrases, and metaphors have begun to appear in psychological literature. The term *stage* has been replaced by *fluid life cycle* (Hirschhorn, 1977), *plateaus* (Mahrer, 1978), *transitions* and *seasons* (Levinson, 1978), and *life cycle* (Neugarten, 1979). The authors of these alternative terms stress that older people continue to develop and struggle. Rather than reinforce the accepted notion that this population has reached the last stage of life and is devoted to preparing for death, these authors emphasize that the elderly also continue to profoundly experience and give meaning to life.

Throughout our lives we give meaning to our environment, our companions, and ourselves. We are forever changing, forever in flux, and forever modifying and transforming the meanings we posit. We are continually living within ambiguities and contrasting life views (Levinson, 1978; McAdams, 1988; Wrightsman, 1988). Influenced by dialectical authors, Levinson (1978) writes that "polarities exist during the entire life cycle. They can never be fully resolved or transcended" (p. 198). We have just begun to explore the meaning structures of later life (Berg & Gadow, 1978; McAdams, 1988; Wonolowski & Davis, 1988; Wrightsman, 1988). To branch out in this exploration, we must affirm that unlike a book that moves logically from a set introduction to a resolved conclusion, we continue to edit and revise the meanings of our lives, even through death.

FROM DISTANCE TO ENCOUNTER

Starr (1983), following Gergen's (1980) lead, urges us to take an "aleatoric" account of aging—one that attends to humans' continuous, improvisational, and flexible development within particular historical, cultural, and interpersonal frameworks that are always imbued with values and meanings. To describe and understand the experiences of an aging person, we must include his or her personal contexts. Berman (1988) reminds us that "understanding a life structure means understanding the meaning of [particular] attachments in the person's life" (p. 55).

Psychology's usual quantitative methods, grounded as they are in logical positivist epistemology, are not adequate to this task. Prematurely collecting data via prestructured inventories bypasses personal context, meaningful ambiguities, and the possibility of encountering unfamiliar themes. Traditionally, interviews, instead of opening to new vistas, are reduced to categories and quantification; presumably qualitative data are transformed into what Fischer (1987) has termed *qualiquantive* data. These data are not particularly helpful to efforts to surpass emphasis on determinants and on stage theory.

Leading gerontologists have begun to emphasize the necessity of working closely with and following the lead of the elders we wish to study (Berman, 1988; Hornstein & Wapner, 1984; Levinson, 1987; Adams, 1988; Neugarten, 1979; Rowles & Reinharz, 1988; Starr, 1983). Many of these authors describe themselves, in part, as biographers. Levinson (1978) notes that "when studying the evolution of life structure, we are being biographical" (p. 43). To write a biography one must collaboratively explore and describe the experiences of older people as they go about their lives. By respectfully and directly addressing those people who are in the midst of the very life world in which we are interested, we may discover the meanings, values, and intentions that constitute the ongoing process of development in the later years of life.

From Quantification to Description

Rowles and Reinharz (1988) term their approach *qualitative gerontology*. In this approach, the researcher attempts to withhold, or bracket, his or her learned attitudes so "patterns that underlie the lifeworlds of individuals, social groups, and larger systems as they related to old age" can naturally emerge (p. 6). These researchers describe specific steps for, as well inherent difficulties in, interviewing the elderly. Generalizability is found in consensus, expressed as reoccurring experiential themes described by the research subjects.

Thomas and Chambers (1989) studied life satisfaction among cohorts of men at least 70 years old in New Delhi, India, and London, England. Standardized measures of well-being were compared with qualitative analyses of transcribed open interviews. There were no differences between the groups on the quantitative instruments, but marked contrasts became apparent in the qualitative data in which personal meanings and life context were preserved. For example, the English sample claimed satisfaction in the sense of having made the best of things, of having adjusted to life. But they also expressed fear of becoming incapacitated, and brooded about their declining powers and prospects. Their focus was on activity, control, and usefulness. In contrast, for the Indian sample, life satisfaction was related to family closeness and to having done one's duty to children and society in consonance with religious belief. The Indian men acknowledged declining physical ability, but few expressed fear of becoming incapacitated. Regrets about decline were related to decreased ability to help the less fortunate. From these findings, Thomas and Chambers stress the problem of "context stripping" in traditional data collection and analysis.

Neugarten (1979) takes a similar methodological approach. Among her findings from qualitative interviewing are: (a) People in the later years of life not only experience problems and losses but also freedoms and gains; (b) most older people do not deteriorate to the point of losing identity; and (c) most older people do not wish to *be* young again although they may wish to *feel* young. The people with whom she spoke wanted to continue to "grow old with equanimity and with the assurance that they will have had a full measure of life's experience" (p. 891).

Wondolowski and Davis (1988), following a phenomenological method, asked, "What is the structural definition of the experience of aging for the oldest old?" From interviewing 100 men and women, ages 80 and up, in parks, community centers, and family homes, they found three prevailing themes. The first was an "unfolding euphony": a harmonious affirming of self by self and others. The second theme was "creative transfiguring": the acknowledgment and appreciation of one's participation in the world of perpetually unfolding possibilities. The third theme was "transcendent voyaging": familiarity with the past, lively connectedness to the present, and excitement in the future.

Other gerontologists have begun to utilize personal diaries to research reflected life events and meanings (Berman, 1986, 1988; McAdams, 1988; Wrightsman, 1988). Berman examined the intimate journal of Florida Scott-Maxwell, an author who in her eighty-fifth year began to document her experiences of later life. Although she faced losses of friends and family and experienced "substantial physical decline," Berman notes her continuing passion for life, "which, if anything, was refined and sharpened by those losses" (p. 322). Woven into this passion for life was her relationship with frailty, particularly her possibilities of invalidism and death. She reported fearing becoming an increasing burden on others and experiencing feelings of helplessness. Berman notes in her experience of old age a theme of gravitating toward "abstract ideas" and toward "an intense involvement with the essence of life, with the nonphysical aspects of humanness, with ideas themselves" (p. 322). This shift paradoxically led to a reactivated involvement with life and sensitivity to the social world.

These firsthand accounts can be appreciated in their own terms even while we relate them to developmental themes. Berman presents Scott-Maxwell's reported experience of being "true to herself" as a process of individuation in which she struggled between the "attachment/separateness" polarities. Borrowing from Levinson, Berman describes Scott-Maxwell's emphasis on being herself as an "extension of the separateness side," which calls for a construction and explanation of one's private inner world.

In her book, *Living and Relating: An Introduction to Phenomenology*, Becker (1992) cites from author Barbara Macdonald's (1983) account of her own old age, *Look Me in the Eye*:

> My hands are large and the backs of my hands begin to show the brown spots of aging. Sometimes lately, holding my arms up reading in bed or lying with my arms clasped around my lover's neck, I see my arm with the skin hanging loosely from my forearm and cannot believe that it is really my own. It seems disconnected from me; it is someone else's, it is the arm of an old woman. It is the arm of such old women as I myself have seen, sitting on benches in the sun with their hands folded in their laps; old women I have turned away from. I wonder now, how and when these arms I see came to be my own—arms I cannot turn away from. (p. 13)

> As we age, we lose the power to outdistance vulnerabilities and to flee from ourselves by cultivating socially valued attributes. We are caught in our bodies and in our lives; we are left facing ourselves, facing our own death. . . . Accepting the inevitability of death can increase appreciation of life. It can also reveal the meanings of ourselves, our lives, and life itself. (1992, pp. 113–114)

COMMENT

Like research into women's development, research into how humans take up their last decades *is* beginning to engage research subjects directly. When we ask directly about life, instead of testing theories through indirect measures, we discover people seeking continuity and meaning, exceeding known stages even while exemplifying them. Remaining at a descriptive level keeps researchers and readers in touch with lives—we *picture and imagine* men and women as they go about their daily lives. Description preserves the particulars and the contexts that allow new understandings and differentiations to arise. Again, like research into women's development, humanistic approaches have demonstrated their promise, but there is much more work ahead than that already accomplished. For example: What are the contexts in which elders remain challenged and inspirational, like Scott-Maxwell? Are there stages within the last decades of life, or does that phase vary too widely for that kind of characterization? In what sense do some men become more nurturant as they age? Does the quality of interpersonal relationships change as we go through our last decades? When do people regard retirement as an end rather than a new beginning? When do people experience old age as involving gains as well as losses? We anticipate that qualitative approaches to actual lives will yield rich and rewarding stories.

SUMMARY

This chapter's account of humanistic psychology's approach to human development was told simply. Research on women's and elders' development was selected to evoke the promise of research that respects individuals as always living in terms of meaning. There *are* related theoretical works on human development, such as Riegel's (1976) dialectical framework, Lerner's (1978) interactionism, Fischer and Alapack's (1987) phenomenological approach to adolescence, and Knowles's (1986) integration of Heidegger and Erikson. There also are nearly a hundred empirical phenomenological studies in educational, nursing, and psychological literature of persons dealing with various developmental challenges, from Alapack's (1984) study of adolescent first love to Holtz's (1984) study of midlife disillusionment. Some of this content has found its way into other chapters of this volume.

For this chapter, however, we opted not to summarize broad research content for fear of underplaying the *approach* of contemporary humanistic psychology. That approach now integrates the qualitative research of human-science and phenomenological psychology, thereby providing both a philosophical framework and methods for meeting postmodernity's invitation and challenge. Before reviewing the themes with which the humanistic literatures on women's and elders' development put us in touch, however, it should be acknowledged that humanistic psychology has not undertaken programmatic study of lifespan development. Because humanistic approaches are descriptive rather than theoretical, there are no agendas for building bodies of knowledge through hypothesis testing. Although human-science research is laudable for its bracketing of assumptions and theory and for its steadfast addressing phenomena as much as possible in their own terms, only now is it maturing to the point of being ready to participate in systematic comparison of qualitative methods and findings. Its historical psychological emphasis on the individual has been at the expense of longitudinal or comparative studies, which it has not undertaken. Nor has it engaged in significant interdisciplinary study. Similarly, most human-science research has not yet attended to the social–economic–political context of individual development, nor to the psychological structures of interpersonal relating, mutuality, and community. Although humanistic psychology has confronted deterministic theories of development, has suggested holistic, interactive, and dialectical corrections, and has accepted both continuity and restructuration as developmental possibilities, a systematic understanding of human development has not yet been constructed.

Humanistic psychology's philosophical alternatives to historically prevailing positivism and reductivism do provide promising directions for psychology and the broader social sciences as they emerge from their developmental crisis and enter the postmodern era. Recognizing that knowledge is inevitably co-authored by *researchers* and their subject matter, postmodern scientists do not seek to identify causal or independent variables. Instead, they strive to find language that expresses individuals' participation in the everyday worlds that they both shape and are shaped by. In this chapter we wrote with metaphors to evoke the structures and depth of particular situations. Metaphors, subjects' quotations, and excerpts from particular lives put writers and readers in personal touch with the diversity and variation of experience and with the constraints and possibilities of growing up female and of growing old.

This connection encourages correction of earlier assumptions about women and elders. It also can lend itself to truly relevant social planning and research questions. But choosing life-based description as a major approach means having to study lives in context, both as seen by observers and as lived by the persons being described. Such research is local, collaborative, and forever open to revision. Validity of new understandings is assessed in terms of consensual agreement among observers and subjects and in terms of everyday practical significance. Addressing actual lives also confronts us with values and engages us in moral questions—what do we believe is good for ourselves and others? Even in the face of inevitable ambiguity, we are responsible to the world that we shape through our concepts, language, research, and teaching. How shall we now foretell the story of lifespan development?

REFERENCES

Aanstoos, C. M. (1987). A comparative survey of human science psychologies. *Methods, 1,* 1–36.
Aanstoos, C. M. (1990a). A brief history of the Human Science Research Conference. *Journal of Humanistic Psychology, 30*(3), 137–145.
Aanstoos, C. M. (Ed.). (1990b). Psychology and postmodernity. *The Humanistic Psychologist, 18*(1), 1–132.

Alapack, R. J. (1984). Adolescent first love. In C. M. Aanstoos (Ed.), *Studies in the social sciences: Vol. 23. Exploring the lived world: Readings in phenomenological psychology* (pp. 101–117). Carrollton, GA: West Georgia College.

Aptheker, B. (1989). *Tapestries of life: Women's work, women's consciousness, and the meaning of daily experiences*. Amherst: University of Massachusetts Press.

Becker, C. S. (1992). *Living and relating: An introduction to phenomenology*. Newbury Park, CA: Sage.

Belenky, M. F., Clinchy, B. M., Goldberger, N. R., and Tarule, J. M. (1986). *Women's ways of knowing: The development of self, voice, and mind*. New York: Basic Books.

Berg, G., & Gadow, S. (1978). Toward more human meanings of aging: Ideals and images from philosophy and art. In S. F. Spicker, K. M. Woodward, & D. D. van Tassel (Eds.), *Aging and the elderly* (pp. 83–92). Atlantic Highlands, NJ: Humanities Press.

Berger, P., & Luckmann, T. (1967). *The social construction of reality*. Harmondsworth: Penguin.

Berman H. J. (1986). To flame with a wild life: Florida Scott-Maxwell's experience of old age. *The Gerontologist, 26*(3), 321–324.

Berman, H. J. (1988). Admissible evidence: Geropsychology and the personal journal. In S. Reinharz & G. D. Rowles (Eds.), *Qualitative gerontology* (pp. 47–63). New York: Springer.

Chodorow, N. (1978). *The reproduction of mothering: Psychoanalysis and the sociology of gender*. Berkeley: University of California Press.

Dychtwald, K. (1989). *Age wave*. Los Angeles: Tarcher.

Eichenbaum, L., & Orbach, S. (1982). *Understanding women: A feminist psychoanalytic approach*. New York: Basic Books.

Erikson, E. H. (1950). *Childhood and society*. New York: Norton.

Fischer, C. T. (1987). The quality of qualitative research. *Theoretical and Philosophical Psychology, 7*, 2–11.

Fischer, C. T., & Alapack, R. J. (1987). A phenomenological approach to adolescence. In V. B. Van Hasselt & M. Hersen (Eds.), *Handbook of adolescent psychology* (pp. 91–107). New York: Pergamon Press.

Fischer, C. T., & Wertz, F. J. (1979). Empirical phenomenological analyses of being criminally victimized. In A. Giorgi, R. Knowles, & D. L. Smith (Eds.), *Duquesne studies in phenomenological psychology* (Vol. 3, pp. 135–158). Pittsburgh: Duquesne University Press.

Gergen, K. J. (1980). The emerging crisis in life-span developmental theory. In P. Bates & D. G. Brim (Eds.), *Life span development and behavior*. New York: Academic Press.

Gergen, K. J. (1985). The social constructionist movement in modern psychology. *American Psychologist, 40*, 266–273.

Gilligan, C. (1982). *In a different voice: Psychological theory and women's development*. Cambridge: Harvard University Press.

Gilligan, C., Lyons, N. P., & Hanmer, T. J. (1990). *Making connections: The relational worlds of adolescent girls at Emma Willard School*. Cambridge: Harvard University Press.

Giorgi, A. (1970). *Psychology as a human science: A phenomenological approach*. New York: Harper & Row.

Gleason, N. (1985). Women's self development in late adolescence. In *Work in progress, No. 17*, (pp. 11–25). Wellesley: Stone Center Working Papers Series.

Hirschhorn, L. (1977). Social policy and the life cycle: A developmental perspective. *Social Service Review, 51*, 434–450.

Holtz, V. A. (1984). Being disillusioned as exemplified by adults in religion, marriage, or career: An empirical phenomenological investigation (Doctoral dissertation, Duquesne University, 1984). *Dissertation Abstracts International, 45*, 3621B.

Horner, M. S. (1968). Sex differences in achievement motivation and performance in competitive and noncompetitive situations. (Doctoral dissertation, University of Michigan, 1968.) *Dissertation Abstracts International, 30*, 407B.

Horney, K. (1967). *Feminine psychology*. New York: Norton. (Original work published 1926)

Hornstein, G., & Wapner, S. (1984). The experience of the retiree's social network during the transition to retirement. *Studies in the Social Studies, 23*, 119–136.

Irigaray, L. (1985). *This sex which is not one*. Ithaca: Cornell University Press.

Knowles, R. T. (1986). *Human development and human possibility: Erikson in light of Heidegger* Lanham, MD: University Press of America.

Kohlberg, L. (1981). *The philosophy of moral development*. San Francisco: Harper & Row.

Kruger, D. (1979). *An introduction to phenomenological psychology*. Pittsburgh: Duquesne University Press.

Lerner, R. M. (1978). Nature, nurture, and dynamic interactionism. *Human Development, 21*, 1–20.

Levinson, D. J. (1978). *The seasons of a man's life*. New York: Ballantine Books.

Luria, A. R. (1973). *The working brain: An introduction to neuropsychology*. New York: Basic Books.

Lyons, N. P. (1983). Two perspectives on self, relationships and morality. *Harvard Educational Review, 53*, 125–145.

Lyons, N. P. (1990). Listening to voices we have not heard: Emma Willard girls' ideas about self, relationships, and morality. In C. Gilligan, N. P. Lyons, & T. J. Hanmer (Eds.), *Making connections: The relational worlds of adolescent girls at Emma Willard School* (pp. 30–72). Cambridge: Harvard University Press.

Macdonald, B., & Rich, C. (1983). *Look me in the eye*. San Francisco: Spinsters/Aunt Lute.

Mahrer, A. R. (1978). *Experiencing: A humanistic theory of psychology and psychiatry*. New York: Brunner/Mazel.

May, R., Angel, E., & Ellenberger, H. (Eds.). (1958). *Existence: A new dimension in psychiatry and psychology*. New York: Basic Books.

McAdams, D. P. (1988). *Power, intimacy, and the life story*. New York: Guilford Press.

Miller, J. B. (1976). *Toward a new psychology of women*. Boston: Beacon Press.

Miller, J. B. (1984). The development of women's sense of self. *Work in progress, No. 12* (pp. 1–15). Wellesley: Stone Center Working Papers Series.

Milner, A., Thomson, P., & Worth, C. (Eds.). (1990). *Postmodern conditions*. Oxford: Berg.

Neugarten, B. L. (1979). Time, age, and the life cycle. *The American Journal of Psychiatry, 136*(7), 887–894.

Parens, H., Pollack, L., Stern, J., & Kramer, S. (1977). On girls' entry into the Oedipus complex. In H. P. Blum (Ed.), *Female psychology: Contemporary psychoanalytic views* (pp. 79–107). New York: International Universities Press.

Randour, M. L. (1987). *Women's psyche, women's spirit*. New York: Columbia University Press.

Riegel, K. F. (1976). The dialectics of human development. *American Psychologist, 31*, 689–700.

Rowles, G. D., & Reinharz, S. D. (1988). Qualitative gerontology: Themes and challenges. In S. D. Reinharz & G. D. Rowles (Eds.), *Qualitative gerontology* (pp. 3–33). New York: Springer.

Sassen, G. (1980). Success anxiety in women: A constructivist interpretation of its sources and its significance. *Harvard Educational Review, 50*, 13–25.

Starr, J. M. (1983). Toward a social phenomenology of aging: Studying the self process in biographical work. *International Journal of Aging and Human Development, 16*(4), 255–270.

Stiver, I. P. (1986). Beyond the Oedipal complex: Mothers and daughters. In *Work in progress, No. 26* (pp. 1–34). Wellesley: Stone Center Working Paper Series.

Stoller, R. J. (1968). The sense of femaleness. *Psychoanalytic Quarterly, 37*, 42–55.

Surrey, J. (1983). The relational self in women: Clinical implications. In *Women and Empathy—Implications for psychological development and psychotherapy. Work in progress, No. 82–02* (pp. 6–11). Wellesley: Stone Center Working Papers Series.

Surrey J. (1984). Eating patterns as a reflection of women's development. *Work in progress, No. 83–06* (pp. 1–8). Wellesley: Stone Center Working Papers Series.

Tesch, R. (1990). *Qualitative research: Analysis types and research tools*. London: Falmer Press.

Thomas, L. E., & Chambers, K. O. (1989). Phenomenology of life satisfaction among elderly men: Quantitative and qualitative views. *Psychology and Aging, 4*, 284–289.

Toulmin, S. (1990). *Cosmopolis: The hidden agenda of modernity*. New York: Free Press.

Vygotsky, L. S. (1962). *Thought and language*. Cambridge, MA: M.I.T. Press.

Wertz, F. J. (1985). Methods and findings in a phenomenological psychological study of a complex life-event: Being criminally victimized. In A. Giorgi (Ed.), *Phenomenology and psychological research* (pp. 155–216). Pittsburgh: Duquesne University Press.

Wondolowski, C., & Davis, D. K. (1988). The lived experience of aging in the oldest old: A phenomenological study. *The American Journal of Psychoanalysis, 48*(3), 261–270.

Wrightsman, L. S. (1988). *Personality development in adulthood*. Newbury Park, CA: Sage.

II

Infants and Toddlers

Social interaction has its genesis almost immediately after birth as the infant and mother begin to bond. During infancy, socialization occurs primarily in the context of the family or between the infant and caretakers, who may not be relatives. For the most part, early socialization transpires during the course of the infant's needs being met. However, as the infant matures and becomes a toddler the influence of siblings increases, and socialization will take place during playlike interactions. In each instance it is important for developmental milestones to be reached in order for socialization to progress to a higher level.

The four chapters in Part II trace the infant's social development through toddlerhood. Inge Bretherton (Chapter 6) examines attachment and bonding from ethological, representational, and societal perspectives. She provides a brief overview of attachment theory and then considers parent–infant bonding, internal working models and attachment, and attachment in the context of family and society. She underscores how "secure attachment requires predictability, responsiveness, intelligibility, supportiveness, and reciprocity of commitment." Heather Walker, Daniel Messinger, Alan Fogel, and Jeanne Karns (Chapter 7) review the social and communicative development of infants in great detail. Describing research from several areas of infant development, the authors document how social and communicative development in the first 18 months of life is markedly affected by the interactive context. Celia A. Brownell and Earnestine Brown (Chapter 8) trace the developmental patterns of the play interactions of infants and toddlers with peers. In examining these issues, it is apparent that the "solitary" and "parallel play" of the first 2 years is of a more complex nature than heretofore understood. Differences in interaction in the first and second years of life are outlined. The authors then consider situational influences and performance factors and the mechanisms of development in peer play. Douglas M. Teti (Chapter 9) reviews the specific factors that contribute to sibling relationships. Despite the numerous interactions that take place between siblings during their development, the author underscores the absence of research that identifies the critical mechanisms of socialization. In this chapter, Teti describes the characteristics of early sibling relationships, sibling behavior and sibling constellation variables, and family influences on sibling relationships.

6

Attachment and Bonding

Inge Bretherton

Introduction

During the 1960s and 1970s, ethological concepts came to hold much fascination for theoreticians of human development. Animal studies on dominance hierarchies and on social bonds were especially influential. Field observations of developing parent–offspring bonds in birds (e.g., Lorenz, 1935/1957; Lorenz, 1957; Tinbergen, 1951) and mammals, especially nonhuman primates (e.g., DeVore, 1965), provided novel ways of thinking about and of studying the human infant's attachment to parents, as well as human parents' attachment to their infants. Previously unfamiliar terms, such as *imprinting, critical period, supernormal stimulus* and *fixed action pattern*, entered developmental psychologists' vocabulary.

Ethological concepts were attractive because they provided a more powerful explanation of phenomena, such as child–mother attachment, separation anxiety, and responses to bereavement than the then-current psychoanalytic theories (Bowlby, 1958, 1959, 1960). Yet psychoanalytic concepts, now dressed in the guise of ethology, remained at the heart of much of the new thinking. Although this is obvious from a close reading of Bowlby's work, it is only recently—with the rise of new theories of mental representation—that attachment researchers have rediscovered and reworked these links to psychoanalytic theory (see Bretherton, 1987, 1990).

In this chapter, I will first discuss Bowlby's (1969) evolutionary-ethological theory of infant–mother attachment. Based on a translation of psychoanalytic into ethological concepts, this theory also incorporates insights from control systems and information-processing theories. Next, I will describe how this work was both supported and extended through empirical studies conducted by Ainsworth and

Inge Bretherton • Department of Child and Family Studies, University of Wisconsin-Madison, Madison, Wisconsin 53706.

Handbook of Social Development: A Lifespan Perspective, edited by Vincent B. Van Hasselt and Michel Hersen. Plenum Press, New York, 1992.

her colleagues and students (see Ainsworth, Blehar, Waters, & Wall, 1978). To discuss parents' attachment to their infants—a topic not well elaborated in attachment theory—I will draw on the work of Klaus and Kennell (1976) and that of other researchers inspired by them. I will then show how current developments in the study of attachment from a representational perspective allow us to gain new understanding of the intergenerational transmission of attachment patterns and of attachment phenomena across the life course. This work highlights attachment theory's link to other psychoanalytic theories of interpersonal relatedness (e.g., Erikson, 1950; Sullivan, 1953; Winnicott, 1965) and is making significant contributions to the field of developmental psychopathology. Finally, I will discuss studies that place the study of attachment within a more comprehensive social framework by demonstrating that the development and maintenance of optimal attachment relations is also influenced by social networks and cultural values.

A BRIEF OVERVIEW OF ATTACHMENT THEORY

At a time when research on the topic was still sparse, Bowlby (1958) postulated that the human infant enters the world preadapted to interact with and respond to a human caregiver. We now have overwhelming evidence that his claim was justified (see Stern, 1985, for an extensive review of this literature). In addition, Bowlby proposed that attachment as an enduring affectional bond to a specific figure or figures emerges fully only during the second half of the first year of life when infants' attachment behaviors become organized into a control system that regulates proximity to a preferred figure or figures. This shift roughly coincides with the onset of locomotor abilities that allow infants to follow their parents about, to search for them when they are gone, and to approach them and seek close bodily contact when they return. It also roughly coincides with the infant's ability to understand that disappearing objects continue to exist (Piaget, 1954). Empirical evidence for a "focalization" of the infant on the primary caregiver came from an important study of foster children by Yarrow (1967), who found that the transition from foster mother to adoptive mother during the first 6 months of life caused only relatively short-lived reactions but that infants tended to have much more severe reactions if this transition was delayed into the second half of the first year.

According to Bowlby (1958, 1969) the evolutionary function of infant attachment behaviors, such as following, clinging, or crying, is proximity to a specific caregiver. Given that human and other primate infants are highly curious and exploratory creatures, chances for survival and leaving progeny are likely to be much increased if the infant is motivated to seek refuge with or call out to a protective figure when frightened. Infants' proclivity not to stray too far from their attachment figure even when at ease has a similar function. Because availability of the caregiver is important for protection, the infant experiences a feeling of security in the presence of that figure and separation anxiety when the attachment figure is physically or psychologically absent. Indeed, the impetus for attachment theory came from a need to explain the effects of maternal separation and deprivation (Bowlby, 1951).

Almost all human infants become attached to their primary caregivers, even in families where parents are abusive or neglectful. Differences in the quality of attachment relations can easily be observed, however, and are held to derive from dyad-specific transactional patterns that—by the end of the first year—become internalized as "internal working models" of self and other in relationships. Bowlby (1969, 1973) defines internal working models of self and attachment figure(s) as dynamic representations with both cognitive and affective components. He derived the term from the writings of Craik (1943), a psychologist involved in the design of intelligent rocket guidance systems. Craik suggested that organisms that carried a small-scale model of reality in their head were thereby enabled to choose among alternative courses of action and to react to anticipated situations before they arise. Bowlby was attracted to this idea of representation as simulation because it was compatible with the psychoanalytic concept of representation as an inner world.

Bowlby, elaborating on the idea of an internal working model, postulated that within an individual's internal working model of the world, working models of self and caregiver in the attachment relationship are of particular salience. Their function is to help forecast and interpret the partner's behavior, as well as to plan one's own behavior in response to the partner. Initially, internal working models of attachment relations encode a person's current patterns of attachment relations encode a person's current patterns of interaction with an attachment figure or figures. However, once formed, old patterns are imposed like templates onto new interactions (Piaget, 1954) and are not readily relinquished, even when a partner's behavior begins to change. Thus an infant who has frequently been rebuffed by a parent and has consequently become more reluctant to seek or accept comfort is not likely to respond in kind when a previously unresponsive parent suddenly becomes responsive (for example, at the end of a prolonged illness that was experienced by the infant as rejection). This, in turn, is likely to make it more difficult for a caregiver to remain responsive. The converse is also likely to be true. If the parent has been consistently responsive, the infant is not likely to abruptly change his or her expectations because of fairly infrequent parental lapses. Over the long term, however, internal working models must be accommodated to developmental and environmental change in order to adequately fulfill their function.

Because of their origin in transactional patterns, internal working models of self and caregiver are complementary to each other so that, taken together, they represent the whole relationship (see also Sroufe & Fleeson, 1986). If the caregiver has acknowledged the infant's needs for comfort and protection and respects the infant's desire to explore the environment, the child is likely to develop an internal working model of self as valued and self-reliant. However, Bowlby envisions a very different process as far as internal working models of inharmonious relationships are concerned. If the parent has frequently rebuffed the infant's bids for comfort or exploration, Bowlby speculates the child is likely to form *two competing* working models that are at odds with each other (Bowlby, 1973). One of these—accessible to awareness and discussion—represents the parent as good and the parent's rejecting behavior as due to the "badness" of the child. The other model—defensively excluded from awareness—represents the rejecting or disappointing side of the parent. Once such dual models become established, later input cannot be flexibly and appropriately processed, resulting in working models that remain ill-adapted to reality, or as Crittenden (1990) has aptly put it, working models that are not working well.

Bowlby's proposal regarding the development of two segregated working models of self and parent in unsatisfying relationships builds on Tulving's (1972) distinction between episodic and semantic memories. Episodic memory stores autobiographical memories of specific events in a person's life history, whereas semantic memory stores generic propositions (general knowledge as opposed to specific memories). Tulving believes that the two memories are based on different storage mechanisms. Be that as it may, Bowlby (1980) emphasizes that autobiographical memory derives from actual experience, whereas generic knowledge (semantic memory) may be based on distorted information supplied by others. Severe psychic conflict is likely to arise when the two sources of stored information (generalizations built on actual experience and on communications from others) are highly contradictory. As a result, defensive processes may be brought to bear on episodically stored memories derived from actual experience as a means of eliminating the conflict.

As Bowlby formulated and elaborated these ideas (1969, 1973, 1980), Ainsworth and her students began to develop methods of observation and coding through which the theory could be put to the empirical test. In so doing, Ainsworth not only validated but also substantially extended attachment theory. Her lengthy longitudinal home observations of mother–infant pairs, conducted in Uganda (Ainsworth, 1967) and later in Baltimore (Ainsworth *et al.*, 1978), yielded detailed narrative records of mother–infant interaction in a variety of contexts. In line with predictions made by Bowlby, Ainsworth and her colleagues found that a mother's sensitive, appropriate responsiveness to infant signals during feeding, physical contact, infant distress, and face-to-face play in the course of the first 3 months was related to a more harmonious (secure) attachment relationship by the end of the first year of life (for a review, see Ainsworth *et al.*, 1978).

At this point, the definition of maternal sensitivity needs clarification. Ainsworth, Bell, and Stayton (1974) termed mothers *sensitively responsive* or simply *sensitive* if they noticed their infants' signals, interpreted them accurately (by taking the infants' perspective), and then responded reasonably promptly and appropriately. Neither Bowlby nor Ainsworth precisely specified the criteria by which one was to judge accuracy of parental interpretation and appropriateness of parental responding, but they can be fairly readily derived from some of the basic assumptions underlying attachment theory (Bowlby, 1969). According to that theory, infants are preadapted to a caregiver who understands their attachment behaviors as bids for comfort, soothing, and protection, but who also permits and supports autonomous action and exploration. The optimal caregiver is one who accepts attachment behavior *and* respects strivings for autonomy. Where a caregiver fairly consistently interprets security seeking as overly demanding, or unimportant, or too often restricts the baby's desire for independent exploration, the infant's attachment behavior will not be effectively assuaged, nor will eagerness to explore be appropriately fostered. This has important sequelae for the development of communication patterns in attachment relationships. Not only is the insensitively mothered infant prevented from reaching his or her immediate goal, but he or she also repeatedly receives the implicit message, "I do not understand you"; "Your communications are not meaningful or important" (see also Stern, 1977, for extensive discussions along similar lines). Note, however, that insensitivity is not necessarily indexed by unpleasant, mean, or nasty maternal behavior. Rather, insensitivity implies that the caregiver is not reading and/or supportively responding to the infant's states or goals.

In Ainsworth's study, mothers who responded sensitively during the infant's early months during feeding (Ainsworth & Bell, 1969), face-to-fact play (Blehar,

Lieberman, & Ainsworth, 1977), physical contact (Ainsworth, Bell, Blehar, & Main, 1971), and distress episodes (Bell & Ainsworth, 1972) had infants who—during the last quarter of the first year—cried less but had a larger communicative repertoire (Ainsworth et al., 1974; Bell & Ainsworth, 1972). These infants were also more obedient (Stayton, Hogan, & Ainsworth, 1973) and demanded close bodily contact less often though they enjoyed it more (Ainsworth et al., 1971). Moreover, sensitively mothered 1-year-olds behaved differently from insensitively mothered infants in a laboratory situation known as the Strange Situation (Ainsworth et al., 1974; Ainsworth et al., 1978). It is because of correlations between the quality of interactions at home and in the Strange Situation that this procedure has now become a shortcut method for assessing the quality of infant–mother attachment, an unfortunately oft-forgotten fact.

The Strange Situation consists of a standard sequence of eight 3-minute episodes in a laboratory playroom where mother and baby are joined by an unfamiliar woman. Of special importance are two sequences during which the mother leaves the room and then returns. Infants whose mothers had responded sensitively to their signals during feeding, crying, holding, and face-to-face episodes at home during the first 3 months of life welcomed their mother's return after a brief separation in the Strange Situation. They approached her readily, sought interaction or close contact, were relatively quickly soothed, and then returned to play. These infants were labeled secure (group B).

Insensitively mothered infants either avoided the returning mother by snubbing her, looking, turning, walking away, or refusing interaction bids (insecure/avoidant, or Group A). Others responded ambivalently when the mother came back, seeking close bodily contact, but also showing angry, resistant behavior. Infants classified into this insecure/ambivalent group (C) wanted to be held but were either too distressed to approach or showed tantrumy as well as contact-seeking behavior during the reunions. At home, mothers of the avoidant babies provided less affectionate holding during the first 3 months and frequently rejected bids for close bodily contact during the last quarter of the first year. These mothers also talked about their dislike of bodily contact in conversations with the observer. Mothers of ambivalent babies, by contrast, were inconsistently sensitive at home. Although they frequently ignored their babies' signals, they did not reject close bodily contact.

More recently, Main and Hesse (1990) identified a fourth group of infants termed insecure/disorganized (group D), whose behavior does not readily fit one of the three categories defined by Ainsworth et al. (1978). The insecure/disorganized classification is given to infants who display a combination of strongly avoidant and resistant reunion behavior, as well as to infants who show a variety of behaviors that did not fit the context (sudden stilling in the midst of a greeting, very fleeting fear responses as the mother returns). Much less is known about this group, and unlike the ABC classifications, the disorganized/disoriented behavior pattern still remains to be validated against home observations during the first year of life. As we will see later, however, parents of infants classified into Group D are known to differ in a number of ways (for further details, see Main and Hesse, 1990). In particular, they often assume a controlling stance in reunions with the parent at 6 years of age (Main, Kaplan, & Cassidy, 1985).

Although both caregiver and baby contribute to reciprocal transactions from the beginning, findings from the Baltimore study indicate that, in the early phases of development, the caregiver's sensitivity to infant signals appears to be more influential in setting the tone of the relationship than are infant characteristics such as temperament (Sroufe, 1985). However, as memory and information-processing capacities improve, the infant gradually assumes a more active role in upholding emerging transactional patterns. Indeed, our understanding of such patterns in attachment relationships has taken a significant step forward through several detailed microanalytic studies of parent–child interactions undertaken in Germany by Escher-Graeub and Grossmann (1983).

In a laboratory playroom, mothers whose infants had been classified as avoidant with them in the Strange Situation joined in when the infants were cheerfully exploring the toys but withdrew when the infants showed evidence of negative feelings. Mothers of secure infants, on the other hand, watched quietly from the sidelines as long as the infants did not need them but joined in supportively when their infants showed signs of stress or distress. In the Strange Situation itself, Grossmann, Grossmann, and Schwan (1986) discovered that avoidant infants tended not to communicate with their parents nor to seek bodily contact when distressed after separation. Secure infants, on the other hand, never stayed away from a parent when they felt unhappy. In other words, once particular patterns of communication are established in a dyad they tend to be maintained by *both* partners.

Corroborating evidence for this line of argument comes from Matas, Arend, and Sroufe (1978), who discovered different communication patterns in dyads earlier classified as secure or insecure at 12 or 18 months. When faced with a difficult problem-solving task, secure 24-month-old toddlers initially worked on their own but asked for mother's assistance when they got stuck. In turn, their mothers intervened only when asked and did so effectively and supportively. Insecure toddlers, by contrast, tended to whine and give up easily, whereas their mothers tended not to offer help. In clinical samples (Lieberman & Pawl, 1990; Radke-Yarrow, Cummings, Kuczynsky, & Chapman, 1985), such mutually maladaptive communication patterns are even more apparent.

These findings not only support Bowlby's theoretical claims but are consonant with microanalytic, process-oriented studies of mother–infant synchrony versus asynchrony in face-to-face play (e.g., Brazelton, Kozlowski, & Main, 1974; Stern, Beebe, Jaffe, & Bennett, 1977; Tronick, Ricks, & Cohn, 1982) and maternal attunement and misattunement to the infant during the latter part of the first year (Stern, 1985). Thus, we now possess ample information about persistent disturbances that can occur in mother–infant communication processes.

In studies of infant–mother attachment and synchrony, the emphasis is on the importance for the developing relationship of the mother's sensitivity to her infant's signals. Researchers and theorists took it as a given that human mothers were or should be motivated to be sensitively responsive to their infants. They did not ask how this motivation arose and whether circumstances surrounding the infant's birth might facilitate or interfere with this commitment. Indeed, they did not study maternal or paternal experiences of bonding with the infant.

Parent–Infant Bonding

In 1972, Klaus, Jerauld, Kreger, McAlpine, Steffa, and Kennell published a provocative paper on maternal–infant bonding that, like Bowlby's and Ainsworth's work, was strongly influenced by ethology. Studies of mammals had shown that newborn infants' appearance and behavior are powerful elicitors of maternal nurturance and protection. For example, Klopfer (1971) had found that female goats whose young are removed immediately after birth will chase them away an hour later. However, a female who has been allowed only 5 minutes of postnatal contact with her young will reaccept it readily as much as 3 hours after removal.

From this and similar animal studies, Klaus and Kennell (1976) concluded that in many mammals there is a sensitive period after birth during which females become bonded to their young, and that, except under special conditions, bonding or adoption will not take place in some species after the sensitive period has elapsed. They cited literature showing that perinatal hormonal changes render mammalian mothers more sensitive to certain offspring stimuli that may be visual, olfactory, or tactile. For example, in goats (Klopfer, 1971) smell seems to be a potent cue, whereas sight is not. Moreover, maternal sensitive behavior quickly wanes if female goats are not given immediate access to their young.

These and related findings led Klaus, Kennell, and their colleagues to ask whether analogous processes might be observed in humans, especially because clinical reports had suggested that the first few hours after birth may be especially significant for a mother's attachment to her infant. They planned a carefully controlled study in which mothers who had given birth to their first babies were given two different types of experiences: (1) early, extended contact and (2) routine care. Routine care in the early 1970s when this investigation was conducted involved a glimpse of the baby after birth, a brief contact after 6 to 8 hours (for identification), and 20 to 30 minute feeding visits every 4 hours.

To determine whether early and extended contact affected later mother–infant interaction, the following outcome variables were used: an interview with the mother, observations of the mother during the first postnatal checkup by the pediatrician, and filmed observations of feeding interactions. During the interview, mothers with extended contact were more reluctant to leave their babies and responded more promptly when they cried. These claims were corroborated by findings from the checkup visit with the pediatrician. Extended contact mothers stood and watched the physical examination and soothed their babies more frequently if they cried. In the filmed feeding observations, extended contact mothers were more affectionate and more often held their babies in a face-to-face position. One year later, extended contact mothers again observed more closely and even helped as the pediatrician examined their babies and soothed them more when they cried. At 5 years of age, the children of extended contact mothers scored higher on IQ tests and language tests than the children of control mothers (though there had been substantial sample attrition at that time).

In a subsequent study of extended contact in Sweden, de Chateau (1976) demonstrated that, 1 year later, extended contact mothers were more affectionate than controls. Extended contact mothers also breastfed until a later age. On the basis of these studies, Klaus and Kennell (1976) proclaimed that in humans, too, there was a sensitive period after birth that was optimal for parent–child attachment. They also pointed out that infants' tendency to be alert during the hour after birth facilitated this process.

Bonding studies meshed well with attachment theory and suggested that the mother's ability to hold her infant and interact with it immediately after birth is a powerful factor in the development of maternal sensitivity. Unfortunately, the original studies had methodological weaknesses, and subsequent studies of bonding yielded more equivocal results. Lamb (1982) criticized the initial findings because personnel collecting data in these studies knew to which group mothers had been assigned. Egeland and Vaughn (1981) found no evidence that mothers with extended early contact were less likely to abuse their infants than mothers without such contact, as had been suggested by Klaus and Kennell (1976). Finally, many subsequent attempts to replicate the original findings either failed (Swejda, Campos, & Emde, 1980; Taylor, Taylor, Campbell, and others, 1979) or showed only short-lived effects (de Chateau, 1980; Grossmann, Thane, & Grossmann, 1981; Hopkins & Vietze, 1977), lasting for days, but not months or years. Indeed, at the International Conference on Infant Studies in 1978, Klaus and Kennell themselves announced that "the epoxy theory of mother–infant bonding is dead." This is not to deny that, when the birth process has gone well, the encounter with the newborn is often a magic moment for mothers and fathers (Bretherton, Biringen, Ridgeway, Maslin, & Sherman, 1989; Greenberg & Morris, 1973). We owe it to Klaus and Kennell's efforts to humanize the birth environment that parents are now able to enjoy these moments.

If sensitive parenting is an index of the quality of parental bonding, we can actually make more robust predictions of this index from knowledge of prenatal measures of parental personality than from early, extended contact. A series of studies has revealed that prenatally assessed personality and marital functioning is correlated with the quality of later mother–infant interaction (e.g., Grossman, Eichler, & Winickoff, 1980; Moss, 1967; Brunquell, Crichton, & Egeland, 1981). For example, Heinicke, Diskin, Ramsey-Klee, and Given (1983) successfully predicted quality of mother–child interaction and of maternal responsiveness from adaptation–competence scales derived from the Minnesota Multiphasic Personality Inventory. Most recently, attachment research has suggested that intergenerational factors have a significant role to play in subsequent parental attachment.

INTERNAL WORKING MODELS AND ATTACHMENT

In their summary of research on maternal–infant bonding (1976), Klaus and Kennell speculated that one important contributory variable might be the mother's care by her own mother. Bowlby, similarly, had acknowledged this idea in his earliest writings (1940) and reiterated it in his volume on separation (1973):

> Because in all these respects children tend unwittingly to identify with parents and therefore to adopt, when they become parents, the same patterns of behaviour towards children that they themselves have experienced during their own childhood, patterns of interaction are transmitted, more or less faithfully, from one generation to another. Thus the inheritance of mental health and of mental ill health through the medium of family microculture is certainly no less important, and may well be far more important, than is their inheritance through the medium of genes. (p. 323)

When these ideas were belatedly taken up by attachment researchers in the 1980s, they yielded provocative findings. These did not strictly support the notion that individuals parent their children as they were parented. Instead of discovering a direct connection between security or insecurity of current parent–child relations and reported quality of the parent's childhood attachments, these studies showed that the content of parental memories was less important than whether the parents were able to discuss these memories with emotional openness and coherence (Main *et al.*, 1985; Ricks, 1985). Sometimes "ghosts" from the nursery (Fraiberg, Adelson, & Shapiro, 1975) can evidently be laid to rest. In addition, Main *et al.* discovered that children classified as secure with their mothers as infants were later able to discuss attachment issues openly and coherently with another adult. Taken together, these studies suggest that attachment partners who can communicate appropriately and with emotional openness *within* relationships are also better able to communicate coherently and openly *about* such relationships with third persons. In this section, I review the new body of literature in detail, linking it to Bowlby's concept of internal working models of self and other in attachment relationships in order to explain the intergenerational transmission of attachment patterns (see also Bretherton, 1990, 1991).

In their ground-breaking study, Main *et al.* (1985) discovered that the quality of children's attachment to parents—as observed at 1 and 6 years of age—is impressively correlated with specific patterns of parental responding to the Berkeley Adult Attachment Interview. This structured, open-ended interview probed for parental recollections of childhood attachment figures as well as for thoughts about the significance of attachment relations in general, including their influence on the parent's own development. To evaluate the interview, Main *et al.* (1985) eschewed the more usual procedure of analyzing responses to each question. Rather, each interview transcript was examined as a whole. Such overall analysis of the interview text revealed that parents of 6-year-olds classified as secure with them in infancy valued both attachment and autonomy and were at ease when discussing the influence of attachment-related issues upon their own development (whether or not they recalled a secure childhood).

Parents of children who were classified as insecure/avoidant with them in infancy, dismissed and devalued attachment, feeling that early attachment experiences had little effect on their own development. They frequently claimed not to remember any incidents from childhood. Specific memories that emerged despite such denial were likely to contradict the generalized (often highly idealized) descriptions of parents.

Parents of children previously classified as insecure/resistant seemed preoccupied with early family attachments. These parents were able to recall many specific, often conflict-ridden incidents about childhood attachments but could not integrate them into an overall picture. In sum, both the dismissing and preoccupied groups found it difficult to discuss attachment relationships in an integrated way.

Finally, parents of children classified as insecure/disorganized in infancy seemed to be struggling with unresolved issues concerning loss of a parent before maturity (see Main & Solomon, 1990). Since 1985, these results have been replicated in two other samples (Eichberg, 1987; Fonagy, Steele, & Steele, 1991; Grossmann, Fremmer-Bombik, Rudolph, & Grossmann, 1991; Ward, Carlson, Altman, Levine, Greenberg, & Kessler, 1990).

One could, of course, argue that correlations between infant–parent attachment and the parent's account of his or her own childhood attachment derive from selective recall cued by the experience with a specific child. The studies by Fonagy *et al.* and by Ward *et al.* were therefore especially important because their Adult Attachment Interviews were conducted before the infant's birth. Selective recall can therefore not explain why insecure (dismissing and preoccupied) interviews predicted insecure attachment classifications at 1 year of age.

In her longitudinal study, Main *et al.* (1985) also discovered that 6-year-olds classified as secure with mother in infancy (on the basis of Strange Situation behavior) gave coherent, elaborated, and open responses to drawings of parent–child separation scenes, graded from mild to stressful. In addition, these children tended to volunteer information about their own separation experiences. In contrast, children earlier judged insecure/avoidant with mother described the pictured children as sad but could not say what they could have done in response to separation. Children classified as disorganized/disoriented (Main & Hesse, 1990) were often completely silent or gave irrational or bizarre responses (Main *et al.*, 1985; for similar findings, see Cassidy, 1988; Slough & Greenberg, 1990).

Building on Main *et al.*'s (1985) findings, Bretherton, Ridgeway, and Cassidy (1990) undertook a study of even younger children. These 37-month-olds were asked to complete attachment doll-story stems. If children addressed the story issues with little hesitation and invented benign resolutions, they were classified as secure. If, on the other hand, they produced irrelevant or very bizarre story resolutions (after a separated family is reunited, they have a car crash), or if they had to be prompted for a response many times, the children were classified as insecure. Secure-insecure classifications of doll story responses were highly concordant with classifications of an actual separation–reunion procedure.

These assessments suggest that children's representations of attachment relations as produced in verbal or enacted narratives reflect actual relationships. In other words, how a child communicates (behaves) *within* an attachment relationship can help predict how that child communicates *about* attachment relationships to a third person. This also holds for parents (Bretherton *et al.*, 1989) and for young adults (Kobak & Sceery, 1988).

Before I go on to discuss how working models mediate the link between quality of communication patterns within attachment relationships and about attachment relationships, I would like to more closely examine Bowlby's notion of working models in the context of current theories of representation.

Note that the concept of internal working model implies a representational system that operates with dynamic event– or agent–action–object structures in order to simulate reality. When Bowlby first incorporated the concept of internal working models into his writings, no existing theory of mental representation dealt with thinking as internal simulation of real-world action. In the meantime, progress in cognitive science has provided some useful hints.

The term *internal working model* can be used in two senses: models that are stored in *long-term memory* and models that are "composed" in short-term or working memory to understand new situations as the need arises. The storage, retrieval, operation, and construction of working models in long-term and working memory would seem to require at least the following: (1) a flexibly and hierarchically organized representational system that stores information in such a way that, when retrieved, it can be operated upon as "inner world"; (2) procedures whereby specific aspects of this information can be located when necessary; (3) procedures whereby this information is retrieved into a temporary "scratch space" in working memory; (4) procedures that operate on information in the "scratch space" (Hendrix, 1979) to generate new information; and (5) procedures whereby new information constructed in working memory is fed back into the long-term representational system or knowledge base.

Different cognitive theorists have concerned themselves with different aspects of this problem. For example, in a recent reworking of Craik's (1943) concept, Johnson-Laird (1983) writes about advantages of being able to construct and test mental models in working memory. He discovered that reasoning ability improves markedly when adults are able to construct a mental model of a concrete problem situation and declines when the same problem is presented in terms of abstract symbols (Wason & Johnson-Laird, 1972). Although he assumes that to construct such concrete models of reality an individual must be able to retrieve from long-term memory relevant elements (representations of people or objects) and relations (spatial, temporal, causal) from which to compose such models, Johnson-Laird does not reflect on what type of long-term memory organization might be required.

Other theorists, by contrast, have concerned themselves with the structure of long-term memory, without paying much heed to issues of retrieval and extrapolation of old information to new situations. For example, building on Bartlett's (1933) work on remembering, Mandler (1979), Neisser (1987), Nelson and Gruendel (1981) and Schank and Abelson (1977), proposed hypothetical entities, termed *event schemata* or *scripts*, that were defined as sequentially organized representational structures with "slots" for specific agent roles, for action sequences motivated by specific goals and emotions, for recipients of actions, and for locales. Schank and Abelson argued that in processing new recurrences of a familiar event, individuals "instantiate" the relevant stored script or event scheme to help predict what might happen next. However, Schank and Abelson do not specify how the relevant script is identified and retrieved, nor do they solve the problem of how an individual might extrapolate to new, never-before-encountered events.

Some conceptual help comes from Schank's (1982) revised formulation of script theory in which he refined his ideas about the organization of long-term memory. In this later work, he argued that components of episodic or autobiographical memories are reprocessed, partitioned, cross-indexed, and summarized into a variety of different schema categories, each of which simulates some aspect of the spatiotemporal-causal-affective-motivational structure of experience. Only some of these schemata organize mini-event representations into coordinated, longer event sequences (such as the "script" of going to a restaurant or putting a baby to bed); others summarize information derived from similar mini-events (e.g., all infant–mother feeding situations regardless of context); and yet others generalize across different event sequences (e.g., all caregiving routines). Note that Schank's new conceptualization blurs the distinction between episodic (autobiographical) and semantic memory (the generic knowledge base) as originally proposed by Tulving (1972, 1983) and substitutes instead a set or web of multiply-interconnected hierarchies composed of schemata that range from being very experience-near to being very general and abstract. There hierarchies are constructed and continually revised and refined on the basis of new input (for related ideas, see Nelson, 1986) and thus provide the building blocks for the recombination of elements of old schemata or part schemata into new mental models, although the question of retrieval is not addressed. Related ideas were proposed by Neisser (1988), who emphasized the obvious fact that humans can remember the same event at many levels of analysis (e.g., the global structure of an event such as a conference; specific talks given during the conference; and sometimes particular pronouncements made during a specific talk), with lower-order events nested in those of higher order.

How does this help us conceptualize internal working models of self and other in attachment relations? Is it not true that theories of event representation were primarily generated in response to a need to explain children's and adult's understanding of common routines such as eating at a restaurant or having lunch at the daycare center? Despite the fact that they were developed with a different aim in mind, I suggest that theories of event representation are entirely consonant with the idea that individuals may develop mental models of relationships with *specific partners*. They accord well with Epstein's (1973, 1980) notion of the self-concept as a hierarchy of postulates (or schemata, as I prefer to call them). At the lowest level would be interactional schemata that are very experience-near ("When I hurt myself, my mommy always comes to comfort and help me"). Above this level would be more general schemata ("My mommy is usually there for me when I need her") that subsume a variety of lower level schemata of need-fulfilling events with mother. Somewhere near the top of the hierarchy would be such schemata as "My mother is a loving person" and "I am loved," each subsuming a variety of lower level schemata.

Note also that there is no need to postulate that all of these schemata are directly accessible to conscious reflection. Some may only be available as procedural knowledge. It may be most fruitful to think of internal working models as composed of hierarchically organized schema systems with an unknown but finite number of levels, rather than as dual-level models composed of episodic and semantic memories as suggested by Bowlby (1980). Current theorizing is also concordant with the notion that internal working models of self and other consist of interlinked web of schema hierarchies, not a single hierarchy as proposed by Epstein (1973, 1980). In fact, an individual's schema hierarchies of self, other, and world are probably not neatly segregated from each other because all schemata (i.e., of the physical environment, of "human nature," of attachment relationships in general, and of specific relationships) are likely to feed back into each other (Guidano & Liotti, 1983).

Finally, whereas Schank (1982) was not specifically concerned with biased or incomplete processing of experience, his revised theory can provide at least some tools for rethinking the operation of defensive phenomena in the construction of working models. If portions of an individual's autobiographical memories enter into cross-referenced schemata at many levels in a variety of schema hierarchies, it is possible to see how defensive processes might selectively interfere in this cross-referencing. For example, one might speculate that material that has been defensively excluded from recall as an autobiographical memory might still influence schema formation at other levels (i.e., general schemata about parenting), thus making the model internally inconsistent and contradictory. The converse might also occur. Autobiographical episodes may be accessible to consciousness but be prevented from extensive further processing and therefore from proper integration into the individual's working model of the world. Once lines of communication within the representational system (working model of the world) are partially or completely severed, later input will not be adequately processed because distorted or dissociated schemata now guide the processing of new experience (Erdelyi, 1985).

I therefore suggest that we get away from the idea that an insecure individual may have two separate but well-organized working models of the same relationship: one based on semantic memory and accessible to conscious reflection and verbal discussion and a second based on episodic or autobiographical memory but defensively excluded from awareness. Instead, I favor the view that insecure individuals have an ill-organized working model of self and attachment figure in which many relevant schemas or schema networks are dissociated from one another across and within hierarchical levels, hence giving rise to contradictory communication with others. In such an ill-organized model, updating of information may occur at one level of the hierarchy but may then not propagate to others; or schemata of what should or might be may not be clearly tagged as such and hence treated as schemata of actual circumstances. The possible confusions, contradictions, and distortions in the interpretation and conduct of attachment relations that such malfunctioning (and hence inflexible) internal working models could generate are endless. Further research on defensive processes will, of course, be necessary to clarify these ideas further, in particular as they pertain to the organizational levels at which biased storage and retrieval of information is taking place. Dismissing adults and avoidant children seem to keep schemata within and across hierarchical levels compartmentalized so that activation of one schema leaves the other unaffected. Preoccupied adults and resistant children, by contrast, seem unable to use autobiographical memories to create summary schemata of their attachment relationships.

Seen from this perspective, recent findings on the intergenerational transmission of secure or insecure attachment patterns become more comprehensible. Even before the birth of an infant, parents have anticipatory working models of themselves as parents and of the unborn infant (Brazelton & Cramer, 1990; Zeanah, Keener, Stewart, & Anders, 1985). When the infant is born, these anticipatory working models must be corrected and fine-tuned to fit the individual baby's temperament and needs (see also Stern, 1985). This task will be relatively easy if the new parents' internal working models are coherent and well organized, and if schemata, whether or not they are accessible to awareness, have not been defensively distorted in a major way. It will be much more difficult if the parent's internal working models are ill organized. In this case, a parent is not only likely to misinterpret attachment signals from an infant but is also likely to provide misleading feedback, thereby making it difficult for the infant to "get it right" (Emde, personal communication). In other words, a parent with a distorted, ill-organized working model of attachment relations is likely, in turn, to communicate with his or her infant in such a way as to interfere with the infant's ability to construct adequate, well-organized internal working models of interpersonal relations. This is likely to have two serious consequences: (1) Both partners will experience continuing difficulties in communicating effectively with each other and (2) both partners' inadequate working models will be difficult to update adequately as the relationships develop and/or the environment demands (for more details regarding developmental implications, see Bretherton, 1987).

Under this view, the converse happens for secure parents whose internal working model of attachment figures and of attachment relationships in general is well organized and reasonably consistent within and across hierarchical levels. Such parents are likely to give the infant helpful and informative feedback, and this will in turn facilitate flexible adaptation to other relationships. Furthermore, both partners' internal working models will be easier to update because the relevant schemata are connected to one another in systematic ways, within and across hierarchical levels of the representational system whether the schemata are directly accessible to awareness or not.

If this approach to working models is correct several things follow: (1) Because reorganization or reconstruction of an ill-organized working model acquired in an unsatisfying attachment relationship will require integration of dissociated or segregated information at many different levels, insight at one level is not automatically followed by insight at another level. The reconstruction of such ill-organized working models will require change at many levels. (2) The developing infant encounters in the parent's behavior the output of the parent's current working model of self in attachment relationships. If a parent with unhappy childhood attachments has been able to rework an initially ill-organized working model into a coherent, well-organized representation of early attachment relationships, whether satisfying or not, and if that parent has also been able to construct a new working model of self in a supportive attachment relationship, the infant will not experience a reenactment of the parent's unhappy childhood relations. On the basis of open and adequate reciprocal communication, such an infant will develop a secure attachment despite the fact that the parent has not experienced secure relations in childhood him- or herself. Main and Goldwyn (in press) as well as other investigators using the adult attachment interview have found corroborating evidence for such a position.

As previously noted, sensitive parental responsiveness (Ainsworth *et al.*, 1974) requires that the parent be ready to take the baby's perspective, to understand the baby's goals, and to respond to them empathically. Without adequate internal working models of self as parent in relation to a specific infant, the parent cannot provide appropriate empathic feedback or acknowledge the infant's signals. If a high proportion of a child's attachment or autonomy signals are not needed or misread, open communication *within* attachment relationships will be impeded because defensively excluded material cannot be used for error-correcting feedback. This in turn will lead the child to develop inadequate internal working models of self.

ATTACHMENT, FAMILY, AND SOCIETY

Although we have made progress in examining mother–child attachment in terms of representation and communication, much work remains to be done in terms of other attachment-related phenomena in the family. For example, we need to gain a much better understanding of child–father attachment, despite studies by Belsky, Gilstrap, and Rovine (1984), Lamb (1978), and Parke and Tinsley (1987) that show fathers to be competent if sometimes less than fully participant attachment figures. In Main *et al.*'s study, infant–father attachment classifications were less strongly related to the father's Adult Attachment Interview classifications than had been found for the mother. Another important topic is sibling attachment, which has been tackled by Stewart and Marvin (1984) as well as Teti and Ablard (1989), but their work is only a beginning. Dunn (1988) has undertaken an interesting study of triadic relations between a mother and two siblings, an important topic that has so far been neglected by attachment researchers. What is more, although triadic studies of parent–child relationships have become more common (for a discussion, see Bronfenbrenner and Crouter, 1982, p. 380; see also Clarke-Stewart, 1979; Lewis & Feiring, 1979), our understanding of family triads is not nearly as advanced as our understanding of dyads. This is especially true when we consider topics, such as loyalty conflicts, alliances by a dyad vis-à-vis a third family member, and enmeshment of a child in the spousal dyad. These topics are highly relevant to attachment theory, though they have not been considered by attachment theorists and researchers, a trend that may be changing. A recent exploratory study (Fish, Belsky, & Youngblade, 1991) shows that parents who violate intergenerational boundaries by inappropriately involving a 4-year-old child in spousal decision making differ from parents who do not, both in terms of earlier attachment classifications with the child and in terms of observed marital interaction.

The well-known work on parent–adolescent communication by Hauser and his colleagues (Hauser, Powers, Noam, Jacobson, Weiss, & Follansbee, 1984) is highly compatible with attachment theory, though it predated work on internal working models. Hauser *et al.* found that adolescent ego development is related to the communication styles adopted by parents toward the adolescent during a familial conflict-resolution task. Adolescent with high levels of ego development had parents both of whom engaged in more enabling versus constraining and devaluing discourse toward the adolescent. This study is also consonant with Kobak and Sceery's (1988) study of young adults, using the Adult Attachment Interview.

Research on marital relations and divorce has been informed by attachment theory since the 1970s (Weiss, 1973, 1977, 1982) but has taken a recent upsurge with work by Shaver and Hazan (1988). These authors translated Ainsworth's infant attachment patterns into the study of adult love relationships, pointing out that adults who describe themselves as secure, avoidant, and ambivalent with respect to romantic relationships report differing patterns of parent–child relations in their families of origin. Finally, Cicirelli (1989, 1991) is applying attachment theory to the study of middle-aged siblings and their elderly parents. Thus, attachment theory and research has been extended to family dyads other than the mother–child couple and is now concerned with all phases of the life course. Future work will be needed to delineate more fully the distinct qualities of child–adult, child–child, and adult–adult attachment relationships and their interplay within the family system as well as to study these relationships from the communication/representation perspective adopted in this chapter.

Finally, although attachment theory speaks to the intergenerational transmission of parenting patterns, it does not explicitly deal with the continued sex-gender differentiation of parenting. Some feminist theorists have interpreted attachment theory as one that supports the traditional view of women as primary caregivers (Chodorow, 1978; Johnson, 1988). This is not strictly justified because attachment theory does not specify that caregiving must be done by mothers or be restricted to females (Marris, 1982). Most central to healthy development, according to attachment theory, is the infant's need for a committed caregiving relationship with one or a few adult figures. Although the majority of attachment studies have focused on mothers because mothers tend to most often fill this role, we do have evidence that infants can be attached to a hierarchy of figures, including fathers, grandparents, and siblings (Schaffer & Emerson, 1964) as well as daycare providers. However, our knowledge about the range of societal options for successfully sharing the task of bringing up children is still woefully inadequate. The recent spate of studies documenting an increased risk of insecure attachment if daycare begins in the first year and is extensive in duration (Belsky & Rovine, 1988) is worrisome, although cross-cultural studies of attachment and daycare in countries such as Sweden or Israel may ultimately provide some reliable answers.

Family and Social Network

Aside from further studies of other attachment dyads across the lifespan, we also need studies that embed attachment in the larger context of family, social network, and society. A prime example of one study that systematically explores family and social network factors as they affect attachment relations was the Pennsylvania Infant and Family Development Project (e.g., Belsky & Isabella, 1988; Belsky, Rovine, & Taylor, 1984). At issue was the prediction of infant–mother attachment security at the end of the child's first year from a set of theoretically guided variables that included not only the mother's evaluation of the social support she received from her spouse and from extrafamilial sources. Interestingly, mother–child attachment quality at the end of the first year was predictable not from *absolute* levels of marital satisfaction before or after the child's birth but from *relative* changes in levels of satisfaction. Marital satisfaction declined in all families, but parents of secure infants reported significantly *less* decline in marital satisfaction than parents of insecure infants.

As for the social network variables, it was not frequency of supportive behaviors but the parents' *rating* of neighbors as friendly and helpful that were significantly correlated with the infant's secure attachment to mother. Belsky had originally planned to ask such complex questions of the data as: "To what extent is being an irritable infant not related to insecure-ambivalent attachment when the mother is mature, with a satisfying marriage and a supportive social network"; or "To what extent is neonatal alertness not related to later security when mothers are psychologically immature and involved in unsatisfying marriages?" The data structure, however, was simpler: It did not matter which specific variables (personality, marital satisfaction, perceived and observed child temperament) were examined. When all factors functioned in a positive, supportive mode, attachment was secure. When all functioned in a nonsupportive mode, attachment was insecure. Finally, Belsky and Isabella (1988) showed that maternal personality was both directly and indirectly related (via marital change) to secure attachment.

Cross-Cultural Studies

Moving from family and social network to the larger societal matrix, studies of Ainsworth Strange Situation classifications in other cultures have sparked a lively debate on the universal versus culture-specific meaning of attachment patterns assessed in the Strange Situation. In a North German study, avoidant Strange Situation classifications were overrepresented (Grossmann, Grossmann, Spangler, Suess, & Unzer, 1985). In Israeli kibbutzim (Sagi, Lamb, Lewkowicz, Shoham, Dvir, & Estes, 1985) and in Japanese samples (Miyake, Chen, & Campos, 1985), on the other hand, ambivalent classifications were overrepresented.

Initial interpretations of these cross-national differences were couched in purely cultural terms. Thus Grossmann *et al.* (1985) proposed that the high incidence of avoidant infants in Germany could not be attributed to a higher incidence of rejection among German parents. Rather, German parents placed more emphasis on self-reliance toward the end of the first year. Hence, avoidant classifications in Germany and the United States did not carry the same meaning for the participants in the relationship. Similarly, the high frequency of ambivalent classifications observed in Israeli kibbutzim and Japan were said to be due to the fact that kibbutz infants were rarely exposed to complete strangers (Sagi *et al.*, 1985) or that Japanese infants were rarely left with a stranger (Miyake *et al.*, 1985). Unfortunately these cultural explanations were neither based on systematic assessments of parental beliefs, nor on close observations of parent–infant interactions.

Since publication of these studies, van IJzendoorn & Kroonenberg (1988) examined frequency distributions of Strange Situation classifications from over a thousand U.S. and cross-national studies, pointing out that valid conclusions about cross-national differences cannot be drawn from single samples. Even within the United States, certain classifications are over- or underrepresented in particular studies. More important, correlations between observed mother–infant interactions and Strange Situation classifications were quite similar in North Germany and the Ainsworth's Baltimore study. Similarly, Sagi, Avizer, Mayseless, Donnell, & Joels (1991) now attribute the abundance of ambivalent Strange Situation classifications to specific nighttime caregiving arrangements in the kibbutzim they studied, rather than to differences in experiences with strangers. Israeli city infants in full-time daycare did not show the same preponderance of ambivalent classifications. Taken in combination, these findings suggest that Strange Situation classifications, and hence the concept of parental sensitivity, may have more cross-cultural validity in industrialized nations than was initially believed.

Systematic work on the more interesting topic of how different cultures—especially non-Western cultures—fit attachment behaviors and relationships into their overall social organization has barely begun. There are, however, some tantalizing suggestions in the ethnographic literature (see Bretherton, 1985, for a review). For example, the Micronesian society of Tikopia (Firth, 1936) deliberately fosters attachment between an infant and its maternal uncle by prescribing that he engage in face-to-face talk with the infant on a regular basis. This maternal uncle is destined to play an important quasi-parental role in the life of the child. Along somewhat different lines, Balinese mothers control their infants' exploratory behavior by using fake fear expressions to bring the infants back into close proximity to them (Bateson & Mead, 1942). In both places, a biological system is molded to a particular society's purposes (fostering specific relationships, controlling exploration).

Especially instructive is a recent study based on observation of everyday parent–infant interaction among the Efe, a seminomadic group whose members live in the African rain forest, subsisting on foraging, horticulture, and hunting (Tronick, Winn, & Morelli, 1985). The Efe's child-rearing system relies on multiple caregiving by the group's adult women. During the first 6 months of life infants receive more care (including nursing) from other adult women than from their own mother, though they sleep exclusively with her at night. Beginning at around 6 months, infants nevertheless insist on more focalized relations with their own mothers, but other female caregivers continue to play a significant role. Caregiving by mother and other adults is sensitive and responsive until the third year of life when growing demands are placed on toddlers, and requests for nursing and comforting increasingly denied, despite the fact that the caregiving adults are quite aware of the stress this places upon the toddler.

Tronick explains Efe caregiving practices in terms of two conflicting requirements. On the one hand, families live in closely spaced dwellings that offer little privacy. For this reason, cooperation and sharing are highly valued behaviors. On the other the Efe move camp frequently, and group composition is flexible, with families moving in and out of the group. Tronick contends that flexibility of group membership calls for an ability to let go of close relationships. Whether or not Tronick's interpretation coincides with the Efe's own, his study demonstrates that attachment behavior is never purely instinctive, but is heavily overlain with cultural prescriptions even in a society that much more closely resembles the conditions of human evolution than our own. To better explore cultural variations in attachment organization attempted by societies with different living arrangements and value systems, the field needs ecologically valid, theory-driven observational and interview measures, tailored to these specific cultures and based on a deeper knowledge of parents' and children's folk theories about family relationships in these cultures.

Concluding Remarks

The discussion of cultural specificity in attachment patterns raises a larger question concerning the societal support for attachment relationships. In a thought-provoking chapter, Marris (1991) points to the fundamental tension between the desire to create a secure and predictable social order and the desire to maximize one's own opportunities at the expense of others. The opportunity to provide optimal support to a developing child is not equally open to all parents. A good society, according to Marris, would be one that, as far as is humanly possible, minimizes disruptive events, protects each child's experience of attachment from harm, and supports family coping. Yet in order to control uncertainty, individuals and families are tempted to achieve certainty at the expense of others (i.e., by imposing a greater burden of uncertainty on them; by providing fewer material and social resources). Secure attachment requires predictability, responsiveness, intelligibility, supportiveness, and reciprocity of commitment. Where powerful groups in society promote their own control over life circumstances by subordinating and marginalizing others, they make it less possible for these groups to offer and experience security in their own families. Valuing of attachment relations thus has political and moral implications for society, not just psychological implications for attachment dyads.

References

Ainsworth, M. D. S. (1967). *Infancy in Uganda: Child care and the growth of love.* Baltimore: The Johns Hopkins University Press.

Ainsworth, M. D. S., & Bell, S. M. (1969). Some contemporary patterns in the feeding situation. In A. Ambrose (Ed.), *Stimulation in early infancy* (pp. 133–170). London: Academic Press.

Ainsworth, M. D. S., Bell, S. M., Blehar, M. C., & Main, M. (1971, April). *Physical contact: A study of infant responsiveness and its relation to maternal handling.* Paper presented at the biennial meeting of the Society for Research in Child Development, Minneapolis.

Ainsworth, M. D. S., Bell, S. M., & Stayton, D. (1974). Infant–mother attachment and social development. In M. P. Richards (Ed.), *The introduction of the child into a social world* (pp. 99–135). London: Cambridge University Press.

Ainsworth, M. D. S., Blehar, M. C., Waters, E., & Wall, S. (1978). *Patterns of attachment: A psychological study of the strange situation.* Hillsdale, NJ: Erlbaum.

Bartlett, F. C. (1933). *Remembering: A study in experimental and social psychology*. London: Cambridge University Press.

Bateson, G., & Mead, M. (1942). *Balinese character: A photographic analysis*. New York: New York Academy of Sciences.

Bell, S. M., & Ainsworth, M. D. S. (1972). Infant crying and maternal responsiveness. *Child Development, 43*, 1171–1190.

Belsky, J., Gilstrap, B., & Rovine, M. (1984). The Pennsylvania Infant and Family Development Project, I: Stability and change in mother–infant and father–infant interaction in a family setting at one, three, and nine months. *Child Development, 55*, 692–705.

Belsky, J., & Isabella, R. (1988). Maternal, infant, and social-contextual determinants of attachment security. In J. Belsky & T. Nezworski (Eds.), *Clinical implications of attachment* (pp. 41–94). Hillsdale, NJ: Erlbaum.

Belsky, J., & Nezworski (1988). *Clinical implications of attachment*. Hillsdale, NJ: Erlbaum.

Belsky, J., & Rovine, M. (1988). Nonmaternal care in the first year of life and the security of infant–parent attachment. *Child Development, 59*, 157–167.

Belsky, J., Rovine, M., & Taylor, D. (1984). The Pennsylvania Infant and Family Development Project II: Origins of individual differences in infant–mother attachment: Maternal and infant contributions. *Child Development, 55*, 706–717.

Blehar, M. C., Lieberman, A. F., & Ainsworth, M. D. S. (1977). Early face-to-face interaction and its relation to later infant–mother attachment. *Child Development, 48*, 182–194.

Bowlby, J. (1940). The influence of early environment in the development of neurosis and neurotic character. *International Journal of Psycho-Analysis, XXI*, 1–25.

Bowlby, J. (1951). *Maternal care and mental health*. Geneva: World Health Organization.

Bowlby, J. (1958). The child's tie to his mother. *International Journal of Psycho-Analysis, XXXIX*, 1–23.

Bowlby, J. (1959). Separation anxiety. *International Journal of Psycho-Analysis, XLI*, 1–25.

Bowlby, J. (1960). Grief and mourning in infancy. *The Psychoanalytic Study of the Child, XV*, 3–39.

Bowlby, J. (1969). *Attachment and loss. Vol. 1: Attachment*. (2nd revised ed., 1982). New York: Basic Books.

Bowlby, J. (1973). *Attachment and loss. Vol. 2: Separation*. New York: Basic Books.

Bowlby, J. (1980). *Attachment and loss, Vol. 3: Loss, sadness and depression*. New York: Basic Books.

Brazelton, T. B., & Cramer, B. G. (1990). *The earliest relationship*. Reading, MA: Addison Wesley.

Brazelton, T. B., Kozlowski, B., & Main, M. (1974). The origins of reciprocity in mother–infant interactions. In M. Lewis & L. A. Rosenblum (Eds.), *The effect of the infant on its caregiver*. New York: Wiley.

Bretherton, I. (1985). Attachment theory: Retrospect and prospect. In I. Bretherton & E. Waters (Eds.), Growing points of attachment theory and research. *Monographs of the Society for Research in Child Development, 50*, Serial No. 209 (1–2), 3–35.

Bretherton, I. (1987). New perspectives on attachment relations: Security, communication, and internal working models. In J. Osofsky (Ed.), *Handbook of infant development* (pp. 1061–1100). New York: Wiley.

Bretherton, I. (1990). Open communication and internal working models: Their role in the development of attachment relationships. In R. A. Thompson (Ed.), *Socioemotional development. Nebraska Symposium on Motivation 1988* (pp. 59–113). Lincoln: University of Nebraska Press.

Bretherton, I. (1991). Pouring new wine into old bottles: The social self as internal working model. In M. Gunnar & L. A. Sroufe (Eds.), *Self processes in development* (pp. 1–41). Hillsdale, NJ: Erlbaum.

Bretherton, I., Biringen, Z., & Ridgeway, D., Maslin, C., & Sherman, M. (1989). Attachment: The parental perspective. *Infant Mental Health Journal, 10*, 203–221.

Bretherton, I., Ridgeway, D., & Cassidy, J. (1990). Assessing internal working models of the attachment relationship: An attachment story completion task for 3-year-olds. In D. Cicchetti, M. Greenberg, & E. M. Cummings (Eds.), *Attachment during the preschool years* (pp. 272–308). Chicago: University of Chicago Press.

Bronfenbrenner, U., & Crouter, A. (1982). Work and family through time and space. In S. B. Kamerman & C. D. Hayes (Eds.), *Families that work: Children in a changing world* (pp. 39–83). Washington, DC: National Academy Press.

Brunquell, D., Crichton, L., & Egeland, B. (1981). Maternal personality and attitude in disturbances of child rearing. *American Journal of Orthopsychiatry, 51*, 680–691.

Cassidy, J. (1988). The self as related to child-mother attachment at six. *Child Development, 59*, 121–134.

Chodorow, N. (1978). *The reproduction of mothering: Psychoanalysis and the sociology of gender*. Berkeley: University of California Press.

Cicirelli, V. G. (1989). Feelings of attachment to siblings and well-being in later life. *Psychology and Aging, 4,* 211–216.

Cicirelli, V. G. (1991). Attachment theory in old age: Protection of the attached figure. In K. Pillemer & K. McCartney (Eds.), *Parent-child relations across the life course* (pp. 25–42). Hillsdale, NJ: Erlbaum.

Clarke-Stewart, K. A. (1979). And daddy makes three: The father's impact on mother and young child. *Child Development, 49,* 466–478.

Craik, K. (1943). *The nature of explanation.* Cambridge: Cambridge University Press.

Crittenden, P. (1990). Internal representational models of attachment relationships. *Infant Mental Health Journal, 11,* 259–277.

de Chateau, P. (1976). *Neonatal care routines: Influences of maternal and infant behaviour and on breastfeeding.* Unpublished thesis, Umea, Sweden.

de Chateau, P. (1980). Early post-partum contact and later attitudes. *International Journal of Behavioral Development, 3,* 273–286.

DeVore, I. (1965). *Primate behavior: Field studies of monkeys and apes.* New York: Holt, Rinehart & Winston.

Dunn, J. (1988). *The beginnings of social understanding.* Cambridge: Harvard University Press.

Egeland, B., & Vaughn, B. (1981). Failure of "bond formation" as a cause of abuse, neglect, and maltreatment. *American Journal of Orthopsychiatry, 51,* 78–84.

Eichberg, D. (1987, April). *Quality of infant-parent attachment: Related to mother's representation of her own relationship history.* Paper presented at the biennial meetings of the Society for Research i n Child Development, Baltimore.

Epstein, S. (1973). The self-concept revisited or a theory of a theory. *American Psychologist, 28,* 404–416.

Epstein, S. (1980). A review and the proposal of an integrated theory of personality. In E. Staub (Ed.), *Personality: Basic aspects and current research* (pp. 82–131). Englewood Cliffs, NJ: Prentice-Hall.

Erdelyi, H. M. (1985). *Psychoanalysis: Freud's cognitive psychology.* San Francisco: W. H. Freeman.

Erikson, E. (1950). *Childhood and Society.* New York: Norton.

Escher-Graeub, D., & Grossmann, K. E. (1983). *Bindungssicherheit im zweiten Lebensjahr-die Regensburger Querschnittuntersuchung* [Attachment security in the second year of life: The Regensburg cross-sectional study]. Research Report, University of Regensburg.

Firth, R. (1936). *We, the Tikopia.* London: Allen & Unwin.

Fish, M., Belsky, J., & Youngblade, L. (1991). Developmental antecedents and measurement of inter-generational boundary violation in a nonclinic sample. *Family Psychology, 4,* 278–297.

Fonagy, P., Steele, H., & Steele, M. (1991). Maternal representations of attachment during pregnancy predict the organization of infant–mother attachment at one year of age. *Child Development, 62,* 891–905.

Fraiberg, s., Adelson, E., & Shapiro, V. (1975). Ghosts in the nursery: A psychoanalytic approach to the problems of impaired infant-mother relationships. *Journal of the American Academy of Child Psychiatry, 14,* 387–421.

George, C., Kaplan, N., & Main, M. (1984). *Adult Attachment Interview for Adults.* Unpublished manuscript, University of California, Berkeley.

Greenberg, M., & Morris, N. (1973). Engrossment: The newborn's impact upon the father. *American Journal of Orthopsychiatry, 4,* 520–531.

Grossman, F. K., Eichler, L. S., & Winickoff, S. A. (1980). *Pregnancy, birth and parenthood.* San Francisco: Jossey-Bass.

Grossmann, K., Fremmer-Bombik, E., Rudolph, J., & Grossmann, K. E. (1991). Maternal attachment representations as related to patterns of infant–mother attachment and maternal care during the first year. In R. A. Hinde & J. Stevenson-Hinde (Eds.), *Relationships within families: Mutual influences* (pp. 241–260). Oxford: Oxford University Press.

Grossmann, K. E., & Grossmann, K. (1990). The wider concept of attachment in cross-cultural research. *Human Development, 33,* 31–47.

Grossmann, K. E., Grossmann, K., & Schwan, A. (1986). Capturing the wider view of attachment: A reanalysis of Ainsworth's Strange Situation. In C. E. Izard & P. B. Read (Eds.), *Measuring emotions in infants and children* (Vol. 2, pp. 124–171). New York: Cambridge University Press.

Grossmann, K. E., Grossmann, K. Spangler, G., Suess, G., & Unzner, L. (1985). Maternal sensitivity and newborns' orientation responses as related to quality of attachment in Northern Germany. In I. Bretherton & E. Waters (Eds.), *Growing points of attachment theory and research, Monographs of the Society for Research in Child Development, 50,* Serial. No. 209 (1–2), 223–256.

Grossmann, K., Thane, K., & Grossmann, K. E. (1981). Maternal tactual contact of the newborn after various post-partum conditions of mother–infant contact. *Developmental Psychology, 17,* 158–169.

Guidano, V. F., & Liotti, G. (1983). *Cognitive processes and emotional disorders.* New York: Guilford Press.

Hartmann, H. (1958). *Ego psychology and the problem of adaptation*. New York: International Universities Press.

Hauser, S., Powers, S. I., Noam, G. G., Jacobson, A. M., Weiss, B., & Follansbee, D. J. (1984). Familial contexts of adolescent ego-development. *Child Development, 55*, 195–213.

Heinicke, C. M., Diskin, S. D., Ramsey-Klee, D., & Given, K. (1983). Pre-birth parent characteristics and family development in the first year of life. *Child Development, 54*, 194–208.

Hendrix, G. G. (1979). Encoding knowledge in partitioned networks. In N. V. Findler (Ed.), *Associative networks: Representation and use of knowledge by computer* (pp. 51–92). New York: Academic Press.

Hopkins, J. B., & Vietze, P. M. (1977, April). *Postpartum early and extended contact: Quality, quantity or both?* Paper presented at the meetings of the Society for Research in Child Development, New Orleans.

Johnson, M. M. (1988). *Strong mothers, weak wives*. Berkeley: University of California Press.

Johnson-Laird, P. N. (1983). *Mental models*. Cambridge: Harvard University Press.

Klaus, M. H., Jerauld, R., Kreger, N. C., McAlpine, W., Steffa, M., & Kennell, J. H. (1972). Maternal attachment: Importance of the first postpartum days. *New England Journal of Medicine, 286*, 460–463.

Klaus, M. H., & Kennell, J. H. (1976). *Maternal-infant bonding*. St. Louis: C. V. Mosby.

Klopfer, P. (1971). Mother-love: What turns it on? *American Scientist, 49*, 404–407.

Kobak, R. R., & Sceery, A. (1988). Attachment in late adolescence: Working models, affect regulation, and perceptions of self and others. *Child Development, 59*, 135–146.

Lamb, M. E. (1978). Qualitative aspects of mother-infant and father-infant attachments in the second year of life. *Infant Behavior and Development, 1*, 265–275.

Lamb, M. E. (1982). Early contact and maternal–infant bonding: One decade later. *Pediatrics, 70*, 763–768.

Lewis, M., & Feiring, C. (1979). The child's social network: Social objects, social functions, and their relationship. In M. Lewis & L. A. Rosenblum (Eds.), *The child and its family* (pp. 9–27). New York: Plenum Press.

Lieberman, A. F., & Pawl, J. H. (1990). Disorders of attachment and secure base behavior in the second year of life: Conceptual issues and clinical intervention. In M. T. Greenberg, D. Cicchetti, & E. M. Cummings (Eds.), *Attachment in the preschool years* (pp. 375–397). Chicago: University of Chicago Press.

Lorenz, K. Z. (1935). Der Kumpan in der Umwelt des Vogels. *Journal für Ornithologie, 83*, 137–213. (English translation in C. H. Schiller [1957] *Instinctive behavior*. New York: International Universities Press).

Lorenz, K. Z. (1957). *King Solomon's ring*. New York: Thomas Y. Crowell.

Main, M., & Goldwyn, R. (in press). Interview-based adult attachment classifications: Related to infant-mother and infant-father attachment. *Developmental Psychology*.

Main, M., & Hesse, E. (1990). Parent's unresolved traumatic experiences are related to input attachment status: Is frightened and/or frightened parental behavior the mechanism? In M. Greenberg, D. Cicchetti, & E. M. Cummings (Eds.), *Attachment during the preschool years: Theory, research, and intervention* (pp. 161–182). Chicago: University of Chicago Press.

Main, M., Kaplan, K., & Cassidy, J. (1985). Security in infancy, childhood and adulthood: A move to the level of representation. In I. Bretherton & E. Waters (Eds.), *Growing points of attachment theory and research, Monographs of the Society for Research in Child Development, 50*, Serial No. 209 (1–2), 66–104.

Main, M., & Solomon, J. (1990). Procedure for identifying infants as disorganized/disoriented during the Ainsworth Strange Situation. In M. Greenberg, D. Cicchetti, & E. M. Cummings (Eds.), *Attachment during the preschool years: Theory, research, and intervention* (pp. 121–160). Chicago: University of Chicago Press.

Mandler, J. H. (1979). Categorical and schematic organization in memory. In C. R. Puff (Ed.), *Memory organization and structure* (pp. 259–299). New York: Academic Press.

Marris, P. (1982). Attachment and society. In C. M. Parkes & J. Stevenson-Hinde (Eds.), *The place of attachment in human behavior* (pp. 185–201). New York: Basic Books.

Marris, P. (1991). The social construction of uncertainty. In J. Stevenson-Hinde, C. M. Parkes, and P. Marris (Eds.), *Attachment across the life cycle*. London: Routledge.

Matas, L., Arend, R. A., & Sroufe, L. A. (1978). Continuity and adaptation in the second year: The relationship between quality of attachment and later competence. *Child Development, 49*, 547–556.

Miyake, K., Chen, S., & Campos, J. (1985). Infants' temperament, mother's mode of interaction and attachment in Japan: An interim report. In I. Bretherton & E. Waters (Eds.), *Growing points of attachment theory and research, Monographs of the Society for Research in Child Development, 50*, Serial No. 109 (1–2), 276–297.

Moss, H. (1967). Sex, age and state as determinants of mother-infant interaction. *Merill Palmer Quarterly, 13,* 19–36.

Neisser, U. (1987). What is ordinary memory the memory of? In U. Neisser & E. Winograd (Eds.), *Remembering reconsidered* (pp. 356–373). New York: Cambridge University Press.

Nelson, K. (1986). *Event knowledge: Structure and function in development.* Hillsdale, NJ: Erlbaum.

Nelson, K., & Gruendel, J. (1981). Generalized event representations: Basic building blocks of cognitive development. In M. E. Lamb & A. Brown (Eds.), *Advances in developmental psychology* (Vol. 1, pp. 131–158). Hillsdale, NJ: Erlbaum.

Parke, R. D., & Tinsley, B. J. (1987). Family interaction in infancy. In J. D. Osofsky (Ed.), *Handbook of infant development* (pp. 579–641). New York: Wiley.

Piaget, J. (1954). *The construction of reality in the child.* New York: Basic Books.

Radke-Yarrow, M., Cummings, E. M., Kuczynsky, L., & Chapman, M. (1985). Patterns of attachment in two- and three-year olds in normal families and families with parental depression. *Child Development, 56,* 884–893.

Ricks, M. H. (1985). The social transmission of parenting: Attachment across generations. In I. Bretherton & E. Waters (Eds.), *Growing points of attachment theory and research, Monographs of the Society for Research in Child Development, 50,* Serial No. 209 (1–2), 211–227.

Sagi, A., Aviezer, O., Mayseless, O., Donnell, F., & Joels, T. (1991, April). *Infant–mother attachment in traditional and nontraditional kibbutzim.* Paper presented at the biennial meetings of the Society for Research in Child Development, Seattle.

Sagi, A., Lamb, M. E., Lewkowicz, K. S., Shoham, R., Dvir, R., & Estes, D. (1985). Security of infant-mother, -father, and -metapelet attachment among kibbutz reared Israeli children. In I. Bretherton & E. Waters (Eds.), *Growing points of attachment theory and research, Monographs of the Society for Research in Child Development,* Serial No. 209 (1–2), 257–275.

Schaffer, H. R., & Emerson, P. E. (1964). The development of social attachments in infancy. *Monographs of the Society for Research in Child Development, 29,* Serial No. 94.

Schank, R. C. (1982). *Dynamic memory: A theory of reminding and learning in computers and people.* Cambridge: Cambridge University Press.

Schank, R. C., & Abelson, R. P. (1977). *Scripts, plans, goals and understanding.* Hillsdale, NJ: Erlbaum.

Shaver, P. R., & Hazan, C. (1988). A biased overview of the study of love. *Journal of Social and Personality Relations, 5,* 473–501.

Slough, N., & Greenberg, M. (1990). 5-year-olds' representations of separation from parents: Responses for self and a hypothetical child. In I. Bretherton & M. Watson (Eds.), *Children's perspectives on the family* (pp. 67–84). San Francisco: Jossey-Bass.

Sroufe, L. A. (1985). Attachment classification from the perspective of infant caregiver relationships and infant temperament. *Child Development, 56,* 1–14.

Sroufe, L. A. (1988). The role of infant-caregiver attachment in development. In J. Belsky & T. Nezworsky (Eds.), *Clinical implications of attachment* (pp. 18–38). Hillsdale, NJ: Erlbaum.

Sroufe, L.A., & Fleeson, J. (1986). Attachment and the construction of relationships. In W. Hartup & K. Rubin (Eds.), *Relationships and development* (pp. 51–71). Hillsdale, NJ: Erlbaum.

Stayton, D., Hogan, R., & Ainsworth, M. D. S. (1973). Infant obedience and maternal behavior: The origins of socialization reconsidered. *Child Development, 42,* 1057–1070.

Stern, D. N. (1977). *The first relationship: Infant and mother.* Cambridge: Harvard University Press.

Stern, D. N. (1985). *The interpersonal world of the infant.* New York: Basic Books.

Stern, D. N., Beebe, B., Jaffe, J., & Bennett, S. (1977). The infant's stimulus world during social interaction. In H. R. Schaffer (Ed.), *Studies in mother–infant interaction.* London: Academic Press.

Stewart, R. B., & Marvin, R. S. (1984). Sibling relations: The role of conceptual perspective-taking in the ontogeny of sibling caregiving. *Child Development, 55,* 1322–1332.

Strage, A., & Main, M. (1985). *Attachment and parent-child discourse patterns.* Paper presented at the symposium "Attachment: A move to the level of representation," (M. Main, chair), during the biennial meetings of the Society for Research in Child Development, Toronto, Canada.

Sullivan, H. S. (1953). *The interpersonal theory of psychiatry.* New York: Norton.

Swejda, M., Campos, J. J., & Emde, R. N. (1980). Mother-infant "bonding": Failure to generalize. *Child Development, 51* 775–779.

Taylor, P. M., Taylor, F. H., Campbell, S. B. G., and others (1979, April). *Effects of extra contact on early maternal attitudes, perceptions, and behaviors.* Paper presented at the meetings of the Society for Research in Child Development, San Francisco.

Teti, D. M., & Ablard, K. E. (1989). Security of attachment and infant-sibling relationships: A laboratory study. *Child Development*, 60, 1519–1528.

Tinbergen, N. (1951). *The study of instinct*. London: Clarendon Press.

Tronick, E. Z., Ricks, M., & Cohn, J. F. (1982). Maternal and infant affective exchange: Patterns of adaptation. In T. Field & A. Fogel (Eds.), *Emotion and early interaction* (pp. 83–100). Hillsdale, NJ: Erlbaum.

Tronick, E. Z., Winn, S., & Morelli, G. A. (1985). Multiple caretaking in the context of human evolution: Why don't the Efe know the Western prescription to child care? In M. Reite & T. Field (Eds.), *The psychobiology of attachment and separation* (pp. 293–321). New York: Academic Press.

Tulving, E. (1972). Episodic and semantic memory. In E. Tulving & W. Donaldson (Eds.), *Organization of memory* (pp. 382–403). New York: Academic Press.

Tulving, E. (1983). *Elements of episodic memory*. New York: Oxford University Press.

Van IJzendoorn, M. H., & Kroonenberg, P. M. (1988). Cross-cultural patterns of attachment: A meta-analysis of the Strange Situation. *Child Development*, 59, 147–156.

Ward, M. J., Carlson, E. A., Altman, S., Levine, L., Greenberg, R. H., & Kessler, D. B. (1990, April). *Predicting infant–mother attachment from adolescents' prenatal working models of relationships*. Paper presented at the Seventh International Conference on Infant Studies. Montreal, Canada.

Wason, P. C., & Johnson-Laird, P. N. (1972). *Psychology of reasoning: Structure and content*. Cambridge: Harvard University Press.

Weiss, R. S. (1973). *Loneliness: The experience of emotional and social isolation*. Cambridge: M.I.T. Press.

Weiss, R. S. (1977). *Marital separation*. New York: Basic Books.

Weiss, R. S. (1982). Attachment in adult life. In C. M. Parkes & J. Stevenson-Hinde (Eds.), *The place of attachment in human behavior* (pp. 171–201). New York: Basic Books.

Winnicott, D. W. (1958). *Through paediatrics to psycho-analysis*. London: Hogarth Press.

Winnicott, D. W. (1965). *The maturational process and the facilitating environment*. New York: International Universities Press.

Yarrow, L. J. (1967). The development of focused relationships during infancy. In J. Hellmuth (Ed.), *Exceptional Infant* (Vol. 1, pp. 227–242). Seattle: Special Child Publications.

Zeanah, C. H., Keener, M. A., Stewart, L., & Anders, T. F. (1985). Prenatal perception of infant personality: A preliminary investigation. *Journal of the American Academy of Child Psychiatry*, 24, 204–210.

7

Social and Communicative Development in Infancy

Heather Walker, Daniel Messinger, Alan Fogel, and Jeanne Karns

Introduction

The evidence presented in this chapter suggests that infant communicative action is highly context specific, showing remarkable variability to even subtle alterations of the social and physical settings in which interaction occurs. The chapter includes reviews of research on affective communication during face-to-face interactions between infants and their social partners, gestural communication in adult–infant interaction, differences in mother versus father interactive patterns with infants, and finally, research on how infants interact in group settings in the family and with peers. These areas reflect the research interest and expertise of the authors and are not intended to cover the scope of work in infant social and communicative development. Rather, our purpose is primarily conceptual: To show by example that *infant social and communicative action is constituted by the dynamic interplay between individuals and the social contexts and physical settings in which that interaction occurs.*

The model of social behavior we propose goes beyond simple notions of the mutual influence of the partner on the infant and vice versa. In our view infant–partner interaction is constantly being created and updated in a process that defies attempts to prescribe a direction of cause and effect. Thus untangling such

Heather Walker, Daniel Messinger, and Alan Fogel • Department of Psychology, University of Utah, Salt Lake City, Utah 84112.   Jeanne Karns • Department of Human Development and the Family, University of Nebraska, Lincoln, Nebraska 68588.

Handbook of Social Development: A Lifespan Perspective, edited by Vincent B. Van Hasselt and Michel Hersen. Plenum Press, New York, 1992.

associations requires consideration of the interaction history of the infant and his/her partner. Patterns of social action—such as games with a parent—emerge and dissolve spontaneously and often in the absence of any explicit or implicit intention of either participant. This idea of emergent patterns of action, occurring without plan or intent and constituted only in the act of performance, has only recently been recognized as a fundamental factor in social development (Camaioni, De-Castro, Campos, & DeLemos, 1984; Fogel, 1990a; Fogel, Nwokah, & Karns, in press; Fogel & Thelen, 1987; Lock, 1980).

How are we to understand the development of infant communication? In broad sweep, infants acquire increasingly subtle forms of expression that eventually approximate the communicative style of the adult culture. How this happens is a matter of considerable theoretical and practical importance. It is also a developmental puzzle that evokes strongly divergent explanations. In reviewing current views deriving from ethological and sociocultural perspectives, we argue that infant communicative action cannot be understood as a simple readout of innate expressive movements nor as being shaped entirely by adult contingencies.

Conceptual Framework

Ethological Theories

Ethologists assume that members of a species—both adults and infants—share a common repertoire that includes the movements and expressions necessary for social interaction. In one theoretical scenario, infants are genetically predisposed to display actions that adults can readily interpret. Via processes of maturation, expressive abilities gradually improve, and the infant uses these new skills to better model the adult forms of communication. Some mechanism for mutually synchronizing these social interactions must also be assumed (Trevarthen, 1986).

In ethologically based attachment theory, for example, not only behavior but social perceptions and expectations become linked to produce synchronized dyadic actions. The internal working model is a concept designed to capture an individual's representations of relationships with particular persons that influence their patterns of social interactions with those persons (Bowlby, 1980; Bretherton, 1985; Stern, 1985).

Contrary to the premises of ethological theories, research suggests that parents and children do not have the same repertoire, goals, or expectations of the relationship (Kaye, 1980; Lock, 1980). Adult behavior during interactions with infants is not similar to infant behavior, and the social behavior that infants gradually acquire does not resemble the forms of exaggerated actions used by adults.

Another problem with ethological theory is that it presumes that all social behavior has a specific function. Smiling is functional because it leads to positive interaction and play; play is functional because it provides opportunities for cultural learning and skill practice. The theoretical fallacy is in thinking that because we can communicate in specific ways, we are "meant" to do so because of an evolved structure dedicated to social interaction, deemed necessary to our species survival. There are a number of elegant arguments against this position (Bates, 1979; Burghardt, 1984; Gould, 1977) that are beyond the scope of this presentation. However, many examples of even highly ritualized social interaction can be explained as spontaneous accidents of local circumstances, maintained for a variety of purposes, not all of which would be beneficial to the individuals. These include patterns of insecure attachment or "games" involving physical or sexual abuse (cf. Fogel, 1990a; Fogel, Nwokah, & Karns, in press).

Sociocultural Theories

The theorists that may be collected under this heading are typically silent regarding the biological constraints on behavior and development. Instead, they focus on describing the sociocultural interactions presumed to shape the development of cognition and action (cf. Bruner, 1983; Kaye, 1982; Rogoff, 1990; Vygotsky, 1978). Bruner (1983), for example, illustrates how complex hierarchical structures of parent–infant games like "peek-a-boo" and "pat-a-cake" provide a structure external to the infant, a scaffold, in which the infant's actions are embedded. The infant is not required to have a cognitive scheme or model for all of the structures necessary to learn a game or acquire a cultural skill. The adult, by carefully regulating the infant's participation in the game, can guide the infant's "uptake" (Bruner, 1983) or "appropriation" (Rogoff, 1990) of cultural skills. Thus, external social structure eventually becomes internal individual structure in this developmental perspective (Vygotsky, 1978).

One contribution of sociocultural theory is the recognition that social interaction has regularities and that culture is transmitted via active participation in these routines. These theorists assume that infants and children have an intrinsic interest in the life of the society around them and some basic skill with which they begin to participate. Sociocultural theories view children as active and motivated participants (not mere recipients of contingent reinforcements). And these theories recognize a complex role for adults that is different from that of the children. Adults are required to recognize the child's intrinsic motivation, alter the cultural activity to fit the child's level (such as by making work into a game), and gradually provide opportunities for the child to expand the scope of participation. Thus the concepts of nurture, planning, developmental perspective, and coparticipation extend the role of adults beyond mere model or reinforcer (Rogoff, 1990).

However, functional thinking of the sort discussed in relation to ethological theory also burdens sociocultural theory. From a sociocultural perspective, social routines presuppose goal-directed behavior on the part of the participants, even though sociocultural theory recognizes that the goals of the child and the adult are often dissimilar. It is difficult, therefore, to account for social interactions that are generated without plans or goals at the outset. The imposition of meaning and structure at the outset of an interaction may be a *post hoc* representation as construed by the observer, having little to do with the actual process by which the interaction emerged and was maintained (Lock, 1980).

The Dynamics of Social Interaction

In essence, we propose that social interaction generally cannot be prescribed in advance or defined simply as the additive sum of its components. Rather, *interaction is a dynamically creative process, emergent from the active discourse between two different individuals, or more, in a particular cultural and physical context.* Our argument is related to Gibsonian perspectives describing action as direct and context specific, without an explicit prescription for the final form of the action (Newell, 1986; Reed, 1982). Our view is similar to constructivist perspectives that do not require the genetic material to have foreknowledge of all the possible outcomes and pathways for developmental change (Fischer & Bidell, 1990; Piaget, 1952). We also recognize a sociocultural component to social development similar to that of Vygotsky (1978). Finally, we propose that human social behavior—including both verbal and nonverbal forms of communication—has not evolved phylogenetically as a manifestation of a dedicated genetic or neurological structure. Instead, communication is an emergent process that partakes of lower level components, none of which contains explicit representations of its final form (Bates, 1979; Burghardt, 1984; Lock, 1980).

In contrast to other perspectives, the dynamic interaction approach suggests that we focus on the contextual constraints that give social action its particular form, rather than appealing to social schemes assumed to represent the action within the infant's partner or to genetic information assumed to be blueprints for the action within the infant (Fogel, 1990b; Thelen, 1989). In the studies reviewed in this chapter, we show that all of the components of an interaction influence the forms and development of social discourse. These include traditional cognitive and affective factors as well as less obvious factors such as the mutual physical posturing of partners and their physical context. Thus our perspective requires one to examine the whole system—individuals in their physical and cultural setting—in order to comprehend how and why they communicate.

Research on Social Systems in Infancy

Face-to-Face Interactions in Early Infancy

As our first research example, we review differences in the social interaction that result from alterations of individuals and settings during face-to-face play between mothers and infants between 3 and 6 months of age. One of the earliest demonstrations of the effects of social context came from research using the "still-face" paradigm, which involves a sudden cessation of maternal participation while the mother continues to gaze at the baby. Although infants rarely cry, they gradually reduce the rate of smiling and gazing at the mother over the time period in which she is asked to remain still-faced, usually 1 to 3 minutes (Cohn & Elmore, 1988; Fogel, Diamond, Langhorst, & Demos, 1982; Gusella, Muir, & Tronick, 1988; Mayes & Carter, 1990; Stoller & Field, 1982; Tronick, Als, Adamson, Wise, & Brazelton, 1978). In related research, mothers were asked to simulate depression and reduce their affect, and their infants correspondingly become more sober after only a few minutes (Cohn & Tronick, 1983).

The experimental setting of these manipulations makes it appear that the mothers' change of behavior causes the infants' behavior to change. Our interpretation is that the infants' actions are also a product of their prior interactive engagement with mother and her history of interaction with them. One of us (Fogel, 1982a; Fogel *et al.*, 1982) and Stoller and Field (1982) showed that the type of behavior infants demonstrated during the period of spontaneous interaction prior to the still face was predictive of their response to the still face. In particular, infants who were smiling prior to the still face were less disturbed by the still face than infants who were not smiling. More recently, others have shown that maternal positivity affects subsequent behavior during the still face: Boys with positive mothers are more positive during still face, whereas girls display more depressed affect (Mayes & Carter, 1990).

Thus the 3-month-old infant's actions are not dependent simply on a halo effect from an earlier affective state nor on the mother's prior actions. Rather, infant responses to the still face probably reflect the state of the *dynamically constituted interactions between mother and infant over time*. How this process happens and the degree to which infant expectations of the interaction need to be ascribed to the infant will need to be resolved by further research (cf. Fogel, 1982a; Gusella *et al.*, 1988; Mayes & Carter, 1990). Our point is merely that the infant's communicative action in this situation must be understood as an emergent result of the whole system: The behavior of each individual in the context of the prior flow of interactive events.

There are significant cultural differences in the dynamics of face-to-face play that can be understood as extensions of this contextual perspective. Mothers in Japan, for example, respond less actively to infant vocalizations than mothers from the United States (Fogel, Toda, & Kawai, 1988). Japanese mothers use upper body movements physically to loom in and out abruptly and their hands to tap the infant and create visual displays. Mothers in the United States use their hands and bodies more tonically, by staying in one position (closer, on average, to the infant's face than the Japanese mothers) and by holding and touching the infant's body for continuous periods. American mothers make phasic use of their voice with many short utterances and questions and respond more to the infant's vocalizations. The result is a very different quality of play interaction in each culture. Japanese mothers use physical modalities to express themes and variations, whereas Americans use vocal modalities (Fogel *et al.*, 1988). In contrast, Bambara mothers from Kenya express themes and variations through postural motor games (Bril, Zack, & Nkoumkou-Hombessa, 1989).

These cross-cultural differences cannot be explained merely on the basis of the culture-specific styles of adult interaction nor even of adult interaction with infants. These styles have developed over centuries of interactions with the infants themselves. In each interaction and within each family, these patterns of interaction are reinvented and reconstituted, based on the dynamic interaction of cultural values and parental and infant proclivities and behaviors. Lock's (1980) concept of the guided reinvention of language is a particularly insightful description of these cultural dynamics and their recreation in the action contexts of the family. Reinvention does not mean a simple reenactment of a cultural script; infants do not know what the script is, and it is doubtful that many adults could articulate such a script except in the most abstract terms. Rather, the concept of reinvention implies a creative and spontaneous process that emerges from action in the context of family and culture.

Even small changes in the local context of parent–infant interaction can affect the form of social behavior that emerges. For example, in one study the total duration of mutual gazing between mother and infant was doubled when the infant's seat was moved from an upright position to a supine position (Fogel, 1988; Fogel, Dedo, & McEwen, in press). Although we are still investigating why a change in postural position alters the face-to-face interaction, we know that the effect is not due to a change in the mother's behavior or style of interaction nor to the infants' inability to hold their heads upright (the youngest infants in the study were 3 months, and all had head control). Clearly, nonobvious changes in physical setting can have unforeseen effects on infant behavior.

With an interactive partner other than the mother, infant social play behavior is also altered. For example, when with peers, 3-month-olds become more intense, abrupt, active, and less facially expressive than when they are with their mothers (Fogel, 1979). Similar intensity has also been observed during infant interactions with a doll (Legerstee, Corter, & Kienapple, 1990; Legerstee, Pomerleau, Malcuit, & Feider, 1987), although the specific behaviors of infants with dolls are different than those with peers. Finally, infant behavior with a peer differs from that seen when the infant is presented with a mirror or with a closed-circuit TV image of himself or herself (Field, 1979).

In these studies, the infants did not simply change a single behavior, such as less gazing or less smiling between conditions. Rather, painstaking microanalyses have revealed complex and systematic patterns of reorganization of the infant's entire body movements including vocalization, gaze, facial expression, and hand and arm movements. What is the source of such systematic reorganizations? Clearly infants do not need sophisticated, scaffolding partners to engage in the systematic organization of their behavior that is apparent in their interaction with partners other than their mothers. Moreover, many of the mothers in our study of infant peers reported their 3-month-olds had never seen another baby (Fogel, 1979). Yet the behavior of all the infants with peers was similar and significantly different from behavior with their mothers. Similarly, infants inexperienced with dolls, still faces, and maternal depression showed similar and characteristic patterns of interactions. Despite the infants' lack of experience, genetically based schema clearly could not anticipate all these possibilities and their variants. Our genes do not have prescriptions for behavior with dolls, televisions, and mirrors. Instead, the infant's actions in these different social contexts seem to be a product of a dynamic interaction between the infant's proclivities and the particularities of the situation.

In a study in which infants were observed weekly between 1 and 6 months while interacting with mothers during a face-to-face play situation on the mother's lap without toys, we found that mothers changed the way they held their infant's bodies as a function of the infant's gazing and affective engagement (Fogel, Nwokah, Hsu, Dedo, & Walker, 1990). Following a 6- to 8-week period in which infants prefer to gaze at mother, infants acquire a visual preference for inanimate, graspable objects and gaze less at their mother. After infants' interest in mother declined developmentally, mothers turned their infants' bodies away from them and toward the direction of the infants' visual interest. This was true, however, only for dyads in which the infant and mother had engaged in mutually positive affective exchange prior to gazing away. For infants who were developmentally late smilers (i.e., they smiled in the weeks following the developmental onset of gazing away from the mother), mothers persisted in trying to attract their infant's attention to themselves until the infants began smiling, which led to positive play exchanges. For these late smilers, mothers did not support the infant's intended gaze preference until the infant had acquired reaching. In the absence of positive interaction, gaze away plus reaching was necessary as a communicative signal to cue the mother's shift in attention management strategies.

The mother's behavior in this study was not caused by the infant's in any strict or simple sense. Rather, the mother's particular actions were contingent on the history of interactions with her particular infant. The participants' actions were constituted by the form and timing of each other's behavior. Therefore, research presented in this section suggests that infant behavior during face-to-face interaction depends on both the current social context and on the history of the particular relationship. In the next section, we discuss interactive and developmental processes in the emergence of intentional gestural communication at the end of the first year of life.

CONTEXTUAL DYNAMICS IN THE DEVELOPMENT OF COMMUNICATIVE GESTURING

Most infants first communicate intentionally by using manual gestures rather than speech. Once regarded as an unimportant precursor to language, gestural interchange—which first appears around 10 months—is currently seen as a separate avenue of communication with a distinct developmental history (Camaioni *et al.*, 1984; Franco & Butterworth, 1989). Communicative gesturing can be defined as the intentional use of gestures to elicit or respond to a partner's actions, when those gestures have a conventional form that both infant and partner can recognize. Examples include pointing to request or indicate an object, nodding the head "yes," and enacting a sign for an object (e.g., bouncing a pretend ball).

This section focuses on how infants' communicative gesturing is affected by the social and physical contexts in which the infants interact. A subsection is devoted to each of two major issues: (1) the effects of physical context on the *comprehension* of gestures; and (2) the effects of social contexts such as partner, concurrent activity, and gestural input on the *production* of gestures. In these subsections, we will hypothesize about elements that may be necessary to these communicative achievements; we will also highlight what is known and not known about the processes through which these developments occur.

Physical Context Affects 9-Month-Olds' Comprehension of Gestures

How do infants begin to understand what others are communicating to them? An important developmental achievement is comprehending that an extended index finger directs one's attention to other objects in the visual environment. At 9 months, infants may see the extended index finger primarily as an interesting display; however, at 14 months they actively search out the object being pointed at. Lempers (1979) and Murphy and Messer (1977) have identified two visual-contextual parameters that affect whether 9-month-olds can use a partner's manual point to direct their attention to an object (see also Schaffer's review, 1984).

Lempers (1979) had experimenters point at objects that were either a half-meter or 2½m away from their extended fingers. At 9 months, the majority of infants could follow the experimenters' points to the near object but not the far object. The close physical proximity of a gesture to the object to which it referred was necessary for the 9-month-olds' comprehension. By 12 months, the majority of infants followed points to both the near and the far objects.

Murphy and Messer (1977) had mothers seated to the left of their infants point at toys that were either (1) across the infant's field of vision to the right; (2) in front of the infant; or (3) to the left of the infant on mothers' side. Only when mothers' points and the toys they referred to were both on the same side of the infants, did 9-month-olds gaze at the toys at above chance levels. Only two of twelve 9-month-olds gazed across from their mothers' hand on their left to an object to their right. The greater the angle that the 9-month-olds had to gaze across from the referring point to the toy, the less likely they were to do so. By 14 months, most infants could follow all three types of points.

In both studies, the less 9-month-olds had to shift their visual fields from the extended index finger to the target, the more likely they were to do so. This finding may shed light on the process through which infants come to comprehend communicative points. Infants may learn that points refer to objects by gradually associating the pointing gesture with objects close to or within the same visual field as the extended index finger. The hypothesis is that a necessary component in initially comprehending the meaning of a partner's referential gesture is seeing the point and the object in proximity without having to switch gaze from one to another. Indirect support for the hypothesis is provided by Murphy and Messer's (1977) observations that early maternal points often actually touch the object being pointed at.

At least in the case of points and probably in comprehending other manual gestures as well, the infant's social partners construct physical contexts that scaffold the infant's developing comprehension of the conventional message. As will be seen in the following sections, social context is also an important factor in infant gestural production.

Social Context Affects the Production of Gestures

In what types of social contexts are infants likely to gesture communicatively? Bakeman and Adamson (1984, 1986) addressed this question with data from videotaped home visits of 28 infants playing with mother, with a familiar peer, and alone when the infants were 9, 12, and 15 months old. Bakeman and Adamson (1986) found that, when infants were with their mothers, they made more conventional gestures such as offers of objects and ritualized requests than when with a peer or alone. When with mother, infants spent more time in states of *coordinated joint engagement*, either actively gazing back and forth between an object and a partner or simply attending to the same object as the partner, and infants spent more time involved in *conventional routines*, such as playing with a toy phone or pretend eating ("action formats" in Bakeman & Adamson, 1984). The percentage of time the infant spent in coordinated joint engagement and conventional routines and the infants' rate of communicative gesturing increased from 9 to 15 months.

What was it about interaction with mother that facilitated communicative gesturing? In general, communicative gesturing tended to occur at times when the infant was jointly engaged with mother and an object and involved in a conventional routine. However, joint engagement and conventional routines also had rather different effects on offering and pointing. At both 12 and 15 months, joint engagement was associated with a high rate of showing and offering objects, whereas conventional routines had no independent effect. However, at 15 months, both conventional routines and joint engagement were associated with increased pointing.

From a social-dynamic perspective, it is not surprising that different gestures are facilitated in the context of diverse social activities. Although offers and requests both involve joint engagement, they seem to involve very different infant goals. In preliminary results from a longitudinal study, Messinger and Fogel (1990) found that infant offers were more likely to cooccur with coordinated joint engagement and were more likely to involve smiling than infant requests, indicating that offers may be occasions for "making contact" with mother by visually engaging her or smiling. In contrast, requests (e.g., points) were more likely to take place during the table condition where mother could control access to the toys rather than during the floor condition. Thus infants seemed to offer objects to become more engaged with mother and seemed to request objects from mother to become more engaged with an object.

The results of the Messinger and Fogel (1990) study, together with those of Bakeman and Adamson (1986), suggest that the conditions under which infants offer and point are likely to differ and to reflect different social dynamics. Regarding offers, Reinecke (1987) noted that shortly after voluntarily releasing objects to mothers, the two infants he studied began to extend objects in offers. Although such detailed description is helpful, these observations need to be codified and employed with larger numbers of subjects. Moreover, more precise descriptions of play routines and conventional routines, which appear to be the site of some early referential offers (Reinecke, 1987), would also be helpful.

Following Vygotsky (1978), detailed work has been carried out on the origins of conventional requests. Vygotsky hypothesized that points develop out of the infant's unintentional finger extensions when reaching for objects. Partners respond by giving the object *as if* the infant's gesture were communicative, providing the conditions for the infant to point with the intention of eliciting the partner's offer. This is reminiscent of Lock's (1980) description of how a partner's responses to an infant's requests at 12 months were associated with increasingly clear gestural requests that culminated in a point at 14 months. In a more systematic, but less developmental treatment, Lock, Young, Service, and Chandler (1990) found that mothers who were less responsive to their infants' requests had infants who requested less than infants who had more responsive mothers. However, Bruner (1983) found that requests for objects began at 9 months as responses to mother offering the object. The degree to which requests are facilitated by responding to the infant and the degree to which they are scaffolded by mothers presenting the object needs further investigation.

To summarize, infants are more likely to gesture conventionally when they are with adult social partners, particularly when the infants integrate their awareness of the adult and the physical environment. It should be noted, however, that as conventional gestures do occasionally occur outside of these contexts, the contexts do not appear to be *necessary* to infant gesturing. Instead more abstract features, which may often be created within these social contexts, could be necessary to various gestures. Thus we hypothesize that offers involve awareness of both object and partner (as indexed by joint visual engagement) as well as a desire to engage the partner (as indexed by involvement in games and smiling). Conventional requests are hypothesized to involve a desire for an object and a social partner who can reliably be signaled to give the object (as indexed by increased requests when infants are dependent on their partners for objects and when the partners tend to respond to requests by providing objects). To ask how infants begin to gesture communicatively, then, is to ask about the social history of a particular gesture: the pattern through which it becomes conventionalized in the context of other social activities.

An area of research in which attention has been devoted to the acquisition of specific gestures (such as making a particular sign for an object or referring with a point) is the study of gestural "input." The literature reviewed on this topic (see also Acredolo & Goodwyn, 1990) indicates that the extent of gestural input an infant receives affects the extent of his or her early gestural "vocabulary."

Acredolo and Goodwyn (1990) trained the parents of six infants to encourage gestures in their infants. Parents were provided with five new toys, each of which they were instructed to embed in a daily routine with their infants, while modeling an iconic gesture and providing a verbal label for the toy. From approximately 11 to 18 months, 120 symbolic gestures were reported for the six infants. Though there was no control group, the mean of 20 signs per infant was severalfold higher than the means of between four and five signs for untrained groups assessed in earlier retrospective and diary studies (Acredolo & Goodwyn, 1988). These results suggest the degree to which social context may facilitate gesture use. Some combination of factors, including embedding the object in a daily routine (e.g., bath time), and providing both gestural and verbal input, appears to have increased the range of gestures that infants employed and probably the frequency with which they were used as well.

Similar studies have shown that deaf and hearing children, exposed to American Sign Language (ASL), develop gestural signs earlier than hearing children develop spoken words. For example, Orlansky and Bonvillian (1985) report that the average age for first sign production among 13 hearing infants who received ASL input was 8.6 months, which is substantially earlier than the average age of onset of spoken words (11 to 14 months).

It appears that infants regularly exposed to large amounts of gestural input develop, and use more, communicative gestures and use them earlier than other infants. However, it is not clear whether everyday gestural input (e.g., parental pointing) is *necessary* to the development of infant gesturing (Goldin-Meadow & Mylander, 1990). It is also important to note that Acredolo and Goodwyn (1990) found no strong evidence in the literature that social context can catalyze *symbolic* gesture use, in which the infant manifests understanding that referents refer to things in a variety of contexts, earlier than 1 year.

Nevertheless, increased gestural input that is embedded in everyday contexts increases the number of gestures that infants use with their partners. Whether these gestures are more likely to be produced in the same social contexts that facilitated the communicative gesturing discussed earlier, such as conventional routines and joint visual engagement, remains open to investigation.

Conclusion

At 9 months, both infants' receptive and expressive gestural communication is limited. However, the provision of contextual components can facilitate increased performance. Nine-month-olds will look from a referring index finger to an object only if the two are, from the infant's perspective, in proximity to one another. It may be that to comprehend early communicative gestures, the conventional meaning of the gesture must be made manifest by the social and physical contexts in which it is presented. Similarly, Bakeman and Adamson (1986) found that only one-seventh of their infants made one or more gestures with mother at 9 months. However, concentrated gestural input (i.e, ASL) seems to catalyze communicative gesturing as early as nine months.

Between 9 and 12 months, infants' production of communicative gestures increases, as does the amount of time spent in communicative activities such as coordinated joint attention and conventional routines. The social scaffolding of infant communication through joint activity, coordinated joint attention, explicit demonstration of gestural models, and appropriate response to infant gestures, all seem to increase the rate or broaden the range of infant communicative gesturing. However, the mechanisms through which these elements affect gesturing remains unclear.

By 15 months, infants spend an average of one-tenth of their time interacting with mother in states of coordinated attention, four-tenths of the time in conventional routines, and produce an average of almost one communicative gesture per minute. Infants have also begun to use gestures (and words) spontaneously as symbolic referents for classes of objects. The social context of joint engagement with mother remains a facilitating context for infant communicative gestures. Yet the rate of communicative infant gestures with peers increases, suggesting that the gestures have become more robust and can be generalized to other social contexts.

From 9 to 15 months, physical and social context facilitate the comprehension, production, and development of communicative gestures. However, we lack an understanding of the dynamic mechanisms through which social context facilitates gesturing. Research to address this question must use more infants than a case study format allows; yet observations must be detailed and frequent so that the *process* of development can be described (e.g., Fogel *et al.*, 1990). Relevant coding variables include (1) detailed coding of different types of infant gestures at various levels of conventionality, in temporal relation to partner gestures coded at the same level of detail; (2) patterns of partner and infant gaze; (3) precisely defined play sequences that include information on infant activity or passivity; and (4) pragmatic coding of the infants' partners' activities. Log-linear techniques that analyze at the level of gesture are recommended. These analyses can determine whether infant gestures are likely to occur prior to, concurrent with, and/or subsequent to patterns of events in all of the modalities listed. Log-linear techniques can also be used to document how facilitating conditions change with age, providing a contextual history of the comprehension and development of infant gestures.

The next sections will highlight the complexity of social context. We first discuss how the different interactive styles of mothers and fathers influence communicative development and conclude with a section on the influence of triads and larger groups on infant communicative development.

DIFFERENCES IN MOTHER– VERSUS FATHER–INFANT INTERACTION

In an attempt to understand the role of family context on infant development, researchers have looked at the differences in communicative strategies between mothers and fathers in various situations. However, the effects of these differential strategies on infants' communicative and social development is not clearly understood. Unlike the process-oriented research reported for face-to-face play and gestural communication, researchers studying between-parent differences have focused on the global styles of parents and infant outcome variables rather than on the process of social interaction and infant development. In order to see a more complete picture of parent–infant social interactions, we need investigations that track the patterns of behavioral changes within these contexts. We focus the following review on a critique of the literature from a process perspective.

Background

The influence of fathers has been studied in the development of gender roles (McGuire, 1982), cognitive development (Parke, 1981), social competence (Easterbrooks & Goldberg, 1984; Sagi, 1982), and independence (Parke, 1981). Even though fathers seem to serve important functions in their infants' development, the process by which fathers contribute to these outcomes is unclear. Why and what are fathers doing during interactions with their infants that is different than mothers? How are infants responding to their mothers versus their fathers?

Studies comparing mothers and fathers have examined a variety of behavioral differences—from responsiveness to cries (Donate-Bartfield & Passman, 1985) to play behavior. In this review, we focus on parent–infant play for several reasons. First, play is increasingly being recognized as a context in which infants can learn and develop a variety of cognitive and social skills such as turn taking (Stern, 1977, 1985). As Fogel, Nwokah, and Karns (in press) point out, parent–infant play is a creative process that emerges from the dynamics of social discourse between two or more individuals, within a particular cultural and physical context. Second, play is one of the most extensively studied areas in which parental differences have been observed. Kotelchuck (1976) reports that mothers spend approximately 25.8% of their time with infants in play activities, whereas fathers spend 37.5% in play. Thus play provides a natural arena for looking at the differential effects of parents on infants.

This section has two objectives. First, we describe major investigations on parent–infant play. Second, we attempt to convey what is missing from each report that would be needed to understand the multiple facets of infant social development. The approach we take is to determine what answers the studies can provide to the following five questions: (1) What do we learn about fathers' actions versus mothers'? (2) How close does this study come to describing social interaction? (3) What is missing from the study? (4) What do we learn about infants' behaviors? (5) What do we learn about the process of infant social development?

Father–Infant Play Research

In a classic study using play observations, Clarke-Stewart (1978) observed families when their infants were 15, 20, and 30 months of age. First, the investigator observed infants within the natural family context. Second, parents were asked to choose between activities that were either social/physical (e.g., playing little piggy), intellectually stimulating (reading a story), or independent activities (child plays with toy on own). Clarke-Stewart found that, in the forced choice condition, father–infant play was more likely to be physical and arousing and less likely to be didactic, intellectual, or mediated by objects as mother–infant play. However, in the naturalistic observations, there were no significant differences between mothers and fathers in the frequency or quality of social/physical play. Clarke-Stewart reported that children seemed to prefer fathers' play over mothers', and they were more responsive to play initiated by their fathers, but only during the forced choice condition.

Power and Parke (1982) videotaped mothers and fathers playing with their 8-month-old infants. They reported that parents engaged in three main types of play activity bouts: attention/arousal-regulating bouts, exploratory bouts, and communicative bouts. The results indicated that fathers engaged in more physical bouts (i.e., toy touching and lifting infant) than mothers. Fathers treated male and female infants more differently than did mothers. Fathers were more likely to encourage visual, large motor, and fine motor exploration in their sons while encouraging vocal behavior in their daughters. Mothers tended to watch more and engage in toy play that "successfully engaged in the infant behavior that defined the bout" (Power & Parke, 1982). For example, an illustration of a behavior in a large motor bout would be retrieving a toy. The investigators suggested that fathers turned to physical play because their toy play was not usually successful. Power and Parke contended that their results indicate that fathers' engagement in physical bouts may lead to their playing a major role in infant social development and that mothers' greatest influence is in the realm of early exploratory and cognitive development.

Belsky, Gilstrap, and Rovine (1984) conducted a longitudinal study of patterns of mothering and fathering when infants were 1, 3, and 9 months of age. Though this study did not focus on play but rather on naturalistic home observations, it provides valuable information on parental differences and similarities. They reported that fathers tended to watch more television and read, whereas mothers responded to, stimulated, and took basic care of infants more frequently. However, Belsky et al. (1984) noted that fathers are as sensitive to the developing nature of their infants as mothers. For both parents, frequency of responding to and stimulating the infant increased over time. As the infants grew older (3 months), mothers and fathers alike frequently directed the infant's attention to objects. Belsky et al. (1984) found that by 9 months of age, the frequency of infants' smiling and positive displays are correlated with measures of father involvement and marital interaction (defined as intensity of engagement between spouses).

Crawley and Sherrod (1984) conducted a cross-sectional study of 7-, 10- and 13-month-old infants in their homes. Infants were observed either with their mothers or with their fathers (not with both). Results indicated that regardless of infant age, both parents spent the majority of the time manipulating objects in play. Fathers used physical rough play more, and their play showed developmental changes that were similar to mothers. As infants grew older, both parents played games that were more sophisticated and that allowed the infant to use coordinated schemes, such as object manipulation. However, fathers increased their use of this type of play between 7 and 10 months, whereas mothers increased gradually over the 7- to 13-month period.

In summary, the studies described provide some information about differences in parents' play styles. Overall, it appears that fathers' play with infants is more social and physical. On the other hand, mothers' play is generally believed to be object mediated and more intellectually focused. Even though the investigations presented in this section were not designed to provide the answers to the five questions previously posed, we can begin to determine what needs to be done to further understanding about infant social development.

First, even though we have learned something about mothers' actions versus fathers', in some cases this information was constrained by factors such as using forced-choice play procedures or observing only one parent in a family. The most important problem, however, is that in two of the studies (Belsky *et al.*, 1984; Clarke-Stewart, 1978) it is uncertain whether direct effects of the father were ever assessed. In both efforts, when fathers were home, they were observed within a triadic situation. Thus any direct effects are obscured by the presence of the other parent. For example, within a triadic context, fathers may not be using intellectual play as they could be leaving it up to mothers to play in this style. Also, fathers would not be as likely to watch as much television or read if mothers were not present. If fathers were alone with their infants, they may be just as responsive and stimulating as mothers.

A second complication with these studies is their statistical methods. Most studies use analyses of variance or correlational methods that do not describe the process or dynamics of social interactions. Because no contingency or other types of process analyses were conducted, we do not know what type of events precipitated or followed particular behaviors, such as fathers' changes from toy to physical play. Thus it is difficult to determine how infants and parents coregulate each others' behaviors within social interactions.

A third problem with this research is that information on infants' behaviors with each parent individually is not provided, thus making it difficult to determine the sequence of developmental events. Do particular infant behaviors occur more with one parent than the others and does this pattern change over time? For example, Belsky *et al.* (1984) reported that fathers' involvement resulted in more smiling. Does this correlation exist due to direct effects, such as games fathers play, or is it due to an indirect effect such as a good marital relationship? When fathers use toys, what do infants do when their father's toy play is unsuccessful? Do infants cry or look away? Because members of a dyad coregulate each other's behaviors, what happens within the context to cause father to start physical play? Does the infant become engaged or redirect the father's attention? More data concerning infant behaviors during play interactions are needed because infants may play a role in encouraging fathers' use of proximal play. As we cannot answer these questions with the available research, we are learning very little about infants' social development or the interactional contexts.

The final concern with this work is that cross-sectional studies do not allow inferences about developmental processes, particularly when little is reported about infant behaviors. Due to cross-sectional procedures, dyadic and triadic history effects are neglected, such as how a mother typically constructs a play situation with her child alone versus how she does it when the father is present.

Parental Effects on Infant Behavior

One common feature of the investigations described is that they do not report how infants' behaviors differ between maternal and paternal play contexts. In a few studies we catch some glimpses of infant behavior during play with either parent that will be described next.

Yogman (1982) studied both parents' and strangers' weekly interactions with

3-month-old infants. An analysis of mutual regulation revealed that there are similarities in joint regulation during dyadic interactions of infants with their mothers and fathers. The author reported that fathers' interactions were more arousing and playful than mothers', whose interactions were more contained and smooth. Infants vocalized more with mothers than fathers. It appears that fathers' physical games resulted in aroused, attentive 3-month-old infants who remained still (immobile) more than with their mothers (Yogman, 1982).

By using longitudinal techniques, Yogman was able to present us with the most descriptive work done on infants and parents' interactions within a laboratory context. However, the author analyzed the monadic phases, or temporal structures of the interactions, by using a system developed by Tronick (1977). Fogel (1988) argues that the use of monadic phase scaling distorts the temporal organization of interactions as it clumps different types of behaviors together. Thus this system ignores discrete behaviors that defeats any functional significance of the interactions for parents and infants. Once again, developmental process is being obscured, this time by a statistical technique.

Field, Vega-Lahr, Goldstein, and Scafidi (1987) examined face-to-face interactions between 8-month-old infants and their employed mothers and fathers. They found that mothers smiled, vocalized, and touched their infants more than fathers. In turn, the infants tended to smile more and were more active with their mothers. However the investigators do not provide any information regarding how the infant was behaving in the presence of their fathers. They do point out that because the infants were in high chairs, this may have restrained fathers' usual mode of physical play. Field *et al.* (1987) did not conduct any sequential analyses; rather, repeated measure analyses of variance were employed. The problems with these approaches to infant communicative and social development have been discussed many times in this chapter.

In the last study to be discussed, Teti, Bond, and Gibbs (1988) compared play behaviors of mothers, fathers, and firstborn siblings with infants aged 12 months and later at 18 months. They reported that mothers and fathers were more alike than different in the amounts of play experiences they provided. In interactions with infants, mothers played with objects more than fathers, who in turn played with objects more than siblings. Teti *et al.* (1988) reported that mothers did more nonsocial object play than fathers, who used objects more socially. However, fathers' play involved language as much as mothers'. Thus they suggest that their results support Power and Parke's (1982) assumptions that mothers' object play contributes to cognitive competence, whereas fathers' social play with objects may have an impact on social and communicative development.

This study provides some insight into how parents may be structuring their infants' environment. For example, the fact that parents choose different activities with toy play (social with fathers vs. nonsocial with mothers) offers some information about how their respective interactions differ. However, we need more description of the interactions and more information about the infants' affect and behaviors within parental contexts to draw any conclusions.

Conclusion

The aforementioned investigations suggest that fathers provide a qualitatively different play context than mothers. Researchers are consistent in their reports that fathers play and act differently than mothers, particularly with toys. There is also the implicit assumption that fathers are insensitive to infant cues. Ninio and Rinott (1988) found that fathers tended to underestimate their infants' needs for, and capacities to engage in, more complex, cognitively demanding activities. In contrast, Crawley and Sherrod's (1984) results indicate that fathers may overestimate infants' abilities because they start more complex interactive play in an earlier timespan than mothers.

Many researchers report that mothers play in a consistent, contingent manner with their infants (Clarke-Stewart, 1978; Power, 1985; Yogman, 1982). The implication is that fathers and others do not play in this manner. Fathers may be providing a context that is less contingent on infant behaviors during play. However, high levels of contingency in play may be a culturally restricted phenomenon associated with American mothers. Carlile and Holstrum (1989) found that both mothers and fathers of the Chamorros of Guam treated infants more like American fathers in terms of involvement and play style.

Fathers could be following their own agenda in play, such as choosing toys *they* like to play with themselves, rather than what the infant prefers. It could be that fathers introduce more objects and "interfere" in order to encourage the infant to play with *him*. Further support for this hypothesis comes from Crawley and Sherrod's (1984) finding that fathers urge infants to play more interactive games at an earlier age than mothers. Also, fathers could be motivated to play in a physical manner because infants appear to like this as they smile and laugh more during this type of play (Clarke-Stewart, 1978; Power & Parke, 1982). Thus fathers' actions may be tapping different developmental processes than mothers. For example, within at least a partially noncontingent play context, infants may have to learn different types of social skills (e.g., gesturing or reaching) that will enable them to obtain what they need or want in such social situations. In summary, fathers may provide a different type of social experience that affords opportunities for infants to develop unique communicative strategies.

It becomes apparent that the studies described provide us with some insight into how the social context might influence infant communicative development. However, they do not give us the detail we need to adequately describe the process of infant social development. We need more descriptive, longitudinal investigations with frequent observation intervals that include analyses that capture the dynamic interactions between individuals in a social context. In the next section, we examine how the addition of others to the infants' social interactions complicates and changes the communicative system.

INFANTS IN GROUPS

Polyadic interactions, which include more than two participants, involve a host of interactive possibilities to infants. For example, in a triadic situation, two participants may form a dyadic interaction while the nonparticipant may engage in behavior nonrelated to the dyad, direct interaction attempts toward one or both participants of the dyad, or may monitor the interaction occurring in the dyad. It is this host of interactional possibilities that makes the study of polyads potentially amenable to a dynamic interactional perspective.

Nevertheless, most polyadic research has remained focused on either individual participant behaviors or on dyadic interactions. This is probably due to the daunting number of interaction possibilities and indirect effects that accompany the addition of each interactant. Two major types of investigation have been popular within the polyadic context. Between-dyad comparisons ask, assuming a common participant (A), what are the behavioral differences between dyad AB and dyad AC? The second type of investigation concerns indirect effects. The behaviors of participants A and B in a dyad are contrasted with the behaviors of the same dyad AB placed in a polyadic context. Differences in behavior between the two contexts within the same dyad are interpreted as evidence of the indirect influence of an additional participant, C, found only in the polyadic context.

Lewis and Feiring (1981) suggest several types of indirect effects that the members of a polyad may have on the interactions of other members. Infants may model or imitate behaviors observed in dyadic interactions among other members, may monitor the interactions of dyads to learn appropriate behaviors, and may experience dyadic interactions altered by the relationships and interactions of the dyadic partner with nondyadic members of the polyad. For example, infants may refrain from behaviors from which they have observed their siblings being punished.

Few studies, however, have focused on how infant communication is affected by the polyadic context. In reviewing research on infant social interaction in group contexts, we can ask similar questions to those posed earlier in reviewing the effects of mothers and fathers on infant social interaction. How well does the study describe social interaction and infant behavior? Does the study provide us with information on how infant action interfaces with those of other participants and on how this process affects infant development?

Siblings in the Family

Murphy (1988) used longitudinal family observations to study the developing relationship between a newborn infant and an older sibling. Families displaying strong sibling mutuality, defined as siblings who were especially sensitive in reading infant cues and responding contingently and empathically to the infant, were the same families where parents showed mutuality with the older siblings. The parents' communication with the sibling reflected a view of the older child as a person of value with unique needs and feelings. In families where the parent–sibling dyad did not display mutuality, the sibling–infant dyad also lacked this quality. Murphy's research, which built on the parallel findings of Kreppner, Paulsen, and Scheutze (1981), reveals that the relationship between parent and sibling influences the sibling's subsequent interaction with the infant. However, these studies provide little information on infant actions, nor do they address how infant actions interface with those of siblings and parents.

Teti and Ablard (1988) used a structured laboratory playroom situation to examine how the attachment of the infant's sibling to mother would influence the interaction of the triad in a play situation. Infants were 1 to 2 years old, and siblings ranged from 2 to 7 years old. Securely attached siblings spent more time consoling distressed infants than did insecurely attached siblings. Infants displayed more positive behavior with securely attached siblings than with insecurely attached siblings.

Both Murphy's (1988) and Teti and Ablard's (1988) investigations illuminate how the quality of an infant's relationship with her siblings is affected by the sibling's prior interactive history with the parent. Unfortunately, these studies do not adequately describe the interactional accompaniments of mutuality and secure attachment. What, for example, was the secure sibling's role in the interactions in which the infant was positive with them?

Kendrick and Dunn (1980) have gone further in investigating actual, real-time differences in polyadic interaction. They compared parent–sibling interaction when the mother was (1) not caretaking the infant or involved with household tasks, and with (2) situations when the mother was actively involved with either the infant's needs or household activities. When mothers were interacting with infants or involved with household tasks, there was both increased confrontation and increased positive involvement between siblings and mothers. This was a triadic interaction in which mother participated simultaneously in both the parent–infant dyad and the parent–sibling dyad, displaying differences in each. When the mother was not involved with the infant or household tasks, the parent–sibling dyad was likely to be less active. Mother's degree of involvement with the infant affected the mother–sibling dyadic interaction within the mother–sibling–infant triad.

The studies of Murphy (1988) and Teti and Ablard (1988) exemplify how the quality of interaction of one polyad (parent–sibling) can have unforeseen positive results on another polyad (sibling–infant). Moving in a different direction, Kendrick and Dunn (1980) have shown that mother's interaction with the infant also has an effect on her interactions with an older sibling. Involvement with the infant (or household tasks) had the unforeseen consequence of intensifying mother's relationship with the sibling. However, as with the other investigations, Kendrick and Dunn (1980) offer little information on what the infants were doing or on how their actions impacted and were impacted by the behaviors of siblings and parents. One wonders, for example, what impact the infants Kendrick and Dunn observed had on maternal activity and how that in turn affected the mother's increased confrontation and positive involvement with the sibling.

Twin Infants in the Family

Mothers with infant twins are a naturally occurring triad with an extensive interactive history. A small number of studies have focused on the process of interaction within families with twins (e.g., Karns & Fogel 1990; Tomasello, Mannle, & Kruger, 1986). However, most of the research on triadic interactions that includes twins focuses on outcome measures. For example, the behaviors of twins are often compared to those of singletons.

Dickman and Clark (1985) found that certain interactive behaviors emerged early for twins. In a study of social competence, one pair of twin boys and their mother were videotaped monthly in a lab playroom from age 8 months to 2½ years. The twins showed interactive behaviors at an earlier age than the norms for singletons. In a similar vein, Goshen-Gottstein (1986) observed 14 sets of twins, triplets, and quadruplets in their homes, beginning in infancy. These multiple-birth infants generally began visual interactions during the fifth or sixth month. Interactions involving touching and taking were common by 8 months. Goshen-Gottstein (1986) observed examples of even more precocious interaction, such as a set of twins interactively touching at 5 months and copying each other's vocalizations at 7 months. Larger subject pools and comparison with control groups of singletons are clearly needed. However, the findings of Dickman and Clark and Goshen-Gottstein suggest that the history of interaction infants of multiple births experience with their birthmates may facilitate the development of sophisticated patterns of social interaction.

Interestingly, from a linguistic perspective, the division of maternal attention toward each twin can be viewed as a deficit. Each infant receives less interaction with mother because mother's interactive behaviors may be divided between the two infants. The linguistic environment of twins was the focus of a longitudinal study carried out by Tomasello *et al.* (1986). They compared triadic interactions of mother–twins with the dyadic interaction of mother–singleton pairs. Mothers in both contexts displayed the same levels of speech and interaction. The twins scored lower on tests of language development than singletons. However, both the language learning environment of the twins and their language development differed from those of the singletons. When analyzed from the infant's point of view, each individual twin received less speech directed specifically to him or her. The individual twin had fewer and shorter episodes of joint attentional focus with mother and had fewer and shorter conversations with her. The twins' mothers were also judged to be more directive in their interactional style. These differences between triadic mother–twin interactions and dyadic mother–singleton interactions were positively correlated with the language development of the children (Tomasello *et al.*, 1986).

These twin studies show clear outcome differences for infants whose social development occurs within a group context. The studies exemplify the sensitivity of communicative skills to the particular features of the social contexts in which they emerge. Children of multiple births are likely to show interactive behaviors with peers earlier than singletons, presumably because of the quantity and regularity of their interactions with each other. However, the language development of the infants of multiple birth may be retarded because having a same-age sibling limits opportunities for direct linguistic input from the adult. Thus differences in everyday interactive context between infants of multiple births and singletons may be associated with different patterns of social and communicative development. With respect to singletons, infants of multiple births appear to be precocious in their interactive competence with each other and somewhat retarded in their linguistic development.

One wonders, however, about the processes of social interaction that yielded these outcomes: What is the developmental history of between-twin patterns of interaction? How does the onlooking twin respond when mother directs attention or speech to his or her twin? It was in order to address these process-oriented questions that some of us (Karns & Fogel, 1990) coded the interaction patterns of triads and then calculated how these patterns changed over time.

Using two mother–twin triads observed weekly during the first year of life, Karns and Fogel (1990) found that more than half of the interaction time of triads was spent in fully triadic interactions or with one infant attending to one or both of the other members of the triad. Triadic interaction was significantly likely to follow interaction patterns in which mother and one infant interacted as a dyad while the second infant attended to the interaction but did not participate. On the other hand, triadic interaction was not likely to follow periods in which mother and one infant interacted while the second infant was engaged in solitary activity. Triadic interactions, in turn, were likely to be followed by the pattern of an interacting dyad with an onlooker or by a double dyad pattern in which mother interacted with both infants but with different activities.

By viewing twin infants and mothers as an interactive system, Karns and Fogel (1990) found that triads do not simply duplicate dyadic behaviors. Over one-half the interactions observed in these structured play sessions involve at least some participation from all three partners. Use of sequential analyses revealed some of the dynamics of the interactions of groups of infants with a caregiver. If the noninteracting twin is attending to the interaction of mother and sibling, she or he is more likely to be incorporated into a traidic activity than if she or he is engaged in solitary play. Thus the actions of the noninteracting twin have a dramatic effect on the other two partners. Approaches that focus only on the interaction of the twins, or only on the interaction of the mother and one twin, are missing the decisive but nonobvious impact of the third partner.

Infants in Group Play

Relatively few investigators have considered group sizes larger than triads because of the technical difficulties involved in observing infant interaction in large groups. The few studies that contribute to our knowledge of the dynamics of group behaviors have examined pairs of peers and established peer groups.

Ross, Tesla, Kenyon, and Lollis (1989) observed the peer conflicts of 20- and 30-month-old infants that occurred when the mothers of both infants were present. When conflicts occurred, mothers were found to support the rights of the peers rather than of their own infants. However, mothers' interventions were directed toward their own infants rather than towards peers, even if the peers were the challengers. Hay and Ross (1982) examined the process of conflict of 21-month-old infants in the same context and found a relationship between conflict roles and order. The loser of a conflict was more likely than the winner to initiate the next conflict. Additionally, some individuals were more likely to engage in conflicts than others. When play partners were rotated, the levels of conflict in the previous play group were predictive of conflict in the new play group.

Lee (1973) found that infants as young as 9 months patterned their interaction with respect to individual differences. Nine-month-olds in an established play group were least likely to approach an infant who had more negative responses, such as grabbing at a peer or a peer's toy. However 9-month-olds displayed a stronger preference for social interaction with peers who had more positive social responses such as smiles.

The findings of Hay and Ross (1982) indicate that in real time, previous losers are likely to initiate the next conflict and that there are individual differences in proclivity to be involved in a conflict. Lee (1973) found that in an ongoing social interactional context, 9-month-olds took account of these proclivities. They were less likely to approach peers who exhibited more negative social responses and were more likely to approach peers who exhibited more positive social responses. By 9 months of age, infants in group settings have developed varied patterns of interaction with different peers. An integration of Hay and Ross's (1982) analysis of the order of events with Lee's focus on peer response might provide a methodological setting for asking how infant peers' patterns of social response change with age.

Infants in polyadic contexts interact in patterns that cannot be derived from a linear transformation of the interactive patterns that occur in a dyadic context. Attending to the cooccurring interaction of a dyad, early complex interaction with a peer and avoiding a peer who is likely to grab toys are all examples of interactive patterns that are specific to (polyadic) interactions with peers. With respect to dyadic interaction with a caregiver, these patterns represent not only a quantitative increase in the number of interaction possibilities open to an infant but also a qualitative change in which new interactive patterns become possible.

These patterns of polyadic interactions have important and particular effects on infant social and communicative development. Although the quality of parents' relations with siblings are reflected in the quality of the siblings' relations with infants, maternal attention to the infant unexpectedly intensifies her interactions with the sibling. Although infants of multiple births develop early complex interactive patterns among themselves, linguistic development often suffers the deficits of reduced directed speech from mother. Triadic interaction of infant twins and their mother is likely to be preceded and followed by a pattern of one dyad interacting while the lone infant attends to this interaction. By 9 months, infant interaction with peers is shaped by a shared interactive history in which infants avoid certain peers and approach others based on their interactive style.

A dynamic interactive perspective asks about the social contexts, the interactive processes, and the physical settings that constitute these effects. Although no prefabricated research agenda can ever be provided, certain issues are clear. Research on infant interaction in polyadic contexts would do well to systematically describe infant behavior in temporal relation to the behavior of partners in naturalistic contexts. Such description could be used relatively frequently to document changes in these interactive patterns over time.

Summary

In this chapter we have presented research from four areas of infant development in an attempt to illustrate the quantity and complexity of interactive effects on infant social and communicative development. In particular, the research demonstrates that different aspects of interactive context have different effects on infant behavior and development and that infant behavior and development is contingent upon the infant's shared interactive history with his or her partner.

Research on mother–infant face-to-face interaction has shown that infant social behaviors are multiply determined by the dyad's shared interactive history. Both infant behavior at the onset of a maternal still face *and* mother's historical level of positive affect predict how infants cope with the maternal still face. Maternal positioning of infants is associated with the history of their interactions. Only when dyads experience bouts of positive affect in conjunction with mutual attention will mothers respond to their infants' changing outward focus of attention by turning the infants away.

Research on communicative gesturing and on the infant interactions with mother, father, and groups of partners demonstrate how different facets of the interactive context are associated with different types of infant social and communicative development. Visual engagement with an object and the social partner is associated with offering objects, whereas participation in conventional routines is often associated with requests and other types of points. Parental demonstration of gestures for objects in everyday settings seems to facilitate acquisition of these gestures, whereas presenting a gesture and its referent in proximity (from the infant's perspective) may catalyze an infant's comprehension of gestures.

In a similar vein, different aspects of interaction with disparate partners may have particular effects on infant social development. Fathers may tend to use less contingent interactive styles with their infants and engage in more physical play than mothers. Infants seem to enjoy this type of interaction and may learn to cope with extremes of positive affect such as excitement. Research on multiple partners has shown that infants' interactions affect and are affected by other interactions in a group context in unexpected ways. For example, twins' extensive social contact with each other may be related to their early interactive competencies, whereas the relative paucity of exclusive maternal speech and attention may retard language development.

This evidence illustrates that infant social and communicative development in the first 18 months of life is profoundly affected by interactive context. Both the history of the infant's interactional patterns and particular features of those patterns, such as type of interaction, partner, and number of partners, profoundly affect infant social and communicative development.

What is lacking is detailed description of the process through which these developmental patterns emerge in interactive context. Ultimately, the process of interaction is coconstituted by all partners in a situation. Partners are exquisitely sensitive both to each other and are affected by nonobvious elements of the physical situation. Moreover, because partners' actions cooccur and because interaction can always be coded in finer detail, turn taking is not an apt metaphor. Instead, partners weave an interaction together; their moment-to-moment actions constitute the warp and weft out of which relationships are created and maintained.

ACKNOWLEDGMENTS This work was supported by an NIH grant R01 HD21036 and by a grant from the University of Utah Research Council.

REFERENCES

Acredolo, L. P., & Goodwyn, S. W. (1988). Symbolic gesturing in normal infants. *Child Development, 59,* 450–466.

Acredolo, L., & Goodwyn, S. (1990). Sign language in babies: The significance of symbolic gesturing for understanding language development. In R. Vasta (Ed.), *Annals of child development* (Vol. 7, pp. 1–42). London: Jessica Kingsley.

Bakeman, R., & Adamson, L. B. (1984). Coordinating attention to people and objects in mother–infant and peer–infant interaction. *Child Development, 55,* 1278–1289.

Bakeman, R., & Adamson, L. B. (1986). Infants' conventionalized acts: Gestures and words with mothers and peers. *Infant Behavior and Development, 9,* 215–230.

Bates, E. (1979). Intentions, conventions, and symbols. In E. Bates, L. Benigini, I. Bretherton, L. Camaioni, & V. Volterra (Eds.), *The emergence of symbols: Cognition and communication in infancy* (pp. 33–68). New York: Academic Press.

Belsky, J., Gilstrap, B., & Rovine, M. (1984). The Pennsylvania Infant and Family Development Project, I: Stability and change in mother–infant and father–infant interaction in a family setting at one, three and nine months. *Child Development*, 55, 692–705.

Bowlby, J. (1980). *Attachment and loss. Vol. 3: Loss, sadness and depression*. New York: Basic Books.

Bretherton, I. (1985). Attachment theory: Retrospect and prospect. *Monographs of the Society for Research in Child Development*, 50 (serial 209), 3–35.

Bril, B., Zack, M., & Nkounkou-Hombessa, E. (1989). Ethnotheories of development and education: A view from different cultures. *European Journal of Psychology of Education*, 4, 307–318.

Bruner, J. (1983). *Child's talk: Learning to use language*. New York: Norton.

Burghardt, G. M. (1984). On the origins of play. In P. K. Smith (Ed.), *Play in animals and humans* (pp. 5–42). Oxford: Basil Blackwell.

Camaioni, L., DeCastro Campos, M. F. P., & DeLemos, C. (1984). On the failure of the interactionist paradigm in language acquisition: A reevaluation. In W. Doise & A. Palmonari (Eds.), *Social interaction in individual development* (pp. 93–106). New York: Cambridge University Press.

Carlile, K. S., & Holstrum, W. J. (1989). Parental involvement behaviors: A comparison of Chamorro and Caucasian parents. *Infant Behavior and Development*, 12, 479–494.

Clarke-Stewart, K. (1978). And daddy makes three: The father's impact on mother and young child. *Child Development*, 44, 466–478.

Cohn, J. F., & Elmore, M. (1988). Effect of contingent changes in mothers' affective expression on the organization of behavior in 3-month-old infants. *Infant Behavior and Development*, 11, 493–505.

Cohn, J. F., & Tronick, E. Z. (1983). Three-month old infants' reaction to simulated maternal depression. *Child Development*, 54, 185–193.

Cohn, J., & Tronick, E. Z. (1988). Mother-infant face-to-face interaction: Influence in bidirectional and unrelated to periodic cycles in either partner's behavior. *Development Psychology*, 24(3), 386–392.

Crawley, S. B., & Sherrod, K. B. (1984). Parent-infant play during the first year of life. *Infant Behavior and Development*, 7, 65–75.

Dickman, Z., & Clark, P. M. (1985). Social interaction between a pair of infant twins. *South African Journal of Psychology*, 15, 119–125.

Donate-Bartfield, E., & Passman, R. (1985). Attentiveness of mothers and fathers to their baby's cries. *Infant Behavior and Development*, 8, 385–393.

Easterbrooks, M. A., & Goldberg, W. A. (1984). Toddler development in the family: Impact of father involvement and parenting characteristics. *Child Development*, 55, 740–752.

Field, T. (1979). Differential behavioral and cardiac responses of 3-month-old infants to mirror and peer. *Infant Behavior and Development*, 2, 179–184.

Field, T., Vega-Lahr, N., Goldstein, S., & Scafidi, F. (1987). Interaction behavior of infants and their dual-career parents. *Infant Behavior and Development*, 10, 371–377.

Fischer, K. W., & Bidell, T. R. (1990). Constraining nativist inferences about cognitive capacities. In S. Carey & R. Gelman (Eds.), *Constraints on knowledge in cognitive development*. Hillsdale, NJ: Erlbaum.

Fogel, A. (1979). Peer vs. mother directed behavior in 1- to 3-month old infants. *Infant Behavior and Development*, 2, 215–226.

Fogel, A. (1982). Affect dynamics in early infancy: Affective tolerance. In T. Field & A. Fogel (Eds.), *Emotion and early interaction* (pp. 15–56). Hillsdale, NJ: Erlbaum.

Fogel, A. (1990a). The process of developmental change in infant communicative action: Using dynamic systems theory to study individual ontogenies. In J. Colombo & J. Fagen (Eds.), *Individual differences in infancy: Reliability, stability and prediction* (pp. 341–357). Hillsdale, NJ: Erlbaum.

Fogel, A. (1990b). Sensorimotor factors in communicative development. In H. Bloch & B. Bertenthal (Eds.), *Sensorimotor organization and development in infancy and early childhood* (pp. 75–88). NATO ASI Series. Amsterdam: Kluwer.

Fogel, A., Dedo, J. Y., & McEwen, I. (in press). Effect of postural position on the duration of gaze at mother during face-to-face interaction in 3-to-6-month-old infants. *Infant Behavior and Development*.

Fogel, A., Diamond, G. R., Langhorst, B. H., & Demos, V. (1982). Affective and cognitive aspects of the two-month old's participation in face-to-face interaction with its mother. In E. Tronick (Ed.), *Social interchange in infancy: Affect, cognition, and communication* (pp. 37–57). Baltimore: University Park Press.

Fogel, A., Nwokah, E., Hsu, H., Dedo, J., & Walker, H. (1990). *Posture and the development of social action*. Paper presented at International Conference on Infant Studies, Montreal.

Fogel, A., Nwokah, E., & Karns, J. (in press). Parent-infant games as dynamic social systems. In K. B. MacDonald (Ed.), *Parents and children playing*. New York: State University of New York Press.

Fogel, A., & Thelen, E. (1987). Development of early expressive and communicative action: Reinterpreting the evidence from a dynamic systems perspective. *Developmental Psychology, 23,* 747–761.

Fogel, A., Toda, S., & Kawai, M. (1988). Mother–infant face-to-face interaction in Japan and the United States: A laboratory comparison using 3-month-old infants. *Developmental Psychology, 34,* 398–406.

Franco, F., & Butterworth, G. (1989). *Is pointing an intrinsically social gesture?* Paper presented at the Annual Conference of the British Psychological Society–Developmental Psychology Section, Guilford.

Goldin-Meadow, S., & Mylander, C. (1990). Beyond the input given: The child's role in the acquisition of language. *Language, 66,* 323–355.

Goshen-Gottstein, E. R. (1986). On whose needs does mother focus? Mother- or child-centered care and the self-other differentiation of maternal needs. *Psychiatry, 49,* 54–68.

Gould, S. J. (1977). *Ontogeny and phylogeny.* Cambridge: Harvard University Press.

Gusella, J. L., Muir, D., & Tronick, E. Z. (1988). The effect of manipulating maternal behavior during an interaction on three- and six-month-olds affect and attention. *Child Development, 59,* 1111–1124.

Hay, D. F., & Ross, H. S. (1982). The social nature of early conflict. *Child Development, 53,* 105–113.

Jennings, K.D., Curry, N. E., & Connors, R. (1986). Toddlers' social behaviors in dyads and groups. *The Journal of Genetic Psychology, 147,* 515–528.

Karns, J. (1986). *Dyadic and group play of toddlers.* Poster presented at the Biennial Conference on Human Development, Vanderbilt University, Nashville, TN.

Karns, J., & Fogel, A. (1990). *Sequential organization of mother–twin infant interaction.* Poster presented at the Seventh International Conference on Infant Studies. Montreal, Canada.

Kaye K. (1980). Why we don't talk 'baby talk' to babies? *Journal of Child Language, 7,* 489–507.

Kaye, K. (1982). *The mental and social life of babies.* Chicago: University of Chicago Press.

Kaye, K., & Fogel, A. (1980). The temporal structure of face-to-face communication between mothers and infants. *Developmental Psychology, 16,* 454–464.

Kendrick, C., & Dunn, J. (1980). Caring for a second baby: Effects on interaction between mother and firstborn. *Developmental Psychology, 16,* 303–311.

Kotelchuck, M. (1976). The infant's relationship to the father: Experimental evidence. In M. E. Lamb (Ed.), *The role of the father in child development* (pp. 329–344). New York: Wiley.

Kreppner, K., Paulsen, S., & Schuetze, Y. (1981). *Infant and family development: From triads to tetrads.* Paper presented to the Society for Research in Child Development, Toronto, Canada.

Lamb, M. E. (1986). The changing roles of fathers. In M. E. Lamb (Ed.), *The father's role: Applied perspectives* (pp. 3–27). New York: Wiley.

Lee, L. C. (1973). Social encounters of infants: The social strategies of two individual infants. *Dornell Journal of Social Relations, 8,* 234–255.

Legerstee, M., Corter, C., & Kienapple, K. (1990). Hand, arm and facial actions of young infants to a social and nonsocial stimulus. *Child Development, 61,* 774–784.

Legerstee, M., Pomerleau, A., Malcuit, G., & Feider, H. (1987). The development of infants' responses to people and a doll: Implications for research in communication. *Infant Behavior and Development, 10,* 81–95.

Lempers, J. D. (1979). Young children's production and comprehension of nonverbal deictic behaviors. *The Journal of Genetic Psychology, 135,* 93–102.

Lewis, M., & Feiring, C. (1981). Direct and indirect interactions in social relationships. In L. Lipsitt (Ed.), *Advances in infancy research* (Vol. 1). Norwood, NJ: Ablex.

Lewis, M., Feiring, C., & Kotsonis, M. (1984). The social network of the young child: A developmental perspective. In M. Lewis (Ed.), *Beyond the dyad.* New York: Plenum Press.

Lock, A. (1980). *The guided reinvention of language.* New York: Academic Press.

Lock, A., Young, A., Service, V., & Chandler, P. (1990). Some observations on the origins of the pointing gesture. In V. Volterra & C. Erting (Eds.), *From gesture to language in hearing and deaf children.* New York: Springer-Verlag.

Mayes, L. C., & Carter, A. S. (1990). Emerging social regulatory capacities as seen in the still-face situation. *Child Development, 61,* 754–763.

McGuire, J. (1982). Gender-specific differences in early childhood: The impact of the father. In N. Beail & J. McGuire (Eds.), *Fathers: Psychological perspectives* (pp. 95–125). London: Junction Books.

Messinger, D., & Fogel, A. (1990). *The role of referential gazing in object exchange.* Poster presented at the annual convention of the American Psychological Association, Boston.

Murphy, S. O. (1988). *Newborns and school age siblings.* Paper presented to the International Conference on Infant Studies, Washington, DC.

Murphy, C. M., & Messer, D. J. (1977). Mothers, infants, and pointing. In H. R. Schaffer (Ed.), *Studies in mother–infant interaction* (pp. 325–354). London: Academic Press.

Newell, K. M. (1986). Constraints on the development of coordination. In M. G. Wade & H. T. A. Whiting (Eds.), *Motor development in children: Aspects of coordination and control* (pp. 341–360). NATO ASI Series. Dordrecht: Martinus Nijhoff.

Ninio, A., & Rinott, N. (1988). Fathers' involvement in the care of their infants and their attribution of cognitive competence to infants. *Child Development, 59,* 652–663.

Orlansky, M. D., & Bonvillian, J. D. (1985). Sign language acquisition: Language development in children of deaf parents and implications for other populations. *Merril-Palmer Quarterly, 31,* 127–143.

Parke, R. D. (1981). *Fathers.* Cambridge: Harvard University Press.

Piaget, J. (1952). *The origins of intelligence in children.* New York: International Universities Press.

Power, T. G. (1985). Mother- and father-infant play: A developmental analysis. *Child Development, 56,* 1514–1524.

Power, T. G., & Parke, R. D. (1982). Play as a context for early learning: Lab and home analyses. In L. M. Laosa & I. E. Sigel (Eds.), *Families as learning environments for children* (pp. 147–178). New York: Plenum Press.

Reinecke, M. A. (1987). The development of referential communication in infancy: An analysis of "point," "grasp," and "show." Dissertation. Purdue University.

Rogoff, B. (1990). *Apprenticeship in thinking: Cognitive development in social context.* New York: Oxford University Press.

Ross, H., Tesla, C., Kenyon, B., & Lollis, S. (1989). *Maternal intervention in toddler peer conflict and the socialization of principles of justice.* Manuscript submitted for publication.

Sagi, A. (1982). Antecedents and consequences of various degrees of paternal involvement in child rearing: The Israeli project. In M. E. Lamb (Ed.), *Nontraditional families: Parenting and child development.* Hillsdale, NJ: Erlbaum.

Schaffer, H. R. (1984). *The child's entry into a social world.* New York: Academic Press.

Stern, D. (1977). *The first relationship: Infant and mother.* Cambridge: Harvard University Press.

Stern, D. (1985). *The interpersonal world of the infant.* New York: Basic Books.

Stoller, S., & Field, T. (1982). Alteration of mother and infant behavior and heart rate during a still-face perturbation of face-to-face interaction. In T. Field & A. Fogel (Eds.), *Emotion and early interaction* (pp. 57–82). Hillsdale, NJ: Erlbaum.

Teti, D. M., & Ablard, K. E. (1988). *Infant-sibling relationships and child-parent attachment.* Paper presented to the International Conference on Infant Studies, Washington DC.

Teti, D. M., Bond, L. A., & Gibbs, E. D. (1988). Mothers, fathers, and siblings: A comparison of play styles and their influence upon infant cognitive level. *International Journal of Behavioral Development, 11,* 415–432.

Thelen, E. (1989). The (Re)discovery of motor development: Learning new things from an old field. *Developmental Psychology, 25,* 946–949.

Tomasello, M., Mannle, S., & Kruger, A. C. (1986). Linguistic environment of 1- to 2-year old twins. *Developmental Psychology, 22,* 169–176.

Trevarthen, C. (1986). Development of inter-subjective motor control in infants. In M. G. Wake & H. T. A. Whiting (Eds.), *Motor development in children: Aspects of coordination and control* (pp. 341–360). NATO ASI Series. Dordrecht: Martinus Nijhoff.

Tronick, E. (1977). *An ontogenetic structure of face-to-face interaction and its developmental functions.* Paper presented to the Society for Research in Child Development, New Orleans.

Tronick, E., Als, H., Adamson, L., Wise, S., & Brazelton, T. B. (1978). The infant's response to entrapment between contradictory messages in face-to-face interaction. *Journal of the American Academy of Child Psychiatry, 17,* 1–13.

Vygotsky, L. (1978). *Mind in society: The development of higher psychological processes.* Cambridge: Harvard University Press.

Yogman, M. W. (1982). Observations on the father–infant relationship. In S. Cath, A. Gurwitt, & J. M. Ross (Eds.), *Father and child: Developmental and clinical perspectives* (pp. 101–122). Boston: Little, Brown.

8

Peers and Play in Infants and Toddlers

CELIA A. BROWNELL AND EARNESTINE BROWN

INTRODUCTION

By the preschool years, children spend long periods in play with other children. Their social play is jointly managed, complex, and facile. There also are identifiable and relatively stable individual differences in the affect, skill, and motivation to play with age-mates. These competencies set the stage for much of subsequent socioemotional and cognitive development (Hartup, 1983).

But where do these abilities come from? Only in the last decade and a half have scholars systematically explored the peer play and interaction skills of infants and toddlers. What can we conclude? That in their first 2 years, children are not asocial with their peers, in contrast to many interpretations of Parten's (1932) early, classic, and oft-cited findings; that rudiments of virtually all the sophisticated skills we can observe in older children's social play emerge in the first 2 years; that individual differences in sociability become obvious in peer contexts during the first 2 years, and appear to remain stable thereafter; that individual differences in some affective dimensions of peer play may also emerge early and remain stable into childhood; that toddlers' peer play reveals remarkable, and heretofore unsuspected, social-cognitive competencies. Finally, despite these important conclusions, we know relatively little at this point about the developmental mechanisms involved in normative changes in very early play skills or in the early emergence of individual differences.

CELIA A. BROWNELL AND EARNESTINE BROWN • Psychology Department, University of Pittsburgh, Pittsburgh, Pennsylvania 15260.

Handbook of Social Development: A Lifespan Perspective, edited by Vincent B. Van Hasselt and Michel Hersen. Plenum Press, New York, 1992.

CELIA A.
BROWNELL and
EARNESTINE
BROWN

This chapter will review what we have learned in recent years about the interaction skills of very young children in play with each other. How sociable are infants and toddlers with peers? What skills do they have available for initiating and sustaining play with age-mates? Do very young children share, cooperate, and empathize with one another? Or are their interactions characterized primarily by conflicts over possessions? How do they manage conflict? Do they have friends, and what does friendship mean for a toddler? What do experience and particular interaction contexts contribute? When do individual differences in interaction style or peer competence begin to emerge, and what are the implications? Finally, what developmental mechanisms have been proposed or might be proposed to explain acquisition and growth of interaction skills and individual differences in interaction style or skill?

We will first discuss the major developmental patterns in a variety of peer play skills, then turn to individual differences. We will also consider influences on the performance of peer competencies and potential mechanisms for change and/or continuity.

DEVELOPMENTAL PATTERNS

The traditional picture of infants and toddlers playing with each other represents them as interested in peers as objects, but lacking the social skill or interest to engage one another as social partners (e.g., Bridges, 1933; Buhler, 1933; Maudry & Nekula, 1939; Parten, 1932; Shirley, 1933). Indeed, brief informal observations of infants in playgroups or child care settings would seem to confirm such a representation. Babies approach one another with little eye contact or other clearly social behavior, toy with one another's clothing, hair, limbs, or playthings, and depart with nary a glimmer of recognition. Toddlers often appear little better. They mostly play solitarily, busy with toys or individual pretend scenarios, or they engage their mothers or other adults in social play. When they do engage one another it often appears accidental, fleeting, and centered around the taking or keeping of favored play objects.

But these informal observations belie remarkable motivations and competencies in peer social play. Although peer play is infrequent in the first 2 years (as well it should be when the infant's major developmental task is to establish an adaptive and functional relationship with parents), when peer play does occur it is clearly socially motivated and directed. That "solitary" and "parallel" play exist in the early years is unquestioned. But these forms of play do not represent the full complement of peer social skills or propensities of very young children. This has been recognized since the mid-1970s (Appolloni & Cook, 1975; Becker, 1977; Bronson, 1975; Eckerman, Whatley, & Kutz, 1975; Finkelstein, Dent, Gallagher, & Ramey, 1977; Goldman & Ross, 1978; Lamb, 1977; Lee, 1973; Lewis, Young, Brooks, & Michalson, 1975; Moore, 1978; Mueller & Lucas, 1975; Mueller & Brenner, 1977; Ross & Goldman, 1977; Rubenstein & Howes, 1976; Vincze, 1971). A rereading of the research conducted earlier in the century reveals that these pioneers observed infant–infant play as well. Moreover, the opportunity to play with peers during the toddler years appears to stimulate more mature activity with both the physical and social worlds (Cohen & Tomlinson-Keasey, 1980; Gunnar, Senior, & Hartup, 1984; Rubenstein & Howes, 1976, 1979; Vandell, 1979).

Researchers have documented several aspects of development in infants' and toddlers' peer play. Some descriptions have focused on the specific social content of young children's overtures to peers, such as gestures, offers of toys, affect displays, and so on. Others have focused on the complexity of children's social overtures and interactions. Still others have focused on the forms that peer play takes, such as imitative, reciprocal, cooperative, or symbolic. Finally, some have assessed particular kinds of skills such as game-playing, group entry, or friendship formation.

The First Year

In the first year, infants' interest in peers is marked by heightened arousal and high rates of mutual visual regard beginning as early as 2 months (Eckerman, 1979; Field, 1979; Fogel, 1979), but relatively low amounts of real engagement. By 6 to 9 months, infants direct looks, vocalizations, smiles, or touches to one another as frequently as once or twice per minute; and up to 40% of the time such overtures get a response from the peer (Becker, 1977; Eckerman *et al.*, 1975; Finkelstein *et al.*, 1978; Hay, Nash, & Pederson, 1983; Vandell *et al.*, 1980; Vandell & Wilson, 1982). Nevertheless, in one exemplary study, out of 15 minutes of observation, only 23 seconds, on average, involved peer interaction (Vandell & Wilson, 1982).

By 10 to 12 months, children's interest in their peers has become more evident, with 60% of brief observation periods including some kind of peer-directed behavior, although half of those are still simple watching (Eckerman, 1979; Eckerman *et al.*, 1975). Interestingly, imitation of peer activities begins to appear at this point also. However, the majority of young infants' peer contacts occur around toys, with smiles and vocalizations to one another next most frequent (Eckerman, 1980), and complex interactions (e.g., imitation) occurring rarely. Whether infants become more responsive to one another's social behavior in the latter half of the first year remains unresolved; reported response rates to a peer's initiation are approximately 50%, with some as low as 12% and some as high as 67% (see Hay *et al.*, 1982, for a more detailed discussion). Nevertheless, by the end of the first year, infants have an impressive repertoire of peer-directed social signals that function to get infants involved in social play with one another, even if infrequently and only briefly.

It should be noted that estimates of interaction rates between very young children depend on how interactions are defined and identified (Bronson, 1981; Hay *et al.*, 1982). For example, interactions might be counted only when specified interactive behaviors occur, such as attempts to imitate a peer's behavior or attempts to join another's play. Alternatively, interaction might be credited whenever any response occurs contingent on a peer's behavior within a preselected time interval. Although the former may underestimate peer responsiveness in infants, the latter may overestimate it. As Vandell *et al.* (1980) have noted, peer social behavior can evoke a variety of responses, some quite undifferentiated and not always clearly social. Yet as Hay *et al.* (1982, 1983) also argue, nonrandom temporal contingencies or statistical dependencies between peers' behaviors reflect the operation of some kind of social influence. For example, they found few instances of strict temporal contingency between 6-month-olds' distress and their peers' distress; however, they did find statistical dependencies cumulated over time intervals. This suggests that 6-month-olds can socially influence one another even if they lack the social and/or cognitive skills to engage one another intentionally in social play. The distinction between "social influence" and "interaction" is an important one, albeit seldom recognized in the research on early peer play. It may be that the former sets the stage for the latter.

The Second Year

In the second year, toddlers make significant strides in peer play. Their interest in and motivation to engage one another in play increases, evidenced by higher rates of engagement. Affect accompanying peer play is also more evident, particularly positive affect (Adamson & Bakeman, 1985; Bronson, 1981; Mueller & Vandell, 1979; Ross & Goldman, 1977). Peer play can be maintained for longer periods, with increases especially marked after 18 months (Bronson, 1981; Eckerman et al., 1975; Eckerman & Whatley, 1977; Finkelstein et al., 1978; Gunnar et al., 1984; Jacobson, 1981; Mueller & Brenner, 1977).

Children's play also becomes more complex as it becomes organized around consistent themes (Brenner & Mueller, 1982; Eckerman, Davis, & Didow, 1989; Goldman & Ross, 1977; Ross, 1982) and exhibits increasingly coordinated role relations between the players (Eckerman & Stein, 1982; Eckerman et al., 1989; Howes, 1987; Mueller & Lucas, 1975; Ross, 1982). These are not the sophisticated social roles like "Mommy," "Daddy," and "Baby" we can observe in preschoolers' social pretend play (Bretherton, 1984; Howes, 1987; Watson & Fischer, 1980). Rather, they are simpler, perhaps foundational behavioral or interactive roles wherein one child's role is to imitate the other or to be the one chased in a game of chase, for example. Such peer "games" or bouts of thematic social play almost never occur in the first year. However, after the middle of the second year, they occur regularly, even among unacquainted children (Brenner & Mueller, 1982; Eckerman et al., 1989; Ross, 1982).

Such coordinated play activity depends, in part, on what Eckerman & Stein (1982) have called *interactive skills*. That is, social behavior must be keyed to the peer's behavior so that it is timed to occur when the peer is attending and so that its content matches appropriately the content of the peer's behavior and the peer's current interests (see also Bronson, 1981; Finkelstein et al., 1977; Ross, 1982). There is ample evidence that such skills do not emerge until the latter half of the second year (cf. Brownell, 1986; Eckerman & Stein, 1982; Eckerman et al., 1989).

There are several kinds of interactive skills available to the toddler for coordinating behavior with a peer partner. One primary strategy is imitating the peer's play (Eckerman et al., 1989). Between 15 and 28 months, toddlers engage in increasing numbers of social games with one another; and the most common strategy for establishing and maintaining them is imitation (Eckerman et al., 1989; Ross, 1982). However, even this strategy entails particular subskills if it is to be effective in coordinating play. These include communicating to the peer one's own intentions as well as understanding the peer's behavior and communications, managing the turn-taking structure, coping with disruptions in the flow of behavior, and so on (Eckerman & Stein, 1982; Ross, 1982). Several studies of toddlers' games and communicative exchanges have documented that 1-year-olds possess a variety of nonverbal means for conveying communicative intentions (Brenner & Mueller, 1982; Eckerman & Stein, 1982; Goldman & Ross, 1978; Ross, 1982; Ross, Lollis, & Elliott, 1982) and that they comprehend and respond appropriately to their peers' communicative overtures.

Corresponding to growth in interactive skills, several distinct dimensions of peer play become evident late in the second year. Toddlers begin to cooperate in problem solving as well as in play (Brownell & Carriger, 1990), regulate possession and conflict episodes (Bakeman & Brownlee, 1982; Bronson, 1981; Brownell & Brown, 1985), and share and exhibit empathy (Radke-Yarrow, Zahn-Waxler, & Chapman, 1983; Zahn-Waxler, Iannotti, & Chapman, 1982). Children's responsiveness to peer behavior also becomes more differentiated over the second year. They begin to respond differently to affiliative versus agonistic overtures from peers (Bronson, 1981; Kavanaugh & McCall, 1982), to age and sex differences in peer partners (Brownell, 1990; Howes, 1988; Jacklin & Maccoby, 1978), and to individual differences in one another's behavior (Brown & Brownell, 1990; Howes, 1988; Ross & Lollis, 1989b).

In conjunction with more differentiated play skills, toddlers also begin to exhibit playmate preferences in the second year. These have been described in two ways. On the one hand, toddlers as a group prefer to play with peers who are sociable and are less likely to play with peers who are relatively seldom socially involved (Brown & Brownell, 1990; Howes, 1988). Individually, toddlers also begin to exhibit preferences for particular playmates (Howes, 1983; Ross & Lollis, 1989b). Although these social preferences have been referred to as "friendships" and they remain stable over the toddler and early preschool years (Howes, 1983, 1988), toddler friendships possess few of the markers of friendships found among older children (see Hartup, 1983). Nevertheless, it is unknown whether the "friendships" of toddlers serve different functions from friendships among older children or whether the differences are due more simply to the nonreflective nature of very young children's relationships.

The differentiation of play types and partner preferences in the second year may mark a qualitative transition in children's social competence. Distinct forms of play as well as sensitivity to partner differences require a variety of social-cognitive and symbolic skills that emerge during this period (see Brownell, 1986a; Howes, 1987; McCune-Nicolich, 1981; Radke-Yarrow et al., 1983). These early skills and preferences also provide the context for the rapid growth and further differentiation of peer play over the preschool years and beyond.

Despite such clear and important differentiation of peer play skills in the second year, we must be careful not to overstate the very young child's social competence with peers. There remain years of development in the peer social system (Hartup, 1983) with corresponding acquisition of a multitude of specific competencies, as well as growth in the sophistication of the rudimentary abilities we observe by 24 months.

First, peer interaction is still infrequent, even by the end of the second year. Twenty to 30% of social behavior directed by one child to another is ignored, and another large proportion is responded to with visual attention only (Bronson, 1981; Holmberg, 1980; Mueller & Brenner, 1977). Adult–child interaction and/or object play occur at greater rates than child–child interaction (Bronson, 1975; Field, 1979; Finkelstein et al., 1978; Mueller, 1979; but see Rubenstein & Howes, 1976).

Second, peer play is still very much object centered during the second year, much as in the first year. Toy- or object-related behaviors constitute up to 60% to 80% of observations of peer social play (Eckerman, 1979; Mueller & Brenner, 1977). It is toy-related social behavior that exhibits the very large increases in frequency over the second year, and object-related social play still occurs more often than social involvement without toys, even by the end of the second year.

Third, very young children remain limited in their abilities to coordinate behavior with one another. Although complementary, reciprocal roles are adopted in some exchanges and although 24-month-olds can share, cooperate, and behave empathically toward one another, these skills require much more environmental support than they will later, even a short 6 months later (Bronson, 1981; Eckerman et al., 1989).

SITUATIONAL INFLUENCES AND PERFORMANCE FACTORS

Understanding of toddler social play is incomplete without considering the variety of influences on children's expression of their social competence. In particular, the roles of toys, partner familiarity, and peer experience in children's peer play reveal that even the youngest children's social play is sensitive to characteristics of the physical and social setting. Some investigators have argued, in fact, that a focus on the child's general, cross-situation abilities limits our picture of development. They suggest that part of development involves flexibility in the conditions under which the child can function, and the variety of partners and settings to which children can respond (Eckerman, 1979; Turkewitz, 1980). We turn, then, to examine young children's social play as a function of selected setting influences.

Toys

Given the high rates of toy- and object-related social play in the first 2 years, a legitimate question is whether the peer-directed behavior observed is truly social or whether it is an artifact of common interest in the same materials. One obvious way to test this possibility is to remove toys from the play situation and look for changes in the frequency or quality of peer-directed social behavior.

Several investigators have taken this approach, and they concur that infants are more sociable with one another in the absence of toys. As early as 1939 (Maudry & Nekula), toys were found to depress rates of social behavior among infants between 6 and 13 months, and to increase negative affect. Similar findings have been reported in more recent investigations with infants (Hay et al., 1983; Ramey, Finkelstein, & O'Brien, 1976; Vandell et al., 1980). Likewise, toddlers are more interactive when toys are absent. They produce more complex interactions, positive affect, physical contact, and imitation when they play together without toys (Eckerman & Whatley, 1977).

In addition to the presence or absence of toys, some research suggests that the size and portability of toys affect the sophistication and affective valence of peer interaction (DeStefano & Mueller, 1982). Specifically, large, nonportable objects encourage more frequent interaction, whereas small toys foster exploration and conflict. Additionally, there is more positive affect expressed in interaction around large toys and more negative affect around small toys.

Finally, longitudinal work has clarified the role that toys play in the growth of peer play (Jacobson, 1981). Early investigators suggested that peer contacts around toys foster the discovery of interpersonal contingencies, hence growth in social skill (Eckerman et al., 1975; Mueller & Lucas, 1975; Mueller & Vandell 1979). Although the data above suggest that objects may serve to distract or undermine peer interaction in some instances, it is possible nevertheless that discovery of the peer as a social being occurs first out of mutual object play (Eckerman, Whatley, & McGhee, 1979). However, upon following a group of infants longitudinally from 10 to 14 months, Jacobson found no evidence that social play emerges out of object play. Instead, he found that most social interaction did not occur in an object-centered context for the youngest infants, even when toys were available. Between 10 and 14 months, children's social play showed similar growth patterns in both object-centered and nonobject centered contexts. It does not appear then that very young children are dependent on the object world to induce or support peer play. Indeed, some scholars of infant development argue that coordinating attention to both object and social partner is a more difficult task than attending to either one alone, and develops only slowly over the first two years (Adamson & Bakeman, 1985; Bakeman & Adamson, 1984). Thus, although toys become more attractive if played with by another (Eckerman *et al.*, 1979), peers do not appear to become either more interesting or more available by virtue of their play with objects.

Peer Experience and Partner Familiarity

By 9 months of age, experience with toddlers or with older siblings depresses sociability among infant peers; however, experience with other infants increases sociability with age-mates (Vandell *et al.*, 1981; see also Becker, 1977; Hay *et al.*, 1982). During the second year, however, experience with siblings appears unrelated to peer social play (Bronson, 1975; Eckerman *et al.*, 1975; Goldman & Ross, 1978; Lewis *et al.*, 1975). As in the first year, though, experience with age-mates generally, as well as familiarity with particular play partners, facilitates peer sociability and skill (Mueller & Brenner, 1977; Howes, 1988; Lewis *et al.*, 1975; Schindler, Moely, & Frank, 1987). For example, toddlers who are familiar with one another are much more likely to touch each other, exhibit more positive affect, initiate play with one another more often (Lewis *et al.*, 1975), and engage in more complex forms of social play (Howes, 1988). Some investigators have speculated that peers become more predictable to one another with increasing familiarity (Bronson, 1975). At ages where it is difficult to establish "shared meanings" or thematic social play, knowing when and how a playmate is likely to respond can be instrumental in facilitating joint play. Even among experienced and familiar toddlers, however, age differences in peer social play remain (Mueller & Brenner, 1977; Brownell, 1990; Eckerman, 1979; Finkelstein *et al.*, 1977; Howes, 1988; Holmberg, 1980). Thus, while experience and familiarity with peers contribute to more frequent and sophisticated interactions, there remain other, perhaps more fundamental developmental mechanisms that contribute to early growth in peer skill.

INDIVIDUAL DIFFERENCES IN PEER PLAY

By the preschool years, there are regular and stable individual differences in children's interest in peer play, in the strategies they use to initiate play with age-mates, in the affective components of their social play, and in the consequences of such differences as seen in other children's preferences for particular playmates. At what point in the acquisition of peer play skills do such individual differences begin to appear? When do they become stable? And when do children recognize and act upon such differences in one another's interaction styles?

CELIA A.
BROWNELL and
EARNESTINE
BROWN

Individual differences in peer play have been relatively little studied in the first 2 years of life. However, a handful of existing investigations are consistent in finding marked differences among children in their earliest peer encounters. In a classic and often-cited unpublished study, Lee (1973) followed a small group of 9- to 12-month-olds as they played with one another. She found that two of the infants stood out, both for their different styles of interacting with their peers, and for the degree to which they were preferred as playmates by their peers. "Jenny" was quiet and unobtrusive in her interactions and was easily engaged by her peers; "Patrick" often grabbed others' toys and failed to respond or terminated interactions with the other infants. In turn, Jenny was most often the recipient of her peers' social bids, whereas Patrick was least often chosen as a playmate. But Jenny was also the frequent victim of many "grabs" and "toy takes"; therefore, it is not altogether clear whether she should be considered "popular" among her infant age-mates or whether she was simply an easy victim.

Vandell (1978, cited in Vandell & Mueller, 1980) reported a slightly different pattern in a playgroup of older toddlers between 16 and 22 months. She found that the most quiet and passive child in the group was the *least* preferred as a playmate. The most active child, who was also "grabby" like Patrick in Lee's analysis, was not shunned by the others as Patrick had been.

Other research since these early reports has also documented individual differences in children's sociability—their motivation to engage peers—and in their play styles as affiliative or agonistic. Bronson (1981), Howes (1988), and Vandell (1979) have found stability in interaction rates over the second year. Children who initiate frequently to peers early in the second year continue to do so throughout the ensuing year. Vandell and Wilson (1982) found similar stability for frequency of social interaction between 6 and 9 months of age, with both mothers and peers.

There is also empirical evidence that peer play *style*, in addition to interaction frequency, is stable over the second year. Bronson (1981) found that differences in rates of agonistic and conflict initiations to peers are stable over the second year, though prosocial and neutral initiations are not. Similarly, Hay & Ross (1982) reported that toddlers' tendency to initiate conflict with peers was stable over a shorter timespan.

Whether these early individual differences are important theoretically or empirically depends on whether they carry any consequences for these young children and whether they continue beyond the second year. Continuity into the preschool years has been reported for rates of play initiations to peers (Bronson, 1981; Howes, 1988), rates of involvement in age-appropriate social play (e.g., simple social play, social pretend play; Howes, 1988), and rates of aggression (Cummings, Ianotti, Zahn-Waxler, & Radke-Yarrow, 1989). Thus individual differences in pre-schoolers' play with peers can be predicted from patterns of peer play in toddlerhood.

By preschool age, individual differences in peer play have important consequences for children's success and standing in the peer group. In other words, preschoolers can differentiate their peers in terms of their social behavior and systematically respond to one another accordingly. Given our understanding of toddlers as relatively unskilled socially and as constrained by egocentrism, added to their relatively low rates of peer interaction, we would not expect them to be able to distinguish individual differences in their peers' play patterns. Accordingly, we would also not expect them to be able to accommodate their own social behavior to such differences among their potential partners. Nevertheless, recent research building on the earlier findings of Lee (1973) and Vandell (1979) suggests that toddlers do, indeed, make such differentiations among their peers. Brown and Brownell (1990) found that the most socially active toddlers were also the most preferred as playmates by peers (see also Bronson, 1981). Like previous investigators, they also found that sociable toddlers were the most "agonistic" in style, often taking toys from others, for example. In contrast, the least preferred toddlers were both less active socially and more friendly or prosocial in their approaches to peers. These quiet, friendly children were seldom approached by playmates, and when they were approached, initiations to them were often agonistic. So toddlers can and do react differently to one another's interaction styles. Further, individual differences in toddlers' social play predicts preschoolers' popularity with their peers (Howes, 1988).

Although small, and in need of replication and greater detail, this literature has important implications. The suggestion is that individual differences in peer sociability and in agonism appear during the second year, are stable over both the short and long term, and are salient enough to systematically affect children's responses to one another. Hence, children's peer group experiences are partly a function of their own social styles, inclinations, and preferences from very early on.

MECHANISMS OF DEVELOPMENT IN PEER PLAY

We have described the developmental patterns in early social play with agemates, as well as several setting influences on the forms that social play takes and individual differences in styles of peer play along with their consequences for the young child. But the real question for developmental psychologists is the question of cause. Knowing that age differences exist does not offer an explanation; it only offers a marker. Similarly, knowing the diversity of factors that influence the performance of early peer competencies does little for helping us to understand their origins and genesis.

Although few have been well tested, explanations have been offered in several forms for both developmental patterns and for individual differences. One class of mechanisms derives from the parent–infant relationship: (a) the security of the child's relationships with parents or (b) concrete interaction skills learned in the scaffolded relationship with parents. A second class of mechanisms derives from factors within the child, such as temperament generally, or sociability specifically. A third class of mechanisms calls on specific experiences outside the parent–infant relationship, particularly experiences with peers. And a fourth class of mechanisms appeals to developments in other domains that might facilitate or constrain the acquisition of social skills.

Developmental Patterns

Although each of these classes of explanation may be a source of individual differences in peer social competence, they are not all relevant for explaining age-related changes. Explanations proposed for normative changes in peer play include generalization of skills learned in parent–infant interaction, acquisition of peer skills directly through peer experience, and cognitive or social-cognitive changes that permit advances in social behavior. These will be considered in turn.

Is it the case "that Freud was correct—that the mother–child relationship is the birthplace of social meaning itself" (Mueller, 1989, p. 323)? Or, as a number of authors have argued, is it more likely that the mother–infant play system and the peer play system are distinct with respect to both skill and motivation (Eckerman, 1979; Hartup, 1983; Lee, 1975; Lewis et al., 1975; Vandell & Wilson, 1982)? Infants and toddlers direct different kinds of social behaviors to mothers than to peers, with vocalizations and looking directed to peers whereas touching and turn-taking characterize interactions with mothers (Lewis et al., 1975; Mueller & Vandell, 1979; Vandell, 1981; Vandell & Wilson, 1987). Nevertheless, there are similarities in the toddlers' developmental trajectories with peer and mother. Growth in time spent in interaction, number of interactions, and the role of objects in interaction occurs in parallel across the two systems (Vandell, 1980). In fact, according to Vandell, no behavior appears first in the mother–infant repertoire, then subsequently in the peer repertoire. These data suggest that development in the mother–infant and infant–infant interaction systems may proceed independently, albeit similarly; it does not fit the hypothesis that the infant generalizes skills from the former to the latter (see also Hartup, 1983, 1989; Hay 1985).

However, Vandell and Wilson (1987) also found that infants with mothers who engaged them in longer turn-taking exchanges were more skilled in infant–infant social interaction. But the implications of these data are less clear when we consider that infants are not always more likely to respond to adult overtures than to peers'. Nor for that matter are adults more likely to respond to infants' overtures than are other infants (Finkelstein et al., 1978; Holmberg, 1980). It remains unclear, therefore, whether infants' social experiences with adults are likely to be any more instrumental than are experiences with peers for acquiring fundamental peer skills. Further, the hypothesis is unexamined that the direction of cause is the reverse—that infants may themselves drive or structure their social interchanges whether with adults or peers (cf. Hay, 1985; Vandell 1980).

In that light, recent research on mother–infant interaction raises the quite intriguing possibility that mothers' social behavior differs in *reaction* to early-appearing differences in infant sociability and person- versus object-orientation (Lewis & Feiring, 1989). Perhaps development of social skill proceeds apace in the mother–infant and infant–infant systems because it is the infant who is in common between the two systems. Indeed, from an ethological perspective it would probably have been unwise (given that we are a social species and depend on the social group for important adaptive functions) for a developmental system to have evolved that required the mother to inculcate such centrally important adaptive skills as those involved in social interaction. This is not to suggest that social experiences are not necessary for the development of social skill. Language experience is necessary to the development of linguistic competence. However, there is little convincing evidence that children are taught language in any explicit way by adults. Similarly, it may be that infants are built to induce normative social skills from even a minimally responsive social environment and that these skills are applied similarly to mothers and peers.

Some investigators have argued that certain aspects of peer skill, such as carrying on a sustained interaction, are directly caused by peer experience specifically (Mueller & Brenner, 1977). However, although there is no doubt that peer experience influences peer play, all the evidence (reviewed before) is that age-related differences in peer social competence remain even among peer-experienced, acquainted children. This suggests that there are other factors operating on the acquisition of peer skill besides experience with age-mates. Moreover, young infants direct different kinds and amounts of social behavior to peers and to mothers prior to peer experience. Thus, although there may be some kinds of skills that can be acquired only in the peer system (see Hartup, 1983), the rudimentary interactive and play skills that we observe in the first 2 years do not appear to belong in that category.

What other age-related factors might be involved in early development of peer social play? There are a wide variety of specific cognitive and perceptual developments over the first two years that correspond to specific advances in social skills (cf. Brownell, 1986a,b; Bullock & Lutkenhaus, 1988; Dunn, 1988; Kagan, 1981; Kopp, 1982; Radke-Yarrow *et al.*, 1983; Sherrod, 1981). In the first year, these include increasing visual acuity early on, followed by changes in contingency perception, memory, causal relations, and object permanence.

In the second year, relevant cognitive changes include the ability to produce mental combinations of symbolically represented real-world events, to plan and monitor one's activity, to subordinate one's activity to external goals or standards, and self–other differentiation. For example, evidence shows relations between increases in the complexity of toddlers' social overtures to peers and growth in their ability to produce more complex sentences and imitate more complex behavior sequences (Brownell, 1988). There is also evidence that growth in self–other differentiation, particularly the recognition that other people are independent agents of their own behavior, relates to development of toddlers' efforts to coordinate their behavior with a peer during the second year (Brownell & Carriger, 1990). The transitions in peer play between 18 and 24 months do not involve simply greater motivation for social engagement. Rather, they feature growth in coordinated actions and roles between peers and in complex overtures directed to peers. It is interesting and telling that these kinds of changes in peer play occur in tandem with similar changes in other domains, including language, imitation, symbolic play, and so on.

What underlies these converging developments is unknown at present. One possibility is advances in the underlying memory and representation system (cf. Brownell, 1986a,b). Another explanation is that children's changing experiences in their social systems induce corresponding changes in cognitive and social-cognitive systems, rather than vice versa. Such possibilities await further scientific inquiry.

Individual Differences

In addition to discerning the contributions to normative developmental changes in peer play, researchers are also interested in the origins and growth of individual differences in peer play. How do some children become more, or less, sociable than others? More or less aggressive or affiliative? More or less the leader or the follower? What accounts for some young children's popularity with other children and some children's lack of success with their peers? Hypotheses here have centered on sources of influence external to the child, as well as intrinsic, child-specific characteristics.

Two sources of influence external to the child are usually posited as sources of individual differences in peer competence: experience with age-mates and experi-

CELIA A.
BROWNELL and
EARNESTINE
BROWN

ences in the parent–infant relationship. Although peer experiences do not appear to contribute a great deal to the development of normative patterns of peer play, they do contribute to individual differences in peer social competence (Howes, 1988). There is nevertheless some dispute over just how much of the variation in peer play styles might be accounted for by experience with age-mates (see Bronson, 1981).

Probably the most likely external source of individual differences in children's developing play style is the parent–infant relationship, if only because of its pervasiveness and its intensity. But there is also conceptual reason to hypothesize that parenting affects children's developing peer competencies (Jacobson, Tianen, Wille, & Aytch, 1986; Lamb, 1978; Maccoby & Martin, 1983; Radke-Yarrow et al., 1983; Sroufe & Fleeson, 1986). There are two main ways that parental influence on early peer competence has been conceptualized. One perspective posits that a variety of particular interaction skills are learned (or not learned) in the parent–infant interaction context and then generalized to peers (e.g., Eckerman et al., 1975; Lamb, 1978; Radke-Yarrow et al., 1983; Vandell & Wilson, 1987). The second perspective emphasizes that the quality of the relationship between infants and parents influences the later acquisition of skills in other social systems (Sroufe & Fleeson, 1986). Thus the security and trust established in the parent–infant relationship (or its failure to be established) is hypothesized to affect fundamental motivations to engage the social environment (Lamb, 1978; Lieberman, 1977) or to affect the infants' affective expressiveness. This, in turn, alters others' social responses to the infant (Jacobson & Wille, 1986; Sroufe & Waters, 1977) or is reproduced by the infant in other social relationships out of a motive to maintain coherence of self over social systems (Sroufe & Fleeson, 1986).

A third perspective has received relatively little empirical attention and so will not be reviewed in detail here. It nevertheless deserves note. It is that parents differentially reinforce particular patterns of peer behavior. For example, Fagot and colleagues (1985) found that parents differentially attended to boys' and girls' assertive and communicative behavior at 13 months when there were no sex differences in the children's behavior. By 24 months children's behavior with peers corresponded to the differential attention previously paid to him or her by parents. Boys were more assertive and girls more communicative.

Empirical test of the first hypothesis, generalization of particular skills from the parent–infant relationship, involves identifying relations between specific maternal behaviors with their infants (and infants with their mothers) and infants' specific behaviors with their peers. Firm conclusions concerning such relations are not yet possible. Some researchers have found parallels in behavior in the peer system and the mother–infant system, with differences in developments in the latter preceding similar differences in the former. This lends support to the notion that skill differences in the peer system are first acquired in the mother–infant system (Eckerman et al., 1975; Vandell & Wilson, 1987). Yet others have found few or no such relations or have found associations that suggest that the common element of the infant carries the parallel developments in the two systems (Lewis et al., 1975; Vandell, 1980; Vandell & Wilson, 1982). One possibility is that the variations in findings are a function of the molecular levels of analysis and the specific behaviors chosen to study. With molecular coding of behavior, there is the risk that either the wrong behaviors are identified by the observation system or that the level of analysis is inappropriate for the question. That is, the source of influence may lie at the level of the interaction or even the relationship, and not at the level of individual, discrete social behaviors (see Jacobson *et al.*, 1986).

Therefore, a second, and more common approach conceptualizes parental influence as acting more generally. The quality of the infant's relationships with parents, broadly defined, is hypothesized to mediate individual differences in other relationships. Here, the supposition is not that different infants learn different specific skills from the parent, but rather that sensitive, responsive parenting provides the infant with the psychological wherewithal to meet new interactive challenges successfully, as well as providing the infant with a generally positive social orientation (Sroufe & Fleeson 1986). Conversely, insensitive parenting leaves the infant poorly prepared to master the peer system.

The literature on infant–parent attachment has consistently shown relations between security of infants' relationships with their mothers and preschool peer competence (LaFreniere & Sroufe, 1984; Lieberman, 1977; Sroufe, 1983; Waters, Wippman, & Sroufe, 1979). Securely attached infants become preschoolers who exhibit greater peer leadership, less caution and withdrawal, more reciprocity in interaction, less negative affect in peer play, and who are judged by their teachers to be more socially competent with peers.

There is also support for similar relations between the quality of the mother–infant relationship and peer competence during the toddler years. Pastor (1981) found that securely attached toddlers were more interested in their peers and were more friendly and prosocial in their peer-directed behaviors than were insecurely attached toddlers. Toddlers who were securely attached as infants were also more attractive as playmates, receiving more positive responses and fewer agonistic initiations, resistance, or disruptive responses from peers than their insecurely attached counterparts (Jacobson & Wille, 1986). Finally, although their attachment relationships were not assessed, toddlers with a manic-depressive parent (and presumably, therefore, less optimal relationships with both parents) exhibited less social play with peers, less sharing and helping, and more frequent and intense aggression toward their playmates following a brief separation from their mothers (Zahn-Waxler, Cummings, McKnew, & Radke-Yarrow, 1984). The research is quite consistent, then, in showing that the quality of the parent–infant relationship has important correlates in peer social behavior both in the toddler years, and beyond. What is transmitted from parenting relationships to peer relationships is, however, unknown at present and will no doubt become a major area of inquiry over the next decade (Jacobson *et al.*, 1986; Lamb, 1978; Maccoby & Martin, 1983; Sroufe & Fleeson, 1986).

Although the most often hypothesized source of individual differences in early peer competence is the parent–infant relationship, constitutional variables may also be at work. Kagan and his colleagues have documented that a small proportion of children are unusually behaviorally inhibited. Their wariness and uncertainty in response to the unfamiliar characterizes their interactions with unfamiliar playmates as well as with unfamiliar objects and events. These children are lower in sociability with unfamiliar peers as early as 21 months, and continuing into middle childhood (Garcia-Coll, Kagan, & Reznick, 1984; Kagan, 1984; Kagan, Reznick, & Gibbons, 1989; Kagan, Reznick, Snidman, & Gibbons, 1988). Although Kagan's research strategy of following a small, extreme group of children is meant to maximize our ability to identify stability and continuity in this aspect of behavioral style, there may also be a lesson for our study of average children.

Namely, if inhibited children's responses to peers can be predicted by early temperament characteristics, perhaps more subtle differences in children's peer play also grow out of individual differences in temperament within the average range. Indeed, Bronson and Pankey (1977) concluded that a within-child dispositional factor accounted for predictability from 2-year-olds' differential reactions in a challenging nonsocial situation to their peer social orientation at 3½ years. And Vandell (1980) found that early in infancy, some infants were more sociable with both mothers and peers than were other infants. Although it is possible that by 6 months mothers have already influenced their infants' sociability with other people, including infant playmates, a more parsimonious explanation would implicate infant temperament. Moreover, even if the quality of the parent–child relationship is formational in early peer relations, it also is fundamentally affected by the child's dispositions (Belsky & Rovine, 1987; Lewis & Feiring, 1989). Despite these intriguing findings, the role of temperament in the development of individual differences in early peer play remains unexplored.

SUMMARY

In this very cursory overview of the major findings and issues in the growth of peer play in the first few years, we hope to have demonstrated the remarkable social competencies of very young children. At the same time, there is much left yet to develop.

During the first year, infants exhibit interest but relatively little skill in interaction with one another. In the second year, and particularly after 18 months, dramatic and pervasive changes begin to occur. Not only does interest in peers and affectivity during peer interaction rise, but a wide variety of interactional skills begin to emerge. These include specific skills for initiating and maintaining interactions as well as more general abilities to coordinate interaction around a theme, goal, or plan, to behave reciprocally, and to communicate effectively. Toddlers also begin to exhibit a variety of prosocial behaviors during interaction with one another, and they begin to differentiate among playmates with different play styles and to have playmate preferences.

There are many influences on the form and frequency of peer play among young children, including the age mixture of the peer group, the familiarity and peer experience of the children involved, the toys available, and so on. There are also many potential influences on the growth of peer play and the emergence of individual differences in play style and skill. Although relatively unexplored, these include characteristics of the parent–infant relationship, children's interaction history with peers, contributions from cognitive or social-cognitive developments, and the child's own temperament or sociability.

It is recognized now that the first 2 years of life are both foundational and formational for later development, whether we focus on normative developmental changes or individual differences in peer play. Future research will continue to detail the particular skills and subskills that are part of successful play exchanges. It will also more directly address issues surrounding the consequences of early emerging individual differences in interactional competence and style as well as questions about origins and mechanisms in the growth of peer social competence.

Adamson, L., & Bakeman, R. (1985). Affect and attention: Infants observed with mothers and peers. *Child Development, 56,* 582–593.

Appolloni, T., & Cook, T. (1975). Peer behavior conceptualized as a variable influencing infant and toddler development. *American Journal of Orthopsychiatry, 45,* 4–17.

Bakeman, R., & Adamson, L. (1984). Coordinating attention to people and objects in mother–infant and peer–infant interaction. *Child Development, 55,* 1278–1289.

Bakeman, R., & Brownlee (1982). Social rules governing object conflicts in toddlers and preschoolers. In K. Rubin & H. Ross (Eds.), *Peer relationships and social skills in childhood* (pp. 99–112). New York: Springer-Verlag.

Becker, J. (1977). A learning analysis of the development of peer oriented behavior in nine-month olds. *Developmental Psychology, 13,* 481–491.

Belsky, J., & Rovine, M. (1987). Temperament and attachment security in the Strange Situation. *Child Development, 58,* 787–795.

Brenner, J., & Mueller, E. (1982). Shared meaning in boy toddlers' peer relations. *Child Development, 53,* 380–391.

Bretherton, I. (Ed.). (1984). *Symbolic play: Development of social understanding.* Orlando, FL: Academic Press.

Bridges, K. (1933). A study of social development in early infancy. *Child Development, 4,* 36–49.

Bronson, W. (1972). Competence and the growth of personality. In K. Connolly & J. Bruner (Eds.), *The growth of competence* (pp. 241–264). New York: Academic Press.

Bronson, W. (1975). Developments in behavior with agemates in the second year of life. In M. Lewis & L. Rosenblum (Eds.), *Friendship and peer relations* (pp. 131–152). New York: Wiley.

Bronson, W. (1981). Toddlers' behavior with agemates: Issues of interaction, cognition, and affect. *Monographs on Infancy,* Vol. 1. Norwood, NJ: Ablex.

Bronson, W., & Pankey, W. (1977). *The evolution of early individual differences in orientation toward peers.* Paper presented at meetings of the Society for Research in Child Development, New Orleans.

Brown, E., & Brownell, C. (1990). *Individual differences in toddlers' interaction styles: Profiles and peer responses.* Paper presented at International Conference on Infant Studies, Montreal.

Brownell, C. (1986a). Convergent developments: Cognitive-developmental correlates of growth in infant/toddler peer skills. *Child Development, 57,* 275–286.

Brownell, C. (1986b). Cognitive correlates of infant social development. In G. Whitehurst (Ed.), *Annals of Child Development, 56,* 275–286.

Brownell, C. (1988). Combinatorial skills: Converging developments over the second year. *Child Development, 61,* 838–848.

Brownell, C. (1990). Peer social skills in toddlers: Competencies and constraints illustrated by same-age and mixed-age interaction. *Child Development, 61,* 838–848.

Brownell, C., & Brown, E. (1985). *Toddler peer interaction in relation to cognitive development.* Paper presented as part of symposium, E. Mueller, Chair, "Early Peer Relations: Ten Years of Research," Society for Research in Child Development, Toronto.

Brownell, C., & Carriger, M. (1990). Changes in cooperation and self-other differentiation during the second year. *Child Development, 61,* 1164–1174.

Buhler, C. (1933). *The first year of life.* New York: John Day.

Bullock, M., & Lutkenhaus, P. (1988). The development of volitional behavior in the toddler years. *Child Development, 59,* 664–674.

Cohen, N., Tomlinson-Keasey, C. (1980). Effects of peers and mothers on toddlers' play. *Child Development, 51,* 921–924.

Cummings, M., Ianotti, R., Zahn-Waxler, C., & Radke-Yarrow, M. (1989). Aggression between peers in early childhood: Individual continuity and developmental change. *Child Development, 60,* 887–895.

DeStefano, C., & Mueller, E. (1982). Environmental determinants of peer social activity in 18 month old males. *Infant Behavior and Development, 5,* 175–183.

Dunn, J. (1988). *The beginnings of social understanding.* Cambridge: Harvard University Press.

Eckerman, C. (1979). The human infant in social interaction. In R. Cairns (Ed.), *The analysis of social interactions: Methods, issues, and illustrations* (pp. 163–178). Hillsdale, NJ: Erlbaum.

Eckerman, C., Davis, C., & Didow, S. (1989). Toddlers' emerging ways of achieving social coordinations with a peer. *Child Development, 57,* 275–276.

Eckerman, C., & Stein, M. (1982). The toddler's emerging interactive skills. In K. Rubin & H. Ross (Eds.), *Peer relationships and social skills in childhood* (pp. 41–72). New York: Springer-Verlag.

Eckerman, C., & Whatley, J. (1977). Toys and social interaction between infant peers. *Child Development, 48,* 1645–1656.

Eckerman, C., Whatley, J., & Kutz, S. (1975). Growth of social play with peers in the second year of life. *Developmental Psychology, 11,* 42–49.

Eckerman, C., Whatley, J., & McGhee, L. (1979). Approaching and contacting the object another manipulates: A social skill of the 1-year-old. *Developmental Psychology, 15,* 585–593.

Fagot, B., Hagan, R., Leinbach, M., & Kronsberg, S. (1985). Differential reactions to assertive and communicative acts of toddler boys and girls. *Child Development, 56,* 1499–1505.

Field, T. (1979). Infant behaviors directed toward peers and adults in the presence and absence of the mother. *Infant Behavior and Development, 2,* 47–54.

Field, T. (1979). Differential behavior and cardiac responses of 3-month old infants to a mirror and a peer. *Infant Behavior and Development, 2,* 179–184.

Finkelstein, N., Dent, C., Gallagher, K., & Ramey, C. (1978). Social behavior of infants and toddlers in a daycare environment. *Developmental Psychology, 14,* 257–262.

Fogel, A. (1979). Peer vs. mother directed behavior in 1 and 3 month old infants. *Infant Behavior and Development, 2,* 215–226.

Garcia-Coll, C., Kagan, J., & Reznick, J. (1984). Behavioral inhibition to the unfamiliar. *Child Development, 55,* 1005–1019.

Goldman, B., & Ross, H. (1978). Social skills in action: An analysis of early peer games. In J. Glick & A. Clarke-Stewart (Eds.), *The development of social understanding* (pp. 177–212). New York: Gardner.

Gunnar, M., Senior, K., & Hartup, W. (1984). Peer presence and the exploratory behavior of 18- and 30-month olds. *Child Development, 55,* 1103–1109.

Hartup, W. (1983). Peer relations. In E. M. Hetherington (Ed.), P. Mussen (Series ed.), *Handbook of child psychology. Vol. 4, Socialization, personality and social development* (pp. 103–196). New York: Wiley.

Hartup, W. (1989). Social relationships and their developmental significance. *American Psychologist, 44,* 120–126.

Hay, D. (1985). Learning to form relationships in infancy: Parallel attainments with parents and peers. *Developmental Review, 5,* 122–161.

Hay, D., Nash, A., & Pedersen (1982). Dyadic interaction in the first year of life. In K. Rubin & H. Ross (Eds.), *Peer relationships and social skills in childhood* (pp. 11–40). New York: Springer-Verlag.

Hay, D., Nash, A., & Pedersen, J. (1983). Interaction between 6-month-old peers. *Child Development, 54,* 557–562.

Hay, D., & Ross, H. (1982). The social nature of early conflict. *Child Development, 53,* 105–113.

Holmberg, M. (1980). The development of social interchange patterns from 12 to 42 months of age. *Child Development, 51,* 448–456.

Howes, C. (1983). Patterns of friendship. *Child Development, 54,* 1041–1053.

Howes, C. (1984). Sharing fantasy: Social pretend play in toddlers. *Child Development, 56,* 1253–1258.

Howes, C. (1987). Social competence with peers in young children: Developmental sequences. *Developmental Review, 7,* 252–272.

Howes, C. (1988). Peer interaction of young children. *Monographs of the Society for Research in Child Development, 53*(1, Serial No. 217).

Jacklin, C., & Maccoby, E. (1978). Social behavior at 33 months in same-sex and mixed-sex dyads. *Child Development, 49,* 557–569.

Jacobson, J. (1981). The role of inanimate objects in early peer interaction. *Child Development, 52,* 618–626.

Jacobson, J., Tianen, R., Wille, D., & Aytch, D. (1986). Infant-mother attachment and early peer relations: Assessment of behavior in an interactive context. In E. Mueller & C. Cooper (Eds.), *Process and outcome in peer relationships* (pp. 57–78). Orlando, FL: Academic Press.

Jacobson, J., & Wille, D. (1986). Influence of attachment patterns on developmental changes in peer interaction from the toddler to the preschool period. *Child Development, 57,* 338–347.

Kagan, J. (1981). *The second year: Emergence of self-awareness* Cambridge: Harvard University Press.

Kagan, J. (1984). Behavioral inhibition to the unfamiliar. *Child Development, 55,* 2212–2225.

Kagan, J., Reznick, S., & Gibbons, J. (1989). Inhibited and uninhibited types of children. *Child Development, 60,* 838–845.

Kagan, J., Reznick, J., Snidman, N., & Gibbons, J. (1988). Childhood derivatives of inhibition and lack of inhibition to the unfamiliar. *Child Development, 59,* 1580–1589.

Kavanaugh, R., & McCall, R. (1982). Social influencing among two year olds: The roles of affiliative and antagonistic behaviors. *Infant Behavior and Development, 6,* 36–52.

Kopp, C. (1982). Antecedents of self-regulation. *Developmental Psychology, 18,* 199–214.

LaFreniere, P., & Sroufe, L. A. (1984). Profiles of peer competence in the preschool: Measures, social ecology, and attachment history. *Child Development, 21,* 56–68.

Lamb, M. (1977). A re-examination of the infant social world. *Human Development, 20,* 65–85.

Lee, L. (1973). *Social encounters of infants: The beginnings of popularity.* Paper presented at the International Society for the Study of Behavioral Development, Ann Arbor, MI.

Lee, L. (1975). Toward a cognitive theory of interpersonal development: Importance of peers. In M. Lewis & L. Rosenblum (Eds.), *Friendship and peer relations* (pp. 204–222). New York: Wiley.

Lieberman, S. (1977). Preschoolers' competence with a peer: Relations with attachment and peer experience. *Child Development, 48,* 1277–1287.

Lewis, M., & Feiring, C. (1989). Infant, mother, and mother–infant interaction behavior and subsequent attachment. *Child Development, 60,* 831–837.

Lewis, M., Young, G., Brooks, J., & Michalson, L. (1975). The beginnings of friendship. In M. Lewis & L. Rosenblum (Eds.), *Friendship and peer interaction* (pp. 27–66). New York: Wiley.

Maccoby, E., & Martin, J. (1983). Parent–child interaction. In E. M. Hetherington (Ed.), *Handbook of child psychology, Vol. 4. Socialization, personality, and social development* (pp. 1–102). New York: Wiley.

Maudry, M., & Nekula, M. (1939). Social relations between children of the same age during the first two years of life. *Journal of Genetic Psychology, 54,* 193–214.

McCune-Nicolich, L. (1981). Toward symbolic functioning: Structure of early pretend and potential parallels with language. *Child Development, 52,* 785–797.

Moore, S. (1978). Child–child interactions of infants and toddlers. *Young Children, 33,* 64–69.

Mueller, E. (1979). Toddlers + toys = an autonomous social system. In M. Lewis & L. Rosenblum (Eds.), *The social network of the developing infant* (pp. 51–73). New York: Plenum Press.

Mueller, E. (1989). Toddlers' peer relations: Shared meaning and semantics. In W. Damon (Ed.), *Child development today and tomorrow* (pp. 312–331). San Francisco: Jossey-Bass.

Mueller, E., & Brenner, J. (1977). The origins of social skills and interaction among playgroup toddlers. *Child Development, 48,* 854–861.

Mueller, E., & Lucas, T. (1975). A developmental analysis of peer interaction among toddlers. In M. Lewis & L. Rosenblum (Eds.), *Friendship and peer relations* (pp. 223–258). New York: Wiley.

Mueller, E., & Vandell, D. (1979). Infant–infant interaction. In J. Osofsky (Ed.), *Handbook of infant development* (pp. 591–622). New York: Wiley.

Parten, M. (1932). Social participation among preschool children. *Journal of Abnormal and Social Psychology, 27,* 243–269.

Pastor, D. (1981). The quality of mother–infant attachment and its relationship to toddlers' initial sociability with peers. *Developmental Psychology, 17,* 326–325.

Radke-Yarrow, M., Zahn-Waxler, C., & Chapman, M. (1983). Children's prosocial dispositions and behavior. In E. M. Hetherington (Ed.), *Handbook of child psychology: Vol. 4. Socialization, personality, and social development* (pp. 469–545). New York: Wiley.

Ramey, C., Finkelstein, N., & O'Brien (1976). Toys and infant behavior in the first year of life. *Journal of Genetic Psychology, 129,* 341–342.

Ross, H. (1982). Establishment of social games among toddlers. *Developmental Psychology, 18,* 509–518.

Ross, H., & Goldman, B. (1977). Establishing new social relations in infancy. In T. Alloway & P. Pliner (Eds.), *Advances in communication and affect, Vol. 3.* (pp. 61–79). New York: Plenum Press.

Ross, H., & Lollis, S. (1989a). Communication within infant social games. *Developmental Psychology, 23,* 241–248.

Ross, H., & Lollis, S. (1989b). A social relations analysis of toddler peer relationships. *Child Development, 60,* 1082–1091.

Ross, H., Lollis, S., & Elliott, C. (1982). Toddler–peer communication. In K. Rubin & H. Ross (Eds.), *Peer relationships and social skills in childhood* (pp. 73–98). New York: Springer-Verlag.

Rubenstein, J., & Howes, C. (1976). The effects of peers on toddler interaction with mother and toys. *Child Development, 47,* 597–605.

Rubenstein, J., & Howes, C. (1979). Caregiving and infant behavior in daycare and in homes. *Developmental Psychology, 15,* 1–24.

Schindler, P., Moely, B., & Frank, A. (1987). Time in daycare and social participation of young children. *Developmental Psychology, 23,* 255–261.

Sherrod, L. (1981). Issues in cognitive-perceptual development: The special case of social stimuli. In M. Lamb & L. Sherrod (Eds.), *Infant social cognition: Empirical and theoretical considerations* (pp. 5–25). Hillsdale, NJ: Erlbaum.

Shirley, M. (1933). *The first two years*. Minneapolis: University of Minnesota Press.

Sroufe, L. (1983). Infant–caregiver attachment and patterns of adaptation in the preschool. In M. Perlmutter (Ed.), *Minnesota Symposium on Child Psychology* (Vol. 16, pp. 41–83). Hillsdale, NJ: Erlbaum.

Sroufe, L., & Fleeson, J. (1986). Attachment and the construction of relationships. In W. Hartup & Z. Rubin (Eds.), *Relationships and development* (pp. 51–72). Hillsdale, NJ: Erlbaum.

Sroufe, L., & Waters, E. (1977). Attachment as an organizational construct. *Child Development, 48*, 483–494.

Turkewitz, G. (1980). The study of infancy. *Canadian Journal of Psychology, 33*, 408–412.

Vandell, D. (1979). Effects of a play group experience on mother–son and father–son interaction. *Developmental Psychology, 15*, 379–385.

Vandell, D. (1981). Sociability with peer and mother in the first year of life. *Developmental Psychology, 17*, 335–361.

Vandell, D., & Mueller, E. (1980). Peer play and friendships during the first two years. In H. Foot, A. Chapman, & J. Smith (Eds.), *Friendship and social relations in children* (pp. 181–208). New York: Wiley.

Vandell, D., Wilson, K., & Buchanan, N. (1980). Peer interaction in the first year of life: Its structure, content, and sensitivity to toys. *Child Development, 51*, 481–488.

Vandell, D., Wilson, K., & Whalen, W. (1981). Birth order and social experience differences in infant–peer interaction. *Developmental Psychology, 17*, 438–445.

Vandell, D., & Wilson, K. (1982). Social interaction in the first year: Infants' social skills with peers vs. mother. In K. Rubin & H. Ross (Eds.), *Peer relationships and social skills in childhood* (pp. 187–208). New York: Springer-Verlag.

Vandell, D., & Wilson, K. (1987). Infants interactions with mother, sibling, and peer: Contrasts and relations between interaction systems. *Child Development, 58*, 176–186.

Vincze, M. (1971). The social contacts of infants and young children reared together. *Early Child Development and Care, 1*, 99–109.

Waters, E., Wippman, J., & Sroufe, L. (1979). Attachment, positive affect, and competence in the peer group: Two studies in construct validation. *Child Development, 50*, 821–829.

Watson, M., & Fischer, K. (1980). Development of social roles in elicited and spontaneous behavior during the preschool years. *Developmental Psychology, 16*, 483–494.

Zahn-Waxler, C., Cummings, M., McKnew, A., & Radke-Yarrow, M. (1984). Altruism, aggression and social interactions in young children with a manic-depressive parent. *Child Development, 55*, 123–136.

Zahn-Waxler, C., Iannotti, R., & Chapman, M. (1982). Peers and prosocial development. In K. Rubin & H. Ross (Eds.), *Peer relationships and social skills in childhood* (pp. 133–162). New York: Springer-Verlag.

9

Sibling Interaction

Douglas M. Teti

Introduction

The study of sibling relationships is an underdeveloped and challenging arena in social and personality development. The dearth of research and theory about siblings is likely owed to traditional emphases on the parent–child relationship, in particular the mother–child dyad, and to the enormous diversity that characterizes sibling behavior. This diversity can create confusion among behavioral scientists who attempt to characterize siblings' behavior along well-defined, conceptual themes. In part, this is because sibling relationships vary along a power–status continuum, which might be expected to influence both structural and qualitative aspects of sibling behavior. In addition, sibling relationships have frequently been described in terms of what are traditionally termed *constellation* variables, such as gender, family size, birth order, and birth spacing, each of which has played a role in discussions of sibling behaviors and influences (e.g., Wagner, Schubert, & Schubert, 1979; Zajonc & Markus, 1975). Finally, sibling relationships, especially in the early years, cannot be understood without consideration of the family contexts in which siblings develop.

Early conceptualizations of sibling behavior as predominantly rivalrous (Levy, 1934; Sewall, 1930; Smalley, 1930) have since yielded to more recent documentation of the remarkable variation in sibling relationships (Dunn, 1983; Dunn & Kendrick, 1982a,b; Furman & Buhrmester, 1985; Teti, Bond, & Gibbs, 1986; Vandell, Minnett, & Santrock, 1987). Indeed, the multidimensional nature of sibling relationships is apparent from interviews with young children, who tend to perceive their relation-

Douglas M. Teti • Department of Psychology, University of Maryland Baltimore County, Baltimore, Maryland 21228.

Handbook of Social Development: A Lifespan Perspective, edited by Vincent B. Van Hasselt and Michel Hersen. Plenum Press, New York, 1992.

ships with their siblings in terms of relative power/status, warmth/closeness, conflict, and rivalry (Furman & Buhrmester, 1985). When young siblings are particularly close in age, their behavior seems to resemble that seen in same-aged peer relationships because of the tendency of each child to create similar experiences for the other. However, siblings' behavior can also take on elements of parent–child relationships in that the younger, less experienced child may be taught, nurtured, or "punished" by the older, more experienced, "wiser" sibling.

In noting the similarities that sibling relationships have to both peer and parent–child relationships, Dunn (1983) invoked the work of Piaget (1965), Hinde (1979), and others to characterize sibling behavior in terms of *reciprocity* and *complementarity*. A reciprocal relationship is one in which each individual creates similar experiences for the other because of commonalities in developmental statuses and interests. Like same-aged peers, young siblings may create reciprocal experiences for each other in imitative, rough-and-tumble, and toy play activities. Complementarity, by contrast, is characteristic of any relationship between two individuals who differ in developmental histories, competencies, and interests. Areas of complementarity include teaching and caregiving, which are more often displayed by older siblings, and monitoring and imitation of play activities, which are more characteristic of younger children. Researchers have yet to elucidate how the reciprocal and complementary features of sibling interaction influence children's development. Dunn (1983) has argued that the reciprocal features of early sibling interaction are of greater developmental import than the complementary features, especially in cultures in which older children are called upon only occasionally to care for and teach their younger siblings. Yet, Rosenberg (1982) has found that personality features and interests seem to vary in relation to the sex composition among sibling dyads. Thus complementary features of sibling interactions may still prove to be important, especially, perhaps, in later childhood and adolescence.

These complexities make siblings particularly compelling subjects to study. In addition, exploring sibling relationships seems important if only because they are likely to be the longest lasting of all family relationships, persisting into old age (Cicirelli, 1982). Thus siblings have many opportunities, perhaps more than parents, to serve as important sources of support, comfort, companionship, and/or antagonism over the lifespan. Even siblings of low access may share salient aspects of their environment and thus may provide validating information of childhood experiences and new avenues for self-reflection and growth. The many years of shared experience are likely to foster bonds between siblings, even though some siblings may not necessarily "get along" at low stress times. Family crises may precipitate the expression of such affectional bonds, or, at the very least, some intensification of the sibling relationship (Bank & Kahn, 1982).

Studying sibling relationships is also justified by the great *differences* that exist among siblings in personality, intellect, and abilities, differences that prevail despite the fact that siblings on average share 50% of their genes (Scarr & Grajek, 1982). So striking are these differences that several behavior geneticists have called attention to the importance of siblings' *nonshared* environmental experiences that stem from differences in such sources as parental treatment, the environments siblings create for each other, and developmental histories. Conceivably, nonshared environmental differences may play a critical role in shaping siblings' abilities (Daniels, 1986; Daniels, Dunn, Furstenberg, & Plomin, 1985; Daniels & Plomin,

1985; Plomin & Daniels, 1987; Rowe & Plomin, 1981). Thus, whereas a sense of shared history and genetic relatedness may foster the development of emotional bonds between siblings, these individuals may yet experience very different environments while growing up. In the early years, the age difference between siblings will inevitably result in each child's creating substantially different environments for the other (e.g., Abramovitch, Corter, & Lando, 1979; Dunn & Kendrick, 1982a; Gibbs, Teti, & Bond, 1987; Lamb, 1978a,b). Differences in sibling-created environments may be reinforced by parental expectations associated with birth order status (Baskett, 1985), gender, and parental labels, which may differentially shape children's behavior toward each other in subtle yet predictable ways (Bank & Kahn, 1982). Further, by late childhood siblings may actively try *not* to be like each other, a process that has been termed *sibling deidentification* (Schacter, 1982; Schacter & Stone, 1987). Thus siblings may represent important reference points against which they can judge and evaluate their behavior and may contribute in important ways to identity formation.

The purpose of this chapter is to examine the extant literature on sibling relationships in infancy and early childhood among normal families. The reader is referred to Lobato (1983), Gallagher and Vietze (1986), and Powell and Ahrenhold (1985) for excellent reviews of sibling relationships within families with a handicapped child. Discussions center first on the more commonly reported interactional characteristics of such relationships from research groups in the United States, Canada, and Great Britain. Relations between these characteristics and sibling constellation variables (e.g., birth spacing, sex) are examined next, in particular because the impact of sibling relationships on personality and intelligence traditionally has been examined in those terms (Sutton-Smith, 1982; Sutton-Smith & Rosenberg, 1970; Wagner *et al.*, 1979). Interactions between young siblings are then discussed in relation to the family context, with specific emphasis on the parent–child relationship in organizing and mediating the development of early sibling relationships. The chapter ends with a broader discussion of what appear to be the salient theoretical issues underlying early sibling relationships and some pressing questions about siblings that remain to be explored.

CHARACTERISTICS OF EARLY SIBLING RELATIONSHIPS

General descriptions of interactions between very young siblings are now available from several research groups, including the United States (Lamb, 1978a,b; Vandell, 1982), Canada (Abramovitch *et al.*, 1979; Abramovitch, Corter, & Pepler, 1980; Abramovitch, Corter, Pepler, & Stanhope, 1986; Pepler, Abramovitch, & Corter, 1981), and Great Britain (Dunn, 1989; Dunn & Kendrick, 1979, 1981a,b, 1982a,b,c). All of these investigations were of two-child families; some were laboratory-based (Lamb and Vandell), others were home-based (Abramovitch and Dunn). Despite the differences in the settings in which the children were observed, a number of consistent findings emerged. First, the complementary nature of early sibling interactions was evident in all studies. Older siblings were typically the leaders in interactions with their younger siblings, directing a disproportionately larger number of social behaviors to the infants than vice versa. In Lamb's studies, which involved the same sample of infants and their preschool-aged siblings when the infants were 18 and 24 months of age, older children were much more likely to vocalize and offer toys to their infant siblings; the infants were much more likely to observe what the older siblings were doing, to imitate the older siblings, and to "take over" the toys with which the older children had played. Abramovitch's longitudinal, home-based observations of young siblings (when the younger children were 20 months, 3 years, and 5 years of age) revealed older siblings to be more likely to initiate prosocial (e.g., give/share, cooperate, request) and agonistic behaviors (e.g., physical aggression, object struggles, verbal threats) to their younger siblings, whereas the toddlers were more likely to imitate their older siblings and to submit to (rather than counterattack) their siblings' aggression. Similar complementarity in interactions was reported by Dunn and Kendrick (1979, 1982a,b), who observed mothers and their preschool-aged firstborns shortly before the secondborn's birth and again when infants were 8 and 14 months of age. Again, older siblings appeared to be important modeling influences for their 14-month-old infants, as evidenced by the infants' strong tendency to imitate the activities of their older siblings. It was also clear from Dunn and Kendrick (1979) and Pepler (1981) that older preschoolers were much more likely to direct and teach their younger siblings than the reverse. As Pepler (1981) described, the brunt of this teaching involved physical, verbal, and conceptual skills. More reciprocal features of infant–sibling interaction were also documented by Dunn and Kendrick (1982a,b), who noted frequent instances of communication in which one child joined the other in an imitativelike game or sequence. These instances they termed *coaction* rather than imitation because of the enjoyment expressed by both children to each other in commonly shared activities.

Interestingly, laboratory studies reported that children spent relatively little time actually interacting with one another in comparison to the time spent interacting with parents (Lamb, 1978a,b) or in nonsocial play (Vandell, 1982). These findings are in marked contrast to home-based observations. The Canadian studies revealed very high rates of interactions between the children at all age points, a difference that is likely attributable to the familiarity of the settings in which the siblings were observed. The absence of extended social exchanges between siblings in laboratory settings may be a simple function of the novelty and diversion that such settings offer both children. In addition, young children in these settings may be predisposed to interact with parents versus siblings when both are available because parents are more inclined to serve a secure-base function for each child in an unfamiliar environment. Dunn and Kendrick's (1979, 1982a,b) further noted that a great range of affect characterized sibling interactions in the home. Some sibling pairs were predominantly prosocial and nurturant, others hostile and rivalrous. Variability in affect was also a cornerstone of many individual sibling dyads, perhaps indicative of ambivalence. Over time, two siblings could direct nurturant or hostile behavior to each other, depending on particular circumstances. Clearly, characterizing early sibling relationships as either "rivalrous" or "prosocial" did no justice to the range of affect observed across and within dyads.

Several of these studies reported stability in siblings' behavior over time and what appeared to be mutual influences between the siblings in their behavior. Lamb (1978b) found significant autocorrelations between 12 and 18 months of the infants' ages for specific interactive behaviors displayed by both children. These behaviors included smiles, vocalizations, looks, laughs, approaches, touches, hits, imitations, accepting toys, taking over toys, struggles, and nonsocial play involving the same materials. Further, a variety of corresponding infant and preschooler behaviors were intercorrelated at the same points in time, and virtually all 12-month infant behaviors directed to preschoolers appeared to relate strongly to preschoolers' corresponding behaviors to infants at 18 months of age. Thus the amount of smiling, vocalizing, looking, laughing, and so forth directed by preschoolers to their infant siblings at 18 months was positively related to the amount of these same social behaviors shown by infants 6 months earlier. Preschoolers' behavior to infants at 12 months also predicted infants' behavior to their older siblings 6 months later, although the associations were less consistent.

Similar stability in sibling interaction during the secondborns' first year was observed by Dunn and Kendrick (1982a,b). Specifically, firstborns who were accepting of and friendly to infant siblings during the first month after the infants' births were more likely to behave prosocially to infants at 14 months of age than were firstborns who were uninterested in or hostile to the infants shortly after birth. Stability in the affective quality of the children's relationships was also apparent over the first 4 to 5 years after the birth of the secondborn, employing maternal reports, interviews with the older siblings, and independent observations of behavior (Stillwell & Dunn, 1985). In addition, when firstborns' behaved prosocially to their infant siblings shortly after birth, the infant appeared to reciprocate in kind at 14 months of age.

Somewhat less longitudinal stability in frequencies of prosocial and agonistic behaviors was reported by Abramovitch *et al.* (1986), although stability in prosocial behavior was improved when such behavior was expressed as a proportion of the total amount of prosocial and agonistic behavior. Like Lamb's and Dunn and Kendrick's findings, Abramovitch *et al.* (1986) found the prosocial and agonistic behavior of both children to be intercorrelated, particularly when the secondborns were 5 years of age (see also Pelletier-Stiefel *et al.*, 1986).

Dunn's British studies are especially noteworthy in that they document the existence of social-cognitive abilities at much earlier ages than what prevailing theories of social-cognitive development would predict. Thus, the sibling dyad appears to be an important vehicle in the study of emerging social-cognitive skills. Dunn and Kendrick (1982a,b) reported that firstborn siblings as young as 2 to 3 years of age appeared capable of correctly interpreting the feelings and intentions of their younger siblings. For example, firstborns commonly remarked to their mothers about their infant siblings' emotional states, why they were in these states, what they liked and disliked, and what they could and could not do, and so forth. These remarks clearly were not projections of the firstborns' own feelings, nor did they reflect confusion in firstborns' ability to distinguish self from other. These findings were contrary to predictions of prevailing theories of social-cognitive development (e.g., Hoffman, 1975), which held that such abilities among 2- to 3-year-olds were rare.

Dunn and Kendrick (1982c) gave further evidence of young firstborns' perspective-taking abilities from observations of firstborns' speech in a study of 13 mother–infant–sibling triads. When addressing the infants, older children consistently simplified their speech, using shorter utterances, more words designed to elicit and maintain attention, and more repetition of utterances in comparison to their speech with mothers. That the older children took pains to make these adjustments indicates that firstborns as young as 2 to 3 years of age are aware of and react to the less advanced developmental status of their infant siblings. There were, of course, still clear differences between firstborns' and mothers' infant-directed speech. Firstborns' attention-getting words and repetitions were almost always used when firstborns were prohibiting the infants, whereas mothers' use of such utterances were typically used in more positive interactive contexts. In addition, mothers were much more likely to incorporate questions and vocal turn-taking sequences during verbal exchanges with their babies than were firstborns, perhaps reflecting mothers' greater concerns about the infants' wishes, intentions, and needs. Interestingly, the firstborns who did use questions typically had close, affectionate relationships with their infant siblings. These firstborns may have been especially concerned with the feeling states of their infant siblings. A more recent study of second-year infants and 3- to 5-year-old older siblings (Tomasello & Mannle, 1985) replicated Dunn and Kendrick's (1982c) findings that older siblings adjusted their speech when addressing their infant siblings, although the quality of this adjustment was again inferior to that of mothers.

Interestingly, Dunn and her colleagues (Dunn & Kendrick, 1982a,b; Dunn, Bretherton, & Munn, 1987; Dunn & Munn, 1985, 1986a) also noted that some *secondborn* children had, by 14 to 15 months of age, a rudimentary ability to understand the feeling states of their older siblings. In one particular case (Dunn & Kendrick, 1982a), a 15-month-old toddler responded to the distress of his older brother by displaying to his brother a behavior (pulling up his shirt to show his stomach) that had always amused his parents. Although this behavior was not appropriate for consoling his older brother, it was apparent that the toddler was aware of his older brother's discomfort and felt his distress might be alleviated by some behavior on his part. Importantly, Dunn and Kendrick (1982a; see also Dunn, 1989) noted that the growth in social-cognitive abilities of 18- to 24-month-old secondborns was not necessarily paralleled by a growth in motivation to respond nurturantly. Older siblings were much more likely to share toys with, help, and comfort their younger siblings than the reverse. Secondborns, by contrast, demonstrated their social-cognitive skills by cooperating with the older siblings during bouts of pretend play and engaging in actions specifically tailored to tease, provoke, and/or annoy.

Two laboratory studies have specifically examined the propensity of preschool-aged children to provide caregiving and nurturance to distressed infant siblings. In a study of 54 mothers and their 30- to 58-month-old children, Stewart (1983) reported that slightly over half of the children attempted to relieve the distress of their infant siblings when mothers were absent from the playroom. In a subsequent study of similarly aged children and their mothers, Stewart and Marvin (1984) replicated the earlier finding that slightly over half of the older children provided caregiving, but also reported that the tendency of the older children to do so was related to their perspective-taking abilities. In addition, infants appeared to use older siblings as subsidiary attachment figures (i.e., approaching and maintaining proximity) in the absence of their mothers only when the older siblings were caregivers. Interestingly, when a mother left their two children alone in the playroom, she was more likely to ask her older child to help take care of the baby when the older child was classified as a perspective taker. Perspective-taking skills presumably are related to the preschoolers' ability to relate and respond to the infants' distress. A more recent study (Howe & Ross, 1990) did not replicate the relation between perspective taking and caregiving in a laboratory playroom among preschool-aged siblings, although the authors noted that a substantially lower proportion of infants were distressed in the laboratory setting.

Sibling constellation variables are germane to any discussion of young sibling relationships for the simple reason that such markers are commonly used to refer to, describe, and "explain" young children's behavior (e.g., "My kids play rough because they're both boys," or "He follows her around because she's the older"). Traditionally, there has been tremendous interest in the role of sibling constellation variables in the development of personality and intelligence (see reviews by Cicirelli, 1967, 1982; Pfouts, 1980; Rosenberg, 1982; Schooler, 1972; Sutton-Smith & Rosenberg, 1970; Wagner, Schubert, & Schubert, 1979). This chapter will not concern itself with this vast literature, except to point out that there is some evidence that firstborns *tend* to score more highly on intelligence and achievement tests and also tend to be overly represented in positions of high prestige. More inconsistent are findings relating sibling constellation variables to personality characteristics and sociability. Most of the studies of young siblings' *behavior* and sibling constellation variables have emerged in the last 15 years. As we shall see, equivocality exists in the findings of these studies as well.

Birth Order

Perhaps the most consistent finding of this literature, and one that was previously discussed, is that firstborns' direct and lead interaction with second-borns. Thus reports in the United States (Gibbs, Teti, & Bond, 1987; Lamb, 1978a,b; Teti, Gibbs, & Bond, 1989; Vandell, 1982), Great Britain (Dunn & Kendrick, 1979, 1982a,b), and Canada (Abramovitch *et al.*, 1979 1980; Pepler, 1981) collectively report that firstborns engaged in greater frequencies of positive, negative social behaviors, and teaching, and that infant siblings were more likely to follow, imitate, and take over the toys of the older sibling regardless of whether the older siblings were actually interacting with the infants. Similar complementarity in the interactions of preschool- and school-aged siblings have been reported (Brody, Stoneman, & MacKinnon, 1982; Brody, Stoneman, MacKinnon, & MacKinnon, 1985; Stoneman, Brody, & MacKinnon, 1984), who found that older siblings took on teacher, managerial, and helper roles more frequently than did younger siblings, who in turn took on observer, managee, and helpee roles more frequently than did older siblings.

The fact that an older sibling evidences her enhanced social competence during interactions with an infant sibling and that the infant sibling seems to find this fascinating is not especially surprising. However, Lamb (1978a,b) speculated that infants may benefit cognitively by observing and imitating the play activities of their older siblings, and a study by Wishart (1986) supported this hypothesis. Specifically, first-year infants' performance in an object concept task improved after observing a preschool-aged sibling demonstrate the task, relative to a no-demonstration control group. In a more recent study of 5- to 6-year-olds, Hesser and Armitzia (1989) reported that a younger sibling looked at and imitated his or her older sibling more than a same-aged friend of the older sibling during triadic object play. These results suggest that an older sibling is more likely to influence the behavior of a younger sibling than is an older peer. Koester and Penny (1987) have provided further support for this view with their findings that 3-year-old children were more likely to explore an unfamiliar environment in the presence of their older siblings than in the presence of unfamiliar older children (see also Samuels, 1980). Pepler's (1981) Canadian observations also indicate that younger siblings' response to teaching by their older siblings is typically positive. And an earlier laboratory study of older children (Cicirelli, 1972) revealed that younger siblings learned a task more effectively when taught by their older female siblings versus an unrelated peer. In a later investigation, Cicirelli (1973) further demonstrated that children's performance on a categorization task was facilitated when they were helped by their older siblings than when they worked alone. Thus younger siblings may benefit from the expanded cognitive and social repertoire of their older siblings, although it is unclear how long term these benefits might be.

Birth Spacing

Equally compelling to researchers have been the putative relations between young siblings' behavior and sibling birth space and gender. This interest is based on a variety of earlier studies highlighting either theoretically or empirically the importance of each of these variables. With regard to birth spacing, Koch (1955) argued that children in closely spaced dyads are more strongly affected by each other than are children in widely spaced dyads, in which there are more concentrated opportunities for parents to exert their influence. Some support for this view has been provided by Minnett, Vandell, and Santrock (1983), who found that 7-year-olds in closely spaced sibling dyads had more intense and rivalrous relationships than did 7-year-olds in widely spaced dyads. Thus a wide birth spacing has been considered by some to be socially and intellectually advantageous for both children. For example, in a study of 5- to 15-year-old boys, Pfouts (1980) reported that five siblings of closely spaced dyads manifested poorer adjustment on the California Test of Personality and to have poorer family relations relative to brothers of widely spaced dyads. In addition, fathers of closely spaced brothers reported that their sons related less well to each other, had fewer intellectual qualities, liked school less, and were less successful in school than did the fathers of widely spaced brothers. Further evidence for the positive association between birth spacing and cognitive/intellectual development has been provided by Cicirelli (1973, 1974), who reported that younger children who were taught by siblings who were 4 years older learned a categorization task better than did younger children who were taught by siblings who were 2 years older. It should be noted, however, that the putative influence of birth spacing on intelligence and personality is by no means clear. Some studies have reported no relation between birth spacing and intelligence (Cicirelli, 1967; Schoonover, 1959). Others have reported that birth spacing "effects" on intelligence, attitudes, and personality are dependent on the sex of sibling (Koch, 1954, 1955, 1956; Rosenberg & Sutton-Smith, 1969).

A major impetus in the development of interest in the "effects" of birth spacing was the provocative report by Zajonc and Markus (1975; see also Zajonc, 1976; Zajonc, Markus, & Markus, 1979) that large birth spacing mitigates against the detrimental "effects" of large family size on intellectual performance, especially for laterborn children. Their "confluence model" was an attempt to explain the negative relations, obtained from aggregate data, between intellectual test scores and family size. In brief, Zajonc and Markus (1975) proposed that the intellectual environment for a given child within a family was diluted with the birth of successive children, under the assumption that intellectual climate can be expressed as an average of the intellectual levels contributed by each member of a family. Assuming that each parent contributes 100 intellectual units to the family (using their example) and each child contributes an increasing number of units as she or he gets older (0 units at birth), the intellectual climate of a given family can be calculated by simply averaging the number of intellectual units contributed by all family members. As family size increases, this average will necessarily become reduced as the number of intellectual immature family members increases. For laterborn children, large birth spacings compensate for the negative association between family size and intelligence because such children are born into a family whose intellectual climate benefits from the advanced age and competence of the older children. For firstborns, smaller birth spacings are beneficial in that they provide firstborns with earlier opportunities to function as teachers of the second-borns (to the detriment of the secondborns, however). The importance of sibling teaching to intellectual development was highlighted by the fact that only chil-dren's intellectual performances tended to be lower than what the confluence model would have predicted. Zajonc and Markus (1975) provided impressive support for this model on the basis of data aggregated from a population of Dutch individuals born during the famine of 1944, although subsequent attempts to apply the model to sample data have met with little success (Grotevant, Scarr, & Weinberg, 1977; see Scarr & Grajek, 1982, and Steelman, 1985, for reviews).

This backdrop led to a variety of studies that specifically examined relations between young siblings' birth spacing and behavior. In all studies reported here, small spacings averaged approximately 1 to 3 years, and large spacings averaged 3 to 5 years. Neither the previously described British (Dunn & Kendrick, 1982a,b) nor the Canadian longitudinal studies (Abramovitch et al., 1979, 1980, 1986; Pepler et al., 1981) found relations between sibling interaction and birth spacing. Both of these investigations had focused primarily on the affective quality of sibling interaction (e.g., prosocial and agonistic behaviors) and concluded that qualitative aspects of sibling interaction in the preschool years bore little relation to the number of years separating the children. This may indeed be the case for the particular age ranges studied and the particular variables examined. Importantly, however, other studies have found birth spacing differences in young siblings' interaction. And the failure of Dunn's and Abramovitch's groups to find such differences may have been because their measures of interaction were largely affective in nature and thus did not tap the differences in cognitive development expected between older and younger preschoolers. Indeed, in the Canadian sample, Pepler (1981) found older siblings in widely spaced dyads to engage in more conceptual teaching than did older siblings in closely spaced dyads. This finding is more in line with Cicirelli's (1973, 1974) report that older siblings of widely spaced dyads were more effective teachers of their younger siblings than were older siblings of closely spaced dyads.

Other work that taps more structural aspects of sibling interaction corroborate the premise that 5-year-old firstborns manifest their more advanced cognitive and social skills during interactions with infant siblings relative to their 3-year-old counterparts. In a middle-class Vermont sample of 12-month-old infants and their predominantly preschool-aged siblings examined over a 6-month period, Teti et al. (1986) found that, when infants and their older siblings were together, infants of widely spaced dyads appeared to enjoy a more intellectually and socially stimulat-ing environment than did infants of closely spaced dyads. Specifically, during 10 minutes of infant–sibling free play, firstborns in widely spaced dyads created significantly more language mastery, concrete reasoning-problem solving, expressive-artistic skill mastery, object play, gross motor, and social game experiences for their infant siblings than did firstborns in closely spaced dyads. In addition, infants and older siblings of widely spaced dyads engaged in significantly less parallel play (play in which each child was involved in their own activity and uninvolved with the other) than did infants and older siblings in closely spaced dyads. Interestingly, these birth spacing differences did not relate to infants' scores on the Bayley Mental Developmental Index (MDI; Bayley, 1969). In a subsequent analysis of the same sample, Gibbs *et al.* (1987) found that infants and older siblings of widely spaced dyads directed more social behavior to each other (e.g., unintelligible vocalizations, verbalizations, and gestures) and were generally more reciprocally interactive than were children of closely spaced dyads. Further, children of widely spaced dyads directed more prosocial bids to each other than did siblings in closely spaced dyads, in contrast to the results of the Canadian and British studies that reported no birth spacing differences in prosocial behavior.

Similar to Lamb's (1978b) and Dunn and Kendrick's (1982a,b) findings, Gibbs *et al.* (1987) reported that moderate stability in infants' and older siblings' behaviors were evident between 12 and 18 months of the infants' age. Further, cross-lagged correlations revealed that the sociability of infants and older siblings when infants were 18 months of age was related to the sociability of their sibling partners 6 months earlier. No relations were found between sibling interaction and the MDI scores of the infants, although there was some evidence that infants' overall amount of social behavior directed to their older siblings related contemporaneously (but not predictively) to the latter's scores on the Stanford Binet Intelligence Scale (Terman & Merrill, 1973). Importantly, both Teti *et al.* (1986) and Gibbs *et al.* (1987) reported that infants of widely spaced sibling dyads spent less time with their older siblings and their mothers than did infants of closely spaced dyads. Thus it was conceivable that infants of widely spaced dyads did not benefit from the more stimulating environment created by their older siblings because the amount of time these infants actually spent with firstborns was insufficient to influence cognitive development. Alternatively, the failure to find differences in the cognitive levels of infants of widely spaced versus infants of closely spaced dyads may have been because infants of closely spaced dyads had increased contact with their mothers, which may have had a compensatory effect.

That older firstborns were apparently more capable of creating more stimulating environments for infant siblings and promoting social interaction with their infant siblings than were younger firstborns during free play is likely due to the enhanced social-cognitive repertoire of the older children. Four- to 5-year-old children would also be expected to be more competent at taking the perspective of their infant siblings and thus more adept at fostering more sustained bouts of interaction than would younger siblings. The differences between the Vermont study and the Canadian and British studies are likely due to the specific behaviors chosen for analyses as well as to the methodologies employed. Teti *et al.* (1986) analyzed behaviors that were perhaps more sensitive to differences in older children's social-cognitive levels (e.g., language mastery, concrete reasoning/problem solving, expressive-artistic skill mastery). And Gibbs *et al.* (1987) not only examined molecular social behaviors but also the degree to which children engaged in turn-taking exchanges. By contrast, the Canadian and British groups reduced all behaviors into broad affective categories that may not have been

sensitive to differences in older children's cognitive levels. In addition, the Canadian and British observations were largely unstructured, whereas the Vermont
study examined infant–sibling interaction during behavioral "probes" specifically
designed to capture free play. Thus the birth spacing results of the Vermont group
are relevant if one wished to determine what infants and their preschool-aged
siblings do when *they actually play with each other*.

Sex of Siblings

Interest in sex differences in the interactions of young siblings has been
motivated in part by earlier studies of older children indicating that older female
siblings are more effective teachers of their younger siblings than are older male
siblings (Cicirelli, 1972, 1975) and by findings suggesting that older female siblings
are socialized to be more nurturant and prosocial and are more likely to perceive
themselves as caretakers than are male older siblings, whereas boys are socialized
to be more aggressive than are girls (Koch, 1956; Sutton-Smith & Rosenberg, 1970).
In addition, a variety of earlier reports on older children found sibling sex
differences in intelligence and personality (e.g., Koch, 1954, 1955, 1956; Rosenberg,
1982), although the specific nature of these differences has varied across studies.
Along these lines, the ability to establish consistent sex differences in studies of
actual sibling interaction has been ephemeral at best, and discrepancies among
studies have not been easily interpreted. Lamb (1978a) found no sex differences in
infant–sibling interaction when the infants were 18 months of age; however, when
data from the 12- and 18-month observation points were combined (Lamb, 1978b),
older girls were found to be more social than were older boys. This finding seemed
to be consistent with the general notion that girls are socialized to be more
nurturant and sensitive in their interactions than are boys. Similar sex differences
in the prosocial, nurturant behavior of older siblings were reported by Abramovitch *et al.* (1979, 1980) when the younger siblings were 20 months of age. However,
these sex differences were no longer apparent at later observation points (Abramovitch *et al.*, 1986; Pepler *et al.*, 1981). Very few sex differences in infant–sibling
behavior were found in the Vermont study as well (Gibbs *et al.*, 1987, Teti *et al.*,
1986) and in a recent laboratory study of sibling interaction, attachment, and
caregiving (Teti & Ablard, 1989).

More consistent sex differences have been reported in unstructured observations of sibling interaction involving older children, however. Teaching of younger
siblings was mostly carried out by older sisters (Brody *et al.*, 1985; Stoneman,
Brody, & MacKinnon, 1986); further, regardless of the sex composition of the
sibling dyad, female older siblings took on the "manager" role most frequently
(Stoneman *et al.*, 1986). Minnett *et al.* (1983) reported similar findings with regard
to teaching among 7-year-old children and also noted that older female siblings
praised their younger siblings most often. These findings and those of Cicirelli and
of Brody and his colleagues suggest that the infancy and early preschool period is
too early to find any differential socialization effects of males and females.

Data regarding infant and preschool-aged sibling behavior and the sex composition of the sibling dyad are no less inconsistent. Dunn and Kendrick (1981a)
reported that, by 14 months of the infants' ages, both older and younger children in
same-sex sibling pairs directed more positive behavior toward each other than did
children in mixed-sex pairs. Further, children in same-sex dyads showed increases

in positive, prosocial behavior between 8 and 14 months of the infants' ages. Older children in mixed-sex pairs directed more negative, agonistic behavior toward their infant siblings than did their counterparts in same sex pairs; both children in mixed-sex pairs increased their negative behaviors toward each other between 8 and 14 months of the infants' ages. In their interpretation, Dunn and Kendrick (1981a) speculated that perhaps children of same-sex dyads are more motivated to interact positively and prosocially with their sibling if they share the same gender, or, alternatively, because they are more likely to enjoy similar interests and activities. They also noted that mothers tended to interact and play more with the baby at 14 months if the baby was the opposite sex of the older child, and that, in the full sample, the quality of this mother–infant interaction was negatively related to the quality of the sibling relationship. Thus it was possible that the more negative interactions between opposite-sexed siblings resulted from the older children's feelings of rivalry and competition vis-à-vis the younger children.

Support for these findings was not forthcoming from other research groups, although it should be noted that, in the Canadian sibling study, Pepler *et al.* (1981) found negative, agonistic behavior to increase in mixed-sex dyads between the secondborns' ages of 20 and 38 months, and a concomitant decline in the amount of imitation of the older children by the younger. This study and others, however, either did not observe relations between sibling behavior and dyadic sex composition (e.g., Gibbs *et al.*, 1987), or if they did so, the results were opposite that of Dunn and her colleagues. Stewart's (1983) laboratory study found that older siblings of *mixed-sex* dyads provided more caregiving in response to infants' distress than did older siblings of same-sex dyads. This observation was replicated in a subsequent study (Stewart & Marvin, 1984), but only for males. By contrast, Teti and Ablard's (1989) laboratory study of sibling behavior and attachment failed to find any "effects" of children's sex or dyadic sex composition on older children's caregiving. Finally, in their study of 7-year-olds and their older or younger siblings, Minnett *et al.* (1983) reported that same-sex sibling dyads showed *more* negative behaviors than did mixed-sex dyads.

Thus it remains unclear just what "effects," if any, sibling sex and dyadic sex composition have on sibling behavior in early childhood. Nor is there any clearly explicated theory that could be used to generate hypotheses regarding this question. Dunn and Kendrick (1981a) argued that same-sex siblings are more prosocial perhaps because of shared interests and activities, perceptions of the other child as "like me," or because mothers' increased interest in infants who are opposite in sex to the older children fosters rivalry and ill-feelings in the older children. However, it also seems feasible to argue that shared interests and activities may just as readily foster rivalry and agonistic behavior between two siblings (as reported by Minnett *et al.*, 1983), especially if they lead to competition for the same resources.

Beyond the clearly established findings that birth order plays a major role in the asymmetry and complementarity of early sibling interaction, it may be too ambitious to expect consistent findings relating sibling interaction to sibling birth spacing and gender among infant and preschool-aged siblings. Indeed, birth spacing, gender, and dyadic sex composition represent nothing more than *marker* variables, each of which says little about the actual dynamics of sibling behavior. This point may pertain especially to attempts to relate affective dimensions of sibling behavior to sibling constellation variables. Indeed, whereas birth order and birth spacing may play a role in *structural* aspects of early sibling relationships, such marker variables appear to be of little value in predicting the *quality* of sibling behavior. As the foregoing discussion also suggests, it is unclear whether differential socialization pressures on males and females can be clearly discerned as early as the infancy and preschool periods, or, for that matter, whether such differential pressures will be as prevalent in the future as they purportedly are at present. As more and more men, from sheer economic necessity, are called upon to perform child care and domestic duties, one might expect young boys and girls to view caregiving and nurturance to be as characteristic of the male sex role as the female role. As the next section indicates, affective dimensions of young sibling interaction may be more effectively and consistently documented by examining sibling relationships within the overall context of the family and, in particular, the parent–child subsystems.

FAMILY INFLUENCES ON SIBLING RELATIONSHIPS

Transitions to Siblinghood

Early conceptualizations of sibling relationships as predominantly rivalrous seem to have stemmed in part from psychodynamic interpretations of the impact of the birth of a younger sibling (Levy, 1934; Winnicott, 1964), which depict the event as a major stressor for the older child (see also Moore, 1969). It has been perceived as normal that a preschool-aged child experiences stress, anxiety, and anger as a result of feeling displaced by the new arrival. Thus psychoanalytic theory would predict that young siblings are at a disadvantage from the very beginning in that their relationship is marked by feelings of rivalry and resentment in the older child.

Efforts to provide empirical support for these claims have met with some success. However, it is important to note that transitions to siblinghood are experienced in a wide diversity of ways, and some older children show no outward manifestation of maladjustment at all. To begin, virtually all studies that have examined this phenomenon report increases in some or all of the following problem areas among many preschool-aged children during the first few weeks following the birth of the second child: Dependency/anxiety (e.g., clingyness, whinyness, following mother around the house, sleep disturbances), regressiveness (e.g., demanding a pacifier or bottle at bedtime or developing toileting problems after toilet training had been achieved), withdrawal (becoming quieter or harder to engage in social interaction), and aggressiveness (verbal and/or physical aggression directed toward mothers and/or the new infants) (Dunn & Kendrick, 1980; Dunn, Kendrick, & MacNamee, 1981; Field & Reite, 1984; Kendrick & Dunn, 1980, 1982; Legg, Sherick, & Wadland, 1974; Nadelman & Begun, 1982; Stewart, Mobley, Van Tuyl, & Salvador, 1987; Taylor & Kogan, 1973; Thomas, Birch, Chess, & Robbins, 1961; Trause *et al.*, 1981; see review by Vandell, 1987). These changes are related to concomitant decreases in the amount of maternal attention given to older children after the birth of the new arrivals, and perhaps to the general prenatal-to-postnatal decreases in prosocial interactions and increases in negative, controlling interactions between mothers and firstborns (Dunn & Kendrick, 1980), especially when mothers were occupied with their babies (Kendrick & Dunn, 1980). In addition, these changes seem to coincide with increases in the older children's activity levels, heart rates, fantasy play and talk, and general agitation during mothers' hospital stay (Field & Reite, 1984).

However, several qualifications are in order. First, much variability characterizes the responses of preschoolers to a baby sibling's birth, and responses range from strongly negative to more positive and maturing (Dunn et al., 1981; Legg et al., 1974; Nadelman & Begun, 1982; Thomas et al., 1961). Indeed, Nadelman and Begun (1982) noted from maternal reports that older children were highly involved in the care of the newborn, with 71% of the older children assisting in diapering and dressing the baby; 43% and 38%, respectively, helping to bathe and feed the baby; and 68% holding, touching, and/or hugging the baby. Second, *strong* negative stress reactions among preschoolers such as those noted may in most cases be shortlived. Thomas et al. (1961) reported that, among 10 children who manifested stress reactions shortly after the newborns' births, 6 showed mild, brief reactions, 1 showed a more moderate reaction, and 3 children showed more severe, lasting reactions.

Third, the specific nature of reactions to new siblinghood appears to vary with a variety of additional factors. Thomas et al. (1961) found the stress reactions to the birth of a newborn to be less severe among older children who already had an older sibling than among firstborn children, suggesting that for the latter group the birth of a baby represents a more salient and threatening environmental change. Thomas et al. (1961) also found little distress in response to a newborn's birth among toddlers 18 months of age or younger, whereas Kendrick and Dunn (1980), Nadelman and Begun (1982), Stewart et al. (1987), and Gottlieb and Mendelson (1990) found dependency/anxiety reactions to be higher in younger preschoolers (between 18 months and 4 years of age) relative to older preschoolers.

The temperamental characteristics of the older children also appeared to play a role in the nature of the response to the newborns' birth. Specifically, Thomas et al. (1961) reported that children with generally more difficult and less adaptable temperaments displayed greater distress in response to the birth than did "easier," more adaptable children. Similarly, Dunn et al. (1981) reported that children with more negative moods were more likely, by mothers' reports, prone to increased withdrawal and sleeping problems than were children who scored below the median on this temperamental dimension. In this study, positive relations were also found between children's clingyness and scores on a scale that combined negative mood and intensity of response. There is some evidence that male preschoolers are more prone to manifest withdrawal than are female preschoolers (Dunn et al., 1981; Nadelman & Begun, 1982). And Nadelman and Begun (1982) reported that males scored more poorly on factor dimensions of frustration/ aggression and proximity maintenance, although girls (but not boys) showed prenatal–postnatal increases in proximity maintenance. Interestingly, Stewart et al. (1987) found that mothers of same-sex sibling dyads reported more "regressive" reactions among preschoolers of same-sex sibling dyads at 1 month post partum than among mixed-sex dyads. Nadelman and Begun (1982), however, reported no such sex of preschooler-sex of infant interactions.

Sibling Behavior and the Mother–Child Subsystem

There are now a variety of studies that relate sibling interaction in early childhood to the quality of the mother–child relationship, under the assumption that young sibling behavior cannot be understood in isolation from the family context in which it develops. Indeed, it does appear that the quality of parent-created environments for older siblings makes a difference in the quality of adjustment of older children to the birth of a secondborn, as well as in the quality of the sibling relationships that ensue. Thomas *et al.* (1961) reported that the birth of a sibling was "not an especially disturbing event" among preschoolers whose fathers were active in providing care to the older children before and after the birth. In addition, Dunn *et al.* (1981) reported increased withdrawal among older pre-schoolers shortly after the birth of their baby siblings when mothers suffered from fatigue or depression.

In a systematic study of the role of parental input in the adjustment of firstborn girls to the birth of a baby sibling, Gottlieb and Mendelson (1990) found that the support reportedly provided to the firstborns by mothers 6 to 10 weeks before the babies' birth interacted with firstborns' level of distress to predict adjustment 5 to 6 weeks postpartum. Specifically, prenatally "high distress" firstborns (as gleaned from mothers' reports on rating scales of preschooler behavior) reportedly showed reductions in their level of distress when they received high levels of support from mothers during the prenatal period (indexed by maternal reports of the amount of nurturance, approval, and assistance directed to first-borns). By contrast, prenatally "high-distress" firstborns whose mothers reportedly provided little prenatal support continued to be highly distressed after the babies' birth. Little difference in postnatal distress was observed between prenatally low-distressed firstborns who received high prenatal maternal support and those who received low prenatal maternal support. Fathers' levels of prenatal support to firstborns appeared to have little impact on firstborns' postnatal adjustment. Similar, albeit nonsignificant interactive, trends between firstborns' prenatal distress and mothers' and fathers' postnatal levels of support were also reported. Although they did not measure parental support *per se*, Dunn and Kendrick (1982a,b) also have provided evidence that the quality of the firstborn–parent relationship prior to the baby's birth appears to relate to the firstborn's quality of adjustment. Specifically, they noted that firstborn girls behaved very negatively to the babies' birth when they were observed to experience more confrontations with their mothers before the birth.

Also reported in Dunn's British studies are relations between mothers' inter-actions with firstborn girls and the developing relationship between the siblings. Dunn and Kendrick (1981b, 1982a,b) reported that when mothers and their first-born girls showed high levels of joint play and attention during the secondborn's perinatal period, firstborns were significantly less likely to behave prosocially toward the infant siblings 14 months postpartum. By contrast, high levels of mother–firstborn confrontation during the early postpartum period were associated with positive infant–sibling relationships at 14 months. These patterns did not seem to relate to the quality of the mother–infant relationship when infants were 14 months of age. These patterns were interpreted in terms of sibling rivalry, which Dunn and Kendrick argued was more likely if mothers were highly and equally playful with both children. This interpretation received some support from additional findings that mothers who were highly playful with firstborns tended to be similarly involved with secondborns as well, and by findings that firstborn girls whose mothers were highly involved with their infants at 8 months of age were especially hostile toward their infant siblings at 14 months. Thus, firstborns, especially females, may be prone to feelings of jealousy and competition if they feel that their relationship with their mothers has been displaced by their younger siblings.

Interestingly, these patterns were not replicated among firstborn boys, perhaps because, as Dunn and Kendrick (1981b, 1982b) speculated, boys are somewhat less susceptible to mothers' influence than are girls and thus are less affected by mothers' shift in attention to the baby. If so, it is of interest to examine firstborn boys' reactions to a newborn sibling in relation to prenatal-to-postnatal shifts in fathers' involvement with them. It would be misleading, however, to conclude that mothers had little influence on developing sibling relationships when the firstborn was a boy. Kendrick and Dunn (1983) reported that firstborn boys were more hostile toward infant siblings at 14 months when mothers frequently prohibited firstborn quarrels with the infant at 8 months. By contrast, mothers with firstborn daughters were likely to prohibit firstborn quarrelsome behaviors when the infants were 14 months old if the siblings displayed high levels of aggression 6 months earlier. Further, mothers were much more stable between 8 and 14 months in their responses to firstborn boys' than to firstborn girls' aggression. However, in a subsequent report, no sex differences in correlational patterns were reported among sibling pairs observed when secondborns were 18 and 24 months of age (Dunn & Munn, 1986b). High levels of maternal prohibition at 18 months were associated with higher frequencies and more intense sibling quarreling at 24 months. In addition, however, high levels of maternal intervention were also associated with the younger children's increased use of justifications, conciliations, and references to socially prescribed rules. As Dunn and her colleagues have noted, causality cannot be inferred from correlational analyses. However, these data suggest that mothers may have clearer attitudes and response strategies with regard to the limits of acceptability in aggression displayed by boys than by girls and resulting in more consistent behavior in response to boys' aggressive behaviors from a very early age. In addition, it appears that high levels of parental attention to sibling conflict may contribute to the frequency of such quarrels but also to an increased in children's understanding of social rules.

That the mother–firstborn relationship may play a salient role in the quality of early sibling relationships is further evidenced by Dunn and Kendrick's (1982a,b) findings that the affective quality of the firstborn–infant relationship was fostered when mothers took the time to involve their firstborns in the infants' care and in understanding the feelings and intentions of the babies. Howe and Ross (1990) reported similar relations between frequencies of mothers' references to firstborns about the babies and older preschoolers' affectively positive interaction and play with their 14-month-old siblings. A logical interpretation of this finding is that firstborns who are included by their mothers in the care of the baby may harbor less feelings of competition and rivalry for their mothers' attention and thus may be more capable of developing less ambivalent, more prosocial relationships with their baby siblings. Additional data that appear to tap the quality of the children's relationship with their mothers more straightforwardly also give evidence that sibling relationships may be organized by the parent–child subsystem along affective domains.

Brody, Stoneman, and MacKinnon (1986) reported relations between school-aged siblings' prosocial behavior and mothers' reported enjoyment of the maternal role. In addition, children's antisocial behavior was negatively related to mothers' reported use of nonpunitive disciplinary techniques. In a study of female siblings in middle childhood, Bryant and Crockenberg (1980) found that children whose mothers were sensitively attuned to their children's expressed needs during play were more frequently prosocial and less frequently antisocial during play. Siblings of insensitive and controlling mothers were more frequently antisocial. Interestingly, sibling disparagement and discomforting were low when both younger and older siblings had a high proportion of their needs met by their mothers but equally high when either or both of the children had a low proportion of their needs met. Such a finding is consistent with family therapy accounts that discrepancies in the way parents treat their children fosters agonistic and competitive relationships between the children (Bank, 1987; Bank & Kahn, 1982).

Only two studies to date (Bosso, 1985; Teti & Ablard, 1989) have systematically examined the role of children's security of attachment to mothers in shaping young sibling relationships, in contrast to the variety of studies that have focused on attachment security and sociability with adults and peers (see review by Teti & Nakagawa, 1990). Using an attachment Q-sorting technique (the Attachment Q-Set) developed by Waters and Deane (1985), Bosso (1985) found that more securely attached 18- to 32-month-older siblings were less negative and more positive toward their infant siblings. These relations were present both in the home and in a university laboratory and in and out of mothers' presence. In a subsequent laboratory study, Teti and Ablard (1989) assessed the security of attachment to mother of older, predominantly preschool-aged siblings' with the same Q-sorting technique and the security of attachment of infants to mothers with the Strange Situation procedure. When mothers played only with the older child, infants who were securely attached were less likely to protest and aggress against their mothers and older siblings than were infants who were insecurely attached infants. In mothers' absence, more secure older siblings were more likely to direct caregiving toward distressed infant siblings than were less secure older siblings; and whenever infants ($n = 6$) sought out the older sibling for comfort in mothers' absence, their older siblings were always more secure.

Teti and Ablard (1989) were able to identify four sibling security status groups: secure infants with more secure older siblings, secure infants with less secure older siblings, insecure infants with more secure older siblings, and insecure infants with less secure older siblings. Of these groups, the highest levels of antagonism were observed among insecure-infant–less-secure older sibling dyads, whereas the lowest levels of antagonism were found among secure infant–more secure older sibling dyads. As previous reviews attest (e.g., Teti & Nakagawa, 1990), secure child–mother relationships are fostered when mothers are sensitively responsive to their children's needs, whereas insecure attachments are associated with parental insensitivity and rejection. Thus the results of these two studies are consistent with earlier findings on older children (Brody *et al.*, 1986; Bryant & Crockenberg, 1980), which reported positive relations between sibling prosocial behavior and positive parent–child relations.

THEORETICAL CONSIDERATIONS AND FUTURE DIRECTIONS

The previous section clearly illustrates the importance of the family in the development of sibling relationships. Children who have developed warm, harmonious relationships with their parents appear to be more likely to develop more prosocial and nurturant relationships with their siblings than are children whose relationships with parents are characterized by insensitivity and rejection. Thus with the obvious exception of birth order, which is straightforwardly related to differences in power and status between very young siblings, it seems more fruitful to consider social-ecological influences on siblings in the early years than to continue the search for relations between sibling behavior and sibling gender, sex composition, and birth spacing. This is not to rule out the potential explanatory power of sibling constellation variables at later ages, however. Gender influences on sibling behavior, for example, might be more consistent in later childhood and adolescence, after the effects of differential socialization pressures on males and females have had more time to be established. One might also expect that the form and structure of sibling relationships will be somewhat more dependent on sibling constellation variables in later years, to the extent that such variables influence the siblings' accessibility to each other and the degree of overlap of each child's peer network.

The relations reported between the parent–child and sibling subsystems fit within a modeling/social learning framework as well as within a more dynamic framework. Teti and Ablard (1989) have interpreted these findings from the perspective of attachment theory (Ainsworth, Blehar, Waters, & Wall, 1978; Bowlby, 1969; Bretherton, 1985; Sroufe & Fleeson, 1986), noting that children who develop "secure" relationships with parents are more likely to develop "working models" of their parents as loving and nurturant and of themselves as worthy of love and support. Further, as Sroufe and Fleeson (1986) have speculated, children internalize both the child's and the parent's role in the parent–child relationship, which in turn organizes children's attitudes and behaviors as they enter into new relationships. Thus, although the sibling and parent–child relationships are distinct family subsystems, children's general approach, perception, and behavior toward siblings might be expected to be influenced by the quality of relationship established with a primary attachment figure. Teti, Nakagawa, Das, and Wirth (1990) have found that security of child–parent attachment among older children has similar interactional correlates as that between infants and their mothers. Specifically, mothers of more secure preschool-aged firstborns behave more nurturantly and sensitively toward their children than do mothers of less secure firstborns. In addition, preschool-aged children's security of attachment to parents might be expected to relate to the sensitivity with which parents manage sibling conflict. Although this hypothesis has not yet been tested, parents who intervene in a large proportion of sibling quarrels may foster insecure attachments in one or both children by being overly intrusive and/or by consistently albeit inadvertently showing favoritism for one child over another. Indeed, in a recent study of 3- to 6-year-olds with 5- to 10-year old siblings, Stocker, Dunn, and Plomin (1989) found that the degree to which mothers behaved differently toward their two children was politively related to sibling competitiveness and control and negatively related to positive sibling play.

That secure children might react less negatively in response to shifts in mothers' attention to a sibling seems in keeping with a more commonsense notion of security. Relative to insecure children, secure children are likely to be more sure of their parents' continued emotional availability despite such shifts because of a relationship history characterized by sensitivity and nurturance. Thus secure children may feel less threatened by their siblings. Even among two children who are both secure, however, it would not be unusual to see rivalrous or hostile behavior on occasion, depending on additional circumstances. Fathers, for example, seem to play an important role in the adjustment of firstborns to the birth of a baby (Thomas *et al.*, 1961) and may play an equally important role in fostering sibling relationships in the early years. The importance of considering fathers' influence on the sibling relationship is highlighted by Dunn and Kendrick's (1982a,b) findings that sibling behavior was negatively affected when mothers had intense, playful relationships with firstborn girls but not with firstborn boys. Preschool-aged boys' reactions to the birth of a baby and to the baby over time may be especially dependent on concomitant fluctuations in their relationships with their fathers.

Interpreting the quality of early sibling relationships from the point of view of attachment theory, however, does not preclude a search for straightforward modeling influences on siblings' behavior. For example, it is unclear what impact the relationship between a first- and secondborn child might have on each child's developing relationship with a thirdborn. Of course this question becomes more and more important and more difficult to address as family size increases. It is no surprise that most researchers have attempted to avoid methodological nightmares relating to family size by studying infant–preschooler sibling relationships in two-child families. In most such families, it is likely that a given sibling pair will have high access to each other in the early years because children's early social ecology is expected to be provided mostly by the immediate family. Efforts to study sibling relationships in larger families might focus on sibling pairs who have high accessibility to each other, under the assumption that highly accessible siblings will be more influential to each others development than will low-access siblings (Bank & Kahn, 1982). A study of sibling relationships in (for example) three-child families, and in particular, how the quality of each sibling dyadic relationship is influenced both directly and indirectly by other family members, would be a noble and worthy undertaking.

As the work of Stewart and Marvin (1984) has attested, preschoolers' cognitive level may play an important role in their propensity to show caregiving to distressed infant siblings, and thus perspective-taking abilities may be an important mediator of sibling relationship quality. Perspective-taking children would be expected to have the ability to generate responses that are more appropriately geared to their infant siblings' distress than would nonperspective-taking children. At present, the author and his colleagues are exploring how preschoolers' perspective-taking skills interact with the quality of the parent–child relationship to affect the transition to siblinghood and to the development of the sibling relationship over time. Perspective takers who enjoy warm, nurturant, "secure" relationships with parents might be expected to show the most adaptive response to the birth of a baby, displaying not only the least agonism but also the most instances of appropriately displayed nurturance. By contrast, nonperspective-takers with problematic, "insecure" relationships with parents might be expected to have the most troublesome transition to siblinghood, showing the most clinginess, whinyness, and the most agonism toward both infant siblings and parents. Nonperspective-taking "secure" children might also be expected to adapt successfully to a new sibling, albeit displaying less appropriate caregiving in response to infant distress. Finally, perspective-taking "insecure" children might be expected to adapt negatively to a new baby, perhaps less in terms of clinging and whining and more in terms of agonistic behavior that is appropriately geared to elicit negative responses from their parents and infant siblings.

In addition to the putative influence of parents in shaping early sibling relationships, it is reasonable to expect that children's endogenous temperamental characteristics would play a role in sibling relationship formation. The few research studies of large samples that have examined the construct of temperament in this regard have done so for the older children of the sibling dyad (e.g., Brody, Stoneman, & Burke, 1987; Dunn *et al.*, 1981; Gottlieb & Mendelson, 1990; Stocker *et al.*, 1989; Thomas *et al.*, 1961) or for both children of sibling dyads who are older (e.g., Brody & Stoneman, 1987). In these studies, parents were asked to complete questionnaires having items that belong to traditionally defined temperamental dimensions (activity, emotional intensity, mood, persistence). It is unclear, however, whether such a method actually assesses "temperament," which is assumed to be a constitutionally, biologically based construct (Lerner & Lerner, 1986), or a more global and diffuse set of perceived personality variables resulting from the interplay among child characteristics, child behavior, and parental behavior and disciplinary styles. Indeed, a mother who reports on her child's temperament much beyond the early infancy period may be reporting on her perception of her *relationship* with her child, which arguably is more akin to an attachment than to a temperament construct. A study of how objective assessments of temperament among secondborns in early infancy impinges upon the sibling relationship independent of parent–child influences would thus be of special interest. It is not unreasonable to expect that older siblings, like some adults (e.g., Crockenberg, 1986), would have more trouble adapting to a younger sibling with a difficult temperament than to one with an "easy" temperament. Less clear is how older siblings' relationships with their parents might mediate this expected relation.

Of potential importance in the study of siblings is the impact that parents' social ecologies have on sibling behavior. Both parental life stressors and buffering influences such as social/marital supports have been negatively and positively associated, respectively, with quality of parenting and child–parent attachment (Crockenberg, 1981; Crnic, Greenberg, Ragozin, Robinson, & Basham, 1983; Egeland & Farber, 1984). Parental stressors and supports may affect sibling relationships through their effects on parent–child relationships or by their more direct impact on the siblings themselves. High levels of parental stress and low levels of social support might be expected to impact negatively on the marital relationship and on the parent–child relationship, which in turn would be expected to foster more agonism and less nurturance between siblings. High levels of support might be expected to have an opposite effect. Further, under conditions of high support, children might be expected to avail themselves directly of parental support figures (e.g., nurturant grandparents and other familial figures), which may hold potential benefits for the sibling relationship. Also important in this vein is the determination of how susceptible the young sibling relationship is to longitudinal changes in life stressors and social/marital supports of parents.

Finally, Kramer (1990) has recently argued that children may learn to deal more effectively with their siblings through friendships, perhaps by fostering basic social skills relating to the establishment and maintenance of interactions with a younger child. In her longitudinal study of 30 families, Kramer (1990) found that the quality 3- to 5-year-old children's relationships with their infant siblings could be predicted by examining the quality of the children's relationships with their friends. Results were similar whether the indexes of quality of sibling relationships were independent videotaped observations or maternal reports of sibling acceptance. Interestingly, predictors relating to the quality of peer relationships appeared to be more important than the quality of the mother–firstborn interaction prior to the infants' birth, although straightforward assessments of firstborns' security of attachment to their mothers were not made. However, this study highlights the point that sibling relationships, even in the early years, may be multiply determined, and that one needs to examine children's social ecology beyond that established by the family.

Summary

The present chapter has been concerned primarily with factors influencing the formation of sibling relationships. However, siblings might also be expected to be potent agents of socialization, given the richness and amount of interaction that exists between siblings in the early years. Interestingly, there are very few published studies that focus on the actual processes by which siblings serve as socialization agents, despite early claims regarding the salience of siblings in this regard (Irish, 1964). It is reasonable to expect that the nature and quality of sibling relationships within a given family context will affect patterns of behavior outside that context. For example, a child who intensely rivals a sibling for the affection or attention of a parent may be predisposed to direct rivalrous behavior to peers in the presence of nonparental authority figures. Such influences can only be identified in the context of family dynamics, as suggested by several family therapeutic accounts of sibling relations in dysfunctional families (Bank & Kahn, 1982; Brody & Stoneman, 1987; Dunn, 1988). Several recent efforts have specifically documented similarities in children's behavior with their siblings and with their peers (Berndt & Bulleit, 1985; Vandell, Minnett, Johnson, & Santrock, 1990; Vandell & Wilson, 1987). It is unclear from these studies, however, whether children's relationships with their siblings were influencing their behavior with their peers, or vice versa. In addition, it is unclear if the observed similarities were by-products of the children's relationship histories with their parents and/or dispositional characteristics of the children themselves. It is argued that establishing sibling socialization effects that are clear of parental influence, especially among very young siblings, is a challenging undertaking because it requires systematic, longitudinal examinations of parent–child, child–sibling, and child–peer interaction, and statistical path analyses that attempt to control for the effects of the mother–child relationship prior to assessing potential causal influences between the sibling and peer systems. Such attempts, however, are critical to a real understanding of how development occurs within a family systems framework.

It is expected that, as children grow older, sibling relationships will become more and more independent of the parent–child subsystem and perhaps more susceptible to the growing influences of friendship and peers. The family's organizational influence on siblings should still be apparent, however, to the extent that siblings predispositions to like each other and to seek out each other for support are expected to be dependent on family influences in the early years. Indeed, it is not unreasonable to suppose that siblings, as a function of the quality of their relationships in the early years, develop perceptions, expectations, and/or "working models" of each other that guide their behavior toward each other in predictable ways. In addition, as children grow, the reciprocal features of sibling relationships would be expected to become more and more predominant, as differences between children in developmental status and competencies diminish. Given the salience of sibling relationships across the lifespan, social scientists should intensify efforts to elucidate the factors that influence the quality and intensity of sibling relationships over time and to determine more clearly the ways in which siblings can shape individual differences in personality, social, and cognitive development.

REFERENCES

Abramovitch, R., Corter, C., & Lando, B. (1979). Sibling interaction in the home. *Child Development, 50,* 997–1003.

Abramovitch, R., Corter, C., & Pepler, D. (1980). Observations of mixed-sex sibling dyads. *Child Development, 51,* 1268–1271.

Abramovitch, R., Corter, C., Pepler, D. J., & Stanhope, L. (1986). Sibling and peer interaction: A final follow-up and a comparison. *Child Development, 57,* 217–229.

Ainsworth, M. D. S., Blehar, M. C., Waters, E., & Wall, S. (1978). *Patterns of attachment: A psychological study of the strange situation.* Hillsdale, NJ: Erlbaum.

Ainsworth, M. D. S., & Wittig, B. A. (1969). Attachment and exploratory behavior of one-year-olds in a strange situation. In B. M. Foss (Ed.), *Determinants of infant behavior* (Vol. 4, pp. 113–136). London: Methuen.

Bank, S. P. (1987). Favoritism. *Journal of Children in Contemporary Society, 19,* 77–89.

Bank, S. P., & Kahn, M. D. (1982). *The sibling bond.* New York: Basic Books.

Baskett, L. M. (1985). Sibling status effects: Adult expectations. *Developmental Psychology, 21,* 441–445.

Bayley, N. (1969). *The Bayley Scales of Infant Development.* New York: Psychological Corporation.

Berndt, T. J., & Bulleit, T. N. (1985). Effects of sibling relationships on preschoolers' behavior at home and at school. *Developmental Psychology, 21,* 761–767.

Bosso, R. (1985). Attachment quality and sibling relations: Responses of anxiously attached/avoidant and securely attached 18 to 32 month old firstborns toward their secondborn siblings. *Dissertation Abstracts International, 47,* 1293–B.

Bowlby, J. (1969). *Attachment and loss: Vol. 1. Attachment.* New York: Basic Books.

Bretherton, I. (1985). Attachment theory: Retrospect and prospect. In I. Bretherton & E. Waters (Eds.), *Growing points of attachment theory and research: Monographs of the Society for Research in Child Development* (pp. 3–35), 50, Serial No. 209, Nos. 1–2.

Brody, G. H., & Stoneman, Z. (1987). Sibling conflict: Contributions of the siblings themselves, the parent-sibling relationship, and the broader family system. *Journal of Children in Contemporary Society, 19,* 39–53.

Brody, G. H., Stoneman, Z., & Burke, M. (1987). Child temperaments, maternal differential behavior, and sibling relationships. *Developmental Psychology, 23,* 354–362.

Brody, G. H., Stoneman, Z., & MacKinnon, C. (1982). Role asymmetries in interactions among school-aged children, their younger siblings, and their friends. *Child Development, 53,* 1364–1370.

Brody, G. H., Stoneman, Z., & MacKinnon, C. (1986). Contributions of maternal childrearing practices and interactional contexts to sibling interactions. *Journal of Applied Developmental Psychology, 7,* 225–236.

Brody, G. H., Stoneman, Z., MacKinnon, C. E., & MacKinnon, R. (1985). Role relationships and behavior between preschool-aged and school-aged sibling pairs. *Developmental Psychology, 21,* 124–129.

Bryant, B. K., & Crockenberg, S. B. (1980). Correlates and dimensions of prosocial behavior: A study of female siblings with their mothers. *Child Development, 51,* 529–544.

Cicirelli, V. G. (1967). Sibling constellation, creativity, IQ, and academic achievement. *Child Development, 38,* 481–490.

Cicirelli, V. G. (1972). The effect of sibling relationship on concept learning of young children taught by child-teachers. *Child Development, 42,* 282–287.

Cicirelli, V. G. (1973). Effects of sibling structure and interaction on children's categorization style. *Developmental Psychology, 9*, 132–139.

Cicirelli, V. G. (1974). Relationship of sibling structuring and interaction on younger sibling's conceptual style. *Journal of Genetic Psychology, 125*, 36–49.

Cicirelli, V. G. (1975). Effects of mother and older sibling on the problem-solving behavior of the younger child. *Developmental Psychology, 11*, 749–756.

Cicirelli, V. G. (1982). Sibling influence throughout the lifespan. In M. E. Lamb & B. Sutton-Smith (Eds.), *Sibling relationships: Their nature and significance across the life span* (pp. 267–284). Hillsdale, NJ: Erlbaum.

Crnic, K. A., Greenberg, M. T., Ragozin, A. S., Robinson, N. M., & Basham, R. B. (1983). Effects of stress and social support on mothers and premature and full-term infants. *Child Development, 54*, 209–217.

Crockenberg, S. (1981). Infant irritability, mother responsiveness, and social support influences on the security of infant–mother attachment. *Child Development, 52*, 857–869.

Crockenberg, S. (1986). Are temperamental differences in babies associated with predictable differences in care-giving? In J. V. Lerner & R. M. Lerner (Eds.), *Temperament and social interaction in infants and children* (pp. 53–74). San Francisco: Jossey-Bass.

Daniels, D. (1986). Differential experiences of siblings in the same family as predictors of adolescent sibling personality differences. *Journal of Personality and Social Psychology, 51*, 339–346.

Daniels, D., Dunn, J., Furstenberg, F. F., & Plomin, R. (1985). Environmental differences within the family and adjustment differences within pairs of adolescent siblings. *Child Development, 56*, 764–774.

Daniels, D., & Plomin, R. (1985). Differential experience of siblings in the same family. *Developmental Psychology, 21*, 747–760.

Dunn, J. (1983). Sibling relationships in early childhood. *Child Development, 54*, 787–811.

Dunn, J. (1988). Annotation: Sibling influences on childhood development. *Journal of Child Psychology and Psychiatry, 29*, 119–127.

Dunn, J. (1989). Siblings and the development of social understanding in early childhood. In P. G. Zukow (Ed.), *Sibling interaction across cultures: Theoretical and methodological considerations* (pp. 106–116). New York: Springer-Verlag.

Dunn, J., Bretherton, I., & Munn, P. (1987). Conversations about feeling states between mothers and their young children. *Developmental Psychology, 23*, 132–139.

Dunn, J., & Kendrick, C. (1979). Interaction between young siblings in the context of family relations. In M. Lewis & L. Rosenblum (Eds.), *The child and its family* (pp. 143–169). New York: Plenum Press.

Dunn, J., & Kendrick, C. (1980). The arrival of a sibling: Changes in patterns of interaction between mother and firstborn child. *Journal of Child Psychology and Psychiatry, 21*, 119–132.

Dunn, J., & Kendrick, C. (1981a). Social behavior of young siblings in the family context: Differences between same-sex and different-sexed dyads. *Child Development, 52*, 1265–1273.

Dunn, J., & Kendrick, C. (1981b). Interaction between young siblings: Association with the interaction between mother and firstborn. *Developmental Psychology, 17*, 336–343.

Dunn, J., & Kendrick, C. (1982a). *Siblings: Love, envy, and understanding*. Cambridge: Harvard University Press.

Dunn, J., & Kendrick, C. (1982b). Siblings and their mothers: Developing relationships within the family. In M. E. Lamb & B. Sutton-Smith (Eds.), *Sibling relationships: Their nature and significance across the lifespan* (pp. 39–60). Hillsdale, NJ: Erlbaum.

Dunn, J., & Kendrick, C. (1982c). The speech of two- and three-year-olds to infant siblings: "Baby talk" and the context of communication. *Journal of Child Language, 9*, 579–595.

Dunn, J., Kendrick, C., & MacNamee, R. (1981). The reaction of first-born children to the birth of a sibling: Mothers' reports. *Journal of Child Psychology and Psychiatry, 22*, 1–18.

Dunn, J., & Munn, P. (1985). Becoming a family member: Family conflict and the development of social understanding in the second year. *Child Development, 56*, 480–492.

Dunn, J., & Munn, P. (1986a). Becoming a family member: Family conflict and the development of social understanding in the second year. *Child Development, 56*, 480–492.

Dunn, J., & Munn, P. (1986b). Sibling quarrels and maternal intervention: Individual differences in understanding and aggression. *Journal of Child Psychology and Psychiatry, 27*, 583–595.

Egeland, B., & Farber, E. A. (1984). Infant-mother attachment: Factors related to its development and changes over time. *Child Development, 55*, 753–771.

Field, T., & Reite, M. (1984). Children's responses to separation from mother during the birth of another child. *Child Development, 55*, 1308–1316.

Furman, W., & Buhrmester, D. (1985). Children's perceptions of the qualities of sibling relationships. *Child Development, 56*, 448–461.

Gallagher, J. J., & Vietze, P. M. (Eds.). (1986). *Families of handicapped persons*. Baltimore: Paul H. Brookes.

Gibbs, E. D., Teti, D. M., & Bond, L. A. (1987). Infant–sibling communication: Relationships to birth spacing and cognitive and linguistic development. *Infant Behavior and Development, 10*, 307–323.

Gottlieb, L. N., & Mendelson, M. J. (1990). Parental support and firstborn girls' adaptation to the birth of a sibling. *Journal of Applied Developmental Psychology, 11*, 29–48.

Grotevant, H. D., Scarr, S., & Weinberg, R. A. (1977). Constellations with adopted and natural children: A test of the Zajonc and Markus model. *Child Development, 48*, 1699–1703.

Hesser, J., & Armitzia, M. (1989, April). *The influence of siblings and non-siblings on children's observation and imitation*. Paper presented at the biennial meeting of the Society for Research in Child Development, Kansas City, KS.

Hinde, R. A. (1979). *Towards understanding relationships*. London: Academic Press.

Hoffman, M. L. (1975). Developmental synthesis of affect and cognition and its implications for altruistic motivation. *Developmental Psychology, 11*, 607–622.

Howe, N., & Ross, H. S. (1990). Socialization, perspective-taking, and the sibling relationship. *Developmental Psychology, 26*, 160–165.

Irish, D. P. (1964). Sibling interaction: A neglected aspect in family life research. *Social Forces, 42*, 279–288.

Kendrick, C., & Dunn, J. (1980). Caring for a second child: Effects on the interaction between mother and firstborn. *Developmental Psychology, 16*, 303–311.

Kendrick, C., & Dunn, J. (1982). Protest or pleasure? The response of first-born children to interactions between their mothers and infant siblings. *Journal of Child Psychology and Psychiatry, 23*, 117–129.

Kendrick, C., & Dunn, J. (1983). Sibling quarrels and maternal responses. *Developmental Psychology, 19*, 62–70.

Koch, H. L. (1954). The relation of "primary mental abilities" in five- and six-year-olds to sex of child and characteristics of his sibling. *Child Development, 25*, 209–223.

Koch, H. L. (1955). The relation of certain family constellation characteristics and the attitudes of children toward adults. *Child Development, 26*, 13–40.

Koch, H. L. (1956). Some emotional attitudes of the young child in relation to characteristics of his sibling. *Child Development, 27*, 393–426.

Koester, L. S., & Penny, J. M. (1987, September). *Siblings as facilitators of exploratory play in young children*. Paper presented at the British Psychological Society, Developmental Section Annual Conference, University of York, York, England.

Kramer, L. (1990, April). Becoming a sibling: With a little help from my friends. In M. Mendelson (Chair), *Becoming a sibling: Adjustment, roles, and relationships*. Symposium conducted at the 7th International Conference on Infant Studies, Montreal.

Lamb, M. E. (1978a). Interactions between 18-month-olds and their preschool-aged siblings. *Child Development, 49*, 51–59.

Lamb, M. E. (1978b). The development of sibling relationships in infancy: A short-term longitudinal study. *Child Development, 49*, 1189–1196.

Legg, C., Sherick, I., & Wadland, W. (1974). Reaction of preschool children to the birth of a sibling. *Child Psychiatry and Human Development, 5*, 3–39.

Lerner, J. V., & Lerner, R. M. (Eds.). (1986). *Temperament and social interaction in infants and young children. New Directions for Child Development* (W. Damon, Editor-in-Chief, pp. 53–73). San Francisco: Jossey-Bass.

Levy, D. M. (1934). Rivalry between children of the same family. *Child Study, 11*, 233–261.

Lobato, D. J. (1983). Siblings of handicapped children: A review. *Journal of Autism and Developmental Disorders, 13*, 347–364.

Minnett, A. M., Vandell, D. L., & Santrock, J. W. (1983). The effects of sibling status on sibling interaction: Influence of birth order, age spacing, sex of child, and sex of sibling. *Child Development, 54*, 1064–1072.

Moore, T. (1969). Stress in normal childhood. *Human Relations, 22*, 235–250.

Nadelman, L., & Begun, A. (1982). The effect of the newborn on the older sibling: Mothers' questionnaires. In M. E. Lamb & B. Sutton-Smith (Eds.), *Sibling relationships: Their nature and significance across the lifespan* (pp. 13–37). Hillsdale, NJ: Erlbaum.

Pelletier-Stiefel, J., Pepler, D., Crozier, K., Stanhope, L., Corter, C., & Abramovitch, R. (1986). Nurturance in the home: A longitudinal study of sibling interaction. In A. Fogel & G. F. Melson (Eds.), *Origins of nurturance: Developmental, biological and cultural perspectives on caregiving* (pp. 3–24). Hillsdale, NJ: Erlbaum.

Pepler, D. (1981, April). *Naturalistic observations of teaching and modeling between siblings*. Paper presented at the Biennial meeting of the Society for Research in Child Development, Boston.

Pepler, D. J., Abramovitch, R., & Corter, C. (1981). Sibling interaction in the home: A longitudinal study. *Child Development, 52*, 1344–1347.

Pfouts, J. H. (1980). Birth order, age-spacing, IQ differences, and family relations. *Journal of Marriage and the Family, 42*, 517–531.

Piaget, J. (1965). *The moral judgment of the child*. New York: Free Press.

Plomin, R., & Daniels, D. (1987). Why are children in the same family so different from one another? *Behavioral and Brain Sciences, 10*, 1–59.

Powell, T. H., & Ahrenhold, P. O. (1985). *Brothers and sisters: A special part of exceptional families*. Baltimore: Paul H. Brookes.

Powell, T. H., & Ogle, P. A. (1985). *Brothers and Sisters—A special part of exceptional families*. Baltimore: Paul H. Brookes.

Rosenberg, B. G. (1982). Life span personality stability in sibling status. In M. E. Lamb & B. Sutton-Smith (Eds.), *Sibling relationships: Their nature and significance across the lifespan* (pp. 167–224). Hillsdale, NJ: Erlbaum.

Rosenberg, B. G., & Sutton-Smith, B. (1969). Sibling age spacing effects upon cognition. *Developmental Psychology, 1*, 661–668.

Rowe, D. C., & Plomin, R. (1981). The importance of nonshared (E_1) environmental influences in behavioral development. *Developmental Psychology, 17*, 517–531.

Samuels, H. R. (1980). The effect of an older sibling on infant locomotor exploration of a new environment. *Child Development, 51*, 607–609.

Scarr, S., & Grajek, S. (1982). Similarities and differences among siblings. In M. E. Lamb & B. Sutton-Smith (Eds.), *Sibling relationships: Their nature and significance across the lifespan* (pp. 357–381). Hillsdale, NJ: Erlbaum.

Schachter, F. F. (1982). Sibling deidentification and split-parent identification: A family tetrad. In M. E. Lamb & B. Sutton-Smith (Eds.), *Sibling relationships: Their nature and significance across the lifespan* (pp. 123–151). Hillsdale, NJ: Erlbaum.

Schachter, F. F., & Stone, R. K. (1987). Comparing and contrasting siblings: Defining the self. *Journal of Children in Contemporary Society, 19*, 55–75.

Schooler, C. (1972). Birth order effects. *Psychological Bulletin, 78*, 161–175.

Schoonover, S. M. (1959). The relationship of intelligence and achievement to birth order, sex of sibling, and age interval. *Journal of Educational Psychology, 50*, 143–146.

Sewall, M. (1930). Some causes of jealousy in young children. *Smith College Studies in Social Work, 1*, 6–22.

Smalley, R. (1930). The influences of differences in age, sex, and intelligence in determining attitudes of siblings toward each other. *Smith College Studies in Social Work, 1*, 23–40.

Sroufe, L. A., & Fleeson, J. (1986). Attachment and the construction of relationships. In W. Hartup & Z. Rubin (Eds.), *The nature and development of relationships* (pp. 51–71). Hillsdale, NJ: Erlbaum.

Steelman, L. C. (1985). A tale of two variables: A review of the intellectual consequences of sibship size and birth order. *Review of Educational Research, 55*, 353–386.

Stewart, R. B. (1983). Sibling attachment relationships: Child-infant interactions in the Strange Situation. *Developmental Psychology, 19*, 192–199.

Stewart, R. B., & Marvin, R. S. (1984). Sibling relations: The role of conceptual perspective-taking in the ontogeny of sibling caregiving. *Child Development, 55*, 1322–1332.

Stewart, R. B., Mobley, L. A., Van Tuyl, S. S., & Salvador, M. A. (1987). The firstborn's adjustment to the birth of a sibling: A longitudinal assessment. *Child Development, 58*, 341–355.

Stillwell, R., & Dunn, J. (1985). Continuities in sibling relationships: Patterns of aggression and friendliness. *Journal of Child Psychology and Psychiatry, 26*, 627–637.

Stocker, C., Dunn, J., & Plomin, R. (1989). Sibling relationships: Links with child temperament, maternal behavior, and family structure. *Child Development, 60*, 715–727.

Stoneman, Z., Brody, G. H., & MacKinnon, C. (1984). Naturalistic observations of children's roles and activities while playing with their siblings and friends. *Child Development, 55*, 617–627.

Stoneman, Z., Brody, G. H., & MacKinnon, C. E. (1986). Same-sex and cross-sex siblings: Activity choices, roles, behavior, and gender stereotypes. *Sex Roles, 15*, 495–511.

Sutton-Smith, B. (1982). Birth order and sibling status effects. In M. E. Lamb & B. Sutton-Smith (Eds.), *Sibling relationships: Their nature and significance across the life span* (pp. 153–165). Hillsdale, NJ: Erlbaum.

Sutton-Smith, B., & Rosenberg, B. G. (1970). *The sibling*. New York: Holt, Rinehart & Winston.

Taylor, M. K., & Kogan, K. L. (1973). Effects of birth of a sibling on mother–child interaction. *Child*

Psychiatry and Human Development, 4, 53–58.

Terman, L. M., & Merrill, M. A. (1973). *Stanford-Binet Intelligence Scale: Manual for the third revision, form L-M.* Boston: Houghton Mifflin.

Teti, D. M., & Ablard, K. E. (1989). Security of attachment and infant–sibling relationships: A laboratory study. *Child Development, 60,* 1519–1528.

Teti, D. M., Bond, L. A., & Gibbs, E. D. (1986). Sibling-created experiences: Relationships to birth-spacing and infant cognitive development. *Infant Behavior and Development, 9,* 27–42.

Teti, D. M., Gibbs, E. D., & Bond, L. A. (1989). Sibling interaction, birth spacing, and intellectual/linguistic development. In P. G. Zukow (Ed.), *Sibling interaction across cultures: Theoretical and methodological issues* (pp. 117–139). New York: Springer-Verlag.

Teti, D. M., & Nakagawa, M. (1990). Assessing attachment in infancy: The Strange Situation and alternate systems. In E. D. Gibbs & D. M. Teti (Eds.), *Interdisciplinary assessment of infants: A guide for early intervention professionals* (pp. 191–214). Baltimore: Paul H. Brookes.

Teti, D. M., Nakagawa, M., Das, R., & Wirth, O. (1990). *Security of attachment between preschoolers and their mothers: Relations among social interaction, parenting stress, and the attachment Q-Set.* Unpublished manuscript, University of Maryland Baltimore County.

Thomas, A., Birch, H. G., Chess, S., & Robbins, A. (1961). Individuality in responses of children to similar environmental situations. *American Journal of Psychiatry, 117,* 798–803.

Tomasello, M., & Mannle, S. (1985). Pragmatics of sibling speech to one-year-olds. *Child Development, 56,* 911–917.

Trause, M. A., Voos, D., Rudd, C., Klaus, M., Kennell, J., & Boslett, M. (1981). Separation for childbirth: The effect on the sibling. *Child Psychiatry and Human Development, 12,* 32–39.

Vandell, D. L. (1982). *Encounters between infants and their preschool-aged siblings during the first year.* Unpublished manuscript, University of Texas at Dallas.

Vandell, D. L. (1987). Baby sister/baby brother: Reactions to the birth of a sibling and patterns of early sibling relations. *Journal of Children in Contemporary Society, 19,* 13–37.

Vandell, D. L., Minnett, A. M., & Santrock, J. W. (1987). Age differences in sibling relationships during middle childhood. *Journal of Applied Developmental Psychology, 8,* 247–257.

Vandell, D. L., Minnett, A. M., Johnson, B. S., & Santrock, J. W. (1990). *Siblings and friends: Experiences of school-aged children.* Unpublished manuscript, University of Texas at Dallas.

Vandell, D. L., & Wilson, K. S. (1987). Infants' interactions with mother, sibling, and peer: Contrasts and relations between interaction systems. *Child Development, 58,* 176–186.

Wagner, M. E., Schubert, H. J. P., & Schubert, D. S. P. (1979). Sibship-constellation effects on psychosocial development, creativity, and health. *Advances in Child Development and Behavior, 14,* 57–148.

Waters, E., & Deane, K. E. (1985). Defining and assessing individual differences in attachment relationships: Q-methodology and the organization of behavior in infancy and early childhood. In I. Bretherton & E. Waters (Eds.), *Growing points of attachment theory and research: Monographs of the Society for Research in Child Development* (pp. 41–65), *50,* Serial No. 209, Nos. 1–2.

Winnicott, D. W. (1964). *The child, the family and the outside world.* London: Penguin Books.

Wishart, J. G. (1986). Siblings as models in early infant learning. *Child Development, 57,* 1232–1240.

Zajonc, R. B. (1976). Family configuration and intelligence. *Science, 192,* 227–236.

Zajonc, R. B., & Markus, G. B. (1975). Birth order and intellectual development. *Psychological Review, 82,* 74–88.

Zajonc, R. B., Markus, H., & Markus, G. B. (1979). The birth order puzzle. *Journal of Personality and Social Psychology, 37,* 1325–1341.

III

Children and Adolescence

The continuation of social development that had its inception in infancy and toddlerhood takes place during childhood and adolescence. In this part the six chapters are devoted to a careful examination of the issues of ongoing development and how such development augurs for the kind of social interaction that will result in adulthood. Unfortunately, the ability to predict from childhood and adolescence onto adulthood is more speculative and theoretical than veridical and data-based at this time, and several of the contributors have focused our attention to this pressing research need. However, despite this limitation, a wealth of data do exist on the social interactions seen in childhood and adolescence, and these known facts are reviewed in the succeeding six chapters.

Carolyn Zahn-Waxler and K. Danielle Smith (Chapter 10) examine the question of the development of prosocial behavior, with specific consideration of the affective, cognitive, and behavioral dimensions. The authors point out how in the last few decades there has been research concern about those developmental factors that contribute to caring, connectedness, and commitment to others. Willard W. Hartup (Chapter 11) considers the importance of peer relationships in early and middle childhood. Although parent–child interactions may be construed as the model for other relationships, children appear to develop their own set of "attributions, expectations, motives, and emotions" when interacting with peers. In looking at the aforementioned, Hartup considers the developmental course, social reputations, social networks, shyness withdrawal, friendship formation, intergroup dynamics, and the individual and the group. Kenneth H. Rubin and Linda Rose-Krasnor (Chapter 12) look at interpersonal problem solving and social competence in children. In so doing, they describe conceptual models for processing social information and suggest variables that could be causally related to interpersonal problem solving. Rubin and Rose-Krasnor's Social Information-Processing Model of Social Competence, Dodge's Model of Social Information Processing, and Selmans's Model of Interpersonal Negotiation and Communicative Competence are examined in detail. Marion O'Brien (Chapter 13) reviews the issues of gender identity and sex roles. She specifically details biological and behavioral sex differences, properties of gender roles, theoretical approaches, and the development of gender-role identity in infancy, early childhood, middle

227

childhood, early adolescence, and adolescence. Throughout the chapter she underscores how this topic has become politicized in recent years, given the concerns of feminists over the unequal treatment of females and males in our society. Susan B. Silverberg, Daniel L. Tennenbaum, and Theodore Jacob (Chapter 14) discuss the issue of adolescence and family interaction. The authors have underscored the major research gaps in this area and have directed the reader to future promising directions. They are particularly concerned with studies that take a longitudinal view and that consider varying ethnic backgrounds, family structures, and socioeconomic levels. A thorough evaluation of coding systems used to categorize family interaction is presented. David J. Hansen, Jeanette Smith Christopher, and Douglas W. Nangle (Chapter 15) survey the work on adolescent heterosocial interaction and dating, pointing to a decline in the amount of research effort in this direction. Developmental issues in terms of dating, sexual activity, sexually transmitted diseases, and pregnancy are evaluated. Other important issues reviewed are dating violence and date rape, special populations (physically and mentally handicapped), and jealousy and infidelity in adolescent relationships. Considerable attention is then accorded to the extant assessment procedures for evaluating heterosocial interactions in adolescents.

10

The Development of Prosocial Behavior

Carolyn Zahn-Waxler and K. Danielle Smith

Introduction

There have been energetic debates throughout time regarding the socio-moral nature of human interaction. Centuries ago, theologians and philosophers framed the issues in terms of stark contrasts (e.g., humans were born with the capacity for good *or* evil, and these qualities were either innate *or* learned). Depending upon one's point of view, societal influences could be seen either as corrupting innocent youth or as a means by which aggressive instincts could be subdued over time to produce caring and compassion. Such unidimensional views gradually began to give way, with increased recognition of our multifaceted nature. Research in the last half century has significantly advanced knowledge about biological and environmental contributors to prosocial and antisocial behaviors. Here we review research on prosocial behavior, from a developmental perspective, emphasizing mainly work published in the last decade. By prosocial or altruistic behaviors we mean acts that include provision of comfort or sympathy, helping, sharing, cooperation, rescue, protection, and defense. We also review work on emotions and cognitions that often accompany, and are integral features of, prosocial behaviors. This includes children's empathy or emotional incorporation of the others' emotional experience, as well as their moral reasoning and cognitive comprehension of others' internal states and needs (perspective taking, role taking).

Carolyn Zahn-Waxler and K. Danielle Smith • Laboratory of Developmental Psychology, National Institute of Mental Health, Bethesda, Maryland 20891.

Handbook of Social Development: A Lifespan Perspective, edited by Vincent B. Van Hasselt and Michel Hersen. Plenum Press, New York, 1992.

CAROLYN ZAHN-
WAXLER and K.
DANIELLE SMITH

Reviews of two decades of research of moral development provide a comprehensive historical, theoretical, and empirical background for work described in this chapter (Hoffman, 1970; Radke-Yarrow, Zahn-Waxler, & Chapman, 1983). Hoffman (1970) reviewed research of the 1960s on moral development. At this time, the emphasis was on the "thou shalt nots," or the ways in which children learned to refrain from wrongdoing. Prevailing constructs included conscience, guilt, internalization, superego, and the like. Freudian theory and learning theory represented the predominant theoretical approaches. By the late 1960s, there was more interest in positive aspects of morality, and prosocial behaviors were studied extensively during the 1970s (see review by Radke-Yarrow et al., 1983). Normative patterns of development and socialization, as well as contexts and mediators of caring behaviors, were emphasized. Research on the development of moral reasoning and its relationship to prosocial, moral actions also assumed prominence (Kohlberg, 1969). This interest in cognitive correlates also was evident in work on perspective taking or role taking, and its relation to positive behaviors.

As we began to review research of the past decade, several shifts in emphasis became apparent. There are now fewer studies of normative patterns of development and socialization of prosocial behavior. There are more studies of conditions of risk both within the child and the environment that may deter adaptive patterns of expression. There has been a shift from conceptualizations of prosocial actions as isolated response patterns to more integrative approaches in which such actions are seen as a part of children's more broadly defined social repertoires. Prosocial behavior is viewed as one dimension of social competence that plays a role in children's developing peer relations. Examination of school-age children's goals and strategies for social interactions, for example, now commonly includes efforts to understand why unpopular children not only engage in aggressive behavior but also show fewer prosocial strategies in problem-solving situations (Renshaw & Asher, 1983).

There has been growing appreciation for the need to study prosocial and antisocial behavior patterns in relation to one another, with entire volumes now devoted to this topic (e.g., Block, Olweus, & Radke-Yarrow, 1986; Zahn-Waxler, Cummings, & Iannotti, 1986). There has been an increase in research on empathy or the vicarious affective arousal experienced in the face of another's distress (Eisenberg & Strayer, 1987) as an important mediator or correlate of prosocial behavior patterns (Radke-Yarrow et al., 1983). The issue of sex differences in empathy and prosocial orientations was a dominant theme during the 1980s. The remainder of this chapter is devoted to review and discussion of substantive findings from representative studies during this research era. We begin with work on the development and socialization of prosocial behavior, then shift to research on empathy, sex differences, conditions of risk, and psychopathology.

THE DEVELOPMENT OF PROSOCIAL BEHAVIOR

When do behaviors reflecting concern for others develop, what forms do they take, and how do they change over time? Many studies have demonstrated that young children show low levels of prosocial behavior and that these behaviors increase during the early and middle elementary-school years. In a review of over 75 naturalistic and experimental studies of children's provision of comfort and sympathy, help, cooperation and sharing (Radke-Yarrow *et al.*, 1983), clear increases with age were found about half of the time. Comforting and sympathetic behaviors were less likely than the other types of prosocial behaviors to increase with age. Most of the research paradigms are cross-sectional, rather than longitudinal in design. These patterns from empirical research are consistent with psychodynamic (Freud, 1958) and social-cognitive (Piaget, 1965) theories in which young children were portrayed as primarily egocentric, dependent, oriented toward self-gratification, and socially inept. In both theories, concern for others, as well as internalization of standards, were hypothesized to evolve during middle childhood.

In Freudian theory, altruism and conscience were not possible until early emotional conflicts within the family were resolved, particularly with regard to the child's aggressive and libidinal impulses. In social-cognitive theory, experience with peers in conjunction with slowly maturing cortical structures were required in order to develop reflective self-awareness, sensitivity to the internal states of others, and role taking or perspective taking. This knowledge was considered an essential prerequisite for prosocial actions.

Age Changes in Prosocial Behavior and Empathy

Studies of children of different ages, conducted since the Radke-Yarrow *et al.* (1983) review, though not so numerous, also indicate that prosocial behaviors increase with age. Older preschool children showed more prosocial behavior than younger preschool children, in response to negative emotions simulated by an unfamiliar adult (Denham & Couchard, 1991). In children ranging in age from late preschool to early adolescence, older children were more likely than younger children to provide verbal comfort or physical help to a crying infant and to help an injured adult or an animal in distress (Chapman, Zahn-Waxler, Cooperman, & Iannotti, 1987; Zahn-Waxler, Friedman, & Cummings, 1983). Empathy also increased with age but not consistently. This is in accord with other studies in which age changes in empathy may or may not appear (Eisenberg & Strayer, 1987; Zahn-Waxler, Kochanska, Krupnick, & McKnew, 1990). Most of the studies where empathy increases with age are based on self-report. In one investigation, when indicators of empathy (e.g., facial sadness in response to another's plight) were directly observed rather than self-reported (Fabes, Eisenberg, & Miller, 1990), a significant *decrease* with age was reported from second to fifth grade.

Studies of moral reasoning during middle childhood and adolescence suggest that as children grow older they come to value intrinsic motives for prosocial acts (e.g., an orientation toward the needs of others) more than extrinsic motives (e.g., hedonism and self-interest) (Eisenberg *et al.*, 1987). This has been demonstrated in cross-national studies as well, including samples from the United States, Italy, West Germany, and Poland (Beohnke, Silbereisen, Eisenberg, Reykowski, & Polmonari, 1989). These data inform us of children's stated values and preferred motives; less is known about how values and motives guide children's actions.

Alternative Interpretations of Developmental Patterns

Children often, but not invariably, show more prosocial behaviors, more empathic responsiveness, more mature reasoning and motivations, and better

CAROLYN ZAHN-
WAXLER and K.
DANIELLE SMITH

comprehension of cultural norms as they grow older. This is consistent with expectations based on psychodynamic and social-cognitive theories that we slowly evolve into more caring and committed creatures. However, these are unresolved issues that are not addressed in these approaches. Development does not always indicate improvement. The motives and empathic feelings verbalized by children are sometimes open to question. And as children grow older, they become increasingly sensitive to what socialization agents desire or require. Prosocial behavior sometimes may reflect conformity, and older children may better understand the utility of such behaviors.

In a carefully designed study of first-, third-, and fifth-grade children's generosity, Zarbatany, Hartmann, and Gelfand (1985) examined whether age increases result in increasing altruistic motivation or increasing susceptibility to situational demands and social influence strategies. Older children were more generous than younger children but only under conditions in which there were adult influence attempts. Younger children were no less generous than older children when adult influence attempts were minimal.

The Early Origins of Concern for Others

According to Kagan (Kagan & Lamb, 1987), children begin to display a moral sense during the second year of life. This is evidenced in adherence to standards, the emergence of empathy, and expressions of anxiety in response to social disapproval. The second year of life is emphasized by emotions theorists view as the period during which higher order, self-conscious, "moral" emotions reflecting some capacity for simple role taking emerge (e.g., empathy, guilt, shame) (Campos, Barrett, Lamb, Goldsmith, & Stenberg, 1983; Darwin, 1872; Izard, 1977). Socialization approaches (Emde, Johnson, & Easterbrooks, 1987; Yarrow, Scott, & Waxler, 1973; Zahn-Waxler, Radke-Yarrow, & King, 1979) also focus on this period as a time when the social environment plays a role in shaping differences in children's moral internalization patterns. Each of these approaches suggests that prosocial behavior patterns are present very early in development, well before children reach school age.

Hoffman (1975) postulated a biological preparedness for empathy that later becomes a basis for prosocial action. It is first in evidence in the reflexive crying of infants responding to the cries of other infants. As children begin to develop understanding of others as separate begins, the arousal beings to be transformed from personal self-distress to sympathetic concern for the victim. Comforting interventions are hypothesized to emerge during this period. Supportive empirical evidence has begun to accumulate. From birth onward, infants are responsive to emotions in others. Contagion (Sagi & Hoffman, 1976; Simner, 1971) and imitation of others' emotions (Field, Woodson, Greenberg, & Cohen, 1982; Meltzoff & Moore, 1977) are present in the first days of life, suggesting a biological predisposition. Infants as young as 10 weeks discriminate between mothers' different emotion expressions (Haviland & Lelivica, 1987; Termine & Izard, 1988).

The beginnings of representational thought during the second year of life (Bruner, 1972; Piaget, 1962) and the use of symbols (e.g., McCall, 1979; Nicolich, 1977) have implications for children's abilities to infer others' perspectives (Butterworth, 1980) and feelings (Rheingold & Emery, 1986). During this period, self-recognition and self–other differentiation to develop (e.g., Amsterdam, 1972;

Bertenthal & Fischer, 1978; Lewis, Sullivan, Stanger, & Weiss, 1989; Watson & Fisher, 1977). Children begin to talk about emotions, demonstrating simple (verbal) understanding of others' internal states as well as their own (Bloom, Lightbown & Hood, 1975; also see review by Bretherton, Fritz, Zahn-Waxler, & Ridgeway, 1986). Prosocial behaviors of helping, sharing, and cooperation emerge during the second year of life (Eckerman, Whatley, & Kutz, 1975; Rheingold, Hay, & West, 1976; Ross & Goldman, 1977). These behaviors may have even earlier underpinnings in early bonding processes with the caregiver. Attachments during infancy may prepare the child for later empathic development through the complex interplay of sharing and exchange of emotions, as well as cooperation and turn taking in social interactions between parent and infant (Stern, 1985; Trevarthen, 1989). Secure attachments formed in the first year of life may influence the child's capacity to empathize and care for others later in development (e.g., Teti & Ablard, 1989).

These studies document a broad repertoire of social skills young children bring to relationships with others. Even by 2 years, children have (a) the cognitive capacity to interpret overt physical and psychological states of others, (b) the emotional capacity to affectively experience the other's state (vicarious emotional responsiveness or empathy), and (c) the behavioral repertoire that makes it possible to try to alleviate discomfort in others in simple distress situations. Two longitudinal studies (Zahn-Waxler & Radke-Yarrow, 1982; Zahn-Waxler, Radke-Yarrow, Chapman, & Wagner, 1990) indicate that prosocial responses to someone in distress do emerge during the second year of life. During this time, children also begin to express empathic concern and some understanding of the other's plight.

Most of the research on prosocial development has been done with preschool and elementary-school-age children. The adolescent period has been very understudied. Different aspects of cognitive, social-emotional, and physical development during this time of transition make it difficult to predict developmental trajectories. There are reasons to predict increased altruistic motivation, but there is also increased self-absorption (Francis & Pearson, 1987).

THE ROLE OF SOCIALIZATION IN PROSOCIAL DEVELOPMENT

Adult Influences

Socialization practices implicated in the development of children's altruism and prosocial behavior were studied extensively in the 1960s and 1970s. In some of the work, differences in socialization practices were observed, or parental observation reports of child-rearing practices were obtained. In other investigations, parenting conditions were simulated in the laboratory. Children exposed to the disparate conditions were then provided with opportunities to help, share, or comfort another in structured situations.

Several core dimensions of caregiving have been examined. One concerns variations in the caregiver as a model of altruism (e.g., modeling prosocial behavior across many versus few settings; preaching but not practicing prosocial behavior). Another dimension involves the caregiver as teacher and disciplinarian (e.g., explaining why it is important to help, and not to harm, others; sensitizing children toward the others' feelings; using modulated control strategies versus more authoritarian, power-assertive techniques). A third dimension concerns the quality of the parent–child relationship (close and warm versus remote and cold). The use of specific instructions and rewards also has been investigated. Finally, parents convey norms, values, and expectations about interpersonally appropriate behavior that may bear on whether or not their offspring develop concern for others.

In the research of the 1970s, the different caregiving dimensions tended not to be studied in combination or in ways that would reflect how they were experienced by children under real-life conditions. A notable exception was the landmark study by Rosenhan (1970) that examined the early socialization histories of fully committed versus partially committed civil rights activists (based on retrospective accounts). Fully committed activists reported having warm, positive relationships with at least one parent, and parents themselves had been fully committed activists of an earlier era (i.e., were good models of altruism). Partially committed activists had more negative or ambivalent relationships with their parents, and their parents tended to have preached but *not* practiced altruism. The behavior of the fully committed activists was said to represent autonomous altruism (i.e., help that is internally directed, presumably by genuine concern for the other), whereas that of the partially committed was thought to illustrate normative altruism (more motivated by concern for self and more externally controlled by rewards and punishment).

The effectiveness of warmth in conjunction with modeling of altruism was demonstrated also in research by Yarrow *et al.* (1973). An adult spent several days as "teacher" in a nursery school setting with the children before conditions for eliciting prosocial behavior were implemented. Several dimensions were manipulated, including (a) nurturance versus aloofness of the experimenter with the child and (b) modeling of altruism in symbolic versus real-life situations. Under all conditions, specific information was provided about how to help, and children were praised for being good helpers. Only children (a) who had experienced a nurturant relationship with the adult and (b) who saw this adult model altruism in real as well as symbolic situations were likely themselves to show generalized and enduring altruism.

More recent work by Clary and Miller (1986) with adults provides a conceptual replication of Rosenhan's work. Adult volunteers reporting childhood experiences with nurturant parents, who modeled altruism in the real world, exhibited more long-term helping than volunteers with a history of less nurturant parents who modeled altruism to a lesser degree. Autonomous altruism appears to result from multiple parenting practices that work "in concert." It suggests that strong identification with the parent is one facilitating condition. This has been borne out in earlier work and in more recent short-term longitudinal research on mother–child relations and the development of empathy in first graders (Siegal, 1985).

Barnett (1987) suggests that empathy is most likely to develop within a family environment that (a) satisfies the child's own emotional needs and discourages excessive self-concern, (b) encourages the child to experience and express a broad range of emotion (but presumably not in a dysregulated manner), and (c) provides opportunities to observe and interact with empathic others. Koestner, Franz, and Weinberger (1990) have attempted to trace family origins of empathic concern in a 26-year longitudinal study. Empathic concern was assessed in 31-year-old adults, originally part of a sample investigated by Sears, Maccoby, and Levin (1957). Eleven parenting dimensions, derived from maternal interviews when children were 5 years old, were examined as predictors of empathic concern. Empathy in adults was predicted by early paternal involvement in child care, maternal tolerance of dependent behavior, mother's inhibition of the child's aggression, and mother's satisfaction with her maternal role. Contrary to predictions, parental warmth was unrelated to empathy. Tolerance of dependency in young children may, however, reflect the mother's nurturance, responsiveness, and acceptance of feelings. Maternal inhibition of aggression may reflect the use of other-oriented inductive techniques sensitizing the child to the harmful consequences for others of the child's aggressive acts.

Some studies (e.g., Fabes *et al.*, 1990) but not others (e.g., Strayer & Roberts, 1989) have found that the child's empathy can be predicted by the parent's empathy. Results may be inconclusive for a variety of reasons. A parent could score high on empathy and still not be empathic toward her or his own child. Moreover, different studies use different measures of empathy. Also, the work of Rosenhan (1970) and Clary and Miller (1986) serve as a reminder that parental contributors to children's empathy and altruism represent a complex "package." By attempting to isolate the components, the larger picture may sometimes be lost.

Sibling Influences

The sibling relationship provides another context in which children may learn prosocial, as well as antisocial, behavior patterns. Teti and Ablard (1989) found that older preschool-age siblings attempt to comfort younger siblings in distress. Moreover, older siblings whose attachment relationship with the mother is secure are more likely to help the sibling than insecurely attached children. Number of siblings may play a role. Rehberg and Richman (1989) observed preschool children's social interactions with peers. Children from smaller families had higher comforting scores than did those from larger families, suggesting that under some conditions, sibling relationships may interfere with children's developing prosocial orientations.

Dunn and her colleagues (e.g., Dunn & Munn, 1986) observed how much siblings share, help, comfort, and cooperate with each other during the preschool years. As early as 18 months these behaviors occur, but not frequently, with the exception of cooperation. Cooperation and conciliation showed some stability over time. Siblings, however, also showed considerable understanding of how to upset and provoke each other during conflict. This learning context, then, may contribute both to heightened altruism and aggression, and hence may contain the potential for significant ambivalence as well.

Extrafamilial Influences

Extrafamilial influences on prosocial development exist both within different cultural institutions (e.g., schools, church, day care) and the individuals who function in these institutions (e.g., teachers and playmates). Piaget viewed the peer group as the foremost socializer of the developing child's prosocial inclinations and moral understanding. Reciprocity, cooperation, and mutual understanding were learned mainly through give-and-take in peer interactions. The parents' authority and power over the child were thought to produce an assymetry that made it difficult to learn negotiation and reciprocal exchange in this context. This view of socialization seems greatly oversimplified.

CAROLYN ZAHN-
WAXLER and K.
DANIELLE SMITH

Children can learn to be caring from their parents as well as peers, and the peer group can provide the training grounds for cruelty as well as compassion. The role of peers in children's prosocial development continues to be an active area of research inquiry. Berndt's (1981) research on the effects of peer friendship on prosocial intentions and behavior in elementary-school-age children is one good example. Research is being done with even younger children, as stable peer reputations are now known to emerge very early to influence the more general nature of children's social interactions. Already by preschool, children's understanding of emotions and capacity for prosocial behavior in the peer setting are direct predictors of how well-liked they are by their peers (Denham, McKinley, Couchard, & Holt, 1991).

Teachers, as well as peers and parents, play an important socializing role. They also nurture, educate, discipline, and provide models of compassion, in varying degrees. And they may, under some conditions, serve as deterrents to children's responsiveness to distress in others. Caplan and Hay (1989) interviewed 5-year-old children to assess their understanding of social norms governing bystander intervention. Prosocial behaviors toward peers also were observed. Although children often paid attention to distressed peers and were capable of intervention, rates of prosocial behavior were low. Children did not believe they were supposed to assist when competent caregivers were present. Most often, young children are in the presence of competent adults and hence may be discouraged, directly and indirectly, from helping others. Early helping behaviors often require patience on the part of parents, as children's prosocial efforts sometimes may be unpolished and time consuming.

Television is another socializing influence, and its effects on positive and negative child behaviors have been addressed repeatedly in research, mainly within the literature on modeling, imitation, and contagion. Although the evidence is more dramatic for the effects of aggressive models in eliciting like behavior in children, some studies indicate that prosocial television models can have positive influences on children's behavior patterns (Radke-Yarrow *et al.*, 1983). Research on prosocial television models has diminished during the 1980s. There has been some work on the effects of videogames (e.g., Chambers & Ascione, 1987). Elementary-school children of different ages were exposed to an aggressive videogame, a prosocial videogame, or a control condition. The prosocial videogame did not increase prosocial responding; however, the aggressive videogame tended to suppress it.

The Role of Direct Rewards

The effects of rewards on children's prosocial motivation has been examined in a number of investigations. Fabes, Fultz, Eisenberg, May-Plumlee, and Christopher (1989) assigned grade-school children to one of four experimental conditions. Conditions differed in whether children received rewards for helping and whether children engaged in the helping task or watched other children help. Rewards were found to enhance helping in the immediate situation. However, rewards tended to undermine children's helping in a free-choice period. Rewards were material rather than social.

In naturalistic contexts, rewards are used infrequently as a socialization technique (Grusec, 1991). But if they are used, the form is more likely to be social (e.g., praise) rather than material. The findings of Fabes *et al.* (1989) are consistent with research (see Grusec, 1982) indicating that, although material reward may increase helping, sharing, and comforting in the immediate context, it may undermine subsequent prosocial motivation in situations where rewards are no longer forthcoming. Mills and Grusec (1989) also have distinguished between dispositional praise ("You are a nice and helpful person") and nondispositional praise ("That was a nice and helpful thing to do"). Dispositional praise produces more internalized sharing, possibly because it elicits more self-direction and internalized motives.

THE NATURE OF EMPATHY

Empathy is a complex construct and has been defined in a number of ways (see Eisenberg & Strayer, 1987). Some definitions focus on affective dimensions (e.g., as vicarious affective arousal that involves affect matching or contagion of others' emotions). Or the emotion may not reflect a direct matching of the other's experience but rather may reflect feelings of sympathy or concern for the victim. Other definitions emphasize the more cognitive dimension of empathy (i.e., imagining oneself in the place of the other in order to understand what is being experienced). Empathy, however defined, is not necessarily a component of prosocial behavior. One can help, comfort, or share without experiencing much feeling; and motives can even be mainly self-serving. However, many studies indicate that there is often an interconnection of cognitive, affective, and behavioral dimensions of positive responsiveness to others. This begins early in development (Denham, 1986; Denham & Couchard, 1991; Lennon & Eisenberg, 1987; Zahn-Waxler, Radke-Yarrow, Chapman, & Wagner, 1990; Zahn-Waxler, Robinson, & Emde, 1990) and is present later in development as well (e.g., Chapman, Zahn-Waxler, Cooperman, & Iannotti, 1987; Eisenberg *et al.*, 1989; Fabes *et al.*, 1990). A metanalytic research review by Eisenberg and Miller (1987) indicates that empathy and sympathy are commonly correlated with prosocial behavior.

Within the adult social psychology literature there has been an ongoing debate about the motives for prosocial actions. Cialdini and his associates have contended that all human prosocial behavior can ultimately be understood in terms of motives based on self-interest or egoistic concerns. Batson and coworkers argue for a pluralism of motives for altruism that includes empathically based as well as egoistically based motivations. Both have constructed experimental research designs that attempt to provide tests of their hypotheses. Batson presents compelling evidence for the position that some forms of altruism are empathically based and do not simply emanate from reward–punishment contingencies or efforts to reduce personal distress. However, alternative interpretations are possible, and the controversy continues (e.g., see Batson *et al.*, 1989; Batson *et al.*, 1988; Carlson & Miller, 1987; Cialdini, Shaller, Houlihan, Arps, Fultz, & Beaman, 1987).

Measurement of Empathy in Children

Initially, earlier research on empathy was based mainly on data obtained from questionnaires and other self-report measures of affect experienced by children in response to another's affect. Advances in conceptualization, technology, and meas-

CAROLYN ZAHN-
WAXLER and K.
DANIELLE SMITH

urement have led to more elaborated and differentiated approaches. Facial expressions of emotion in response to others' emotion can now be subjected to microanalytic, detailed coding systems based on muscle action patterns. Moreover, assessments of autonomic functioning (heart rate, blood pressure, skin conductance) provide opportunities to examine psychophysiological arousal in the face of another's distress. Eisenberg and her colleagues have used such approaches, in conjunction with children's self-report and observations of their prosocial behavior, to study the development and socialization of empathically based altruism.

In one study, preschoolers and second-grade children viewed three films portraying others' emotions of anxiety, empathic sadness, and cognitively induced sympathy (Eisenberg, Fabes et al., 1988). Children's heart rate accelerated during the anxiety films and decelerated during the other two films. Heart rate acceleration is thought to reflect personal distress, whereas heart rate deceleration is thought to reflect empathy, or the direction of attention outward. Facial expressions were consistent with film content, and observed emotions correlated with self-reported empathy.

Subsequent studies by Eisenberg and colleagues confirm the distinction between sympathetic distress (indexed by heart rate deceleration) and personal distress (indexed by heart rate acceleration). Heart rate deceleration during exposure to a needy other was associated with increased willingness to help in both children and adults (Eisenberg et al., 1989). Moreover, facial expressions of concerned attention were positively related to prosocial behavior, especially in younger children. Facial expressions of personal distress were unrelated or negatively related to willingness to help. Zahn-Waxler et al. (1983) similarly found that personal distress (seen in facial expressions and body tension) in elementary-school-age children exposed to infant cries was inversely related to actual helping responses toward an infant in distress. In other work with children and adults (Eisenberg, Schaller et al., 1988), heart rate acceleration also was associated with personal distress. Sympathy-inducing conditions tended to elicit facial expressions of sadness and self-reports of sympathy.

Research with adults also demonstrates that personal distress may interfere with adaptive responsiveness to another in distress (Frodi et al., 1978). Self-report and physiological measures were gathered on parents shown videotapes of crying (preterm and full-term) infants. Cries of premature infants elicited greater autonomic arousal and were perceived as more aversive than cries of normal infants. Preterm infants are at risk for child abuse, and the increased negative arousal experienced by caregivers may be a contributing factor.

The relationship between personal distress and sympathetic distress is complex. From a developmental perspective, sympathy appears to evolve from personal distress. Hence it may not be meaningful to construe them as polar opposites. Sometimes sympathy and personal distress are interrelated or have common correlates (Fabes et al., 1990). Preschool children who respond prosocially to peers in distress are children who are likely to cry themselves (Howes & Farver, 1987). Moreover, sympathetic, calm orientation associated with heart rate deceleration could sometimes represent a lack of emotional arousal needed for effective intervention. Little is known about how laboratory demonstrations generalize to altruism in natural settings.

Finally, the work of Wiesenfeld, Whitman, and Malatesta (1984) provides a good example of how *high* physiological arousal may, under some circumstances, reflect empathy. Emotional and physiological responsivity to infant signals was assessed in individuals who differed in empathy. High-empathy subjects, more than low-empathy subjects, had larger electrodermal responses, tended to respond to infant emotions with matching facial expressions, had more extreme emotional reactions, and indicated a stronger desire to hold the infants. The empathic group also showed a trend toward greater cardiac responsiveness to infant signals and held different values about caregiving behavior.

Whenever the distress of another is vicariously experienced, by definition, negative emotion is aroused in the self. Whether this negative emotion is experienced as aversive, personal distress or becomes modulated and redirected outward as sympathy for another will be decided by many factors (e.g., developmental level, constitutional patterns, and socialization experiences, as well as expectations, beliefs, and attitudes about the circumstances and plights of others).

Individuals learn to control vicarious emotional arousal as they grow older. Bengtsson and Johnson (1987) explored cognitions related to empathy in 5- to 11-year-old children. Few kindergartners knew how to control empathic arousal purely by means of thoughts. Older children had mentalistic strategies to maximize or minimize empathy. Older children who could reassure themselves, either by rationalizations or denial, that things might not be so bad for the other showed attenuation of vicariously aroused distress.

Biological Bases of Concern for Others

Hoffman (1970) has argued that reflexive crying of infants in response to other infant cries reflects a primitive precursor of empathy and signals an innate tendency to be socially connected to others. Experimental studies (e.g., Simner, 1971) have confirmed that infants are more responsive to cries of other infants, than to other equally aversive, but nonsocial stimuli. Most sociobiological approaches focus on the selfish nature of man (e.g., Dawkins, 1976), emphasizing concepts of survival value, self-interest, and self-preservation. This is expressed through the biologically based urge to perpetuate the self via reproduction, through future generations. More recent neuroscience and sociobiological perspectives place greater emphasis on empathy as a positive mediator of concern for the welfare of others. There are beginning efforts to understand the neural substrates of empathy (Brothers, 1989) and to examine temperament as a correlate of prosocial behavior (Stanhope, Bell, & Parker-Cohen, 1987).

MacLean (1985) has argued that the capacity for empathy emerged in conjunction with the evolution of mammals 180 million years ago in late Triassic times. Mammals are warm-blooded creatures who nurture, nourish, and protect their young, as opposed to reptilian, cold-blooded creatures who destroy and abandon their offspring. In his view, when mammals opted for "a family way of life," the stage was set for exposure to very distressful forms of pain and suffering in others. Such stimuli are integral to the expression of empathy. In MacLean's analysis of the mammalian, triune brain, he proposes interconnections of the limbic system with prefrontal cortex, linked originally to parental concern for the young from which a sense of responsibility emerged. He argues that through the higher reaches of the brain, parental concern for the young may generalize to other members of the species. Such speculations are thought provoking because they require us to consider, from an evolutionary perspective, how deeply embedded the capacity for empathy may be.

If emotional responsiveness to the distress of others is innately determined, it also raises the question of biologically based individual differences. Adult mono-zygotic (MZ) and dyzygotic (DZ) twins have been compared on empathic concern (Matthews, Batson, Horn, & Rosenman, 1981) and altruism (Rushton, Fulker, Neale, Nias, & Eysenck, 1986). Both studies indicate greater concordance of empathy and prosocial scores in MZ and DZ twins, suggesting a possible heritability component. However, measures are based solely on self-reports, and other than biologically based differences may contribute to concordance patterns.

Segal (1984) has studied cooperation, competition, and altruism *within* MZ and DZ twin sets. These behaviors were observed in IQ-concordant twin pairs between 6 and 11 years of age while they were completing joint projects or tasks. MZ, more than DZ, twins showed evidence of greater cooperation. They worked more effectively on a task together and expended greater effort for their twin partners, suggesting a more altruistic spirit is operative. It is possible that MZ and DZ twins have differential socialization experiences that contribute to such differences. It is nonetheless intriguing to consider the possibility of biologically based origins of individual differences in compassionate behaviors.

The Role of Gender

From both sociobiological and socialization perspectives there might be reasons to expect sex differences in (a) the frequency, quality, and types of compassionate behaviors, (b) the contexts in which they occur, and (c) the underlying motives. If empathic concern is integral to caregiving (and perhaps derives from the caregiving experience as MacLean has argued), then individuals who are biologically prepared to bear and rear children (i.e., females) might be expected to show more of it. Moreover, many cultures and societies emphasize the value for males of behaviors that may be incompatible with empathy (e.g., competition, aggression, assertion, achievement, and independence). In contrast, for females, appropriate gender-role-related patterns such as empathy, compassion, caregiving, emotional connection, commitment, and relationship orientations are likely to be emphasized. And there is evidence for negative sanctions when "nonnormative" behaviors occur. Adolescent females are judged more harshly than males if they do not express sensitivity and emotional responsiveness to someone in need (Barnett, McMinimy, Flouer, & Masbad, 1987). Such cultural expectations may play a significant role in the differential development and socialization of caring orientations in males and females.

Prosocial Behavior

The first comprehensive study of sex differences in prosocial behavior was part of a large-scale investigation of early moral development, conducted by Hartshorne, May, and Mahler (1929). This effort included broad samplings of children's altruistic and prosocial behaviors in the classroom, as well as their reputations for social behaviors. Girls showed more prosocial behavior than boys. However, the strongest effects were seen in differential reputations, with girls reputed to be much more altruistic. These findings were replicated in another large-scale investigation by Shigetomi, Hartmann, & Gelfand (1981). In one review of the literature on prosocial behaviors (comfort, cooperation, sharing, help), clear sex differences were not evident (Radke-Yarrow *et al.*, 1983). Two other reviews (Hoffman, 1977; Rushton, 1976) are more suggestive of sex differences, favoring females.

Patterns of sex differences may depend on the type of prosocial behavior that is required. Situations requiring more action-oriented "agentic" behaviors may elicit patterns of sex differences favoring males (Eagley & Crowley, 1986), whereas distress situations requiring "repair" of relationships or physical or emotional caretaking may favor females. Moreover, situations that require the ability to "read" emotional (distress) signals (sometimes subtle in expression) may favor females (e.g., see reviews by Brody, 1985; Hall, 1978).

There continue to be indications that girls are likely to display more altruism than boys. Berndt (1981) found that young elementary-school-age boys are less prosocial with friends than acquaintances; girls are likely to share with both and hence show less competition with their friends than do boys. Cialdini, Eisenberg, Shell, and McCreath (1987) found that girls were more willing to live up to their commitments to help at an earlier age than boys. In other, recent work (Fabes *et al.*, 1990), girls were observed to be more willing to help an ill child than were boys.

The work of Hartshorne *et al.* (1929) and Shigetomi *et al.* (1981) sometimes has been interpreted to mean that, because of gender stereotypes, females come to be reputed as more helpful and caring than they really are. It also may be that the reputations are accurate and derived from another form of prosocial behavior, typically not defined as such (i.e., the capacity for restraint from aggression or ability to refrain from violating the rights of others). Numerous studies document that boys, more than girls, bring harm to others through acts of aggression (see review by Parke & Slaby, 1983).

Empathy

Previous reviews indicate that females often are better able to read or interpret emotional signals than are males and may be more sensitive to their own emotions as well (Brody, 1985; Hall, 1978). Moreover, their lower levels of aggression, relative to males, may reflect their concern for others and anxiety about hurting them (Frodi, Macaulay, & Thome, 1977). These differences suggest that females may be more empathic as well. Results of numerous investigations support this view. In a comprehensive metanalysis of empathy research (Eisenberg & Lennon, 1983), females were reported to be consistently more empathic than males, but mainly for self-reported measures.

Some have argued that such gender differences reflect a reporting bias (e.g., reflecting social desirability or females' attempts to represent themselves as the way that they "should" be, consistent with their role). It is equally plausible to assume that females veridically report what they feel and, hence, that the motives underlying their behaviors differ as well. Zahn-Waxler, Friedman, and Cummings (1983) observed children's prosocial responses toward an infant in distress. They also measured children's self-reported empathy in response to infant cries (i.e., how sorry they felt for the baby). Girls reported more empathy than boys, yet there were no sex differences in helping and comforting interventions. Affective accompaniments of prosocial behaviors thus may differ for boys and girls.

Observational studies of children between the ages of 1 and 2 suggest that girls show more concerned responses than boys to distresses in others (Robinson, 1989; Zahn-Waxler *et al.*, 1990), also suggesting that sex differences in empathy do not simply reflect reporting bias. In hypothetical situations of interpersonal conflict and distress as well, girls express more empathy themes than boys and emphasize the value of social relationships (Chapman *et al.*, 1987; Zahn-Waxler *et al.*, 1990). In work by Eisenberg *et al.* (1988), girls not only reported more distress than boys but were also observed to exhibit more facial sympathy. In research by Fabes *et al.* (1990), children's observed vicarious emotional responses, and prosocial behaviors were examined in relation to mothers' sympathetic dispositions. Mothers who were more sympathetic and better perspective takers had girls who reported feeling more sympathy, negative mood, and less happiness after exposure to others in need. These girls also showed physiological patterns indicative of sympathy and were more willing to help a distress victim. Fewer, but some, patterns were evident for mothers with their boys.

These data support Feshbach's (1978) conclusion that empathic-related behaviors in girls are correlated with maternal qualities that are also likely to foster prosocial behavior. They are also consistent with the data of Barnett (1987) suggesting that warm, empathic mothers facilitate emotional responsiveness in their offspring. Further research is needed (1) to determine *why* patterns of association between parent and child behaviors sometimes differ as a function of gender and (2) to clarify the role of paternal empathy. Additional work also is needed concerning differential socialization patterns of aggression in boys and girls, in terms of implications for empathy (see Zahn-Waxler, Cole, & Barrett, 1991). In a long-term longitudinal study, mothers who inhibited aggression in their girls had more empathic offspring several decades later (Koestner *et al.*, 1990); however, this pattern was not present for boys.

The motives and meaning of empathy and related altruistic patterns may differ for boys and girls (Bauman, Cialdini, & Kendrick, 1983). Prior research showed that temporary sadness produces reduced altruism in young children (7 to 10 years) and increased altruism in older children (15 to 18 years). Cialdini and Kendrick (1976) have argued that this shift occurs because, increasingly with age, children become sufficiently socialized to find altruism self-gratifying and hence will act altruistically as a way to dispel a sad mood. If girls are socialized to altruism at an earlier age than boys, they should show enhanced altruism when sad, more than same-age boys. This hypothesis was tested by inducing a sad mood in 12- to 13-year-old children who then had an opportunity to behave charitably. Temporary sadness increased altruism in females but decreased it in males, relative to neutral mood controls. Research of Mills and Grusec (1989) also suggests that the motives and dynamics underlying altruism may differ substantially for boys and girls. In one study, girls were actually more generous than boys but perceived themselves as less intrinsically motivated to share. Through different socialization histories, girls and boys may learn to attribute their altruism to different motives. Girls may be less able to attribute their actions internally and to perceive themselves as altruistic, even though their actions appear more internalized.

Moral Reasoning

A comprehensive review of research on the development of moral reasoning is beyond the scope of this chapter. However, one particular aspect of this research regarding gender differences is particularly germane. We review here a major theoretical controversy of the 1980s, in which different moral orientations for males and females, representing justice versus care orientations, respectively, were addressed. The controversy began with Gilligan's (1977, 1982) critique of Kohlberg's stage theory describing the course and processes of moral development. In Kohlberg's theory, individuals progress through several levels, from less mature levels of moral reasoning. Initially, reasoning is based on hedonistic concerns and self-interest. Later, mature forms of reasoning come to include abstract conceptions of justice. Intermediary levels of reasoning focus on concerns with societal rules and conformity to these rules, as well as the importance of interpersonal relationships in reaching decisions about moral issues. Gilligan argued that abstract conceptions of justice may not ultimately reflect the highest level of reasoning about moral conflicts. She described another moral orientation or "voice," concerned with care, relationships, and connection with other people and argued that this orientation is especially salient for women.

Gilligan suggested that Kohlberg's theory, model, and means of assessing moral reasoning places females at a disadvantage because relationship concerns reflect a lower level of moral reasoning than adherence to duty and maintaining the social order. That is, in Kohlberg's theory, Stage 3 traditionally has included "feminine" characteristics of expressiveness and the need to do good to gain approval; Stage 4 accommodates the typical "masculine" role of law and order (Bussey & Maugham, 1982). In Gilligan's view, men tend to organize social relationships in a hierarchical order and subscribe to a morality of rights. Females value interpersonal connectedness, care, sensitivity, and responsibility to people. In Kohlberg's scoring system, interpersonal care orientations (more characteristic of females) would receive lower ratings than responses based on a morality of rights (more characteristic of males).

Kohlberg's stage theory has been challenged as being sexually biased in favor of males on a number of conceptual and procedural grounds (see Donenberg & Hoffman, 1988, for elaboration of these issues). However, a thorough review of moral reasoning studies failed to support Gilligan's claim that females more often end up being categorized at a lower stage of moral reasoning than males by virtue of their valuing of relationships (Walker, 1984). Walker's generalizations have been challenged in turn (e.g., Baumrind, 1986). Complex methodological as well as conceptual issues contribute to interpretive problems. Some research procedures and types of moral dilemmas are more conducive to eliciting sex differences than others. In past work, children were asked to discuss abstract dilemmas of relatively little relevance to their daily lives (e.g., stories about a man stealing medicine from a druggist for his ill wife). In one study that employed dilemmas more salient to children's own experiences, boys adopted more absolute standards, whereas girls' judgments reflected a relativistic approach (Keltikangas-Travinen, 1989).

In a study of prosocial development in middle childhood (Eisenberg et al., 1987), modes of prosocial moral reasoning that most explicitly reflect role taking or empathy increased in use with age for girls but not for boys. In a cross-national study of mainly adolescents (Boehnke, Silbereisen, Eisenberg, Reykowski, & Polomari, 1989), preferences for different types of motives (e.g., hedonism, self-interest, conformity, task-orientation, and empathic other-orientation were assessed). Males valued more developmentally immature motives (e.g., hedonism, self-interest), whereas females valued more developmentally mature motives. These patterns are consistent with earlier generalizations of heightened empathy in females.

Donenberg and Hoffman (1988) found support for Gilligan's position that two distinct ways of thinking about moral problems exist—justice and care—and they are differentially related to gender. Adolescent girls emphasized the morality of care significantly more than justice. However, contrary to Gilligan's claims (1982), boys emphasized the morality of justice and care equally. Findings also were task-dependent. Donenberg and Hoffman (1988) stress the importance of focusing less in future research on gender differences *per se* and more on the processes by which different moral orientations are acquired. The ultimate contribution of the controversy between Kohlberg and Gilligan may rest on the broadening of our assumptions of what is a moral person and how this relates to the integration of concepts of abstract justice and concern for particular others (Muuss, 1988).

CONDITIONS OF RISK AND PSYCHOPATHOLOGY: RELATIONS TO EMPATHY, SOCIAL COGNITION, AND PROSOCIAL BEHAVIOR

Biological and Environmental Risk Conditions

Research recently has placed more emphasis on conditions that may diminish, unduly heighten, or alter in other maladaptive ways children's understanding, sensitivity, and capacity to intervene on behalf of others in need. Early distressful life events may have long-lasting effects on empathic development. Barnett and McCoy (1989) traced the empathic responsiveness of young adults back to distressful events experienced as children. Intensity, but not frequency, or early distress events predicted later empathy. This work did not distinguish between different types of early distresses or examine conditions that might lead to diminished responsiveness. We next review some biological and psychological conditions of the child, as well as familial and societal/cultural conditions implicated in potentially maladaptive patterns.

FAMILIAL CONDITIONS

Marital discord and divorce have been identified as influencing children's premature adoption of a caregiving or nurturing role and engagement in overly prosocial behavior. Emery's (1982) review indicates that parental discord and divorce sometimes result in children's coming to feel responsible for parents' problems and trying to take care of the difficulties. Children as young as 2 have been observed to show anger, distress, and attempts to ameliorate parental distress in such situations (Cummings, Zahn-Waxler, & Radke-Yarrow, 1981).

In a study of family predictors of preschoolers' observed prosocial behavior toward peers (helping and/or comforting), father-absent males were found to have the highest scores for comforting behavior (Rehberg & Richman, 1989). Comforting of peers also was related to the mothers' dependency on their children for emotional support. Helping in the preschool was related to the number of chores children performed at home. One might speculate that these family conditions begin to approximate circumstances where small children are relied on too heavily by their caregivers and begin to assume unduly high levels of responsibility for others.

Parental depression (often correlated with marital discord) also may lead to high levels of prosocial behavior expressed both toward the caregiver and in other distress situations as early as the preschool years (Zahn-Waxler & Kochanska, 1990; Zahn-Waxler, Kochanska et al., 1990). Early overinvolvement in others' problems may become burdensome and contribute also to ambivalent and avoidant styles of relating to others. Adolescent girls who show high interpersonal sensitivity toward depressed parents may be themselves at risk for emotional problems and are likely to have dysfunctional peer relations (Beardslee, Schultz, & Selman, 1987). There is also evidence (Beardslee & Podorefsky, 1988) that some children and young adults work through family difficulties; their heightened patterns of empathy reflect genuinely mature levels of interpersonal sensitivity and commitment to others. Parental depression and discord reflect examples of environments often characterized by physical and emotional distress. They do provide stimuli for learning to be aware of others' feelings and circumstances, to experience empathy, to develop coping mechanisms, and to engage in problem-solving strategies in order to alleviate distress. There may be a variety of adaptive and maladaptive outcomes. Future research is needed to determine why environmental conditions of adversity foster healthy versus unhealthy prosocial patterns in offspring. Empathy may promote a depressive orientation as it can blur the needs of self and other; that is, it may promote treating the problems of others as one's own, and produce excessive feelings of guilt, responsibility, and helplessness (Zahn-Waxler, Cole, & Barrett, 1991).

Parental abuse of the young is another environmental condition associated with maladaptive outcomes for children. Much of the research in this area has been motivated by an interest in belief systems and interaction patterns that repeat across generations to perpetuate abuse and maltreatment. The work of Main and her colleagues (e.g., Main & Goldwyn, 1984) has focused on the quality of the parent–child attachment relationship and its implications for the development of subsequent relationships. It is assumed that the nature and quality of the caregiver's bonding with her own parent will influence the quality of the attachment and empathic ties formed with one's own offspring. The quality of the relationship, as well as the maltreatment per se (i.e., aggression that is modeled and experienced), will influence whether their children maltreat others. There is increasing evidence that children who are securely attached to their caregivers are better able to empathize and share with others.

Studies of toddler and preschool-age children demonstrate the poor quality of the attachment relationship with their caregiver (Cicchetti, 1990). They also suggest that the inadequate, hostile, and unempathic caregiving of maltreating parents, dramatically apparent in clinical work (Haynes-Seman, 1987), may affect children's early developing peer relations. In three observational studies, abused youngsters have been found not only to cause distress and behave more aggressively toward playmates but also to show more inappropriate responses in the face of a peer's distress. Abused children are more likely to withdraw or aggress toward a distressed peer, and they are less likely to show concern or offer help (Howes & Eldridge, 1985; Klimes-Dougan & Kistner, 1990; Main & George, 1985). Thus, even in early interactions with playmates, many abused children appear to adopt behavior patterns similar to those of maltreating parents. These behavior patterns are likely to elicit rejection by peers, which may, in turn, have long-term implications for the quality of later social relations. Peer rejection is a powerful early predictor of later interpersonal difficulties, behavior problems, and psychopathology.

CAROLYN ZAHN-
WAXLER and K.
DANIELLE SMITH

A number of neurological, physical, psychological, cognitive, and psychiatric conditions of children have been linked with atypical patterns of prosocial behavior, empathy, and understanding of another's circumstances. Parmelee (1986) has argued persuasively for the beneficial effects of children's minor illnesses on their own behavioral development. Illnesses provide opportunities for children to increase their knowledge of self, other, empathy, and prosocial behavior, as well as a realistic understanding of the sick role. Such illnesses, in other family members, also provide opportunities to gain knowledge and develop ways of dealing with others' personal and social experiences.

Support for Parmelee's position can be found in the work of Nelms (1989) on emotional behaviors of chronically ill children. When 9- to 11-year-old children with diabetes or asthma were compared with controls, the chronically ill children showed higher levels of empathy and emotional responsiveness. Chronically ill children, because of their illness and its management, encounter many intense emotional experiences. They may learn to attend to both positive and negative feelings, as they are often asked how they feel. If these self-awareness generalizes to awareness of the emotional states of others, conditions for empathy would be enhanced. Childhood illness might also be expected to elicit sensitivity in caregivers, further heightening children's empathy (see review of socialization research by Radke-Yarrow et al., 1983). Chronic illness in children also was associated with higher levels of depression (Nelms, 1989), raising the question of whether too much empathy sometimes may be a causal factor in depression (Zahn-Waxler et al., 1991).

Early childhood autism is a biologically based illness characterized in part by severe deficits in empathy, social skills, and awareness of others as social beings with whom feelings can be shared and interactions achieved. The egocentrism of these children is not evidenced in physical perspective-taking abilities. For example, they do not show impairment on visual–spatial tasks (Hobson, 1984), suggesting that the difficulties may have to do more with taking social perspectives. Efforts to increase the social skills of autistic children have been attempted in many behavior modification studies. In recent work (Redefer & Goodman, 1989), pet-facilitated therapy with autistic children was used to develop social skills. When a friendly dog was used as a component of therapy, prosocial behavior increased, and self-absorption decreased. Children also showed fewer autistic behaviors. However, consistent with other research (e.g., Strain & Odom, 1986), there was continuous erosion of improvement from treatment to follow-up.

Learning disabilities reflect other biologically based problems that produce difficulties for children in interpersonal relations. Learning-disabled children often do not receive social information accurately because of poor discrimination abilities. Poor social perception could make it difficult to predict thoughts and feelings of others, hence making it hard to make appropriate social judgments and adapt to social situations. Learning-disabled boys have been found to be less able to view moral dilemmas from a community or societal perspective (Derr, 1986), when compared with average achieving adolescents. Much of their reasoning was based on an egocentric perspective that focused on the needs and desires of the self. The immature, inappropriate social interactions of these children (that may stem, in part, from their difficulties understanding and predicting others' thoughts and feelings) may escalate to culturally deviant, antisocial behavior (Bryan, Werner, & Pearl, 1982).

Aggressive, antisocial children are relevant to our interests because of their frequent failures to be prosocial, to respect the rights of others, and to experience empathy and guilt. Whether antisocial behavior invariably or inevitably reflects deficits in empathy and compassion is a very complex question. A recent meta-nalysis review (Miller & Eisenberg, 1988) of relations between aggression and empathy reveals low-to-moderate-level inverse correlations. Patterns of association (i.e., of incompatibility between aggression and empathy) tend to be strongest under extreme conditions of antisocial behavior, such as abuse. Earlier reviews of research on relations between prosocial and antisocial behaviors reveal a complex set of patterns (Cummings, Hollenbeck, Iannotti, Radke-Yarrow, & Zahn-Waxler, 1986). Depending on the study, associations can be positive, negative, or nonexistent. McCord (1990) has suggested that altruism and aggression should be viewed as orthogonal factors and that research be devoted to why different patterns of covariation do, or do not, occur. McCord notes that even highly antisocial youth can be quite caring and altruistic toward members of their own peer groups and to effectively engage in mutual aid.

Affective and Cognitive Mediators of Conduct Problems

Research in the 1970s provided indications that antisocial behavior patterns could be linked to failures in perspective taking. Chandler (1973) examined the relation between social perspective taking and deviant behavior in delinquent versus nondelinquent preadolescent boys: Nondelinquents showed significantly less egocentric behavior. Jurkovic (1980) found delinquents were significantly lower than matched nondelinquent peers in their stage of moral reasoning (see review by Blasi, 1980).

Research of the 1980s has explored these issues further. Studies do not uniformly indicate that delinquents are more deficient in empathy or perspective taking. Kaplan and Arbuthnot (1985) measured affective empathy on a structured task, affective empathy on an unstructured task, and cognitive role taking on male and female delinquents and nondelinquents. Differences were found (a) on the unstructured empathy task, with delinquents performing more poorly than non-delinquents, and (b) on the structured affective empathy task with male, but not female, delinquents performing more poorly. The heightened empathy of female, relative to male, delinquents, may serve both (a) to protect females against further antisocial behavior and (b) to increase vulnerability to internalizing problems such as depression, anxiety disorders, and somatic complaints. There is known to be less stability in conduct problems in females over time. Moreover, there is evidence from longitudinal research (Robins, 1986) that aggressive females are likely to experience later internalizing problems.

In a comprehensive study, delinquent and nondelinquent males were compared on several measures of empathy, cognition, and moral reasoning. They were administered two empathy scales, a role-taking task, two Piagetian cognitive tasks, and two of Kohlberg's structured moral dilemmas (Lee & Prentice, 1988). Adolescents were approximately 16 years old, and groups were equated for IQ. Delinquents as a group displayed significantly more immature modes of role taking, logical cognition, and moral reasoning than did nondelinquents. In contrast to the study reported previously, groups did not differ on affective empathy tasks. Three subgroups of delinquents (psychopathic, neurotic, and subcultural) did not differ significantly from one another on any of the dimensions.

CAROLYN ZAHN-
WAXLER and K.
DANIELLE SMITH

Bear (1989) studied sociomoral reasoning in sixth-graders attending regular classrooms. Maturity of sociomoral reasoning was correlated with conduct disorder and socialized aggression (assessed via self-ratings using the Revised Behavior Problem Check List), but only for boys. Girls reported significantly less aggression than boys, perhaps making it more difficult to assess systematic covariations in aggression and sociomoral reasoning. Research by Sigman, Ungerer, and Russell (1983) indicates that difficulties in moral reasoning may also be associated with other types of behavior problems as well. Emotionally disturbed, cognitively delayed youngsters were examined. Adolescents reported by their teachers to be shy and submissive were less capable of reasoning about moral issues than adolescents who were more assertive and socially engaged. Level of moral judgment was not a function of intelligence.

Thus investigations continue to document linkages between deficiencies in role-taking abilities, empathy and moral reasoning, and behavior problems (mainly externalizing) in children. Findings are a function of the types of tests administered, kinds of behavior problems explored, populations studied, whether or not females are included in the sample, whether the interviewer knows the diagnostic status of the child—and a host of other factors. The findings highlight the importance of affective and social-cognitive dimensions as mediators and predictors of antisocial behaviors of children and adolescents. However, they do little to illuminate the more complex questions of etiology (i.e., how children develop the kinds of deficiencies identified). Moreover, we do not know whether some of the dimensions studied result from, rather than contribute to, delinquent, antisocial lifestyles.

Several studies reveal higher moral reasoning in children whose parents use higher moral reasoning, encourage participation, and spend more time in collective problem solving, use induction versus power-assertion in discipline, provide and receive more support, and use less love withdrawal (see review by Arbuthnot & Gordon, 1986). Mothers of nondelinquents have higher moral reasoning stages than mothers of delinquents (Hudgins & Prentice, 1973). Similarly, positive parenting techniques (e.g., nurturance, modeling of altruism, inductive discipline, empathy) have been associated with empathy and prosocial behavior in offspring. Thus, there is some reason to believe that particular socialization practices may contribute to higher levels of social cognition and empathy early in development. This may, in turn, protect children against certain kinds of emotional problems. But this possibility needs to be considered within the broader context of many other biological and environmental conditions that foster behavior problems and diminished interpersonal sensitivity. Moreover, group comparisons often lead to generalizations that are too stark or extreme. Many of the delinquent children studied are not deficient in empathy and social awareness. Why is this so?

Intervention Research

The work of Chandler and his colleagues (1974) demonstrated that delinquents who were taught perspective-taking skills showed fewer problems and fewer repeat offenses for a sustained period of time. The work of the Feshbach's and their colleagues (e.g., Feshbach, 1979) focused on attempts to facilitate empathy and role taking in antisocial youths. There have been some continued efforts in the 1980s to use these known mediators of prosocial behavior to diminish antisocial behavior in youth. Arbuthnot and Gordon (1986) reasoned that because delinquents have been consistently shown to function at lower stages of moral reasoning than non-delinquents, adolescents at risk for juvenile delinquency would benefit both cognitively and behaviorally from an intervention designed to accelerate moral reasoning development.

Adolescents identified by teachers as aggressive and/or disruptive were given 16 to 20 weekly 45-minute sessions and were then compared with matched and randomly assigned nonparticipating controls. The group given moral reasoning training showed (a) advances in moral reasoning stage and (b) improvement on several behavioral indexes, including behavior referrals, tardiness, academic performance, and police/court contacts. For a subgroup followed up 1 year later, positive effects of the intervention were still evident. Although the intervention focused mainly on guided moral dilemma discussion, there were also efforts to (a) build and maintain rapport using warmth and humor and (b) develop feelings of openness, group identity and cohesion, safety, acceptance, and respect for others' views. This aspect of relationship building may have fostered empathy as well as the social-cognitive skill development, hypothesized to contribute to the positive subsequent outcomes.

Dubow, Huesmann, and Eron (1987) utilized different school-based interventions designed to decrease children's aggression and promote prosocial behavior. Boys ranging in age from 8 to 13 from "behavior-disorder" classrooms were assigned to one of four training conditions: cognitive (self-control) training, behavioral (prosocial skills) training, combined cognitive-behavioral training, or attention/play training. Boys were trained in small groups for 10 one-hour sessions. Cognitive-behavioral and attention/play interventions produced the most improvement. Improvement was evidenced through decreased aggression and increased prosocial behavior.

Biologically based interventions have also been used to alter the behavior patterns of children who are disruptive. Hinshaw, Henker, Whalen, Erhardt, and Dunnington (1989), for example, assessed the effects of methylphenidate on aggressive, prosocial, and nonsocial behavior in 6- to 12-year-old hyperactive boys in naturalistic settings. The stimulant medication reduced physical and verbal aggression in hyperactive boys to levels comparable to boys without such attentional and behavioral problems. There were no overall group effects of medication on frequency of prosocial or nonsocial behaviors. A subgroup of medically treated hyperactive children, however, showed increases in prosocial behavior. The authors note, too, that prosocial interventions of these children may be qualitatively different, in ways that are significant but are not always captured by coding systems or by the use of frequency measures.

Thus a variety of different types of interventions have been used with varying degrees of success to diminish antisocial behavior and promote prosocial patterns. Both behavioral and environmental contributors have been identified. The research provides a number of promising leads but also emphasizes the need for a cautionary note, as intervention effects are often not enduring.

Summary

In this overview of work on prosocial behavior in children, we have attempted to focus on the major significant substantive contributions of the 1980s. We have reviewed work on the development and socialization of children's potentials for compassion. Affective, cognitive, and behavioral dimensions have all been considered. In our view, it is somewhat arbitrary to consider the actions that may benefit others independently from the thoughts and emotions implicated in this process. Many issues have received little attention in this review. Prosocial behavior has been treated, in the main, as a unitary construct, and this clearly oversimplifies the meaning of such diverse behaviors as helping, sharing, comforting, cooperation, rescue, protection, defense, and so on. These behaviors may or may not share a common core. Even for a particular type of prosocial behavior, the meaning of the act may vary considerably, depending upon the particular motive. And motives are notoriously difficult to measure. It is difficult to anticipate the trajectories of future work in this area. We consider it a healthy sign that, despite considerable shifts in specific research foci over the past several decades, there has been an abiding interest in exploring those qualities of humankind from a developmental perspective that facilitate our capacity to maintain connectedness, caring, and commitment to others. Conceptual and technological advances of recent years assure the possibility of continued progress in this important area of research.

REFERENCES

Amsterdam, B. (1972). Mirror self-image reactions before age two. *Developmental Psychology*, 297–305.

Arbuthnot, J., & Gordon, D. A. (1986). Behavioral and cognitive effects of a moral reasoning development intervention for high-risk behavior-disordered adolescents. *Journal of Consulting Clinical Psychology*, *54*, 208–216.

Barnett, M. A. (1987). Empathy and related responses in children. In N. Eisenberg & J. Strayer (Eds.), *Empathy and its development* (pp. 146–162). New York: Cambridge University Press.

Barnett, M. A., & McCoy, S. A. (1989). The relation of distressful childhood experiences and empathy in college undergraduates. *Journal of Genetic Psychology*, *150*, 417–426.

Barnett, M. A., McMinimy, V., Flouer, G., & Masbad, I. (1987). Adolescent's evaluations of peers' motives for helping. *Journal of Youth and Adolescence*, *16*, 579–586.

Batson, C. D., Batson, J. G., Griffitt, C. A., Barrientos, S., Brandt, J. R., Spnengelmeyer, P., & Bayly, M. J. (1989). Negative-state relief and the empathy-altruism hypothesis. *Journal of Personality and Social Psychology*, *56*, 922–933.

Batson, C. D., Dyck, J. L., Brandt, J. R., Batson, J. G., Powell, A. L., McMaster, M. R., & Griffitt, C. (1988). Fives studies testing two new egoistic alternatives to the empathy-altruism hypothesis. *Journal of Personality and Social Psychology*, *55*, 52–77.

Bauman, D. J., Cialdini, R. B., & Kendrick, D. J. (1983). Mood and sex differences in the development of altruism as hedonism. *Academic Psychology Bulletin*, *5*, 299–307.

Baumrind, D. (1986). Sex differences in moral reasoning: Response to Walker's (1984) conclusion that there are none. *Child Development*, *57*, 511–521.

Bear, G. G. (1989). Sociomoral reasoning and antisocial behaviors around normal sixth graders. *Merrill-Palmer Quarterly*, *35*, 181–196.

Beardslee, W., & Podorefsky, D. (1988). Resilient adolescents whose parents have serious affective and other psychiatric disorders: Importance of self-understanding and relationships. *American Journal of Psychiatry*, *145*(1), 63–69.

Beardslee, W. R., Schultz, L. H., & Selman, R. L. (1987). Level of social-cognitive development, adoptive functioning, and DSM-III diagnoses in adolescent offspring of parents with affective disorders: Implications for the development of the capacity for mutuality. *Developmental Psychology*, *23*(6), 807–815.

Bengtsson, H., & Johnson, L. (1987). Cognitions related to empathy in five- to eleven-year-old children. *Child Development*, *58*, 1001–1012.

Berndt, T. J. (1981). Effects of friendship on prosocial intentions and behavior. *Child Development*, *52*, 636–643.

Berthenthal, B., & Fischer, K. W. (1978). The development of self-recognition in the infant. *Developmental Psychology*, *14*, 44–50.

Blasi, A. (1980). Bridging moral cognition and moral action: A critical review of the literature. *Psychology Bulletin, 88*, 1–45.

Block, J., Olweus, D., & Radke-Yarrow, M. (1986). *Development of anti-social and prosocial behavior: Research, theories and issues.* New York: Academic Press.

Bloom, L., Lightbown, P., & Hood, L. (1975). Structure and variation in child language. *Monographs of the Society for Research in Child Development,* serial No. 160, Vol. 40, No. 2. Chicago, University of Chicago Press.

Boehnke, K., Silbereisen, R. K., Eisenberg, N., Reykowski, J., & Polomari, A. (1989). Developmental pattern of prosocial motivation: A cross-national study. *Journal of Cross-Cultural Psychology, 20*, 219–243.

Boom, J., & Molenaar, P. C. (1989). A developmental model of hierarchical stage structure in objective moral judgements. *Developmental Review, 9*, 133–145.

Bretherton, I., Fritz, J., Zahn-Waxler, C., & Ridgeway, D. (1986). The acquisition and development of emotion language: A functionalist perspective. *Child Development, 57*, 529–548.

Brody, L. R. (1985). Gender differences in emotional development: A review of theories and research. *Journal of Personality, 53*, 102–149.

Brothers, L. (1989). A biological perspective on empathy. *American Journal of Psychiatry, 146*, 10–19.

Bruner, J. S. (1972). The nature and uses of immaturity. *American Psychologist, 27*, 1–22.

Bryan, T., Werner, M., & Pearl, R. (1982). Learning disabled students' conformity responses to prosocial and antisocial situations. *Learning Disability Quarterly, 1*(1), 33–38.

Bussey, K., & Maugham, B. (1982). Gender differences in moral reasoning. *Journal of Personality and Social Psychology, 42*, 701–706.

Butterworth, G. (1980). A discussion of some issues raised by Piaget's concept of childhood egocentrism. In M. V. Cox (Ed.), *Are young children egocentric?* pp. 17–40. York, England: Batsford Academic and Educational.

Campos, J. J., Barrett, K. C., Lamb, M. E., Goldsmith, H. H., & Stenberg, C. (1983). Socioemotional Development. In P. H. Mussen, M. M. Haith, & J. J. Campos (Eds.), *Handbook of child psychology: Infancy and developmental psychobiology* (Vol. 2, pp. 783–915). New York: Wiley.

Caplan, M. & Hay, D. F. (1989). Preschoolers' responses to peers' distress and beliefs about bystander intervention. *Journal of Child Psychology and Psychiatry, 30*, 231–242.

Carlson, M., & Miller, N. (1987). Explanation of the relation between negative mood and helping. *Psychological Bulletin, 102*(1), 191–208.

Chambers, J. H., & Ascione, F. R. (1987). The effects of prosocial and aggressive videogames on children's donating and helping. *Journal of Genetic Psychology, 148*, 499–505.

Chandler, M. J. (1973). Egocentric and anti-social behavior: The assessment and training of social perspective-taking skills. *Developmental Psychology, 9*(3), 326–332.

Chandler, M. J., Greenspan, S., & Barenboim, C. (1974). Assessment and training of role-taking skills in institutionalized emotionally disturbed children. *Developmental Psychology, 10*(4), 546–553.

Chapman, M., Zahn-Waxler, C., Cooperman, G., & Iannotti, R. (1987). Empathy and responsibility in the motivation of children's helping. *Developmental Psychology, 23*, 140–145.

Cialdini, R. B., Eisenberg, N., Shell, R., & McCreath, H. (1987). Commitments to help by children: Effects on subsequent prosocial self-attributions. *British Journal of Social Psychology, 26*, 237–245.

Cialdini, R. B., & Kendrick, D. T. (1976). Altruism as hedonism: A social development perspective on the relationship of negative mood and state and helping. *Journal of Personality and Social Psychology, 34*, 907–914.

Cialdini, R. B., Schaller, M., Houlihan, D., Arps, K., Fultz, J., & Beaman, A. L. (1987). Empathy-based helping: Is it selflessly motivated? *Journal of Personality and Social Psychology, 52*, 749–758.

Cicchetti, D. (1990). The organization and coherence of socioemotional, cognitive and representational development: Illustrations through a developmental psychopathology perspective on down syndrome and child maltreatment. *Nebraska Symposium on Motivation, 1988: Socioemotional Development,* R. Thompson, (Ed.), Lincoln: University of Nebraska Press, pp. 259–366.

Clary, E. G., & Miller, J. (1986). Socialization and situational influences on sustained altruism. *Child Development, 57*, 1358–1369.

Cummings, E. M., Hollenbeck, B., Iannotti, R. J., Radke-Yarrow, M., & Zahn-Waxler, C. (1986). Early organization of altruism and aggression: Developmental patterns and individual differences. In C. Zahn-Waxler, E. M. Cummings, & R. J. Iannotti (Eds.), *Altruism and aggression: Biological and social origins* (pp. 165–188) New York: Cambridge University Press.

Cummings, M., Zahn-Waxler, C., & Radke-Yarrow, M. (1981). Young children's responses to expressions of anger and affection by others in the family. *Child Development, 52*, 1274–1282.

Darwin, C. (1872). *The expression of the emotions in man and animal*. London: John Murray.

Dawkins, R. (1976). *The selfish gene*. London: Oxford University Press.

Denham, S. A. (1986). Social cognition, prosocial behavior and emotion in preschoolers: Contextual validation. *Child Development, 57*, 194–201.

Denham, S. A., & Couchard, E. A. (1991). Social-emotional predictors of preschoolers' responses to adult negative emotion. *Journal of Child Psychology and Psychiatry and Allied Disciplines, 32*, 595–608.

Denham, S., McKinley, M., Couchard, E. A., & Holt, R. (1991). Emotional and behavioral predictors of preschool peer ratings. *Child Development, 61*, 1145–1152.

Derr, A. M. (1986). How learning disabled adolescent boys make moral judgments. *Journal of Learning Disabilities, 19*, 160–164.

Donenberg, G. R., & Hoffman, L. W. (1988). Gender differences in moral development. *Sex Roles, 18*, 701–717.

Dubow, E. F., Huesmann, L. R., & Eron, L. D. (1987). Mitigating aggression and promoting prosocial behavior in aggressive elementary schoolboys. *Behavior Research Theories, 25*, 527–531.

Dunn, J., & Munn, P. (1986). Siblings and the development of prosocial behavior. *International Journal of Behavioral Development, 9*, 265–284.

Eagly, A. H., & Crowley, M. (1986). Gender and helping behavior: A meta-analytic review of the social psychological literature. *Psychological Bulletin, 100*, 283–308.

Eckerman, C. O., Whatley, J. L., & Kutz, S. L. (1975). Growth of social play with peers during the second year of life. *Developmental Psychology, 11*, 42–49.

Eisenberg, N., Fabes, R. A., Bustamante, D., Mathy, R. M., Miller, P. A., & Lindholm, E. (1988). Differentiation of vicariously induced emotional reactions in children. *Developmental Psychology, 24*, 237–246.

Eisenberg, N., Fabes, P. A., Miller, P. A., Fultz, J., Shell, R., Mathy, R. M., & Reno, R. R. (1989). Relation of sympathy and personal distress to prosocial behavior: A multimethod study. *Journal of Personality and Social Psychology, 57*, 55–66.

Eisenberg, N., & Lennon, R. (1983). Sex differences in empathy and related capacities. *Psychological Bulletin, 94*, 100–131.

Eisenberg, N., & Miller, P. A. (1987). The relation of empathy to prosocial and related behaviors. *Psychological Bulletin, 101*, 91–119.

Eisenberg, N., Schaller, M., Fabes, R. A., Bustamante, D., Mathy, R. M., Shell, R., & Rhodes, K. (1988). Differentiation of personal distress and sympathy in children and adults. *Developmental Psychology, 24*, 766–775.

Eisenberg, N., Shell, R., Pasternack, J., Lennon, R., Belber, R., & Matty, R. M. (1987). Prosocial development in middle childhood: A longitudinal study. *Developmental Psychology, 23*, 712–718.

Eisenberg, N., & Strayer, J. (1987). *Empathy and its development*. Cambridge, Cambridge University Press.

Emde, R., Johnson, W., & Easterbrooks, M. A. (1987). The do's and don'ts of early moral development: Psychoanalytic tradition and current research. In J. Kagan & S. Lamb (Eds.), *The emergence of morality in young children* (pp. 245–276). Chicago: University of Chicago Press.

Emery, R. E. (1982). Interparent conflict and the children of discord and divorce. *Psychological Bulletin, 92*, 310–330.

Fabes, R. A., Eisenberg, N., & Miller, P. (1990). Maternal correlates of children's vicarious emotional responsiveness. *Developmental Psychology, 26*, 639–648.

Fabes, R. A., Fultz, J., Eisenberg, N., May-Plumlee, T., & Christopher, F. S. (1989). Effects of rewards on children's prosocial motivation: A socialization study. *Developmental Psychology, 25*, 509–515.

Fergusion, T. J., & Rule, B. G. (1988). Children's evaluation of retaliatory aggression. *Child Development, 59*, 961–968.

Feshbach, N. D. (1978). Studies of empathic behavior in children. In B. A. Maher (Ed.), *Progress in experimental personality research* (Vol. 8, pp. 1–47), New York: Academic Press.

Feshbach, N. D. (1979). Empathy training: A field study in affective education. In S. Feshbach & A. Fraczek (Eds.), *Aggression and behavior change: Biological and social processes* (pp. 234–249). New York: Praeger.

Field, T., Woodson, R., Greenberg, R., & Cohen, D. (1982). Discrimination and imitation of facial expressions by neonates. *Science, 218*, 179–181.

Francis, L. J., & Pearson, P. R. (1987). Empathic development during adolescence: Religiosity, the missing link? *Personality and Individual Differences, 8*, 145–148.

Freud, S. (1958). *Civilization and its discontents*. New York: Doubleday Anchor Books.

Frodi, A., Lamb, M. E., Leavitt, L. A., Donovan, W. A., Neff, C., & Sherry, D. (1978). Fathers' and mothers' responses to the faces and cries of normal and premature infants. *Developmental Psychology*, *14*(5), 490–498.

Frodi, A., Macaulay, J., & Thome, P. R. (1977). Are women always less aggressive than men? A review of the experimental literature. *Psychological Bulletin*, *84*(4), 634–660.

Gilligan, C. (1977). In a different voice: Women's conception of self and morality. *Harvard Educational Review*, *47*, 481–517.

Gilligan, C. (1982). *In a different voice: Psychological theory and women's development*. Cambridge: Harvard University Press.

Grusec, J. E. (1982). The socialization of altruism. In N. Eisenberg-Berg (Ed.), *The development of prosocial behavior* (pp. 139–166). New York: Academic Press.

Grusec, J. E. (1991). Socializing concern for others in the home. *Developmental Psychology*, *27*(2), 338–342.

Hall, J. A. (1978). Gender differences in decoding nonverbal cues. *Psychological Bulletin*, *85*(4), 845–857.

Hart, D. (1988). A longitudinal study of adolescents' socialization and identification as predictors of adult moral judgment development. *Merrill-Palmer Quarterly*, *34*, 245–260.

Hartshorne, H., May, M. A., & Mahler, J. B. (1929). *Studies in the nature of character* (Vol. 2), *Studies in service and self-control*. New York: Macmillan.

Haviland, J. M., & Lelivica, M. (1987). The induced affect response: 10-week-old infants' responses to three emotion expressions. *Developmental Psychology*, *23*(1), 97–104.

Haynes-Seman, C. (1987). Developmental origins of moral masochism: A failure-to-thrive toddler's interactions with mother. *Child Abuse and Neglect*, *11*, 319–330.

Hinshaw, S. P., Henker, B., Whalen, C. K., Erhardt, D., & Dunnighton, R. E. (1989). Aggressive, prosocial, and nonsocial behavior in hyperactive boys: Dose effects of methylphenidate in naturalistic settings. *Journal of Consulting Clinical Psychology*, *57*, 636–643.

Hobson, R. P. (1984). Early childhood autism and the question of egocentrism. *Journal of Autism and Developmental Disorders*, *14*, 85–104.

Hoffman, M. L. (1970). Moral development. In P. H. Mussen (Ed.), *Carmichael's manual of child psychology*: (Vol. 2) (pp. 261–360). New York: Wiley.

Hoffman, M. L. (1975). Developmental synthesis of affect and cognition and its implications for altruistic motivation. *Developmental Psychology*, *11*, 605–622.

Hoffman, M. L. (1977). Sex differences in empathy and related behaviors. *Psychological Bulletin*, *84*, 712–722.

Howes, C., & Eldridge, R. (1985). Responses of abused, neglected and non-maltreated children to the behaviors of their peers. *Journal of Applied Developmental Psychology*, *6*, 261–270.

Howes, C., & Farver, J. (1987). Toddler's responses to the distress of their peers. *Journal of Applied Developmental Psychology*, *8*, 441–452.

Hudgins, W., & Prentice, N. M. (1973). Moral judgment in delinquent and non-delinquent adolescents and their mothers. *Journal of Abnormal Psychology*, *82*, 145–152.

Izard, C. E. (1977). *Human emotions*. New York: Plenum Press.

Jurkovic, G. J. (1980). The juvenile delinquent as a moral philosopher: A structural-developmental perspective. *Psychological Bulletin*, *88*, 709–727.

Kagan, J., & Lamb, S. (1987). *The emergence of morality in young children*. Chicago: University of Chicago Press.

Kaplan, P. J., & Arbuthnot, J. (1985). Affective empathy and cognitive role-taking in delinquent and nondelinquent youth. *Adolescence*, *20*, 323–333.

Keltikangus-Tarvinen, L. (1989). Moral judgements of aggressive and non-aggressive children. *The Journal of Social Psychology*, *129*, 733–739.

Klimes-Dougan, B., & Kistner, J. (1990). Physically abused preschoolers' responses to peers' distress. *Developmental Psychology*, *26*(4), 599–602.

Koestner, R., Franz, C., & Weinberger, J. (1990). The family origins of empathic concern: A 26-year longitudinal study. *Journal of Personality and Social Psychology*, *58*, 709–717.

Kohlberg, L. (1969). Stage and sequence: The cognitive-developmental approach to socialization. In D. A. Goslin (Ed.), *Handbook of socialization theory and research* (pp. 347–480). New York: Rand McNally.

Lee, M., & Prentice, N. M. (1988). Interrelations of empathy, cognition, and moral reasoning with dimensions of juvenile delinquency. *Journal of Abnormal Child Psychology*, *16*, 127–139.

Lennon, R., & Eisenberg, N. (1987). Emotional displays associated with preschoolers' prosocial behavior. *Child Development*, *58*, 992–1000.

Lewis, M., Sullivan, M., Stanger, C., & Weiss, M. (1989). Self development and self-conscious emotions. *Child Development*, *60*, 146–156.

MacLean, P. D. (1985). Brain evolution relating to family, play, and the separation call. *Archives of General Psychology*, *42*, 405–417.

Main, M., & George, C. (1985). Response of abused and disadvantaged toddlers to distress in playmates: A study in the day care setting. *Developmental Psychology*, *21*, 407–412.

Main, M., & Goldwyn, R. (1984). Predicting rejection of her infant from mother's representation of her own experience: Implications for the abused-abusing intergenerational cycle. *Child Abuse and Neglect*, *8*, 203–217.

Matthews, K. A., Batson, C. D., Horn, J., & Rosenman, R. H. (1981). Principles in his nature which interest him in the fortune of others: The heritability of empathic concern for others. *Journal of Personality*, *49*, 237–247.

McCall, R. B. (1979). Qualitative transitions in behavioral development in the first two years. In M. H. Bornstein & W. Kessen (Eds.), *Psychological development in infancy* (pp. 182–224). Hillsdale, NJ: Erlbaum.

McCord, L. (1990). *Altruism, mutual aid and aggression.* Paper presentation at workshop, hostility and sociability: Developmental and socio-psychological perspectives, Warsaw, Poland.

Meltzoff, A. N., & Moore, M. K. (1977). Imitation of facial and manual gestures by human neonates. *Science*, *198*, 75–78.

Miller, P. A., & Eisenberg, N. (1988). The relation of empathy to aggressive and externalizing/antisocial behavior. *Psychological Bulletin*, *103*, 324–344.

Mills, R. S. L., & Grusec, J. E. (1989). Cognitive, affective, and behavioral consequences of praising altruism. *Merrill-Palmer Quarterly*, *35*, 299–326.

Muuss, R. E. (1988). Carol Gilligan's theory of sex differences in the development of moral reasoning during adolescence. *Adolescence*, *23*, 229–243.

Nelms, B. C. (1989). Emotional behaviors in chronically ill children. *Journal of Abnormal Child Psychology*, *17*, 657–668.

Nicholich, L. (1977). Beyond sensorimotor intelligence: Assessment of symbolic maturity through analyses of pretend play. *Merrill-Palmer Quarterly*, *23*, 89–99.

Nolen-Hoeksema, S. (1987). Sex differences in unipolar depression: Evidence and theory. *Psychological Bulletin*, *101*(2), 257–282.

Olweus, D., Block, J., & Radke-Yarrow, M. (1986). *Development of antisocial and prosocial behavior.* Orlando, FL: Academic Press.

Parke, R. D., & Slaby, R. G. (1983). The development of aggression. In P. H. Mussen & E. M. Hetherington (Eds.), *Handbook of child psychology: Socialization, personality, and social development* (Vol. 4, pp. 547–641). New York: Wiley.

Parmelee, A. (1986). Children's illnesses: Their beneficial effects on behavioral development. *Child Development*, *57*, 1–10.

Pecukis, E. V. (1990). A cognitive/affective empathy training program as a function of ego development in aggressive adolescent females. *Adolescence*, *25*, 59–76.

Piaget, J. (1962). *Play, dreams and imitation in childhood.* New York: Norton.

Piaget, J. (1965). *The moral judgement of the child.* New York: Harcourt, Brace. (Originally published 1932)

Radke-Yarrow, M., Zahn-Waxler, C., & Chapman, M. (1983). Children's prosocial dispositions and behavior. In P. H. Mussen & E. M. Hetherington (Eds.), *Handbook of child psychology: Socialization, personality, and social development* (Vol. 4, pp. 469–545). New York: Wiley.

Redefer, L. A., & Goodman, J. F. (1989). Pet-facilitated therapy with autistic children. *Journal of Autism and Developmental Disorders*, *19*, 461–467.

Rehberg, H. R., & Richman, C. L. (1989). Prosocial behavior in preschool children: A look at the interaction of race, gender, and family composition. *International Journal of Behavioral Development*, *12*, 385–401.

Renshaw, P. D., & Asher, S. R. (1983). Children's goals and strategies for social interaction. *Merrill-Palmer Quarterly*, *29*, 353–374.

Rheingold, H. L., & Emery, G. N. (1986). The nurturant acts of very young children. In D. Olweus, J. Block, & M. Radke-Yarrow (Eds.), *The development of anti- and prosocial behavior* (pp. 75–96). Orlando, FL: Academic Press.

Rheingold, H. L., Hay, D. F., & West, M. J. (1976). Sharing in the second year of life. *Child Development*, *47*, 1148–1158.

Robins, L. N. (1986). The consequences of conduct disorder in girls. In D. Olweus, J. Block, & M. Radke-

Yarrow (Eds.), *Development of antisocial and prosocial behavior: Research, theories and issues* (pp. 385–414). Orlando, FL: Academic Press.

Robinson, J. (1989). *Sex differences in the development of empathy during late infancy: Findings from the MacArthur longitudinal twin study*. Presentation at SRCD, Kansas City, Missouri.

Rosenhan, D. L. (1970). The natural socialization of altruistic autonomy. In J. R. Macaulay & L. Berkowitz (Eds.), *Altruism and helping behavior* (pp. 251–268). New York: Academic Press.

Ross, H. S., & Goldman, B. D. (1977). Establishing new social relations in infancy. In T. Alloway, L. Kramer, & P. Pliner (Eds.), *Advances in the study of communication and affect, Attachment behavior* (Vol. 3, pp. 61–79). New York: Plenum.

Rushton, J. P. (1976). Socialization and the altruistic behavior of children, *Psychological Bulletin, 83*, 898–913.

Rushton, J. P., Fulker, D. W., Neale, M. C., Nias, D. L. B., & Eysenck, H. J. (1986). Altruism and aggression: The heritability of individual differences. *Journal of Personality and Social Psychology, 50*, 1192–1198.

Sagi, A., & Hoffman, M. L. (1976). Empathic distress in the newborn. *Developmental Psychology, 12*, 175–176.

Sears, R. R., Maccoby, E. E., & Levin, H. (1957). *Patterns of child rearing*. Evanston IL: Row and Peterson.

Segal, N. L. (1984). Cooperation, competition, and altruism within twin sets: A reappraisal. *Ethology and Sociobiology, 5*, 163–177.

Segal, N. L. (1988). Cooperation, competition, and altruism in human twinships: A sociobiological approach. In K. B. MacDonald (Ed.), *Sociobiological perspectives on human development* (pp. 168–206). New York: Springer-Verlag.

Shigetomi, C. C., Hartmann, D. P., & Gelfand, D. M. (1981). Sex differences in children's altruistic behavior and reputations for helpfulness. *Developmental Psychology, 17*, 434–437.

Siegal, M. (1985). Mother-child relations and the development of empathy: A short-term longitudinal study. *Child Psychiatry and Human Development, 57*, 355–365.

Sigman, M., Ungerer, J. A., & Russell, A. (1983). Moral judgements in relation to behavioral and cognitive disorders in adolescents. *Journal of Abnormal Child Psychology, 11*, 503–511.

Simner, M. L. (1971). Newborn's response to the cry of another infant. *Developmental Psychology, 5*, 136–150.

Stanhope, L., Bell, R. Q., & Parker-Cohen, N. Y. (1987). Temperament and helping behavior in preschool children. *Developmental Psychology, 23*, 347–353.

Stern, D. (1985). *The interpersonal world of the "infant"*. New York: Basic Books.

Strain, P., & Odom, S. L. (1986). Peer social initiations: Effective intervention for social skills development of exceptional children. *Exceptional Children, 56*, 543–551.

Strayer, J., & Roberts, W. (1989). Children's empathy and role taking: Child and parental factors, and relations to prosocial behavior. *Journal of Applied Developmental Psychology, 10*, 227–239.

Termine, N. T., & Izard, C. E. (1988). Infants' responses to their mothers' expressions of joy and sadness. *Developmental Psychology, 24*, 223–229.

Teti, D. M., & Ablard, K. A. (1989). Security of attachment and infant-sibling relationships: A laboratory study. *Child Development, 60*, 1519–1528.

Thompson, R. A., & Hoffman, M. L. (1980). Empathy and the development of guilt in children. *Developmental Psychology, 16*, 155–156.

Trevarthen, C. (1989, Autumn). Origins and directions for the concept of infant intersubjectivity. *Society for Research in Child Development*. Newsletter, pp. 1–4.

Walker, L. J. (1984). Sex differences in the development of moral reasoning: A critical review. *Child Development, 55*, 677–691.

Watson, M., & Fischer, K. (1977). A developmental sequence of agent use in late infancy. *Child Development, 48*, 828–836.

Wiesenfeld, A. R., Whitman, P. B., & Malatesta, C. Z. (1984). Individual differences among adult women in sensitivity to infants: Evidence in support of an empathy concept. *Journal of Personality and Social Psychology, 46*, 118–124.

Yarrow, M. R., Scott, P. M., & Waxler, C. Z. (1973). Learning concern for others. *Developmental Psychology, 8*, 240–260.

Zahn-Waxler, C., Cole, P., & Barrett, K. C. (1991). Guilt and empathy: Sex differences and implications for the development of depression. In K. Dodge & J. Garber (Eds.), *Emotion regulation and dysregulation* (pp. 243–272). New York: Cambridge Press.

Zahn-Waxler, C., Cummings, E. M., & Iannotti, R. (1986). *Altruism and aggression: Biological and social origins*. New York: Cambridge University Press.

Zahn-Waxler, C., Friedman, S. L., & Cummings, E. M. (1983). Children's emotions and behaviors in response to infants' cries. *Child Development, 54*, 1522–1528.

Zahn-Waxler, C., & Kochanska, G. (1990). The development of guilt. In R. Thompson (Ed.), *Nebraska Symposium on Motivation, 1988: Socioemotional Development* (pp. 183–258). Lincoln: University of Nebraska Press.

Zahn-Waxler, C., Kochanska, G., Krupnick, J., & McKnew, D. (1990). Patterns of guilt in children of depressed and well mothers. *Developmental Psychology, 26*(1), 51–59.

Zahn-Waxler, C., & Radke-Yarrow, M. (1982). The development of altruism: Alternative research strategies. In N. Eisenberg (Ed.), *The development of prosocial behavior* (pp. 109–137). New York: Academic Press.

Zahn-Waxler, C., Radke-Yarrow, M., & King, R. (1979). Child rearing and children's prosocial initiations toward victims of distress. *Child Development, 50*, 319–330.

Zahn-Waxler, C., Radke-Yarrow, M., Chapman, M., & Wagner, E. (1990). *The development of concern for others*. Unpublished manuscript.

Zahn-Waxler, C., Robinson, J., & Emde, R. (1990). *The development and heritability of empathy*. Unpublished manuscript.

Zarbatany, L., Hartmann, D. P., & Gelfand, D. M. (1985). Why does children's generosity increase with age: Susceptibility to experimenter influence or altruism? *Child Development, 56*, 746–756.

11

Peer Relations in Early and Middle Childhood

WILLARD W. HARTUP

INTRODUCTION

Child–child interaction is essentially egalitarian. Some relationships between children are more egalitarian than others, but peer relations are generally understood by children to be structured horizontally rather than vertically. The egalitarian nature of the social exchanges that occur between children and other children distinguish them clearly from the exchanges that occur between children and adults (Furman & Buhmester, 1985; Youniss, 1980).

Infants and toddlers manifest considerable interest in one another; however, coordinated and sustained interaction between children is not common until the beginning of the third year (Brownell, 1990; Eckerman, Davis, & Didow, 1989). Early and middle childhood are then marked by tremendous changes in both the quantity and quality of child–child interaction, the emergence of social reputations, the increasing centrality of friendship relations, and the differentiation of social networks.

Recent studies document both the concurrent and developmental significance of peer relations, and this work will be summarized in this chapter. Children differ enormously from one another in the success achieved in peer relations. Consequently, the developmental implications of these differences will also be considered. The nature and origins of these differences will be discussed as well as the mechanisms through which family relations influence peer interaction. Children's

WILLARD W. HARTUP • Institute of Child Development, University of Minnesota, Minneapolis, Minnesota 55455.

Handbook of Social Development: A Lifespan Perspective, edited by Vincent B. Van Hasselt and Michel Hersen. Plenum Press, New York, 1992.

friendships will also be scrutinized—both their significance and the unique qualities that friendship relations possess. Finally, group relations will be examined. As will be seen, the weight of the evidence supports the notion that children's relations with one another are necessities in social development, not mere niceties.

THE DISTINCTIVENESS AND CENTRALITY OF CHILDHOOD PEER RELATIONS

Time Spent with Other Children

With increasing age, more and more time is committed to relations with other children. The proportion of the child's social activity involving other children rises from about 10% at age 2, to 20% at age 4, to slightly over 40% between ages 7 and 11. Among older children, about one-sixth of this socializing involves siblings; the remainder mainly involves friends (Barker & Wright, 1955).

Because children have been studied most frequently in schools, which are age-graded, we know more about age-mate than non-age-mate interaction. And yet, ecological studies (Barker & Wright, 1955) reveal that 65% of children's interactions with other children involve companions who differ in age by more than 12 months (52%, excluding sibling interaction). Non-age-mate interaction is thus as normative as age-mate interaction. This distinction is important because social interaction between children is differentiated according to the age difference between them. In six cultures (both Western and non-Western), observations showed that (a) aggression and conflict occur more frequently between children who are within 1 year of each other in age than between children who differ in age by more than that; (b) nurturance and sympathy are extended more frequently to younger children than to age-mates or older companions; and (c) help seeking is directed more frequently to older children than to age-mates or younger children (Whiting & Whiting, 1975). Age-mates and non-age-mates also represent different social supports: Among socially isolated preschoolers, for example, contact with younger children increases sociability to a greater extent than contact with either age-mates (i.e., children within 6 months of one another) or children who are 15 months older (Furman, Rahe, & Hartup, 1979).

Developmental Course

Children's exchanges with one another consist mostly of play and "fooling around." During early and middle childhood, the most significant developmental changes revolve around children's increased capacities and motivation for engaging in coordinated interaction—both positive and negative, cooperative and aggressive. Numerous studies demonstrate that associative and cooperative activities increase during the preschool years (Parten, 1932), accounting for a greater and greater percentage of the child's social activity. Even so, solitary activity and parallel play remain at relatively high levels (Roper & Hinde 1978); social maturity does not involve the exclusion of solitary activity from the repertoire. At the same time, though, task involvement and the cognitive maturity of solitary and semi-social activity increase (Rubin, Watson, & Jambor, 1978).

The developmental course of aggression and altruism is not easy to describe.

Although total frequencies of aggression tend to increase during the preschool years and then decline, this gradient does not describe every aggressive act (Parke & Slaby, 1983). Verbal aggression increases during early childhood more than physical aggression (which has been shown to decline in most studies). More important, the form of the aggressive act changes: Although preschool children evidence more frequent aggression than school-age children, the difference derives mainly from their more frequent instrumental aggression (mostly struggles over objects and territory). Older children actually demonstrate *more* hostile, person-oriented aggression than younger ones (Hartup, 1974). Older children also use an elaborate network of causal attributions to evaluate aggressive behavior: Aggression that is unintended, unforeseeable, and unavoidable is generally regarded as less blameworthy and less deserving of retaliation than aggression that is intentional, foreseeable, and avoidable (Ferguson & Rule, 1980; Olthof, 1990).

Prosocial development occurs similarly. Toddlers willingly offer their possessions to others (especially in making new social contacts), but these acts of generosity decline with age. Radke-Yarrow, Zahn-Waxler, and Chapman (1983) summarized the preschool child's dispositions in this way:

> Children of these ages are not only egocentric, selfish, and aggressive; they are also exquisitely perceptive, have attachments to a wide range of others and respond prosocially across a broad spectrum of interpersonal events in a wide variety of ways and with various motives. (p. 484)

And across middle childhood, prosocial activity does not *generally* change. Sometimes children have been observed to be more generous with increasing age; sometimes not. Older children, however, seem to be able to assimilate more subtle cues associated with help giving than younger children (Pearl, 1979) and to utilize causal attributions in evaluating these actions.

Thus one major conclusion can be drawn about developmental change in child–child interaction: Relevant changes seem not to derive from alterations in general dispositions to be aggressive or altruistic but, rather, from changes in cognitive and social abilities for dealing with different social contexts. School-age children live in a different social world from the world inhabited by pre-school-aged children: Different companions, different demands, different issues, and different settings are encountered (Higgins & Parsons, 1983). Developmental changes in peer relations, then, cannot be described solely in terms of changing individuals; they can only be described in terms of changing individuals in changing contexts.

Social Reputations

Among children who know one another, "schemata" or expectations about one another are generated on the basis of earlier encounters. Reputations are acquired for aggression and contentiousness in this way and lead to being disliked by other children (Hymel, Wagner, & Butler, 1990). Prosocial reputations are also based on children's experiences with one another (Jensen & Moore, 1977), constituting one, but only one, reason for being liked by other children. Social reputations, once established, are relatively stable and tend to bias the attitudes and behavior of other children. For example, children anticipate hostility and destructiveness from a child who has an aggressive reputation even when provocation is uncertain

(Dodge, 1980). Such biases are also related to the child's social status: Behavior that is acceptable to other children when displayed by a popular child is less acceptable and less memorable when displayed by an unpopular child (Hymel *et al.*, 1990). Social reputations are also related to self-esteem. Both shy and aggressive reputations are associated with poor self-regard, especially in middle childhood.

Friendships

As they grow older, children's relations with other children are increasingly centered on their friends. Children use the word *friend* during the early preschool years (usually sometime in the fourth year), although specifying an age when friendships first appear is difficult. Mothers sometimes believe that their infants or toddlers have "best friends." However, this may mean only that the child has a regular playmate with whom interaction is harmonious.

Yet among 4- and 5-year olds, stable distinctions are made by most children among their associates. By this time, children reliably identify their best friends in sociometric interviews, parents and teachers identify these same children as best friends, and children spend more time with those classmates whom they designate as friends than with other children (Hartup, Laursen, Stewart, & Eastanson, 1988; Hinde, Titmus, Easton, & Tamplin, 1985; Howes, 1988). School-age children have four or five friends, on the average, and most of their "own time" is spent with them (Epstein, 1989; Medrich, Rosen, Rubin, & Buckley, 1982). Children also differentiate behaviorally between their friends and "other kids," beginning during the preschool years.

Social Networks

Children separate themselves into small groups on playgrounds and in other situations in which large numbers of individuals are gathered together. These networks are based in social attraction and common interests, beginning in early childhood (Howes, 1983). Children continue to interact with one another mainly in dyads and triads throughout middle childhood, preferring the intensity and concentration that one-on-one situations permit (Peters & Torrance, 1972); games often require smaller groups, too.

Social networks vary with the child's sex, age, and social reputation. Children's groups are mainly sex-same and same-age in both early and middle childhood (see Hartup, 1983); girls' networks are both smaller and more exclusive than boys' (Eder & Hallinan, 1978). Socially popular children are members of social networks, and some disliked children are network members, too. Observational studies reveal, however, that the social networks of popular children differ substantially from the social networks of rejected children: They are larger, more likely to include children older than the child, and more likely to include other well-liked children. When aggressive, disliked children have friends, these relationships are likely to be with other aggressive, disliked children rather than with their better liked peers (Cairns, Cairns, Neckerman, Gest, & Gariepy, 1988; Ladd, 1983).

Summary

Children spend more and more time together through early and middle childhood. Thinking and acting in relation to other children become more differentiated, and setting variations are taken into account. Children also acquire stable social reputations. These as well as the emergence of friendships and social networks are among the most important events of the era.

DEVELOPMENTAL SIGNIFICANCE

Striking individual differences are evident in the extent to which children are accepted or rejected by their peers. Status rankings in the classroom are correlated with status rankings obtained in other groups (Coie & Kupersmidt, 1983), and these rankings are relatively stable over time. By the most commonly used criteria, 15% to 20% of children are popular among their classmates and about the same proportion are rejected (i.e., liked least) by their classmates. Among rejected children, approximately 50% remain rejected from year to year, and 30% remain consistently rejected over longer periods, although these rates are somewhat smaller among younger children (third-graders) than among older ones (fifth-graders). At the same time, some children change from being well-liked or disliked to being average. More marked changes (e.g., from being disliked to being well-liked) are relatively rare (Coie & Dodge, 1983).

Considerable interest has been expressed in the connection between childhood peer relations and adult adjustment. Ground-breaking longitudinal studies were published more than 20 years ago, suggesting that psychologically troubled individuals have histories of poor peer relations extending back to early and middle childhood (Cowen, Pederson, Babijian, Izzo, & Trost, 1973; Roff, 1961). Considerable numbers of new investigations (both follow-forward and follow-back studies) support the old ones: Children who have major difficulties with other children (especially school-age children) are at risk in social development.

Among follow-back studies, results nearly universally demonstrate that maladjusted adults are more likely to have had peer difficulties in childhood than better adjusted individuals. Relevant childhood difficulties include being disliked, being aggressive, and being shy/withdrawn. Incidence varies, but between 30% and 70% of maladjusted adults in these studies are shown to have had poor peer relations earlier, as compared to 10% to 15% among control cases (Parker & Asher, 1987). Follow-back studies, of course, only indicate the extent to which these difficulties were experienced by older maladjusted individuals. Such studies do not indicate the extent to which poor peer relations may be predictive of adult disorder. However, a sizable number of follow-forward studies (more than 30) also demonstrate a significant connection between troubled peer relations and subsequent socioemotional difficulties (Kupersmidt, Coie, & Dodge, 1990; Parker & Asher, 1987). Overall, then, the weight of the evidence strongly suggests that poor peer relations are risk factors in social development.

This risk hypothesis, however, must be qualified for several reasons: (a) Peer relations assessments show similar errors of prediction, namely there are few false-negative errors but many false-positive ones. That is, peer relations problems are seldom absent among children who ultimately exhibit problematic outcomes, however, at the same time, indications of early peer difficulties overselect many children who are not actually at risk for later maladjustment. (b) Prediction success varies according to the peer measure one uses. (c) Prediction success also varies according to the disorder being predicted. (d) Prediction success varies according to the age when peer relations are assessed. (e) Correlational results (which these are) can seldom be interpreted definitively. Difficulties arise in determining whether poor peer relations are merely markers indicating individuals who are at risk, but for other reasons; whether children's relations with one another moderate the effects of more basic causal conditions (e.g., constitution or family relations); or whether peer experiences contribute directly and causally to later outcome. We turn briefly to each of these considerations.

Errors in Prediction

Many children identified as unpopular or rejected do not have problems later on, even though others do. Several considerations are relevant.

First, although relatively good measures, sociometric and observational methods are not completely reliable. Among sociometric instruments, test–retest correlations vary according to the type of measure employed as well as the children's ages. Paired comparisons and peer ratings produce reliability coefficients ranging around .75 among both preschool children and school-aged children (based on test–retest intervals ranging from 1 to 3 weeks), with negative (dislike) nominations being somewhat less reliable than positive ones (Asher, Singleton, Tinsley, & Hymel, 1979). Nominations techniques, however, yield more variable and generally lower stability coefficients, especially with younger children (Hymel, 1983). Stability estimates vary directly with age, probably for several reasons. Friendship relations fluctuate more rapidly among younger than among older children, and they may also understand the sociometric procedure less well. Although the reported reliabilities of sociometric instruments are within the range of acceptability used in psychological assessment, they may not be sufficient to ensure minimal errors in long-term prediction.

Second, sociometric instruments may simply not provide the differentiated assessments needed to forecast later difficulties accurately. For example, *being disliked* is not a single condition. Using cluster analysis, French (1988) demonstrated that two distinct subtypes can be identified among disliked elementary-school boys. Psychological dynamics were relatively clear with one subtype that accounts for about 50% of the cases: These are children who are aggressive, impulsive, and disruptive. The other disliked children did not show a clear profile but seemed undercontrolled. Subsequently, other investigators (Cillessen, Van IJzendoorn, Van Lieshout, & Hartup, in press), working with a large sample, differentiated still further among rejected boys. Again, aggression was a major factor in the rejection of 48% of these cases; shyness/withdrawal and the belief that others disliked them were major conditions underlying the social rejection in another 13% of the cases, and the remaining 39% were not especially deviant. The stability of social rejection itself differed among these groups: 58% of the children in the aggressive group remained rejected when tested a year later, but only 34% of the children in the other groups remained rejected after that time. Consistent with these results are earlier findings showing that children who are rejected from year to year, as compared to children who change (i.e., improve) receive lower ratings from other children on cooperation and leadership as well as higher ratings on disruption and starting fights (Coie & Dodge, 1983). The variations existing among rejected children are thus extreme.

Although status variations have been more extensively studied among boys than among girls, French (1990) showed that social rejection does not define a socially homogeneous condition among them either. Cluster analyses showed two main clusters, one more deviant than the other. The more deviant group was characterized by withdrawal, anxiety, and poor academic performance (aggression did not differentiate between the clusters). The other group was characterized by midrange scores that were not greatly different from those of the popular children.

Better understanding of the varieties of peer rejection is urgently needed. Obvious implications exist for the selection of children who should receive early intervention. Already established, in addition to the importance of assessing sociometric status, is the need for obtaining measures of aggression, shyness/withdrawal, self-regard, and the size of the social network among boys as well as measures of shyness/withdrawal, anxiety, and academic performance among girls.

Predictor and Outcome Variables

Long-term prediction varies according to the peer measures and outcome measures selected. Aggression is the most consistent predictor of negative outcome—especially of delinquency and criminality. Follow-back studies (e.g., Conger & Miller, 1966) show that most adolescent offenders were aggressive individuals earlier; follow-forward studies (e.g., West & Farrington, 1973) reveal that to-be-delinquent children are significantly more troublesome and antisocial than those who do not become delinquents. The evidence is very strong: By the second or third grade, aggression and troublesomeness among boys are correlated with difficulties in subsequent social relations and, in adolescence and adulthood, crime and delinquency. Aggression has not been studied extensively in relation to female criminality. However, the available data suggest that it predicts delinquency in girls as well (Roff & Wirt, 1984). Childhood aggression also predicts early school withdrawal, especially among males (Cairns, Cairns, & Neckerman, 1989). Yet, other variables, such as friendlessness, may be more closely tied to this outcome (see later discussion). Aggression is also an antecedent of other forms of adult maladjustment, especially externalizing difficulties, although it does not predict adult mental health status as accurately as it predicts criminal behavior (Parker & Asher, 1987).

Considering that aggression characterizes only about 50% of rejected children, being disliked is not correlated as consistently with criminality as is aggression (Kupersmidt et al., 1990; Parker & Asher, 1987). Indeed, in several investigations, childhood aggression is significantly correlated with adolescent criminality, whereas peer rejection is not (e.g., Kupersmidt & Coie, 1990; West & Farrington, 1973). Being disliked, however, is a strong and consistent predictor of school-related difficulties—having academic problems in school, being truant, having discipline problems, and early school leaving. Early school withdrawal, in fact, occurs among rejected children three to five times more often than among nonrejected children (both girls and boys). Poor peer relations in middle childhood are also predictive of other, nonspecific mental health problems in adolescence and adulthood (see Kupersmidt et al., 1990; Parker & Asher, 1987).

Shyness/withdrawal in early and middle childhood has not been demonstrated consistently to be a risk factor. Follow-back studies suggest that preschizophrenic girls are more socially isolated and socially rejected than comparison cases; this is not true for boys (Watt & Lubensky, 1976). Long-term follow-forward studies are virtually nonexistent, however, making conclusions difficult.

Perhaps shyness neither disrupts peer interaction nor peer reputations as extensively as aggressiveness, or it is unstable developmentally. As mentioned earlier, shy children are not as likely to be rejected or remain rejected as aggressive children. But shyness and withdrawal are also difficult to measure effectively in large-scale studies, and many investigators have not been very systematic about measurement issues. One investigation (Rubin, 1985) assists in clarifying this matter. Results suggest that shyness may be independent of sociometric status in early childhood (even though shy children are recognized as such by both teachers and other children) but becomes increasingly associated with peer rejection in middle childhood— especially when the condition has been stable over time. Because, among older children, social withdrawal is also correlated with loneliness, depression, and low self-esteem, it may be a constellation of shyness and negative self-perceptions that gradually generates negative evaluations of the shy child by other children (Rubin, LeMare, & Lollis, 1990).

Overall, then, externalizing disorders are better predicted by childhood aggressiveness than any other variable. Being disliked more clearly predicts other mental health difficulties and early school withdrawal than aggression. Shyness and withdrawal in child–child relations, however, are yet to be clearly linked to subsequent pathology, although there is some evidence to suggest that shyness becomes correlated with peer rejection as middle childhood progresses. Prediction and outcome centered on childhood peer relations must thus be studied in a carefully differentiated manner.

Developmental Status

Few studies exist to show that peer relations in early childhood (i.e., the years from 3 through 5) actually predict adolescent and adult outcomes. Occasional investigators have followed children from the preschool years into middle childhood (Kagan & Moss, 1962; Richman, Stevenson, & Graham, 1982; Rubin & Daniels-Beirness, 1983). However, the existing literature is much too thin to support more than patchwork guesses concerning the significance of early peer relations for the child's development beyond that. The limited evidence suggests that shyness and withdrawal are not stable across these years (Rubin, 1985). Although boys with extreme restlessness and difficulties with impulse controls at age 3 show conduct disorders at age 8 (Richman et al., 1982), similar continuity has not been reported for girls. Continuities in aggressiveness from early to middle childhood reveal this same-sex difference (Kagan & Moss, 1962).

With respect to the correlates of sociometric status, friendliness, prosocial dispositions, and competent social behaviors are directly related to social acceptance in early childhood. In addition, aggressive and disruptive behavior enhance the likelihood of social rejection among young children, especially among boys. Similar correlations occur in middle childhood. The behaviors distinguishing popular from unpopular children thus vary little from early to middle childhood, except for the greater importance of athletic and academic competence that exists among older children (see Coie, Dodge, & Kupersmidt, 1990; Hartup, 1983).

Few investigators, then, would conclude that social continuities are completely absent through early and middle childhood. To the contrary, stable organizational patterns in social relations, including both adult–child and child–child relations, are being demonstrated with increasing frequency (Sroufe & Fleeson, 1986). Even so, the database inking peer relations to adolescent and adult adjustment does not extend solidly back into the preschool years.

265

PEER RELATIONS

How Shall the Results Be Interpreted?

Although child–child relations are correlated with later disorder, especially antisocial behavior and school-related difficulties, interpreting these correlations is difficult. Does disorder derive more or less directly from constitutional factors and early socialization, with peer difficulties serving merely as markers for later maladjustment? Or, are peer relations causal contributors to subsequent outcome— either indirectly through moderating the effects of disordered family relations or directly through lowering feelings of self-efficacy and restricting opportunities for learning social skills? The current evidence does not favor either scenario, simply because the necessary long-term investigations have not been carried out. Only longitudinal investigations, beginning in early childhood, extending through adolescence, and including continuous assessment of sociometric status, social relations, and self-attitudes will provide this evidence.

Current studies, however, demonstrate that poor peer relations among school-children are *risk markers* at the very least. Children who are disagreeable, impulsive, aggressive, and disruptive typically are disliked and avoided by other children; further, they are at risk for delinquency and criminality. We know that the negative impressions created by the impulsive, aggressive child are maintained and perpetuated in the minds of other children (Hymel *et al.*, 1990). We know that children treat rejected and nonrejected children differently, being less inclined to initiate social contact with rejected children and more inclined to behave negatively toward them (Hartup, Glazer, & Charlesworth, 1967). We know that children behave otherwise toward one another in accordance with social reputations (Feldman & Ruble, 1986). These processes, however, have not been studied as they cycle through time in children's social relations.

Nevertheless, one can suppose that being disliked affects children in several ways: (a) Over time, negative and biased treatment from other children should be anticipated with increasing consistency by disliked children, and their social behavior modified accordingly. (b) Self-esteem should decline and social alienation increase, leading the disliked child to avoid others as well as strike out in reaction to their feelings of anger and frustration. (c) Over time, opportunities for constructive interactions with other children that enhance skills in cooperative problem solving, effective conflict management, communication, and intimacy may decline. (d) Simultaneously, the companions available to the aggressive/rejected child most likely include an ever larger proportion of unskilled, rejected children, that is, children who are similar to the disliked children themselves. Such shopping for social opportunities (Patterson & Bank, 1989) is undoubtedly transactional; children most likely select associates who are similar to themselves at the same time that similar associates select them.

Empirical studies support these hypotheses in limited ways. Rejected children's biases and social behaviors, for example, have been shown to be concordant with the attitudes and biases of other children toward them (Price and Dodge, 1989). On the other hand, nothing is known about the extent to which these concordances change over time. Similarly, disliked children are known to have lower self-esteem (sometimes unrealistically low *or* high self-esteem) than better liked children (Boivin & Begin, 1989; Finn, 1985; Reese, 1961). However, no one knows whether these differences increase over time. Children's social networks also become increasingly differentiated through middle childhood with networks of socially aggressive children being more readily identified among eighth-graders than among fourth-graders, especially among girls (Cairns *et al.*, 1988). Such trends suggest that the associates of the antisocial child slip further and further to the extremes in terms of both social incompetence and antisocial dispositions, thereby increasing the likelihood that the child will remain fixed in the antisocial process. Nevertheless, social networking has not been studied longitudinally.

Summary

Although much remains to be learned about the antecedents and consequences of peer difficulties, the relevant literature is expanding exponentially. One can lament that mainly cross-sectional evidence is available to evaluate our developmental models. More will surely come. Meanwhile, diagnosticians can argue with certainty that children who have trouble relating to their contemporaries not only endure considerable pain but face a more uncertain future than children who are securely anchored in the peer group.

PARENT–CHILD RELATIONS AND PEER RELATIONS

Although parent–child and peer relations differ in many ways, most investigators believe that these two social systems are closely connected (Hartup, 1979; Parke, 1978). Some writers take a different view, arguing that sociability advances *generally* through childhood, with common forces (e.g., temperament) responsible for developmental change in both systems (see Lamb & Nash, 1989). Considerable evidence, however, suggests that parent–child relations are causally linked to child–child relations.

Theories concerning these interconnections can be divided into two groups: *Stage-setting theories* and *intervention theories*. Stage-setting theories, themselves, can be subdivided: (a) Some investigators argue that children carry forward working models of relationships with caregivers into their encounters with other children (Sroufe & Fleeson, 1986). (b) Other investigators suggest that early attachments set the stage for child–child relations by providing the child with a secure base for exploring the environment, thereby bringing about contact with other children (Hartup, 1979). (c) A third group of stage-setting theories stress the social exchanges that occur between parents and their children and that establish behavioral orientations that mediate encounters with other children (Patterson & Bank, 1989). Intervention theories, on the other hand, suggest that parents influence the course of child–child relations directly through managing their children's encounters with other children and through teaching them social skills (Hartup, 1979; Parke, 1978).

Setting the Stage

Numerous investigations indicate that early attachments serve as springboards or secure bases that support children in engaging the environment. Securely attached toddlers range over a greater distance from their mothers than do insecurely attached youngsters (Ainsworth & Wittig, 1969). And this exploration occurs at greater distances when other children are around than when they are not (Anderson, 1972). Toddlers evidence considerable interest in other toddlers when their mothers are near, as well as orient toward them and interact with them (Eckerman, Whatley, & Kutz, 1975). The organization of secure-base behavior with the mother thus accounts, in part, for why children come together in the first place and begin to interact.

Secure attachments may also contribute to the child's success in peer relations through contributions to self-esteem and the disposition to behave prosocially. Working models may be carried forward into these relationships, as suggested earlier. Existing data do not elucidate the relevant mechanisms very well (Lamb & Nash, 1989). However, the quality of the child's early attachments is correlated with the quality of children's encounters with other children in both early and middle childhood. One longitudinal investigation, for example, showed that 2-year-olds with histories of secure attachments to their mothers were more sociable with other securely attached children than children who were resistantly or avoidantly attached (Pastor, 1981). When these same children were 4 years of age, the securely attached subjects were less negative than the avoidantly attached ones and more sociable and socially dominant with other children than the resistantly attached ones. Sociometric evaluations also favored the securely attached children (La Freniere & Sroufe, 1985). Still later assessments of these children indicated that the securely-attached ones maintained their histories of better relations with other children through middle childhood (Sroufe & Fleeson, 1986). Other investigators have reported similar results across shorter time intervals (Booth, Rose-Krasnor, & Rubin, 1991; Vandell, Owen, Wilson, & Henderson, 1988; Waters, Wippman, & Sroufe, 1979). Some replication studies have not yielded similar results (e.g., Jacobson & Wille, 1986). Nevertheless, the weight of the evidence supports the hypothesis that the quality of the early attachment is correlated with the quality of subsequent relations with other children.

Studies dealing with specific parent–child transactions and their contributions to the child's socialization are much too numerous to summarize briefly. In general, parental involvement, warmth, and moderate control are associated with good developmental outcome (cf. Baumrind, 1971), and these same dimensions are associated with good peer relations. Among preschool children, both maternal and paternal involvement as well as affective elicitation have been shown to be positively correlated with sociometric status. Verbal stimulation among mothers and nondirectiveness among fathers are also correlated with peer acceptance (MacDonald & Parke, 1984). Other efforts show that mothers who are positive and agreeable, as well as infrequently demanding and disagreeable, have young children who are well liked (Putallaz, 1987).

Parent–child transactions also account for significant variance in sociometric status among school-aged children. Socially rejected boys, as compared with sociometrically average boys, experience poorer parent management (i.e., poor monitoring of daily activities as well as coercive discipline) and greater family stress. Structural equation modeling reveals, however, that the family variables affect the child's sociometric status indirectly rather than directly (i.e., these effects are mediated by the boys' antisocial activities and low academic achievement) (Dishion, 1990). The results thus support the hypothesis that the children's own behavior mediates the relation between parent behavior and the child's social status. Parent–child relations induce child behaviors that, in turn, set the stage for peer difficulties or successes (Putallaz & Heflin, 1990).

Interventions

Mothers and fathers manage their children, deliberately creating opportunities or making choices that determine what the child will do and with whom (Hartup, 1979; Parke & Bahvnagri, 1989; Rubin & Slomin, 1984). Mothers arrange contacts for their youngsters with other children (fathers initiate these contacts less often). These management decisions enlarge the child's social world and serve as bridges between family and peer relations. Mothers of securely attached 3-year-olds have been shown to arrange contacts more frequently than mothers of insecurely attached children (Lieberman, 1977), thus suggesting a more or less direct connection between mother–child relations and the mother's management decisions. Other research shows that these arrangements have a bearing on the quality of the child's relations with other children. One investigation (Ladd & Golter, 1988), for example, showed that preschool children whose parents frequently arranged peer contacts had more playmates and more frequent play companions outside of school than children whose parents less frequently arranged them. In addition, boys whose parents initiated these contacts were better liked and less often rejected than boys whose parents did not initiate them. Girls, for some reason, did not differ according to the extent that their parents arranged these contacts. Parents also manage their children's social lives in many other ways: by moving from neighborhood to neighborhood expressly for this reason and by enrolling their children in afterschool classes.

Direct tuition also serves as a connecting link between family and peer relations. In one investigation (Parke & Bhavnagri, 1989), mothers and fathers were observed separately under two conditions: (a) when asked to supervise their own child and a playmate, along with being given instructions "to help the children play together"; and (b) when asked not to assist or interfere with them. Supervisory encouragement elicited both direct and indirect instruction by the parents and, among the children, more frequent turn taking, longer play episodes, and more cooperation. The children's behavior toward each other was also correlated with the mother's behavior, including her ability to initiate and sustain interaction, her responsiveness, the extent to which her actions fit the child's actions, and her emotional expression.

Social skills can be induced through modeling and coaching (Putallaz & Heflin, 1990). These skills may then generalize to interactions with other children. Physical play between young children and their parents, for example, enhances the child's encoding and decoding of emotional signals, and these abilities, in turn, are correlated with the child's sociometric status (Parke et al., 1989). Observational data show, too, that mothers of popular children coach their children in group entry skills differently from the mothers of neglected and rejected children. The former suggest group-oriented strategies more often (Russell & Finnie, 1991). And, as mentioned earlier, the mother's use of aversive controls in interacting with the child is positively correlated with the child's aversiveness toward other children and thereby associated with his or her sociometric status (Dishion, 1990; Putallaz, 1987).

Altogether, then, the evidence suggests that parent–child relations are significant sources of variance in peer relations. Further, early peer relations combine with parent–child relations in determining social relations in childhood and adolescence. Several different theories have been advanced to account for these effects; each gains support from empirical research. Clearly, multiple pathways lead from parent–child to peer relations. Whether peer relations, in turn, cycle back to parent–child interaction is a largely unanswered question.

CHILDREN AND THEIR FRIENDS

Why Are Friends Important?

The essentials of friendship are reciprocity and commitment between individuals who see themselves more or less as equals. Children's friendships are not as exclusive as mother– child or father–child relations, and interaction between friends is marked by a more equal power base than interaction between children and their parents. Nevertheless, these relationships serve similar functions in the child's socialization to those served by other close relationships: (a) They are *social contexts* in which basic skills are acquired or elaborated (e.g., social communication, cooperation, and group entry skills); (b) they are *information sources* for acquiring self-knowledge as well as knowledge about others; (c) they are emotional and cognitive *resources* (both for having fun and resolving conflicts); and (d) they are *forerunners* of later relationships (by modeling the mutual regulation and intimacy that most close relationships require).

Children understand the essential themes in friendship relations (a sense of mutual attachment and common interests) beginning in early childhood. Among preschool children, though, expectations center on common pursuits and concrete reciprocities ("We play"). Later on, children expect their friends to display mutual understanding, loyalty, and trust ("You tell them all your secrets and they tell you theirs"). Older children also believe that friends have a special commitment to one another in the management of conflict ("A friend is someone you fight with, but not forever") and also that conflict may actually strengthen these relationships.

Children's friendship expectations have been studied extensively (Bigelow & LaGaipa, 1975; Furman & Bierman, 1984; Selman, 1980) although investigators disagree about the meaning of the age differences that have been observed. Some investigators argue that these differences represent elaborations or extensions of the child's understanding of social reciprocity (Youniss, 1980). Others believe that they reflect structural transformations in the child's understanding of social relations (Selman, 1980). And still others argue that the age differences represent cumulative assimilation of basically unrelated themes or dimensions (e.g., commonalities in play interests and self-disclosure) (Berndt, 1981). These theoretical variations have not been sorted out. However, the evidence reveals clearly that, beginning in early childhood, the child's social world is cognitively differentiated, becoming more so as time goes on (Berndt & Perry, 1986).

Children who have difficulties in social and emotional development commonly have difficulties in forming and maintaining friendships. Among schoolchildren, disliked and aggressive children are not always friendless, and this needs to be understood (Cairns *et al.*, 1988). Nevertheless, these difficulties are twice as common among children referred to child guidance clinics as among nonreferred children (Achenbach & Edelbrock, 1981). Referred children have fewer friends and less contact with them, their friendships are significantly less stable over time (Rutter & Garmezy, 1983), and their understanding of the reciprocities and intimacies involved in friendships is less mature (Selman, 1980).

Longitudinal evidence is not extensive, however, so the meaning of these results is unclear. Being without friends seems to be a risk factor, but one cannot argue that friends are developmental necessities. Good socialization outcomes may not require having friends in the same way that these outcomes require a stable relationship with a caretaker. Other opportunities exist for most children to learn cooperative and group entry skills, for example, as well as strategies to use in conflict resolution. More likely, friendships are developmental advantages. That is, these relationships may be optimal settings for accomplishing various developmental tasks that might also, but with more difficulty, be managed in other ways (Hartup & Sancilio, 1986).

Similarities between Friends

Children and their friends are concordant in age, reflecting the egalitarian nature of these relationships. Children's friendships are also same-sex; cross-sex friends are relatively rare, accounting for only about 5% of these relationships in middle childhood (Duck, 1975). Same-sex children are apparently attracted to one another as friends for the same reasons that sex segregation exists in children's groups generally—common play interests and the attraction that emanates from similarities between self and others. The similarity → attraction hypothesis also accounts for the increase from early through middle childhood in children's choices of same-race individuals as best friends (Singleton & Asher, 1979).

Behavioral concordances are not as great as similarity between friends in age, sex, and race. Occasional investigators have reported significant correlations between friends in IQ and sociability (see Hartup, 1983); however, most studies yield small or nonsignificant correlations. Sociometric status, for example, is generally uncorrelated among best friends (Roff & Sells, 1967), even though the social networks observed on playgrounds are roughly concordant (Ladd, 1983). Good studies concerning the relation between similarities and attraction in early and middle childhood are rare, although this is not the case with adolescence. Younger adolescents are generally not very similar to their friends behaviorally. The greatest similarities occur in two areas: (a) school attitudes, educational aspirations, and school achievement; and (b) orientation toward certain normative behaviors in the contemporary teen culture (e.g., drinking). The relevant investigations show that teenagers are both more likely to choose one another as friends than dissimilar individuals and to become more similar, over time, through the common experiences encompassed by their relations with one another (Kandel, 1978a,b). Similar conclusions about selection and socialization among friends in middle childhood, however, cannot be drawn.

Friendship Formation

Among preschool children, the first indications of social attraction are sustained social exchanges, complementaries in play interaction, and mutually directed affect. Children who are becoming friends can be differentiated from those who are not, mostly in terms of the time they spend together and the reciprocities one can observe in their interactions (Howes, 1983).

Similar sequences can be observed among older children, although friendship formation in middle childhood is a more elaborate process. Furman and Childs (1981) observed third-grade children during one session while they become acquainted. The children usually began by asking questions to determine common ground in their backgrounds and attitudes and followed them with mutually rewarding activities that served, in turn, as friendship content. Gottman's (1983) longitudinal observations extended these revelations. Conversations between children, initially strangers to one another, were recorded during three sessions in one child's home. After 2 months, the mothers were asked whether the children were hitting it off outside the research sessions: Some were and some were not. Results indicated that (a) communication clarity and connectedness in the first session was the best predictor of hitting it off, although information exchange, conflict resolution, and common play activities during this session were also significantly correlated with the criterion; (b) communication clarity in the second and third sessions was even more closely related to hitting it off, and self-disclosure joined the list of significant predictors; and (c) regression analyses showed that this combination of variables accounted for more than 80% of the variance in the children's becoming friends.

Overall, then, friendship formation among children begins with information exchange and communication that is clear and well-connected. The children then move to common-ground activities and talk about play and play materials. Should this not meet with success, the children must return temporarily to exchanging information; otherwise, conflict will occur. Once common ground is attained, the children must strike a balance between the social demands of activity and conflict; the children must work continually to clarify messages as well as work to avoid and resolve conflicts (Gottman & Parker, 1986). To become friends, then, children must discover their similarities and their differences, exploiting the former and resolving the latter.

Behavior between Friends

Once friendships are established, these relationships are cooperative socialization contexts. Preschool friends evidence more frequent positive exchanges (as well as more frequent neutral ones) than unselected partners or children who do not like one another (Masters & Furman, 1981). Friends also cooperate more extensively than nonfriends when working on tasks that require turn taking and mutually regulated effort (Charlesworth & La Freniere, 1983). Similar results have been obtained with school-aged children. When working on novel tasks, friends are more interactive than nonfriends, smile and laugh more, pay closer attention to equity rules in their conversations, and direct their conversations toward mutual rather than idiosyncratic ends. Children also remember more individually about a task solved with a friend than one solved with a nonfriend (Newcomb & Brady, 1982). Cooperation is thus one of the most important *conditions* of children's friendships. That is, children behave cooperatively with one another both to become friends and to remain so. As middle childhood comes to a close, these dynamics also include intimacy and sharing.

Competition and conflict bear complex relations to friendship. Although young children infrequently bargain with one another, friends seek self-serving solutions in zero-sum situations less frequently than nonfriends (Matsumoto, Haan, Yabrove, Theodorou, & Carney, 1986). In nursery-school classrooms, friends disagree with one another *more* often than nonfriends because they spend more time with one another. Conflicts between friends, however, are less heated (although not less aggressive) than the conflicts of nonfriends, mutual disengagements during disagreements are more common, and outcomes are more equal. Friends are also more likely to stay in proximity with each other and to engage in social interaction when the conflict is over (Hartup *et al.*, 1988). The evidence thus suggests that friends make stronger efforts than nonfriends to minimize the damage resulting from those disagreements that are inevitable whenever individuals interact. The motivation underlying this effort is unclear. However, one can guess that it derives from the time, energy, and investment that friends have made in one another.

Among older children, friends and nonfriends resolve conflicts according to the social setting. When competition and disagreements occur in closed situations (i.e., when children cannot change partners or activities), friends disagree more frequently and compete more extensively than nonfriends, especially among boys (Berndt, 1981a; Hartup & Laursen, in press). In these situations, friends may feel freer and more secure in disagreeing with one another than nonfriends, although they may also be more motivated to avoid the negative self-evaluations that result from losing arguments with someone close (Tesser, 1984). In any event, friendship and situational context combine in determining children's conflicts.

Comment

Becoming friends and maintaining these relationships are surely among the most significant social achievements of early and middle childhood. Children spend much time doing these things, but the importance of these relationships transcends the time that children spend on them. These relationships furnish children with socialization opportunities not easily obtained elsewhere, especially in mutually regulated activity and conflict resolution.

GROUP RELATIONS

Children socialize in collectives that range from one or two children to the dozens that come together in classrooms and on playgrounds. Membership in some groups is not determined by choice (e.g., in classrooms). In other instances, membership is a matter determined by the child and his or her associates (e.g., a friendship network). In both cases, groups are social entities in their own right, possessing certain characteristics that individuals do not (e.g., cohesiveness and hierarchical structures). Moreover, groups are more than mere aggregations of individuals; they are aggregations of dyads as well as aggregations of triads and other subdivisions. Because every group member has some kind of relationship with every other member, these entities are best conceived as aggregations of relationships (Hinde, 1976) or as social systems.

Group membership attains significance during early childhood, not merely because adults begin to assemble children in schools and creches. Casual observation in any city park conveys a sure sense that collectives are important to 3- and 4-year-olds apart from whatever importance adults attach to them. And, of course, no one could seriously doubt the importance of group membership to school-aged children.

Intragroup Dynamics

Whenever children come together, their collectives acquire hierarchical structures, and social norms emerge. Organizational structures sometimes become evident rather quickly, sometimes more slowly. Dominance hierarchies, for example, exist in many nursery-school groups, although they vary considerably from group to group in their linearity and rigidity (Strayer, 1980). Dominance structures can be identified among young children on the basis of object struggles, threats, teasing, and conflict outcomes (i.e., who wins and who loses), and the social structure varies somewhat according to the measure used. Children give more attention to dominant members of the group than to other members, although so-called attention structures are not entirely concordant with dominance structures (Vaughn & Waters, 1981). Superimposed on both dominance and attention structures are other networks based on affiliation and altruism. In most instances, these are the friendship networks in which children spend much time (Ladd, 1983). Among school-aged children, social structuring continues to be related, in part, to social dominance (Strayer & Strayer, 1976). Group structures are also based, however, on being good at games and sports, knowing how to organize activities, and social skills—especially skills that are relevant to the normative activities that bind the group together (Sherif & Sherif, 1953). Most classrooms and playgrounds, then, are multidimensionally structured.

Group relations vary according to the setting conditions involved. For example, crowding large numbers of children into small spaces, especially with less than 20 square feet per child, is marked by more aggression than less crowded conditions. More fights (but shorter ones) occur on small playgrounds than on large ones (Ginsburg, 1975). Nevertheless, resource densities have as much to do with preschool children's conflicts as do social densities (Smith & Connolly, 1981).

Reward conditions affect children's interactions according to the nature of the task. Winners-take-all conditions elicit better performance than shared-reward conditions on simple tasks not requiring coordinated interaction (Sorokin, Tranquist, Parten, & Zimmerman, 1930). Shared rewards, on the other hand, elicit better performance on tasks requiring social coordination. Distributing rewards in proportion to each individual's contribution (an individualistic goal structure) is not as effective as shared rewards in enhancing group effort on coordinated tasks (French, Brownell, Graziano, & Hartup, 1977).

Attitudes toward self and others in classrooms are also affected by reward contingencies, with cooperative conditions usually promoting greater solidarity than competitive ones (Johnson, Johnson, Johnson, & Anderson, 1976). Finally, social climate bears on intragroup relations, as a series of well-known investigations shows. Social climates established by authoritarian leadership elevate both aggression and conflict among children, as compared to democratic leadership, also constraining initiative and constricting individual variation. Moreover, these social climates have carryover effects, influencing children's behavior with one another even when their adult leaders are absent (Lewin, Lippitt, & White, 1938).

WILLARD W.
HARTUP

The best known studies of intergroup relations were done 30 years ago, and not many recent advances have been made in this area. Earlier ideas have been applied in schools and community settings, however, in order to test their efficacy in easing tensions created by school desegregation: The results remain robust.

Preeminent among these studies is the so-called Robbers Cave Experiment, named after the site of the summer camp where it was completed (Sherif, Harvey, White, Hood, & Sherif, 1961). Observations were conducted on two groups of 11-year-old boys who were brought together in separate camp sites without knowing the other was present. During the first weeks, common goals, distinctive names, a sense of belonging, and a social organization all evolved from the activities scheduled, many of which had been engineered by the counselors to require cooperative activity among the group members. When the groups accidentally discovered one another and a series of friendly competitions between them were arranged by the counselors, the difficulties began. Conflicts *within* groups increased, including blaming one another and scapegoating, although these perturbations eventually declined; we and they became salient frames of reference. Most important, the competitions between the groups supported continuing and intense conflict *between* the collectives themselves. Only cooperation in seeking common objectives (e.g., repairing the water supply for everyone) ameliorated these disagreements and established intergroup harmony. Preaching cooperation by the camp counselors was to no avail; only cooperative experience between the collectives involving superordinate goals eliminated the competition that had been created.

Other investigators have discovered that the best interventions for integrating diverse individuals in classrooms (e.g., handicapped and nonhandicapped students) encompass the same basic elements identified in this experiment: (a) an active and necessary role for every child; (b) cooperative effort; and (c) a superordinate goal (Aronson, 1978). The widespread application of these results has been generally to good effect, even though the original experiment has some obvious limitations (e.g., the exclusive use of boys).

The Individual and the Group

Within larger groups, children separate themselves into smaller enclaves that are frequently changeable. New children enter them, other children leave them, and the social organization changes accordingly. Group entry, however, is a difficult task for both younger and older children and remains a difficult challenge for many adults. Among preschool children, approximately half of their attempts to enter ongoing play groups are resisted (Corsaro, 1981). Children vary greatly in their success with group entry, and these variations are related to their sociometric status (Putallaz & Gottman, 1981). But even among the most socially competent children, entry attempts are resisted 25% of the time. Thus, group entry exposes nearly everybody to social conflict.

Observational studies rather consistently show that the smoothest transitions from being an outsider to being an insider involve one main scenario, which Garvey (1984) described as follows:

The Don't's: don't ask questions for information (if you can't tell what's going on, you shouldn't be bothering those who do); don't mention yourself or state your feelings about the group or its activity (they're not interested at the moment); don't disagree or criticize the proceedings (you have no right to do so, since you're an outsider). The Do's: be sure you understand the group's frame of reference, or focus (are they playing house?); understand the participation structure of the activity; slip into the ongoing activity by making some relevant comment or begin to act in concert with the others as if you actually were a knowledgeable member of the group; hold off on making suggestions or attempting to redirect until you are well into the group. (Garvey, 1984, pp. 164–165)

Entry success, then, is not a matter of choosing the correct overture but, rather, executing a series of moves, beginning with hovering and ending with making relevant comments in order to enter the group's activity (Dodge, Schlundt, Schocken, & Delugach, 1983).

Group members resist the entry attempts of new children for many different reasons (Putallaz & Wasserman, 1990). Among young children, resistance usually relates to property, sometimes "we're too crowded," and sometimes "we don't like you." Many overtures are turned down without justification. Same-sex groups are difficult to enter by members of the opposite sex; mixed-sex groups are a bit easier for boys to enter than for girls. Strangers have a harder time than acquaintances. Reasons for resisting group entry among older children seem to be centered on the belief that bringing others into an ongoing activity will be disruptive; empirical studies relating to this notion, however, are scarce.

Once a group member, children ascribe to the normative activity that serves the group as a raison d'être—skipping rope on the playground, should this activity be salient, or pilfering from grocery stalls and smoking cigarettes, should these be. The issue is not mere conformity: it is simply that, to enter a group and maintain one's status there, norm sharing must occur. Although new children sometimes effect normative change in the groups they enter, this depends on their social status as well as the normative change proposed.

Both parents and professionals have concerns about peer pressure, (i.e., group demands for conformity) especially involving antisocial norms. Peer pressure, however, is a complex phenomenon. First, children impose many standards on one another that are concordant with the demands of adults. Children pressure one another to be sociable, to share, to behave in accordance with one's sex, to be trustworthy, and to be fun in ways that are concordant with adult pressures. Second, peer pressures in support of antisocial behavior change with age, increasing toward the beginning of adolescence but *declining* thereafter (Berndt, 1979). Third, as mentioned previously, antisocial norms are most likely to be pressed on children who are already disposed to be antisocial and aggressive. Peer pressure may be responsible for an antisocial child's transition from being troublesome to being a hard-core delinquent. Children socialize each other toward criminality as well as select one another on the basis of their antisocial attitudes (Patterson & Bank, 1989). One must understand, however, that criminal socialization within child–child relations varies in its effectiveness according to the child's nature. Children without antisocial inclinations are not as likely to be members of antisocial groups as children with antisocial dispositions, and their exposure to antisocial models is less likely to take.

Comment

WILLARD W.
HARTUP

Children's groups encompass affilitative networks as well as dominance hierarchies. Cooperative and competitive reward structures create different social climates both within and between groups. Among the more difficult challenges for individual children is group entry (i.e., insinuating oneself into an ongoing group). Good entry skills usually characterize children who are generally socially competent. However, everybody must cope with the social conflict engendered by these situations. Peer pressure turns out to be a complex phenomenon involving prosocial as well as antisocial socialization, even though exposure to antisocial norms is especially risky for certain children.

Summary

Establishing and maintaining relationships with other children are achievements of the utmost importance during early and middle childhood. Schoolchildren spend as much time with other children as with adults and think a great deal about their contemporaries. Although parent–child relations set the stage for peer relations and contribute importantly to them, children evolve their own attributions, expectations, motives, and emotions for use in relations with other children.

Peer relations cannot be considered separately from the settings in which they occur. Social interaction varies according to the task as well as who happens to be present. Friends behave differently with one another from nonfriends; these differences vary according to the situation. Sex differences are ubiquitous, but these also vary from situation to situation. Peer pressures themselves vary according to normative demands and which children are being pressured.

Nevertheless, children who have general difficulties in relating to other children should be regarded with concern. Being disliked is not a happy experience and, in combination with aggressiveness, augurs poorly for future development. Although shyness (especially in early childhood) seems to be neither serious nor stable across time, social withdrawal in preadolescence may be more so.

Researchers are not completely certain about the extent to which peer difficulties contribute causally to later outcome. However, they clearly mark individuals who are at risk, and these difficulties appear, in turn, to result in social assortments wherein competent children interact mostly with other competent children, whereas less competent ones interact mostly with each other. At the same time, this segregation has deleterious effects on self-attitudes and social reputations.

Sorting out these complexities is an enormous task. The most sophisticated methodologies are required. Fortunately, investigators continue to be drawn to these issues; current research activity is extensive. Strategies for intervention are being developed in many different laboratories, too, and with considerable success. The significance of peer relations in early and middle childhood is something *established*, then, not a mere guess.

ACKNOWLEDGMENTS   Support in the completion of this manuscript was provided by Grant No. RO1-42888, National Institute of Mental Health; a grant from The

Netherlands Organization for Scientific Research, and a Fulbright Research Scholarship. The author would also like to acknowledge the generous support of the Psychologisch Laboratorium, University of Nijmegen.

REFERENCES

Achenbach, T. M., & Edelbrock, C. S. (1981). Behavioral problems and competencies reported by parents of normal and disturbed children aged 4 through 16. *Monographs of the Society for Research in Child Development, 46* (1, No. 188).

Ainsworth, M. D. S., & Wittig, B. A. (1969). Attachment and the exploratory behavior of one-year-olds in a strange situation. In B. M. Foss (Ed.), *Determinants of infant behaviour* (Vol. 4; pp. 113–136). London: Methuen.

Anderson, J. W. (1972). Attachment behaviour out of doors. In N. Blurton Jones (Ed.), *Ethological studies of child behaviour* (pp. 199–215). London: Cambridge University Press.

Aronson, E. (1978). *The jigsaw classroom.* Beverly Hills, CA: Sage.

Asher, S. R., Singleton, L. C., Tinsley, B. R., & Hymel, S. (1979). A reliable sociometric measure for preschool children. *Developmental Psychology, 15,* 443–444.

Barker, R. G., & Wright H. F. (1955). *Midwest and its children.* New York: Harper & Row.

Baumrind, D. (1971). Current patterns of parental authority. *Developmental Psychology Monographs, 4* (1, Pt. 2).

Berndt, T. J. (1979). Developmental changes in conformity to peers and parents. *Developmental Psychology, 15,* 608–616.

Berndt, T. J. (1981a). Effects of friendship on prosocial intentions and behavior. *Child Development, 52,* 636–643.

Berndt, T. J. (1981b). Relations between social cognition, nonsocial cognition, and social behavior: The case of friendship. In J. H. Flavell & L. Ross (Eds.), *Social cognitive development* (pp. 176–199). Cambridge, UK: Cambridge University Press.

Berndt, T. J., & Perry, T. B. (1986). Children's perceptions of friendships as supportive relationships. *Developmental Psychology, 22,* 640–648.

Bigelow, B. J., & LaGaipa, J. J. (1975). Children's written descriptions of friendship: A multidimensional analysis. *Developmental Psychology, 11,* 857–858.

Boivin, M., & Begin, G. (1989). Peer status and self-perception among early elementary school children: The case of the rejected children. *Child Development, 60,* 591–596.

Booth, C. L., Rose-Krasnor, L., & Rubin, K. H. (1991). Relating preschooler's social competence and their mothers' parenting behaviors to early attachment security and high risk status. *Journal of Social and Personal Relationships, 8,* 363–382.

Bowlby, J. (1969). *Attachment and loss* (Vol. 1). New York: Basic Books.

Brownell, C. A. (1990). Peer social skills in toddlers: Competencies and constraints illustrated by same-age and mixed-age interaction. *Child Development, 61,* 838–848.

Cairns, R. B., Cairns, B. D., & Neckerman, H. J. (1989). Early school dropout: Configurations and determinants. *Child Development, 60,* 1437–1452.

Cairns, R. B., Cairns, B. D., Neckerman, H. J., Gest, S., & Gariepy, J.-L. (1988). Peer networks and aggressive behavior: Peer support or peer rejection? *Developmental Psychology, 24,* 815–823.

Charlesworth, W. R., & La Freniere, P. (1983). Dominance, friendship, and resource utilization in preschool children's groups. *Ethology and Sociobiology, 4,* 175–186.

Cillessen, T., Van IJzendoorn, H., Van Lieshout, K., & Hartup, W. W. (in press). Heterogeneity of rejected boys: Subtypes and stabilities. *Child Development.*

Coie, J. D., & Dodge, K. A. (1983). Continuities and changes in children's social status. A five-year longitudinal study. *Merrill-Palmer Quarterly, 29,* 261–282.

Coie, J. D., Dodge, K. A., & Kupersmidt, J. B. (1990). Peer group behavior and social status, In S. R. Asher & J. D. Coie (Eds.), *Peer rejection in childhood* (pp. 17–59). Cambridge, UK: Cambridge University Press.

Coie, J. D., & Kupersmidt J. A. (1983). A behavioral analysis of emerging social status in boys groups. *Child Development, 54,* 1400–1416.

Conger, J. J., & Miller, W. C. (1966). *Personality, social class and delinquency.* New York: Wiley.

Corsaro, W. A. (1981). Friendship in the nursery school: Social organization in a peer environment. In S. R. Asher & J. M. Gottman (Eds.), *The development of children's friendships* (pp. 207–241). Cambridge, UK: Cambridge University Press.

Cowen, E. L., Pederson, A., Babijian, H., Izzo, L. D., & Trost, M. A. (1973). Long-term follow-up of early detected vulnerable children. *Journal of Consulting and Clinical Psychology, 41,* 438–446.

Dishion, T. J. (1990). The family ecology of boys' peer relations in middle childhood. *Child Development, 61,* 874–892.

Dodge, K. A. (1980). Social cognition and children's aggressive behavior. *Child Development, 51,* 162–170.

Dodge, K. A., Schlundt, D. G., Schocken, I., & Delugach, J. D. (1983). Social competence and children's social status: The role of peer group entry strategies. *Merrill-Palmer Quarterly, 29,* 309–336.

Duck, S. W. (1975). Personality similarity and friendship choices by adolescents. *European Journal of Social Psychology, 5,* 351–365.

Eckerman, C. O., Davis, C. C., & Didow, S. M. (1989). Toddlers' emerging ways of achieving cooperative social coordinations with a peer. *Child Development, 60,* 440–453.

Eckerman, C. O., Whatley, J. L., & Kutz, S. L. (1975). The growth of social play with peers during the second year of life. *Developmental Psychology, 11,* 42–49.

Eder, D., & Hallinan, M. T. (1978). Sex differences in children's friendships. *American Sociological Review, 43,* 237–250.

Epstein, J. L. (1989). The selection of friends: Changes across the grades and in different school environments. In T. J. Berndt & G. W. Ladd (Eds.), *Peer relationships in child development* (pp. 158–187). New York: Wiley.

Feldman, N. S., & Ruble, D. N. (1986). *The effect of personal relevance on dispositional inference: A developmental analysis.* Unpublished manuscript, New York University.

Ferguson, T. J., & Rule, B. G. (1980). Effects of inferential set, outcome severity, and basis of responsibility on children's evaluations of aggressive acts. *Developmental Psychology, 16,* 141–146.

Finn, M. G. (1985). *Being disliked: Self-report and social status.* Unpublished doctoral dissertation, Duke University.

French, D. C. (1988). Heterogeneity of peer-rejected boys: Aggressive and nonaggressive subtypes. *Child Development, 59,* 976–985.

French, D. C. (1990). Heterogeneity of peer rejected girls. *Child Development, 61,* 2028–2031.

French, D. C., Brownell, C. A., Graziano, W. G., & Hartup, W. W. (1977). Effects of cooperative, competitive, and individualistic sets on performance in children's groups. *Journal of Experimental Child Psychology, 24,* 1–10.

Furman, W., & Bierman, K. L. (1984). Children's conceptions of friendship: A multidimensional study of developmental changes. *Developmental Psychology, 20,* 925–931.

Furman, W., & Buhrmester, D. (1985). Children's perceptions of the personal relationships in their social networks. *Developmental Psychology, 21,* 1016–1022.

Furman, W., & Childs, M. K. (1981, April). *A temporal perspective on children's friendships.* Paper presented at the biennial meetings of the Society for Research in Child Development, Boston.

Furman, W., Rahe, D. F., & Hartup, W. W. (1979). Rehabilitation of socially withdrawn preschool children through mixed-age and same-age socialization. *Child Development, 50,* 915–922.

Garvey, C. (1984). *Children's talk.* Cambridge, MA: Harvard University Press.

Ginsburg, H. J. (1975, April). *Variations of aggressive interaction among male elementary school children as a function of spatial density.* Paper presented at the biennial meetings of the Society for Research in Child Development, Denver.

Gottman, J. M. (1983). How children become friends. *Monographs of the Society for Research in Child Development, 48* (3, Serial No. 201).

Gottman, J. M., & Parker, J. G. (1986). *Conversations of friends.* Cambridge, UK: Cambridge University Press.

Hartup, W. W. (1974). Aggression in childhood: Developmental perspectives. *American Psychologist, 29,* 336–341.

Hartup, W. W. (1979). The social worlds of childhood. *American Psychologist, 34,* 944–950.

Hartup, W. W. (1983). Peer relations. In P. H. Mussen & E. M. Hetherington (Eds.), *Handbook of child psychology Vol. 4, Socialization, personality, and social development* (pp. 103–196). New York, Wiley.

Hartup, W. W., Glazer, J. A., & Charlesworth, R. (1967). Peer reinforcement and sociometric status. *Child Development, 38,* 1017–1024.

Hartup, W. W., & Laursen, B. (in press). Conflict and context in peer relations. In C. H. Hart (Ed.), *Children on playgrounds: Research perspectives and applications.* Ithaca, NY: State University of New York Press.

Hartup, W. W., Laursen, B., Stewart, M. A., & Eastenson, A. (1988). Conflict and the friendship relations of young children. *Child Development, 59,* 1590–1600.

Hartup, W. W., & Sancilio, M. F. (1986). Children's friendships. In E. Schopler & G. B. Mesibov (Eds.), *Social behavior in autism* (pp. 61–79). New York: Plenum Press.

Higgins, E. T., & Parsons, J. E. (1983). Cognition and the social life of the child. In E. T. Higgins, D. N. Ruble, & W. W. Hartup (Eds.), *Social cognition and social development* (pp. 15–62). Cambridge, UK: Cambridge University Press.

Hinde, R. A. (1976). On describing relationships. *Journal of Child Psychology and Psychiatry, 17,* 1–19.

Hinde R. A., Titmus, G., Easton, D., & Tamplin, A. (1985). Incidence of "friendship" and behavior with strong associates versus non-associates in preschoolers. *Child Development, 56,* 234–245.

Howes, C. (1983). Patterns of friendship. *Child Development, 54,* 1041–1053.

Howes, C. (1988). Peer interaction of young children. *Monographs of the Society for Research in Child Development, 53* (Serial No. 217).

Hymel, S. (1983). Preschool children's peer relations: Issues in sociometric assessment. *Merrill-Palmer Quarterly, 29,* 237–260.

Hymel, S., Wagner, E., & Butler, L. J. (1990). Reputational bias: View from the peer group. In S. R. Asher & J. D. Coie (Eds.), *Peer rejection in childhood* (pp. 156–186). Cambridge, UK: Cambridge University Press.

Jacobson, J. L., & Wille, D. E. (1986). The influence of attachment pattern on developmental changes in peer interaction from the toddler to the preschool period. *Child Development, 57,* 338–347.

Jensen, R. E., & Moore, S. G. (1977). The effect of attribute statements on cooperativeness and competitiveness in school-age boys. *Child Development, 48,* 305–307.

Johnson, D. W., Johnson, R. T., Johnson, J., & Anderson, D. (1976). Effects of cooperative versus individualized instruction on student prosocial behavior, attitudes toward learning, and achievement. *Journal of Educational Psychology, 68,* 446–452.

Kagan, J., & Moss, H. A. (1962). *Birth to maturity.* New York: Wiley.

Kandel, D. B. (1978a). Homophily, selection, and socialization in adolescent friendships. *American Journal of Sociology, 84,* 427–436.

Kandel, D. B. (1978b). Similarity in real-life adolescent friendship pairs. *Journal of Personality and Social Psychology, 36,* 306–312.

Kupersmidt, J. B., & Coie, J. D. (1990). Preadolescent peer status, aggression, and school adjustment as predictors of externalizing problems in adolescence. *Child Development, 61,* 1350–1362.

Kupersmidt, J. B., Coie, J. D., & Dodge, K. A. (1990). The role of poor peer relationships in the development of disorder. In S. R. Asher & J. D. Coie (Eds.), *Peer rejection in childhood* (pp. 274–305). Cambridge, UK: Cambridge University Press.

La Freniere, P. J., & Sroufe, L. A. (1985). Profiles of peer competence in the preschool: Interrelations between measures, influence of social ecology, and relation to attachment history. *Developmental Psychology, 21,* 56–69.

Ladd, G. W. (1983). Social networks of popular, average, and rejected children in school settings. *Merrill-Palmer Quarterly, 29,* 283–308.

Ladd, G. W., & Golter, B. S. (1988). Parents' management of preschoolers' peer relations: Is it related to children's social competence? *Developmental Psychology, 24,* 109–117.

Lamb, M. E., & Nash, A. (1989). Infant-mother attachment, sociability, and peer competence. In T. J. Berndt & G. W. Ladd (Eds.), *Peer relationships in child development* (pp. 219–245). New York: Wiley.

Lewin, K., Lippitt, R., & White, R. K. (1938). Patterns of aggressive behavior in experimentally created "social climates." *Journal of Social Psychology, 10,* 271–299.

Lieberman, A. F. (1977). Preschoolers' competence with a peer: Relations with attachment and peer experience. *Child Development, 48,* 1277–1287.

MacDonald K., & Parke, R. D. (1984). Bridging the gap: Parent–child play interaction and peer interactive competence. *Child Development, 55,* 1265–1277.

Masters, J. C., & Furman, W. (1981). Popularity, individual friendship selections, and specific peer interaction among children. *Developmental Psychology, 17,* 344–350.

Matsumoto, D., Haan, N., Yabrove, G., Theodorou P., & Carney, C. C. (1986). Preschoolers' moral actions and emotions in prisoner's dilemma. *Developmental Psychology, 22,* 663–670.

Medrich, E. A., Rosen, J., Rubin, V., & Buckley, S. (1982). *The serious business of growing up.* Berkeley, CA: University of California Press.

Newcomb, A. F., & Brady, J. E. (1982). Mutuality in boys' friendship selections. *Child Development, 53,* 392–395.

Olthof, T. J. (1990). *Blame, anger, and aggression in children*. Groningen, The Netherlands: Stichting Kinderstudies.

Parke, R. D. (1978). Children's home environments: Social and cognitive effects. In I. Altman & J. R. Wohlwill (Eds.), *Children and the environment* (pp. 33–81). New York: Plenum Press.

Parke, R. D., & Bahvnagri, N. P. (1989). Parents as managers of children's peer relationships. In D. Belle (Ed.), *Children's social networks and social supports* (pp. 241–259). New York: Wiley.

Parke, R. D., & Slaby, R. G. (1983). The development of aggression. In P. H. Mussen & E. M. Hetherington (Eds.), *Handbook of child psychology, Vol. 4, Socialization, personality, and social development* (pp. 547–641). New York: Wiley.

Parke, R. D., MacDonald, K. B., Burks, V. M., Carson, J., & Bhavnagri, N., Barth, J. M., & Beitel, A. (1989). Family and peer systems: In search of the linkages. In K. Kreppner & R. M. Lerner (Eds.), *Family systems in life span development* (pp. 65–92). Hillsdale, NJ: Erlbaum.

Parker, J. G., & Asher, S. R. (1987). Peer relations and later adjustment: Are low-accepted children "at risk"? *Psychological Bulletin, 102,* 357–389.

Parten, M. B. (1932). Social participation among preschool children. *Journal of Abnormal and Social Psychology, 27,* 243–269.

Pastor, D. L. (1981). The quality of mother-infant attachment and its relationship to toddlers' initial sociability with peers. *Developmental Psychology, 17,* 326–335.

Patterson, G. R., & Bank, L. (1989). Some amplifier and dampening mechanisms for pathologic processes in families. In M. Gunnar & E. Thelen (Eds.), *Minnesota Symposia on Child Psychology,* Vol. 22, (pp. 167–209). Hillsdale, NJ: Erlbaum.

Pearl, R. A. (1979, April). *Developmental and situational influences on children's understanding of prosocial behavior*. Paper presented at the biennial meetings of the Society for Research in Child Development, San Francisco.

Peters, R. W., & Torrance, E. P. (1972). Dyadic interaction of preschool children and performance on a construction task. *Psychological Reports, 30,* 747–750.

Price, J. M., & Dodge, K. A. (1989). Peers' contributions to children's social maladjustment: Description and intervention. In T. J. Berndt & G. W. Ladd (Eds.), *Peer relationships in child development* (pp. 341–370). New York: Wiley.

Putallaz, M. (1987). Maternal behavior and sociometric status. *Child Development, 58,* 324–340.

Putallaz, M., & Gottman, J. M. (1981). An interactional model of children's entry into peer groups. *Child Development, 52,* 986–994.

Putallaz, M., & Heflin, A. (1990). Parent-child interaction. In S. R. Asher & J. D. Coie (Eds.), *Peer rejection in childhood* (pp. 189–216). Cambridge, UK: Cambridge University Press.

Putallaz, M., & Wasserman, A. (1990). Children's entry behavior. In S. R. Asher & J. D. Coie (Eds.), *Peer rejection in childhood* (pp. 60–89). Cambridge, UK: Cambridge University Press.

Radke-Yarrow, M., Zahn-Waxler, C., & Chapman, M. (1983). Children's prosocial dispositions and behavior. In P. H. Mussen & E. M. Hetherington (Eds.), *Handbook of child psychology, Vol. 4, Socialization, personality, and social development* (pp. 469–545). New York: Wiley.

Reese, H. W. (1961). Relationship between self-acceptance and sociometric choice. *Journal of Abnormal and Social Psychology, 62,* 472–474.

Richman, N., Stevenson, J., & Graham, P. J. (1982). *Preschool to school: A behavioural study*. London: Academic Press.

Roff, M. (1961). Childhood social interactions and young adult bad conduct. *Journal of Abnormal and Social Psychology, 63,* 333–337.

Roff, M., & Sells, S. B. (1967). The relation between the status of chooser and chosen in a sociometric situation at the grade school level. *Psychology in the Schools, 4,* 101–111.

Roff, J. D., & Wirt, R. D. (1984). Childhood aggression and social adjustment as antecedents of delinquency. *Journal of Abnormal Child Psychology, 12,* 111–126.

Roper, R., & Hinde, R. A. (1978). Social behavior in a play group: Consistency and complexity. *Child Development, 49,* 570–579.

Rubin, K. H. (1985). Socially withdrawn children: An "at risk" population? In B. H. Schnedier, K. H. Rubin, & J. E. Ledingham (Eds.), *Children's peer relations: Issues in assessment and intervention* (pp. 125–139). New York: Springer-Verlag.

Rubin, K. H., & Daniels-Beirness, T. (1983). Concurrent and predictive correlates of sociometric status in kindergarten and grade one children. *Merrill-Palmer Quarterly, 29,* 337–352.

Rubin, K. H., LeMare, L. J., & Lollis, S. (1990). Social withdrawal in childhood: Developmental pathways to peer rejection. In S. R. Asher & J. D. Coie (Eds.), *Peer rejection in childhood* (pp. 217–249). Cambridge, UK: Cambridge University Press.

Rubin, Z., & Slomin, J. (1984). How parents influence their children's friendships. In M. Lewis (Ed.), *Beyond the dyad* (pp. 223–250). New York: Plenum Press.

Rubin, K. H., Watson, K. S., & Jambor, T. W. (1978). Free-play behaviors in preschool and kindergarten children. *Child Development, 49,* 534–536.

Russell, A., & Finnie, V. (1990). Preschool children's social status and maternal instructions to assist group entry. *Developmental Psychology, 26,* 603–611.

Rutter, M., & Garmezy, N. (1983). Developmental psychopathology. In P. H. Mussen & E. M. Hetherington (Eds.), *Handbook of child psychology, Vol. 4, Socialization, personality, and social development* (pp. 775–911). New York: Wiley.

Selman, R. L. (1980). *The growth of interpersonal understanding.* New York: Academic Press.

Sherif, M., Harvey, O. J., White, B. J., Hood, W. R., & Sherif, C. W. (1961). *Inter-group conflict and cooperation: The Robbers Cave experiment.* Norman, OK: University of Oklahoma Press.

Sherif, M., & Sherif, C. W. (1953). *Groups in harmony and tension.* New York: Harper.

Singleton, L. C., & Asher, S. R. (1979). Racial integration and children's peer preferences: An investigation of developmental and cohort differences. *Child Development, 50,* 936–941.

Smith, P. K., & Connolly, K. J. (1981). *The ecology of preschool behaviour.* Cambridge, UK: Cambridge University Press.

Sorokin, P. A., Tranquist, M., Parten, M., & Zimmerman, C. C. (1930). An experimental study of efficiency of work under various specified conditions. *American Journal of Sociology, 35,* 765–782.

Sroufe, L. A., & Fleeson, J. (1986). Attachment and the construction of relationships. In W. W. Hartup & Z. Rubin (Eds.), *Relationships and development* (pp. 51–72). Hillsdale, NJ: Erlbaum.

Strayer, F. F. (1980). Current problems in the study of human dominance. In D. Omark, F. Strayer, & D. Freedman (Eds.), *Dominance relations* (pp. 443–452). New York: Garland.

Strayer, F. F., & Strayer, J. (1976). An ethological analysis of social agonism and dominance relations among preschool children. *Child Development, 47,* 980–989.

Tesser, A. (1984). Self-evaluation maintenance processes: Implications for relationships and for development. In J. C. Masters & K. Yarkin-Levin (Eds.), *Boundary areas in social and developmental psychology* (pp. 271–299). New York: Academic Press.

Vandell, D. L., Owen, M. T., Wilson, K. S., & Henderson, V. K. (1988). Social development in infant twins: Peer and mother-child relationships. *Child Development, 59,* 168–177.

Vaughn, B. E., & Waters, E. (1981). Attention structure, sociometric status and dominance: Interrelations, behavioral correlates and relationships to social competence. *Developmental Psychology, 17,* 275–288.

Waters, E., Wippman, J., & Sroufe, L. A. (1979). Attachment, positive affect, and competence in the peer group: Two studies in construct validation. *Child Development, 50,* 821–829.

Watt, N. F., & Lubensky, A. (1976). Childhood roots of schizophrenia. *Journal of Abnormal Psychology, 85,* 363–375.

West, D. J., & Farrington, D. P. (1973). *Who becomes delinquent?* London: Heinemann.

Whiting, B. B., & Whiting, J. W. M. (1975). *Children of six cultures.* Cambridge, MA: Harvard University Press.

Youniss, J. (1980). *Parents and peers in social development: A Piaget-Sullivan perspective.* Chicago: University of Chicago Press.

12

Interpersonal Problem Solving and Social Competence in Children

Kenneth H. Rubin and Linda Rose-Krasnor

We secure our friends not by accepting favors but by doing them.
(Pericles, *The Peloponnesian War*)

Do unto others as you would have them do unto you.
(The Golden Rule)

It will be seen that some habits which appear virtues, if adopted would signify ruin, and others that seem vices lead to security and well-being . . . the question arises . . . whether it is better to be loved than feared or feared than loved . . . it is much safer to be feared than to be loved, if one must choose.
(Niccolo Machiavelli, *The Prince*)

The greatest slave is not he who is ruled by a despot, great though that evil be, but he who is the thrall of his own moral ignorance, selfishness, and vice.
(John Stuart Mill, *On Liberty*)

INTRODUCTION

Well-known sayings, quotations, and proverbs help provide us with bases for understanding socially acceptable thoughts and deeds. Generally, in Western cultures, it is believed that adherence to the Golden Rule and acting in a charitable

Kenneth H. Rubin • Department of Psychology, University of Waterloo, Waterloo, Ontario N2L 3G1. Linda Rose-Krasnor • Department of Psychology, Brock University, St. Catharines, Ontario L2S 3A1.

Handbook of Social Development: A Lifespan Perspective, edited by Vincent B. Van Hasselt and Michel Hersen. Plenum Press, New York, 1992.

manner will lead to interpersonal and intrapersonal profit, whereas those who subscribe to Machiavellian rhetoric will suffer because of his or her own moral ignorance, selfishness, and vice. In short, common sense dictates that those whose social behaviors are judged to be skillful, successful, and acceptable over time and across settings will lead productive, honorable, and successful lives. Those judged as incompetent are predicted to suffer a variety of malevolent consequences.

Given the significance of socially competent behavior, it would appear worthwhile asking to what it is that we can attribute its development and display. Obviously this is a question of significant proportion. But the question requires framing before any answers can be offered. First, one needs to know what is meant by *social competence*. Next, one requires a theory or theories in which are described the functional components of the construct. It also helps to know how to study the phenomenon. With the guidance of definition, theory, and method, one can turn to questions of ontogenesis and phenotype.

In the present chapter, we discuss social competence with particular reference to the literature that has emerged, over the past 20 years or so, concerning interpersonal or social problem-solving skills. We have come to believe that these skills, when displayed consistently across settings and time, lead to judgments by others that the actor is socially competent. Thus we begin this chapter with some prototypical definitions of social competence. We then describe how these definitions best fit into the frame of problem solving in the social domain. In subsequent sections, we focus on the ways that social skills are studied, on the development of interpersonal problem-solving skills, and on the contemporaneous correlates and the predictive consequences of competent and incompetent social problem-solving skills in childhood. Finally, we present a brief overview of investigations designed to prevent or to ameliorate difficulties in social problem-solving development in children.

Defining Social Competence within an Interpersonal Problem-Solving (IPS) Framework

A number of years ago, Dodge (1985) wrote that there are probably as many definitions of social competence as there are researchers currently gathering data on the topic. We fear that Dodge's observation was less "tongue in cheekish" than one might have hoped. We offer here a smattering of definitions culled from the many that have been suggested by investigators of social competence: "An organism's capacity to interact effectively with its environment" (White, 1959, p. 297); "the effectiveness or adequacy with which an individual is capable of responding to various problematic situations which confront him" (Goldfried & D'Zurilla, 1969, p. 161); "an individuals' everyday effectiveness in dealing with his environment" (Zigler, 1973); "a judgment by another that an individual has behaved effectively" (McFall, 1982, p. 1); "attainment of relevant social goals in specified social contexts, using appropriate means and resulting in positive developmental outcomes" (Ford, 1982, p. 324); the ability "to make use of environmental and personal resources to achieve a good developmental outcome" (Waters & Sroufe, 1983, p. 81); and "the ability to engage effectively in complex interpersonal interaction and to use and understand people effectively" (Oppenheimer, 1989, p. 45).

The definitions noted share several common properties. First, most of the authors, in defining social competence, refer to "effectiveness." Second, competence appears to involve the manipulation of others to meet one's own needs or goals. It is important, however, to distinguish between the effective manipulation of others in the Machiavellian sense and the effective manipulation of others using conventionally accepted means in accord with "common sense." Thus, McFall's notion that social competence refers to a "judgment call" based on the display of skilled behavior is an important one. Further, Ford's suggestion that competence involves the use of "appropriate means" is significant.

Drawing from the definitions noted, as well as from others found in the work of Attili (1989), Dodge (1986), Strayer (1989) and many others, we will refer to social competence as *the ability to achieve personal goals in social interaction while simultaneously maintaining positive relationships with others over time and across situations.* This definition has, over the years, served as a useful heuristic in guiding our own research program (e.g., Rubin & Krasnor, 1986). It has also served us well in understanding and mentally "filing" the burgeoning numbers of published papers, chapters, and books concerning social skills and social competence in children.

A reexamination of the functional properties of social behavior—a *goal* orientation, the employment of appropriate and acceptable *strategies* to achieve these goals, and the successful and effective *outcomes* of these strategies—are all nicely encapsulated in the literature extant on problem solving. Thus we turn now to a discussion of the significance of social competence for normal development and to a description of several traditional and contemporary models of social competence and interpersonal problem solving.

MODELS OF INTERPERSONAL PROBLEM SOLVING (IPS)

Children regularly face social dilemmas ranging in magnitude from miniscule to overbearing. Take, for example, the following questions that a child may ask herself or himself within any given day: "How can I get that Ninja Turtle toy from my older sister?"; "Should I try to get to know the new kid next door; how can I do it?"; "How can I get the kids in my class to help out with the recycling project?"; "How can I convince my parents that one half hour of playing Nintendo per day won't kill me?"

For children who can solve their interpersonal dilemmas successfully and effectively, the social world is a welcome and reinforcing milieu. For children whose IPS skills are lacking, there may be considerable developmental risk.

Repeated social failure may bring with it the development of negative self-perceptions of competence and effectance (Goetz & Dweck, 1980; Harter, 1982; Hymel & Franke, 1985). It may also promote a maladaptive generalized social response such as aggression or passive withdrawal. Additionally, a child who uses socially unacceptable means to achieve his or her goals may become rejected by peers and adults and thus be unlikely to form supportive social relationships. Given that these relationships and the interpersonal exchanges of ideas, perspectives, and actions experienced within them supposedly *promote* the development of social cognition and social competence, a destructive cycle of negativity may eventuate. If social relationships and social exchange promote the development of social cognition and social skills and if the lack of mature and competent social

KENNETH H.
RUBIN and LINDA
ROSE-KRASNOR

thinking and behavior negate opportunities for the development and maintenance of productive social relationships, one comes quickly to realize what the costs of poor social skills may be, both interpersonally and intrapersonally.

Our description of the dialectical relation between interpersonal exchange and intellectual growth has been part and parcel of the developmental literature for many years. Piaget (1926), for example, believed that intelligent thought and behavior evolved through the experience of discussion, negotiation, and conflict, especially in the company of peers. Considerable research has proved supportive of these early Piagetian premises (Chandler, 1985; Damon, 1977; Doise & Mugny, 1981).

From social negotiation, discussion, and conflict, it was argued that children learn to understand others' thoughts, emotions, motives and intentions. In turn, armed with these new social understandings, the child could think about the consequences of his or her behaviors for both the self and for others, and with this in mind, engage in appropriate and effective social behavior. The bottom line is that from Piaget, the dialectical relation between social cognition and behavior on the one hand and opportunities for experiencing the benefits of interpersonal relationships and exchange on the other, could well be understood.

In a later section of this chapter, we discuss issues concerning the *development* of social competence. To this end, we leave Piagetian and neo-Piagetian theory concerning the relations between social-cognitive development and interpersonal behavior for the time being. Suffice it to say that the development of competent social behavior is critical for normal human growth and development.

We turn now to a discussion of the *processes* involved in the demonstration of social competence. One of the earliest models of social competence was articulated by Goldfried and D'Zurilla (1969). Briefly, these authors outlined a multistep process of problem-solving ability that included, in sequence: (1) the identification of a situation that was problematic; (2) the generation of possible alternatives to solve the problem; (3) the decision of choosing the appropriate alternative for the situation; and (4) strategy implementation.

This particular model was drawn from earlier work on impersonal problem solving (e.g., Miller, Galanter, & Pribram, 1960), but more importantly, it proved influential for the seminal writings of Spivack and Shure (1974). The latter two psychologists proposed that children's social competence can best be defined as a set of interrelated interpersonal cognitive problem-solving (ICPS) skills. These skills included (a) sensitivity to or the recognition of interpersonal problems; (b) the ability to generate alternative solutions to solve these problems; (c) the ability to consider step-by-step means to achieve social goals ("means–ends thinking"); (d) the ability to articulate consequences of social acts for oneself and for others and to generate alternative consequences to acts of social significance before deciding how to behave ("causal thinking"); and (e) the ability to identify and understand the motives and behaviors of others.

Unlike the earlier model of Goldfried and D'Zurilla (1969), the elements of ICPS proposed by Spivack and Shure were cast into a developmental framework. Spivack and his colleagues (Spivack, Platt, & Shure, 1976; Spivack & Shure, 1974) suggested that the ability to produce alternative solutions to alleviate social problems is a developmental prerequisite for "mean–ends" and "consequential thinking," and to sensitivity to social dilemmas. The last three components of ICPS were presumed to require advanced perspective-taking skills and the appreciation of consequences, which following a strictly Piagetian view, are virtually nonexistent in early childhood.

Over the years, the ICPS model of Spivack and Shure has been extremely influential in the development of social skills training and research programs (e.g., Weissberg, 1985, 1989). The conceptual model "driving" contemporary applied programs, however, has undergone considerable elaboration and change. For example, in the 1980s, at least three "new and improved" models of social competence emerged, two with a decidedly information-processing bias, and one with a neo-Piagetian perspective.

Rubin and Rose-Krasnor's Social Information-Processing Model of Social Competence

Borrowing largely from the work of Newell and Simon (1972) and Schank and Abelson (1977), Rubin and Krasnor (1986) have developed an information-processing model of social competence. From the outset, these authors suggested that much, if not most, social behavior reflects automaticity in thinking. Most social *interchanges* are routine; for example, there are standard "scripts" of greeting and leave- taking behavior that are learned quickly. Many social *relationships* "slot" members into particular roles that are played out in highly predictable ways (see Strayer's, 1989, descriptions of dominance and affiliation roles and hierarchies in early childhood).

Thus, borrowing from Schank and Abelson (1977), Rubin and Krasnor assimilated the notion of automaticity and social scripts into their processing model of social competence. Social scripts (e.g., greeting behavior) were posited to be stored awaiting evocation by specific cues that could be produced internally (e.g., anxious anticipation) or externally (e.g., the sight of friends upon arrival at preschool).

The existence of scripts means that children have easy access to sequences of actions corresponding to highly familiar social situations. In familiar social situations, therefore, there is usually no problem in producing routine, script-driven behavior. When appropriate and familiar eliciting conditions are absent, or when an obstacle prevents an action from being completed, a "social problem" or dilemma exists and script-driven behavior is precluded.

Children, by virtue of their relatively limited social experience, regularly find themselves in situations that are novel and/or significant, that violate expectations, and that have led to unsuccessful resolutions in the past. With this in mind, Rubin and Krasnor borrowed the model of information flow from Newell and Simon (1972) and developed the social information-processing model outlined in Figure 1.

To illustrate this model, an example is provided here. Joshua and Nathan are fifth-grade children who are the best of friends. Most of the time, their interactions lead the parents of both children to assume that both partners operate on some type of "cooperative automatic pilot."

JOSH: (as Nathan comes through the front door). Hi Nathan, how're you doin'?

NATHAN: O.k., how're you? (not waiting for an answer) Wanna go upstairs and play Nintendo hockey?

JOSH: Sure, I'll be Team Canada . . . o.k.? You can be Team USA.

NATHAN: O.k., but I'll be Team Sweden, not USA.

KENNETH H.
RUBIN and LINDA
ROSE-KRASNOR

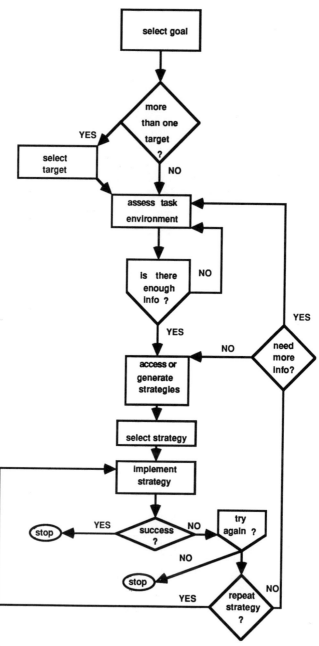

FIGURE 1. An information-processing model of social problem solving (adapted from Rubin & Rose-Krasnor, 1986).

This episode was entirely predictable—from standard greeting behavior, to the request to play ice hockey, to the choice of teams. The behavior of both children appeared to be script driven. After the first 15-minute game, however, script-driven behavior was precluded.

NATHAN: This time I'll be Team Canada . . . you always get to be them.

JOSH: No way! In my house, I'm Canada, and in your house you're always Canada. (Canadian children rarely show nationalistic behavior unless it is in the context of an ice-hockey match.) You can be Russia this time.

NATHAN: Nope. Canada's the best team; we need to take turns. So tomorrow, at my place we'll take turns too.

JOSH: I'll be Team Sweden, you can be Team Canada. But remember, at your house I'll get to be Canada, right?

In this sequence, Nathan had a particular social *goal* that precluded the children's following their usual "Nintendo script." He wanted to gain access to his favorite hockey team. Nathan used the *strategy* of employing the imperative to let Josh know what he wanted. The *outcome* of his initial attempt, however, was a failure. Nathan then produced a *flexible* move to achieve his goal (". . . we need to take turns. So tomorrow, at my place we'll take turns too."), and it proved successful.

Rubin and Krasnor (1986) make use of the components identified by italics to describe their social information-processing model. Children's social goals, the means by which they attempt to achieve these goals, the outcomes of these strategies, and the consequences of strategic failure are all described. Further, Rubin and Krasnor acknowledge the significance of context in their model. For example, how familiar are the social partners? Is the interaction occurring in private or in the company of others? Is the interaction taking place on "neutral ground" or in one of the partner's homes? A discussion of the individual components of their model follows.

SELECTING THE SOCIAL GOAL

The study of social competence involves the analysis of how well children achieve their social goals. These goals may include gaining attention or acknowledgment, information acquisition, giving and/or receiving help, object acquisition, defense, initiating social play, and avoiding anger and/or loss of face. The goal, by definition, is a representation of the end state of the problem-solving process. Goals may be broken down into subgoals, or a goal may be changed during problem solving; however, the operating goal at a particular time provides the basis for outcome feedback.

EXAMINING THE "TASK ENVIRONMENT"

Children are likely to consider contextual factors when choosing goals or the means to achieve their social goals. For example, it is well known that from very early in childhood, different strategies are used to meet given goals in different social contexts. Boys and girls are likely to produce different strategic responses when in the company of same-sex as opposed to opposite-sex peers (Rubin &

Krasnor, 1983). The social status, the familiarity, the type of relationship (e.g., stranger, acquaintance, friend), and the age of the coactors are all likely to influence the strategies chosen by children to deal with their interpersonal dilemmas. These factors are also likely to influence children's choice of social goals. A child who is viewed by his or her peers as aggressive may *elicit* goals of social avoidance or active rejection. In contrast, an older child may elicit goals of information seeking from younger children. In turn, these goals may lead to the demonstration of hostile strategies (e.g., teasing, taunting, and otherwise acting "mean") directed toward aggressive children on the playground, whereas information questions and requests for help may be directed toward older children on that same playground.

Impersonal or inanimate features of the environment must also be taken into account during the problem-solving process. For example, general venue (e.g., school, home, or campground), population density, and visibility (public versus private encounters) are all important factors likely to influence the social goals children have and the strategies they use to meet them.

In summary, children's social goals and the strategies that are selected to achieve these goals are constrained somewhat by the information the actor accesses about the surrounding environment.

ACCESSING AND SELECTING STRATEGIES

Rubin and Krasnor (1986) describe several ways that strategies are chosen to achieve social goals. First, the child may have stored, in long-term memory, a set of strategies. The child retrieves one or more of these strategies and brings them into a "working space" for consideration or implementation.

Strategy *retrieval* may be automatic or deliberate, but the strategies retrieved must already exist in the individual's cognitive repertoire. New strategies may also be constructed by a cognitive transformation of available strategies. Thus, two key factors in accessing strategies appears to be (a) automaticity of recall and (b) the size, complexity, and perceived acceptability and effectiveness of the strategy repertoire.

Strategy *selection* may also be automatic or deliberate. If a script is available to guide behavior, strategy selection is relatively automatic, but only if task environmental concerns fail to put the processing system on "pause." If task environmental factors put the system on "alert," however, there may be a shift to active, conscious processing.

Another selection procedure can best be described as "generate and test." In this case, each available strategy is assessed, sequentially, with regard to preset criteria of acceptability, "performability" (can it be implemented?), and potential effectiveness. The first strategy to match the criteria is implemented.

Strategies may be assessed not only as the singular potential means to achieve a goal but also as a step toward goal attainment. Thus Rubin and Krasnor (1986) describe *partial solutions* as those strategies that move the situation closer to the goal state or that increase the likelihood of achieving a goal. For example, a child may have the goal of object acquisition. Strategies may be selected to first put the target in a "good mood" (affect manipulation); next, strategies might be selected that would not involve the target's giving up the desired object immediately (sharing); and finally, suggestions for singular use by the protagonist may be assessed.

Once selected, the next step in the sequence is to produce the strategy in its relevant context. It may be, however, that the best strategy for a given situation (and one that is in the cognitive and behavioral repertoire of the child) cannot be enacted for some reason. For example, if factors that were not anticipated arise suddenly, the original strategy choice may be abandoned and the processing sequence must be reinitiated.

STRATEGY OUTCOME

After strategy implementation, the protagonist must make a "reading" of the task environment in order to assess the relative success of the problem-solving interchange. Social information is compared to the preestablished criteria for success to examine whether the original goal was fully or partially achieved.

The judgment of success or failure represents an important branching point in the social-problem-solving process. If the strategy is judged to be successful, the problem solving process ends. Information concerning the social interchange is retained in long term memory. If a strategy has been judged as partially successful, the actor may accept the outcome as "successful enough" and proceed as if the outcome was a success. Alternately, the individual may decide to judge the outcome as a failure. Thus, the social problem-solving process operates as a negative feedback system.

If the social interchange is judged to have failed, three general options may be available. First, the child may stop the sequence and leave the goal unattained. Information about the relative ineffectiveness of the strategy, as directed to a particular target, to accomplish a particular goal, is stored for future access. A new or modified goal may be chosen, and the sequence of information processing begins again. Second, the problem solver may choose to repeat the original strategy. Finally, the problem solver may choose to alter the previous strategy while maintaining the same goal; modifications may be subtle or substantive.

Just as the accessing and choice of strategy may involve cognitive reflection or automaticity, so, too, may the individual's response to failure. A child may repeat a failed strategy after spending some time thinking about possible alternatives, or she or he may perseverate without thinking. Similarly, reflection may lead the child to abandon a failed goal attempt. Modification of a failed original strategy would usually entail cognitive reflection. However, in some instances it may proceed automatically, as in when the child has built a scripted sequences of response to failure (e.g., if demands fail, use a politeness marker).

FACTORS ASSOCIATED WITH THE CHOICE AND IMPLEMENTATION OF STRATEGIES AND WITH THE PURSUIT OF GOALS FOLLOWING FAILURE

We have already noted that an assessment of context plays an important role in the choice of goals and strategies. Rubin and Krasnor (1986) cite several other factors that influence strategy choice and the continued pursuit of goals following failure. These factors include children's self-perceptions of competence, the causal attributions generated after failure, an the affect associated with the social target or with the failure experience.

First, some children believe strongly that they lack social skills (Harter, 1985; Rubin & Mills, 1988). Others do not believe that they are socially efficacious (Ladd & Wheeler, 1985). It may be that when these children are in the company of others, they choose social goals of relatively low cost to their social targets (e.g., they might be more likely to try to gain the attention of others than to try to get others to join them in play). The strategies that such children might choose would likely be "softer," perhaps more polite than those used by children with more positive self-appraisals. Finally, in the face of failure, children with negative self-regard may simply give up rather than make an attempt to pursue a failed strategy.

Second, children with stable, internal, or uncontrollable attributions for unsuccessful social outcomes are likely to demonstrate unproductive responses to failure (Goetz & Dweck, 1980; Rubin & Krasnor, 1986). Thus children who attribute their social failures to relatively permanent, personal causes tend to give up more often than those who attribute their failures to external unstable, and/or controllable reasons.

Finally, the social target, the social context, or the experience of social failure may be accompanied by strong negative affect. Such affect may be reflected externally, as in anger directed at the target, or internally, as in sadness or fearfulness directed to the self. In the case of anger, strategy selection may be biased toward agonism, and a response to failure may be a heightened negative strategy of the same form as the original (e.g., yelling louder; hitting harder). In the case of fearfulness, the initial strategy may be overly careful and polite; the response to failure might be one of retreat to terminate an already unpleasant emotional state. In studies of impersonal problem solving, negative affect has generally been found to result in restricted response search and in loss of flexibility (Clark & Isen, 1981).

In summary, Rubin and Krasnor (1986) have developed an information-processing model of social competence that takes into account children's social goals, the means by which strategies are accessed and chosen to achieve these goals, the production of strategic behaviors, the outcome of the initial social attempt, and the sequencing of goals and strategies following failure. These processes are identified within particular social contexts (task environmental factors). Moreover, internalized attributions, self-perceptions, and emotions are considered significant contributors to the display of socially competent behaviors.

The research program derived from this processing model is described in the sections that follow.

Dodge's Model of Social Information Processing

At the same time that Rubin and Krasnor began to develop the information-processing model described, Dodge (1986) outlined a social-cognitive model designed specifically to explain and to predict the consistent demonstration of aggressive behavior in children. Indeed, both models were described formally at the 1983 *Minnesota Symposium on Child Psychology* (see Perlmutter, 1986, for a complete description).

Dodge has proposed five sequential steps necessary for the demonstration of skilled social behavior. The first step involves the *encoding* of social cues. This involves attending to relevant bits of social information such as who it is that is in the social milieu (a friend, a stranger, a popular child, an unpopular child), how it is that this person is expressing him- or herself (affectively happy, angry, or sad), and so on. In many respects, this step is like Rubin and Rose-Krasnor's processing step of examining the task environment. As in their model, the encoding of social information may be reflective or automatic, accurate or inaccurate.

The second step involves the *interpretation* of the encoded cues. This step requires that the child search his or her memory store in an effort to understand the meaning of the encoded information. For example, one of the social cues encoded at Step 1 might be a facial expression denoting anger. Interpreting the facial expression correctly may lead to the assumption that the social situation involves hostility and anger.

In the third step, the child must *access and generate potential responses* to the interpreted social cues. The question asked here is basically, "What are all the things I can do in this situation?" Next, she or he must evaluate each of the accessed alternatives and decide on the optimal response. For example, the individual might consider the potential interpersonal consequences ("Will she still like me?"), the instrumental consequences ("Will I get what I want?"), and the moral value of the strategy (Crick & Dodge, 1989). Finally, the child enacts the chosen response.

In many ways, the models of Dodge and Rubin and Rose-Krasnor are similar. Both assume that the processing steps occur rapidly in real time. Both assume that the steps of information processing follow a particular sequence and that the steps are dynamically interrelated, yet separable. Both assume that processing can proceed automatically at the unconscious level. The research programs of the authors differ quite substantively, however. Although both programs center on the study of competent and incompetent social behavior, Rubin and Rose-Krasnor focus more closely on children with internalizing difficulties; Dodge and his colleagues focus on externalizing disorders. Rubin and Rose-Krasnor tend to examine problem-solving deficiencies by observing social activity; Dodge has been more reliant on the use of interview procedures.

The latter distinction between research programs is rather important. By carefully interviewing children, (Dodge 1986; Dodge, Pettit, McClaskey, & Brown, 1986) has found that he can identify information processing deficits that allow the *prediction* of maladaptive social behavior. For example, deficiencies are found to occur when children respond inappropriately at a particular step (e.g., misinterpreting social cues at Step 2) or when they fail to consider a step entirely (e.g., producing a response without evaluating its consequences at Step 4). Rubin and Rose-Krasnor, on the other hand, have not attempted to predict maladaptive behavior in their research program; rather, they have attempted to describe the particular processing difficulties contemporaneously associated with particular forms of maladaptive behavior.

Although Dodge and Rubin and Rose-Krasnor have discussed developmental issues in the study of social information processing, their writings have been conspicuously vacuous in this area. Thus we turn now to a third model of IPS that has had, as its main focus, developmental issues.

Selman's Model of Interpersonal Negotiation and Communicative Competence

Selman and his colleagues have developed an important theoretical context for understanding and assessing the IPS process; this context is his theoretical model of social perspective taking. In his extensive work on social perspective taking, Selman (1980) has combined Mead's (1934) emphasis on the significance of role taking in the construction of the self, Werner's (1948) ontogenetic principles, and Piaget's (1970) structural-developmental theory. To Selman, social perspective taking progresses from an undifferentiated and egocentric process (Level 0) in early childhood to an indepth, societal-symbolic orientation (Level 4) beginning in adolescence. These stages provide a framework for conceptualizing social-cognitive development in a variety of domains, including a specific stage sequence describing children's understanding of conflict resolution strategies. This latter work has encompassed the study of interpersonal negotiation strategies (INS), which have been defined as "the ways in which individuals in situations of social conflict within ongoing relationships deal with the self and a significant other to gain control over inner and interpersonal disequilibrium" (Schultz & Selman, 1989, p. 123). Interpersonal negotiation strategies, therefore, represent a subset of social problem-solving strategies, differentiated by the context of an ongoing relationship and the presence of emotional disequilibrium.

The assessment of INS *strategies*, as drawn from interviews about hypothetical situations and from observation of actual behavior, has gradually evolved over the past decade, beginning with classification according to perspective-taking stage (e.g., Selman, Schorin, Stone, & Phelps, 1983) and progressing toward complex, interpretive, and multidimensional measurements (e.g., Schultz & Selman, 1989). In fact, the interpretation and classification of INS strategies requires consideration of the sociohistorical context of the relationship (Selman & Schultz, 1989), including aspects of the individual (e.g., personal style), the dyad (relationship history), and of the group (past relationship experience, reference group norms).

Recent assessments of INS combine two major psychological dimensions: developmental level and interpersonal orientation (Selman & Demorest, 1986; Selman & Schultz, 1989). According to Selman and colleagues, the assessment of a strategy's *developmental level* depends on its cognitive, emotional, and motivational components. The *cognitive* component consists of the individual's construal of self and other, beginning with an undifferentiated conception and progressing to a differentiated and integrated view in which both self- and other perspectives are recognized and appreciated. The *emotional* component of a strategy reflects the way in which an individual perceives and manages the disequilibrium that results from conflict and negotiation. At the lowest levels, emotions are conceptualized as diffuse and uncontrollable. With development, the child moves toward a reflective view of emotions, interpreting them in the context of personal and relationship history and coping with disequilibrium through communication and shared reflection. The *motivational* aspect of a strategy is its primary goal. Lower level social goals are those judged to be immediate, material, and egocentric. Higher level goals reflect mutual satisfaction, with priority given to the maintenance of long-term positive relationships.

Interpersonal orientation, the second INS dimension, describes three modes of social control: (a) *other transforming*, in which the individual attempts to alter the actions or thoughts of the target; (b) *self-transforming*, in which the individual attempts to change his or her own actions or thoughts; and (c) *collaborative*, which integrates both self- and other-transforming strategies to the balanced collaborative mode. Developmental changes in interpersonal orientation reflect a movement from the rigid, isolated use of other-transforming and/or self-transforming strategies to the balanced collaborative mode.

The developmental and social orientation dimensions, when taken together, produce a matrix of INS classifications (Selman, 1985; Selman & Schultz, 1989). For example, an impulsive, aggressive act is an other-transforming strategy that reflects an undifferentiated, egocentric level of perspective taking (Level 0) in which the other is treated as an "object," without personal thoughts or feelings. An impulsive withdrawal strategy also reflects level 0 social perspective taking, but it is self-transforming in orientation.

At Level 1, the other is seen as having needs and thoughts distinct from one's own, but the differentiation is subjective. The child views conflict as being inherently "me versus you," with no coordination or compromise of perspectives. Other-transforming strategies would include the use of direct commands and threats, whereas self-transforming strategies include weak initiations and quick submissions.

Level 2, strategies are self-reflective and reciprocal, revealing a psychological view of the self and other. Other-transforming strategies at this level include attempts at changing the other's mind through persuasion (e.g., appeal to feelings of guilt). Self-transforming strategies serve to persuade the self to subordinate one's own goals to those of the other.

Self- and other-transforming strategies can be found at Levels 0, 1, and 2. Level 3 strategies, however, require a collaborative orientation (e.g., the suggestion of a mutually satisfying compromise). At Level 3, the child considers both the perspectives of the self and the other simultaneously. Strategies show sensitivity to the other's feelings; both the self and the other are open to transformation. Protection of the relationship is as much a concern as the immediate goal itself.

Selman's initial theoretical models were developed largely from children's interview responses to hypothetical social situations. However, there was early concern for specifying the relation between children's level of interpersonal understanding as expressed in hypothetical situations and the level reflected in actual behavior observed during naturalistic social interaction (Cooney & Selman, 1978; Jacquette, 1980). In recent work, Schultz and Selman (1989) have attempted to identify factors that may help explain discrepancies between hypothetical and observed INS, including the individual's defense mechanisms and object representations of self and other. Contextual and relationship influences on the relation between INS thought and behavior have also been examined (e.g., Selman & Demorest, 1986). This exploratory work offers considerable promise for both theory and intervention.

The Assessment of Children's Social Problem-Solving Skills

As noted, models of interpersonal competence receive empirical support through the use of different research methodologies. Thus it is useful to describe briefly the typical means by which social problem-solving skills are assessed.

The most often employed assessment procedure involves presenting the child with hypothetical social dilemmas and requesting that she or he think about potential solutions to these problems. Typically, in these hypothetical-reflective interview studies, the social *goal* is clearly presented (e.g., object acquisition, conflict resolution, entering an ongoing playgroup, initiating a friendship, seeking help). *Strategies* to meet these clearly defined goals are then elicited from the child. In some cases, the experimenter informs the child that her or his strategy has failed;

additional responses are thus solicited in an effort to assess the *flexibility* of the child's cognitive repertoire (e.g., Rubin & Krasnor, 1983). In other cases, the child is faced with a provocative incident (e.g., paint is spilled on his or her drawing) produced by a child known to have particular characteristics (e.g., aggressive, popular) and she or he is asked whether the action was carried out accidentally or intentionally (Dodge *et al.*, 1986). This allows an assessment of the relation between cognitions about task environmental properties and the choice of social problem-solving strategies.

The strength of the hypothetical-reflective assessment procedure lies with the control the experimenter has in manipulating responses to particular types of dilemmas that occur rarely naturalistic settings. The interview procedure is also likely to take minutes, not days or hours. In contrast, a much less often used procedure involves the careful monitoring of interpersonal negotiation strategies (Selman & Schultz, 1990) and social goals, strategies, outcomes, and context through observational means (Krasnor, 1985; Krasnor & Rubin, 1983; Sharp, 1981). Although far more time consuming than hypothetical-reflective procedures, observational methods are advantageous for a number of reasons. First, it is difficult to evaluate the likelihood of a strategy's success in an interview context; this is not a problem with observational procedures. Second, the observer can identify the child's "real-life" social goals and the strategies actually chosen for use. One problem with presenting hypothetical dilemmas is that the goals and strategies suggested are only *potentially* representative of competence. It is one thing to be able to produce a hypothetical response to a hypothetical dilemma; it is quite another to actually enact the chosen strategy. Thus, given the pressures of ongoing social exchange, verbally derived goals and strategies may never be observed in the natural setting (Damon, 1977).

Naturalistic approaches also allow the assessment of the environmental influences that might maintain maladaptive social problem solving. In particular, the responsivity of partners can be observed. Finally, the unstructured nature of the observational method allows individual priorities in goals and targets to emerge as reflected by the frequency of particular goals, the emotional intensity with which the strategy is produced, and the child's persistence after a failed attempt. These useful pieces of information are unavailable when the goals are predetermined or when the social situation is tightly structured by the experimenter.

Differences in procedures help investigators address different research questions. From our perspective, both hypothetical-reflective and observations methodologies can help answer important and interesting questions. It is important, however, that the reader keep in mind that the interview data described next generally refer to the ways that children *think about* social dilemmas; the observational data refer to the *production* or *enactment* of interpersonal problem solving behaviors. This is especially important to keep in mind given that social thought and action are often found to be unrelated (Rubin & Krasnor, 1986; Schultz & Selman, 1989; Shantz, 1983).

Developmental Changes in Interpersonal Problem-Solving Skills: A Conceptual and Empirical Analysis

In this section, we briefly review developmental changes in the information-processing steps outlined in Figure 1. From the outset, there is a relatively little published information concerning developmental change in IPS and social competence. Given this lack of attention to such a high profile research topic, we have suggested, below, possible ways in which developmental factors may be implicated in each component of the social problem-solving process. We leave the examination of the veracity of our conjectures to future research programs.

GOAL SETTING

With increasing competence and social experience, the number, breadth, and content of children's social goals are likely to increase (Rubin & Krasnor, 1986). Infant social goals, for example, consist largely of attempts to moderate stimuli, establish contact, seek comfort, and initiate feeding or other forms of caretaking behavior. Older children's social goals are more complex and differentiated. The appearance of self-awareness at around 2 years of age (Kagan, 1989b), for example, marks the emergence of goals reflecting self-presentation. Similarly, goals concerned with enhancing relative status among peers are most likely to emerge in middle childhood, when the child begins to use social comparison to determine self-esteem (Ruble, Boggiano, Feldman, & Loebel, 1980). The development of locomotion skills, the birth of a sibling, school entry, puberty, and other developmental transitions and changes are also likely to alter the content and priorities of children's social goals, but there is little empirical documentation of these potential effects.

Changes in both the complexity and content of goals are also likely to result from the child's increasing capacity for self-regulation and control (Bandura, 1989). A growing ability to inhibit responses enables behavior to become increasingly under the control of long-term social goals. Combined with a developing capacity for complex thinking, self-control allows the child to pursue subgoals and to tolerate delays in the satisfaction of more distant, complex social goals (e.g., to be elected to the student council). In addition, the child's increasing ability to understand the perspectives of others is likely to result in goals that are more "other oriented" or prosocial in nature. These progressions in self-control and perspective taking are described in Selman and Demorest's (1986) assessment of interpersonal negotiation strategies. The developmental level of a strategy is determined partially by its goal or motivational component. Cognitively lower level goals have an egocentric orientation and an immediate, material character, whereas higher level goals show integration of self- and other perspectives and are oriented toward relationship enhancing results.

In summary, although researchers have not examined developmental differences and changes in children's interpersonal goals, a reading of the extant literature suggests that changes do occur. Goals appear to become more numerous, more complex, more other oriented, and more likely to involve social comparison as children grow older.

EXAMINING THE "TASK ENVIRONMENT"

With development, children are expected to demonstrate significant increases in the amounts and types of social information they can process. Researchers have shown, for example, that the abilities to scan task environments, sustain attention, detect relevant information, and retain greater amounts of information in large chunks are related to age and social experience (see Bjorkland, 1989, for a review).

It is also noteworthy that the development of operational thinking (Piaget,

1970) allows the child to examine task-relevant information by going beyond the surface features of the information given. Thus, whereas young preschoolers tend to perceive individuals in terms of their physical characteristics, those of concrete or formal operational competence are better able to make use of psychological attributes when assessing social input (Barenboim, 1981). This results in the encoding of social information that would be more useful than a simple understanding of physical features alone when attempting to deal with interpersonal dilemmas. In addition, the ability of older children to decenter (i.e., to consider simultaneously more than a single aspect of a given person or situation) should result in more complex encoding of information.

To summarize, the ability to encode task-relevant information changes with age and development. We have suggested several factors that likely influence developmental change; these include the ability to go beyond that which is directly observable, the ability to decenter, and the ability to encode greater amounts of social information with age.

ACCESSING AND SELECTING STRATEGIES

Age differences in the quantity and quality of social strategies can be predicted from a number of theoretical orientations. From *social learning theory*, one would predict that an increasing amount and diversity of social experience will increase the number of strategies to which the child is exposed. With experience, then, there should be an increased likelihood of learning strategies through observation and direct teaching by peers and adults. From *cognitive-developmental theory*, it would be predicted that children generate more strategies with age. The increasing abilities to think hypothetically, and to perspective-take should, by all accounts, extend the strategy repertoires of developing children.

Although it seems reasonable to expect a broadening of the strategy repertoire with age, researchers have actually reported few age-related changes and differences. For example, Rubin and Krasnor (1983, 1986) found no differences in the *numbers* of different strategies suggested by preschoolers, kindergarteners, and first-grade children to solve hypothetical object acquisition dilemmas. Guerra and Slaby (1989) reported no increases in the social strategy repertoire between Grades 2–3 and Grades 5–6. Similar nonsignificant differences in strategy breadth have been reported by Cowan, Drinkard, and MacGavin (1984), who studied children in Grades 6, 9, and 12.

The lack of age-related changes in the *quantity* of strategies that children can produce stands in marked contrast to findings concerning developmental differences in the *types* of strategies that children generate. First, children's strategies become less physical and more verbal over the preschool period; this reflects the child's growing ability to communicate verbally (e.g., Evans & Rubin, 1979).

Second, social strategies become more cognitively complex with age. This results from the growing ability to integrate simple bits of information (e.g., single strategies) into larger units and to perform mental operations on strategies within working memory. Practice and experience with less complex strategies, combined with neurological maturation, results in an increased ability for higher order mental operations (Case, 1987).

Third, the strategies that children can access and generate are increasingly reflective of the ability to understand the social target's needs, thoughts, and feelings. In short, the child's developing ability to cognitively decenter (Piaget, 1970) is mirrored by the increasing suggestion of strategies that reveal an appreciation of others' perspectives (Selman & Demorest, 1986).

STRATEGY SELECTION

Once strategies are generated, they must be evaluated against situational demands and constraints; evaluation then leads to the production of the perceived "best solution" to the social problem. Operationally, the evaluation process can be deduced from children's ratings of strategies along a number of evaluative dimensions, from their ability to judge the consequences of the strategies and from their ability to systematically vary strategies on the basis of relevant social or task characteristics. The ability to effectively match behaviors to task is an important component of competence (Nakamura & Finck, 1982) and has been related to IPS success (Krasnor, 1982).

As a result of increased experience in situations that allow children to observe the consequences of different strategies and as a function of children's growing ability to perceive others in cognitively complex ways, to use perspective-taking to make accurate inferences about likely consequences, and to use abstract, hypothetical thinking to consider outcomes, one would expect age-related changes in the ability to accurately determine the outcomes of strategy selection. This developmental expectation is supported in the literature. For example, Downey and Walker (1989) found an increase in age (from 7 to 14 years) in children's ability to select appropriate social strategies and to generate consequences for suggested social actions. Berg (1989) reported an age-related increase in Grades 5, 8, and 11 children's accuracy in judging strategy effectiveness during interpersonal dilemmas.

In addition, there is evidence that the ability to match strategy to task requirements increases with age. Rubin and Krasnor (1983) found that kindergarten children showed greater differentiation of strategies by target age and sex than a preschool comparison group. Berg (1989) and Piché, Rubin, and Michlin (1978) have also reported greater strategic variety in response to target characteristics among young adolescents than among elementary-school-age children.

To summarize, the existing data indicate that children become better able to evaluate the probable success of strategies as they get older; they are also better able to vary their strategies in concert with task demands.

STRATEGY SEQUENCING

The ability to respond adaptively to social failure is one of the critical skills in the social problem-solving processing model. One initial assumption has been that flexibility after failure is an appropriate response, leading to a higher probability of success than simply repeating an already unsuccessful strategy (Rubin & Krasnor, 1986). It has been expected also that flexibility in strategy sequencing would increase with age, reflecting both elaboration and growth of strategy repertoires and developing tendencies to be sensitive to cues given by the social target. Although some observational studies of strategic flexibility have been reported, researchers have most commonly chosen hypothetical-reflective approaches, using the introduction of obstacles after the child's first strategic response to elicit sequencing (e.g., "What else might you do or say if your first strategy didn't work?").

In general, support for the predictions has been mixed. In one of the few observational studies of a developmental nature, Levin and Rubin (1983) found an age-related increase in flexibility after noncompliance in 4-, 5-, and 6-year old children. Flexibility after a hypothetical-reflective obstacle was introduced also increased with age in preschool and kindergarten children (Rubin & Krasnor, 1983).

Berg (1989), however, has found few age changes in flexibility after the introduction of obstacles in children from grades 5, 8, and 11. If anything, she reported that flexibility decreased with age. These findings occurred within the context of a negative correlation between strategy knowledge and flexibility, indicating that children with a more accurate understanding of strategy effectiveness were more likely to repeat or only slightly modify a failed strategy than were children with less strategic knowledge. Berg suggested that the knowledgeable children knew how to subtly alter strategies, whereas children with less sophistication jumped to a new strategy type.

It may be possible that the appropriateness of being flexible after failure has a curvilinear function, in which a moderate degree of flexibility is more effective than either a simple repetition or a dramatic change in approach. Another possibility is that children's flexibility after failure reaches a plateau in early elementary school, as seems to be the case with strategy repertoire size. After this level is reached, developmental change may largely center on better consideration of the initial strategy choice. Made with care and confidence, the older child's selection may not dramatically change in the face of a hypothetical obstacle.

INTEGRATION OF SOCIAL PROBLEM-SOLVING COMPONENTS

In the preceding pages, we have examined developmental differences in each of several social problem-solving components independently. In fact, this is often how it has been studied (Dodge's 1986 research program being a notable exception). It is also important, however, to take an integrated, dynamic view of the process. A dynamic approach better approximates how social problem solving operates in "real" interaction and may yield alternate insights into areas of individual strengths and weaknesses.

The social problem-solving process can be viewed as the sequential flow of activity along the steps outlined in our model (Figure 1). Each step receives the information it requires from the step that precedes it. Successful social problem solving, therefore, requires that the information passed between steps is valid and appropriate for the step that follows. A well-functioning process is characterized by completeness, efficiency, and flexible adaptation to environmental feedback (Krasnor, 1988). Feedback about environmental conditions and the effects of social actions is essential for this process, and poor social problem-solving processing may occur from a breakdown of the feedback loops between the individual and the environment.

Feedback loops operate in three basic steps (Miller *et al.*, 1960). First, the system senses environmental conditions then compares these conditions to a reference standard. Results from this comparison are used to determine the next step—whether to act to reduce the discrepancy, continue to monitor conditions, or exit the loop entirely. For example, a common social goal is attention seeking, in which a child attempts to get another person to watch an event or observe an object. In order to judge success, the child must have a criterion for what constitutes "watching" (e.g., eyes and body oriented toward a specific point for at least a few seconds with a verbal acknowledgment). Once such a goal is set, the child assesses the situation to determine if the target person is already watching (success). If a discrepancy between the current situation and the criterion exists, an action may be taken to reduce the discrepancy (e.g., the child may request the target to "Look!"). Information is then gathered from the environment to see if the discrepancy has been eliminated or reduced, and the feedback cycle begins again.

Feedback systems can be disrupted or distorted in a number of ways, including the absence or inappropriateness of reference criteria, inability to perform actions needed to eliminate the discrepancy, inadequate or distorted information needed for effective feedback, and a breakdown in the comparison process (Carver & Sheier, 1981). In addition, strong emotions may interrupt information processing and lead to distortion or breakdown (Dodge, in press; Simon 1967). Each of these problems is less likely to occur as children develop (Krasnor, 1988).

First, as a child gains social experience and observational skills, he or she is likely to develop more precise and appropriate social reference standards. Second, older children have a wider range of available strategies due to their increased verbal, physical, and cognitive abilities and thus are less likely to show a performance failure. Third, older children's more sophisticated attention and social information-processing skills will generally result in more appropriate feedback information, and therefore distortions will be less frequent than for younger children. In addition, the child's increasing role taking and social comparison processes will result in self-initiated feedback, making the child less dependent on external input. Fourth, the more efficient processing abilities of older children (e.g., Case, 1987) make it possible for them to better perform the complex mental operations involved in comparison processes. Finally, developmental increases in emotional control and self-regulation are likely to reduce the frequency of affectively overwhelming experiences.

Most developmental studies of social problem solving have focused on the study of one or more components, but in a relatively static framework. In itself, this approach is insufficient because a child may show appropriate processing at almost every processing step and yet be unable to coordinate these thoughts in such a way as to produce appropriate behavior (Dodge et al., 1986; Krasnor, 1988). Consequently, much work is necessary, at present, to examine, not only the developmental course of children's social goals, strategies, outcomes, response flexibility, and ability to attend to task-relevant features but also the coordination of these essential steps in the information-processing flow.

FACTORS ASSOCIATED WITH THE DEVELOPMENT OF INTERPERSONAL PROBLEM-SOLVING SKILLS

We have suggested that there are developmental changes in social information-processing skills with age. We have suggested further that these changes are largely associated with concomitant growth in cognitive skills and operations. It is likely, however, that the development of IPS skills is a function, not only of cognitive developmental factors, but of many other factors as well. In the following section, we provide some speculation about the identification of these other influential forces.

Conceptualizing the Relation between Temperament and IPS Skills

There have been few attempts to examine the contributions of dispositional or biological factors to the development of social problem-solving skills and social competence in childhood. Yet, it is not difficult to imagine how such factors may be influential. Take, for example, three infant dispositional characteristics that have received a good deal of attention in recent years—inhibition/sociability, difficult temperament, and activity level (e.g., Bates, Maslin & Frankel, 1985). *Inhibition* refers basically to a timid, fearful, vigilant, and restrained behavioral style when faced with socially novel stimuli (Kagan, 1989a). *Sociability* refers to an open, outgoing, spontaneous response to novelty. *Difficult temperament* refers to the frequent and intense expression of negative affect (Thomas & Chess, 1977; Thomas, Chess, & Birch, 1968). Fussiness and irritability would be two characteristics of an infant who is described as being "difficult." Finally, there are some infants and toddlers who can best be described as *excessively active* and highly excitable.

Each of these temperamental characteristics appears to have some stability, and each bears a continuous, long-term relation with variables that have some conceptual association with them. For example, infant inhibition is a highly stable construct (Kagan, Reznick, & Snidman, 1990) that appears to predict socially withdrawn behavior in early and middle childhood. Difficult temperament has long been associated with the development of behavior problems in childhood, particularly those of an externalizing nature (Thomas & Chess, 1977; Thomas, Chess, & Korn, 1982). High activity level, especially in concert with difficult temperament, also appears to predict developmental difficulties of an under-controlled nature (Bates *et al.*, 1985; Campbell, 1991).

How then could one conceive of a relation between these reasonably stable individual characteristics or traits and the development of IPS skills? In recent years, Rubin and colleagues have suggested a number of possible scenarios (e.g., Rubin, LeMare, & Lollis, 1990; Rubin & Lollis, 1988). They posit, for example, that social reticence or an inhibited social behavioral style may preclude the child from (a) the possibilities of establishing normal social relationships; (b) the experience of normal social interactive play behaviors; and (c) the development of those social and cognitive skills that are supposedly encouraged by peer relationships and social play. Moreover, given the belief that social-cognitive knowledge (or the "thinking" steps of the information-processing models described above) is prerequisite to the production of competent social behavior (the "enactment" step of the information-processing model), it is easy to envision a circular effect with the failure to develop effective IPS skills leading to further anxiety and withdrawal from the social arena. In short, the aforementioned dialectical relation between social cognition and behavior on the one hand, and opportunities for experiencing the benefits of interpersonal relationships and exchange, on the other hand, might be a function, *in part*, of the child's inhibition or sociability.

Difficult temperament and high activity level may also be related conceptually to the development of social competence. The child who has difficulty inhibiting responses is easily distracted and who is irritable may be less likely to think through his or her social dilemmas in the competent manners described in the information-processing models described. As a consequence, social response selection for this child may be overly "automatic," or it may result from not focusing on any or all of the processing steps required for the production of effective and acceptable social behavior. Rubin *et al.* (1990) suggest that unthinking, unacceptable social behaviors lead to the isolation of the child by the peer group. Once isolated, the child will be precluded from the social-cognitive and social "gains" brought on by normal peer relationships and peer interactive experiences; thus, as in the scenario described regarding the socially inhibited child, a similar pathway can be described for the temperamentally difficult and overactive child.

Conceptualizing the Significance of Parent–Child Relationships and Socialization Experiences

Clearly, individual traits or disposition do not develop *in vacuo*. Children grow up in homes, often with two parents and one or more siblings. Moreover, their families are not immune to societal and cultural influences or to stressors impinging on them from time to time. As such, it should not be surprising that the link between parent–child relationships, parenting behavior, and children's social competence has received a good deal of attention over the years.

According to Hartup (1985), parent–child relationships serve at least three functions. First, they represent contexts within which competencies can develop. Second, they constitute emotional and cognitive resources that allow the child to explore his or her social and nonsocial worlds. Third, the early parent–child relationship may serve as the precursor of all subsequent relationships (e.g., Sroufe, 1983). Given these perspectives, it is not difficult to understand how parent–child relationships contribute to the development of social competence and IPS skills.

Most toddlers and preschoolers develop *secure* relationships with their parents (Ainsworth, Blehar, Waters, & Wall, 1978; Belsky & Nezworski, 1988; Sroufe, 1983). These relationships appear to be caused and maintained, in part, by sensitive and responsive parenting (Spieker & Booth, 1988). The sensitive and responsive parent is one who is in tune with the child's behaviors. She or he is a competent processor of social information that derives from the child. She or he interprets signals correctly and responds effectively and appropriately to the child. Moreover, although the sensitive and responsive parent may, from time to time become irritated by the child's behavior, she or he is accepting of the child and does not remain angry, hostile, or resentful. In short, from our perspective, the competent parent is a good interpersonal problem solver within the context of the parent–child relationship.

Within the context of a *secure* relationship, then, we suggest a conceptual link to the development of social problem-solving skills. This link draws its conceptual underpinnings from the belief that the attachment relationship results in the child's development of an internal working model of the self in relation to others. For example, we posit that the child who believes that his/her parent is available and responsive to his or her needs will feel secure, confident, and self-assured when introduced to novel settings. Felt security is thought to result in active exploration of the social environment (Sroufe, 1983). In turn, exploration (which addresses the questions, "What are the properties of this person? What is she like? What does she do?") of the social environment is likely to lead to the experience of peer play

KENNETH H.
RUBIN and LINDA
ROSE-KRASNOR

("What can I do with this person?") and to the development of healthy, growth-supporting peer relationships. As noted earlier, these play experiences are likely to result in the development of social competencies, and more specifically, in the ability to manage competently and independently one's interpersonal dilemmas (see Hutt, 1966, for an early description of the exploration, play, problem-solving sequence; see also Rubin, Fein, & Vandenberg, 1983).

We suggest further that the child's display of cognitively and socially mature behavior in extrafamilial settings will be nurtured consistently by the competent parent. It has been long thought, for example, that the sensitive parent can "provoke" the child to think through and display problem solving at levels just beyond that which the child can handle on his or her own (e.g., Vygotsky, 1978). Rather than directly telling the child how to deal with his or her social milieu, the competent parent uses "distancing" strategies (Sigel, 1982) that focus the child on alternative means to tackle given problems ("What are all the things you can do in order to. . .?"). The parent also queries the child about potential consequences of his or her suggested strategies and helps the child deal flexibly with his or her social failures. In short, the competent parent is one who is emotionally available, sharply attuned to social situations and the thought and emotions of her or his child, able to anticipate her/his child's behaviors and the consequences of the child's actions, and able to predict the outcomes of her/his own actions.

The competent parent thus provides the child with an appropriate social problem-solving model. Further, she or he encourages the independent development of the processing skills required for effective and appropriate problem-solving behavior.

On the other hand, there are some children who do not develop secure relationships with their parents. The internal working models of insecurely attached children may conjure up cognitions of a comfortless and unpredictable social universe. These cognitive representations may lead to the insecure child's behaving in the peer group "by shrinking from it or doing battle with it" (Bowlby, 1973, p. 208). Children who follow the pathway of shrinking anxiously away from the world of peers preclude themselves from the positive outcomes associated with exploration and peer play. Children who do battle with their peers will likely engage in inappropriate exploration and play, thereby leading to rejection and isolation by the peer group. Such rejection and isolation will thus preclude the child from experiencing the benefits of cooperative peer play and of peer negotiation and competition.

Insecure attachment relationships are developed and maintained, in part, by insensitive and unresponsive caregiving (Spieker & Booth, 1988). As noted earlier, incompetent parents may be described as poor problem solvers within the context of the parent–child relationship. They are likely to be adult centered in their goals, their range of available alternatives with regard to proactive socialization strategies and reactive behaviors to the display of inappropriate child behaviors may be limited, and their choice of problem-solving strategies may be highly power assertive (Booth, Rose-Krasnor, & Rubin, 1991; Rubin & Mills, 1990).

This description of the insensitive, unresponsive parent is similar to that of the "authoritarian" parent (Baumrind, 1967). Of particular interest is Baumrind's finding that children of "authoritarian" parents are, in many ways, less socially competent than children of "authoritative" parents. These children were more conflicted and irritable and more passively hostile than those of competent parents. The bottom line is that we posit significant relations between the quality of the parent– child relationship, the sorts of socialization behaviors produced by parents, and the development of IPS skills.

Temperament, Parent–Child Relationships, Parenting, and Children's IPS Skills: The Empirical Evidence

Are there actually data concerning the posited relations between temperament, parent–child relationships, parenting, and children's social-problem solving skills *per se*? Basically, the data are severely limited. This is particularly surprising given the long-held assumption that personality actors, parent–child relationships, and socialization behaviors play a strong role in the development of children's IPS skills.

From the outset, we know of no studies in which are examined the long-term relations between infant or toddler temperament and the subsequent development of IPS skills. There is a literature, however, on the problem-solving concomitants of social withdrawal and of aggression, two suggested "outgrowths" of temperamentally based inhibition and difficultness overactivity, respectively. We review this work in a later section.

Insofar as the relation between the quality of the parent–child relationship and children's social problem-solving skills is concerned, the database is likewise scarce. Arend, Gove, and Sroufe (1979) reported that insecurely attached infants were less able than their securely attached counterparts 4 years, to produce numerous alternative solutions and more likely to choose forceful (agonistic) solutions to hypothetical social problems presented to them in an interview format. More recently, Goldberg, Lojkasek, Gartner, and Corter (1989) found that insecure infant attachment predicted preschoolers' lesser response flexibility and the greater suggestion of aggressive strategies to hypothetical social problems. These findings have been replicated by Rubin, Rose-Krasnor, and Booth (1990). Taken together, these data suggest that the *response repertoires* of preschoolers who have had insecure infant attachment relationships are more constrained than those of securely attached children. Moreover, the *selection of alternatives* is less likely to be adaptive and the *response to strategic failure* less flexible in insecurely attached youngsters.

In the only study of *observed social problem solving skills to date*, Booth et al. (1991) reported significant differences between pre-school-age children who, as infants, were classified as securely versus insecurely attached to their mothers. The securely attached children were less likely to use aggressive means to achieve their social goals than were their insecurely attached age-mates. Further, the problem-solving strategies used by securely attached children from middle-class, low-risk families were more likely to meet with successful outcomes than were the strategies employed by insecurely attached children from low-risk backgrounds. On the other hand, insecurely attached children from high-risk families were *more* successful than their secure counterparts in meeting their social goals; this high success rate appears to have stemmed from the fact that clearly one-quarter of the high-risk, insecure children's strategies were of an agonistic nature. Thus immediate success must be judged against the longer term consequences of displaying culturally unacceptable behaviors. Taken together with the data produced by children's responses to hypothetical-reflective interviews, the observational data indicate that insecure infant attachment relationships predict maladaptive cognizing about resolving interpersonal dilemmas, maladaptive production and enactment of maladaptive strategies, and the experience of negative social problem-solving outcomes.

Given that insecure attachment and negative parent–child relationships supposedly emanate, in part, from insensitive and unresponsive parenting behaviors, it behooves us to examine relevant data relating "parenting" behaviors and children's IPS skills. Pettit, Dodge, and Brown (1988) postulated that early family experience, as assessed by retrospective maternal reports of the use of authoritarian discipline strategies, the child's exposure to aggressive models, parental endorsement of aggression, and maternal beliefs that their children purposely (rather than unintentionally) caused negative interactive outcomes would be associated with social problem-solving deficits in preschoolers. In general, the number of alternative solutions to hypothetical social dilemmas was strongly predicted by these family experience variables. Thus the child's social-cognitive response repertoire appeared associated with the child's experience of maladaptive parenting.

In an earlier set of studies, Shure and Spivack (1978) reported that maternal choice of inductive techniques (suggesting solutions, explaining consequences) to socialize children's interpersonal problem-solving skills was associated significantly with their daughter's production of numerous alternatives to hypothetical social dilemmas. Similar findings were not discovered for mothers and their sons. Carlson-Jones, Rickel, and Smith (1980) indicated that mothers who reported using restrictive, authoritarian child-rearing strategies had children who often chose evasive strategies in dealing with hypothetical interpersonal dilemmas. A negative association was found between maternal nurturance and children's suggestions that they would turn to an adult to help resolve an interpersonal dilemma.

More recently, Brown (1989) asked mothers of 5-year-olds how they would feel and respond if they observed their child behaving aggressively with peers. She also interviewed the children and asked them to generate alternatives to hypothetical social dilemmas involving entry to an ongoing playgroup and responses to peer provocation. Brown reported that the maternal strategic choice of reasoning was associated with children's generation of competent responses to the hypothetical dilemmas. She also reported that the limited use of power assertion in concert with high concern about children's aggressive behavior was associated with the children's ability to produce competent responses.

The studies described are fairly typical of research concerning the relations between socialization techniques and children's social competence. That is, for the most part, there has been extensive use of questionnaire and interview data; limited attempt has generally been made to associated observed parent and child behavior or to relate interview/questionnaire data on the one hand, with observed social behavior on the other. In fact, the only observational study we were able to trace in our literature search was produced in our own labs.

Recently, Rubin, Mills, and Rose-Krasnor (1989), summarized the results of a study concerning the relations between mothers' proactive beliefs, that is, when it is they expected their children to learn specific social skills, how it is that they believed these skills are developed, and what they believed should be done to aid in the development of these skills and their children's observed social problem-solving behavior in preschool. The mothers were interviewed and asked a series of questions concerning the development of three social skills: (a) making friends,

(b) sharing possessions, and (c) leading or influencing others. Mothers were first asked to rate, on a 5-point scale, the importance of attaining each of the three skills. Next, each mother was asked the reasons why she thought children might succeed or why they might fail in attaining these social goals. They were also asked to describe what parents should or should not do to help their child learn the three social skills.

In order to assess the children's social problem-solving skills, each child was observed during free play for an extended period of time. Observers used a microcomputer to record the child's social problem-solving goals, strategies, targets, and outcomes. The data indicated that mothers who believed strongly that social skills are important had children who were more likely to have prosocial goals, who employed a relatively high frequency of indirect requests to achieve their goals, and who experienced a high degree of strategic success. Mothers who felt that the attainment of these skills was not so important had children who were more likely to have many intrusive, stop-action goals, and to cry in order to achieve their goals. In short, it was discovered that mothers who viewed the attainment of social skills as highly significant tended to have children who were socially competent.

Second, mothers who believed that it would be difficult to change their children's poor social performance had youngsters who demonstrated a number of difficulties. The children were more likely to attempt to stop the behaviors of others, they were less likely to use indirect requests to meet their social goals, and they were relatively unsuccessful in reaching their social goals.

Third, insofar as attributions are concerned, mothers who suggested more *external/direct* causes for the development or nondevelopment of social skills (e.g., "Children learn social skills because of parenting behaviors"), tended to have children who showed a relatively high overall frequency of directive attempts. In particular, the number of external-direct attributions offered by mothers was positively associated with their children's goals to begin social action and negatively associated with their children's attention-seeking goals. Children of these mothers also showed higher success levels.

On a hypothetical internal-external continuum of control and causality, external-direct and child-centered attributions are at opposite ends. Maternal child-centered attributions (e.g., "Some children have personalities that make them more or less socially skilled") across tasks and outcomes were negatively correlated with children's direct and indirect commands. These children also had higher social failure percentages than their peers.

Finally, insofar as parental beliefs concerning socialization strategies were concerned, Rubin *et al.* (1989) reported that children whose mothers suggested the use of *high power* to socialize social skills were more likely to have assistance-seeking goals, to approach teachers rather than peers as social targets, and to use indirect and questioning social strategies. These children were less likely to try to stop others' actions and less likely to use aggressive social strategies to meet their goals.

In summary, mothers who were more strongly committed than others to aid in the development of their children's social skills, who attributed the development of social skills to external factors, and who did not subscribe to the use of highly directive, power assertive strategies had children who demonstrated well-developed social problem-solving skills. That is, these children had social *goals* that were prosocial and sociable, they used indirect requests (*strategies.*) to achieve these goals, and they were more often *successful* in achieving these goals than children whose mothers were less committed to the development of social skills, who attributed skills to internal causes, and who suggested the use of high power-assertive techniques to socialize social skills.

To conclude, it is clear that the study of the relations between child temperament, parent–child relationships, socialization behaviors, and the development of children's interpersonal problem solving skills is in its infancy. Little, if any, work exists concerning the contributions of temperament to the development of children's social skills. The data indicate that parents are *indirectly* influential in helping their children develop socially competent behavior by reinforcing, maintaining, and sharing a positive, secure relationship with their children. Surprisingly little effort has been made to assess the *direct* means by which parents attempt to influence the development of their children's interpersonal problem-solving skills and the associations between these socialization attempts and children's·production of skilled social thought and behavior. For the most part, researchers have relied heavily on interview/questionnaire data to the neglect of observational methodology. From our perspective, this general lack of information leaves the field open for the development of interesting and important research programs concerning the interface between parent and child competence.

Individual Differences in Children's IPS Skills

The study of IPS skills began, not so much, with an eye on the development of the phenomenon, but rather with an eye on deviations from the normal and prospects for intervention (e.g., Spivack & Shure, 1974). For example, from the outset, psychologists regarded inadequate social problem solvers, regardless of age, as being "at risk" for psychological adjustment problems (Goldfried & D'Zurilla, 1969; Jahoda, 1953; Muus, 1960). Spivack and Shure (1974) were sensitive to these speculations and suggested that the well-broadcast problem-solving deficiencies of socioeconomically lower-class children (e.g., Sigel & McBane, 1967) were evident not only in the impersonal domain but also in the interpersonal domain. Their research program was reinforced by arguments presented by early Head Start education advocates that social competence should be a major focus of early intervention efforts (e.g., Zigler, 1973).

Another early source responsible for the proliferation of IPS research in the 1970s and 1980s stemmed from concerns that children who experience qualitatively impoverished peer relationships are "at risk" for a variety of social, psychological, and educational ills when they reach adolescence (see Parker & Asher, 1987, for an extensive review of this literature). Given that a lack of IPS skills was thought to contribute extensively to the development of poor peer relationships (specifically to rejection and isolation by the peer group' see Hartup, Chapter 11, this volume), it became important to demonstrate empirically that such connections existed.

In the sections that follow, we describe the IPS characteristics of two groups of children who deviate from peer group norms in that they evidence relatively high rates of either aggressive or withdrawn behavior, two of the major patterns of behavioral disturbance in childhood (Moskowitz, Schwartzman, & Ledingham, 1985). The goal of this particular review is to highlight potential areas of difficulty that may provide the applied psychologist with useful information when instituting preventative or ameliorative programs for children.

Socially Withdrawn Children

We begin first with a description of the interpersonal problem-solving characteristics of children who have been described by psychologists as socially inhibited (Kagan *et al.*, 1990) or passively withdrawn (Rubin, Hymel *et al.*, 1991). We do so because it is these children who, for whatever reason, preclude themselves from the opportunities of experiencing peer interaction, negotiation, persuasion, and conflict that purportedly influence the growth and development of social-cognitive and social skills (Doise & Mugny, 1981; Piaget, 1970).

Data concerning the interpersonal problem-solving skills and deficits of extremely withdrawn children emanate almost entirely from one laboratory at The University of Waterloo. Thus it is important that readers recognize the importance of replication and extension research in future years. At any rate, Rubin and colleagues have gathered interview and observational data concerning the developmental course of interpersonal problem-solving skills of extremely withdrawn children.

Extremely withdrawn kindergarten and Grade 2 children appear to evidence some differences from socially average children in terms of their choice of problem-solving strategies to hypothetical social dilemmas (Rubin, 1982; Rubin, 1985; Rubin, Daniels-Beirness, & Bream, 1984). For example, they suggest more adult dependent and nonassertive problem-solving strategies with regard to object conflict (kindergarten) and friendship initiation dilemmas (Grade 2). However, an examination of the problem-solving repertoires of those children identified as *continuously* withdrawn from kindergarten to Grade 2 suggests no cumulative effect of social inactivity on hypothetical-reflective reasoning. Perhaps, then, a relatively low level of peer interaction is sufficient to stimulate social problem-solving development in the early years; perhaps, too, children may acquire *knowledge* of social strategies by observing others or through conversations with and instructions from parents and other adults.

Another possibility suggested by our data is that young, withdrawn children may experience difficulties in areas other than the processing of social information. It is possible that the withdrawn child has the cognitive repertoire necessary for successful problem solving; however, as a function of the causes of withdrawal (i.e., feelings of insecurity, anxiety; negative thoughts about the self's abilities to be socially successful) (Rubin & Lollis, 1988), the child may have problems translating competent cognitions into adaptive social behaviors. Indeed, this appears to be the case.

In The Waterloo Longitudinal Project, socially withdrawn and nonwithdrawn children were paired with same-sex, same-age, nonwithdrawn play partners (e.g., Rubin & Borwick, 1984; Rubin *et al.*, 1984) and observed during free play. The data revealed that the distribution of children's goals, the means by which they attempted to meet these goals, and the success rates of these strategies varied in accord with the child's sociability. Concerning *goals*, withdrawn children were more likely to attempt to gain their partners' attention and were less likely to attempt to gain access to objects or to elicit action than their more sociable counterparts. The attention-seeking goals, which comprised over 50% of the socially withdrawn children's goals, required that their targets simply glance momentarily at the requestor; object acquisition and elicit action goals required active compliance from the targets and, as such, could be considered more "costly" to the targets. Thus the social goals of withdrawn children could be considered "safer" or of lower "cost" to their play partners than those of their more sociable age-mates.

Given the high proportion of low-cost goals, one might have predicted that the requests of withdrawn children would be more successful than those of non-withdrawn children. This was not the case. Success rates for the withdrawn versus nonwithdrawn children were 54% and 65%, respectively.

Other between-group differences were found for the total number of requests directed at targets (withdrawn children made fewer) and the proportion of direct requests (imperatives) produced (withdrawn children made fewer). Thus these data reinforce classroom-derived data that the withdrawn children were less sociable and less assertive than their nonwithdrawn age-mates. Finally, withdrawn children were more likely than their average counterparts to modify their initial requests after failure; consequently, they could be conceived as quite resilient following initial social failure.

In summary, the young, withdrawn child can be characterized as nonassertive, responsive to feedback from social partners, and yet relatively unsuccessful in his or her social problem-solving attempts. It is important to note that an analysis of the IPS goals, strategies, and outcomes for the *play partners* of the withdrawn children (compared with the partners of nonwithdrawn children; Rubin & Borwick, 1984) revealed a number of interesting differences. First, the goals of the partners of withdrawn children were more costly than those of the partners of nonwithdrawn children; second, the strategies directed to withdrawn children were more direct; third, the outcomes were more successful. These data confirm the emerging picture of the withdrawn child as a nonassertive, compliant youngster. They also suggest that children appear to regard socially withdrawn children as "easy marks." Further support for this picture is drawn from a subsequent examination of the peer management attempts of withdrawn versus nonwithdrawn second-grade children.

In a second study, Rubin (1985) observed the role relationships of children playing dyadically for two 15-minute sessions. As in the study described above socially withdrawn and nonwithdrawn children were paired with a nonwithdrawn, same-sex, same-age play partner. The data were coded so as to allow an analysis of the peer management attempts of the children; in short, it was noted each time a child requested (verbally or nonverbally) his or her playmate to perform or not to perform a behavior (Brody, Stoneman, & MacKinnon, 1982). Rubin also coded when the child asserted his or her own rights, thus attempting to influence the behavior of the partner. Finally, the success or failure of each behavior management attempt was coded.

Data analyses revealed that the withdrawn Grade 2 children were less likely to attempt to manage the behaviors of their partners; furthermore, their attempts were proportionally less likely to result in success than those of nonwithdrawn children.

Taken together, the data described paint an interesting portrait of socially withdrawn children. In early and middle childhood, withdrawn children do not appear to have major difficulties in producing strategies in response to hypothetical social dilemmas. The only consistent difference found between withdrawn and nonwithdrawn children concerned the former group's greater reliance on adult intervention and nonassertive strategies. In all other respects (number of strategies produced; response flexibility), they did not differ from their more sociable peers. When observed in the natural setting, however, socially withdrawn children were less assertive and less successful in attaining their social goals. Thus the cognitive repertoire or social cognitions of withdrawn children do not appear lacking; rather, it is in the arena of behavioral enactment and interchange that their problems are evidenced.

Aggressive Children

The association between IPS and aggressive behavior has been of interest to researchers for two decades. Much of the early work involved the study of the numbers and types of solutions children offered in situations that varied with regard to the social goals. For example, in the first programmatic set of studies on this topic, Spivack and colleagues (e.g., Spivack & Shure, 1974) indicated that children identified by teachers as aggressive generated fewer solutions to hypothetical dilemmas involving peer and parent conflict than their nonaggressive age-mates. For goals that involved the acquisition of objects or access to desired activities, Rubin and Clark (1983) found that preschoolers rated by teachers as aggressive offered as many relevant solutions as their nonaggressive counterparts to hypothetical problems. However, the aggressive youngsters were more likely to suggest agonistic or bribe strategies and less likely to offer prosocial strategies to the set of hypothetical problems.

More recent studies of elementary schoolchildren have produced somewhat similar results. Rubin, Moller, and Emptage (1987) found that children rated as aggressive by their Grade 1 teachers were not less likely to produce fewer strategies than their nonaggressive age-mates; however, their choice of particular solutions did vary from the norm. Aggressive children were more likely to suggest bribe and affect manipulation as strategies and were less likely to offer the possibility of prosocial strategies. With regard to the goal of friendship initiation, aggressive youngsters not only produced fewer relevant strategies overall, but they also had a higher proportion of bizarre/abnormal strategies and offered fewer invitations to potential friends than did the nonaggressive children. Further, when informed by the interviewer that the initial strategy would not work, aggressive children were less able to provide alternate methods to resolve the social dilemma. As such, these children could be described as less cognitively flexible than their nonaggressive counterparts. Finally, with regard to the goal of seeking help from another, aggressive youngsters were more likely to suggest strategies that involved commanding their targets ("You better help.") or using bizarre/abnormal strategies; they were also less likely to offer prosocial strategies such as asking politely.

In a study of Grades 2 to 6 children, Walters and Peters (1980) found that teacher-rated aggressive boys did not produce quantitatively fewer relevant solutions to goals involving object possession, peer group initiation, and the resolution of peer provocation; however, the quality of their solutions deviated from the norm in different ways across the three different types of dilemmas. For example, across all problems, aggressive boys were the most likely to suggest aggressive solutions as a first response. This finding suggests the primacy of an aggressive response across social situations. Aggressive boys were also more likely to seek help from others (adults) when asked how they would go about initiating a friendship, and they were more likely to suggest physically aggressive strategies in response to peer provocation.

The investigations described concern the social problem-solving concomitants of teacher-rated aggression. According to Deluty (1981), *peer*-identified aggressive elementary-school children are more likely than nonaggressive children to suggest more aggressive solutions in hypothetical situations involving the resolution of peer conflict. In this study, aggressive children did not differ from others concerning the overall number of solutions offered. Finally, Rubin, Bream, and Rose-Krasnor (1991) have discovered that in both Grades 1 and 2, peer-nominated aggressive children are less likely to offer prosocial solutions and more likely to suggest bribery as resolutions to object acquisition dilemmas; they are also more likely to suggest abnormal/bizarre resolutions to friendship initiation dilemmas (e.g., "I'd buy him a belt"; "I'd sneak into her room at night").

Taken together, these studies suggest that for certain goals (e.g., object acquisition, the resolution of peer conflict, friendship initiation), aggressive children, from the preschool through elementary-school years, are more likely than their nonaggressive age-mates to suggest that they would employ agonistic or other, nonnormative strategies to deal with interprsonal dilemmas. Interestingly, the breadth of their cognitive repertoires (as assessed by the number of suggested alternatives) do not appear lacking except perhaps during the preschool years.

Given these findings, it would appear reasonable to ask *why* it is that aggressive children offer agonistic solutions to hypothetical-reflective interviews concerning solutions to their interpersonal dilemmas. One answer may derive from research that has concerned the assessment of the task environment. According to Dodge (1986; Dodge *et al.*, 1986), children can interpret social situations and interactions in ways that are biased and/or deficient. Such misguided and potentially inaccurate perceptions may predict the strategies children choose to resolve their interpersonal dilemmas. For example, if a child has not received an invitation to a classmate's party, he or she may conclude that this negative consequence was intentional. The attribution of negative consequences to hostile, malevolent intent may evoke anger and ultimately the selection of an inappropriate, aggressive solution to the dilemma (e.g., physically attack the party giver).

Interestingly, Dodge (1986) has demonstrated that aggressive children *do* misperceive the intentions and/or thoughts of others in their social milieus. Thus when negative circumstances befall them and when the intentions of the provocateur are clearly ambiguous, aggressive children are more likely than their nonaggressive peers to insist that the negative circumstances were caused by malevolent intent. One consequence of this biased perception is that aggressive youngsters are likely to react with hostility when the believe they have been intentionally harmed (Dodge, 1980; Dodge & Frame, 1982).

The cycle of violence that aggressive children find themselves in may be exacerbated by the ways in which their age-mates interpret their intentions in socially provocative situations. For example, Dodge (1980, 1986; Dodge & Frame, 1982) has found that when negative circumstances of ambiguous intent are experienced by nonaggressive youngsters and when the perpetrator is an aggressive child, negative, hostile intentions are attributed to the provocateur. This negative attribution is much less likely to occur when the provocateur is a nonaggressive child. Needless to say, when hostile intentions are attributed to a social "outcome," nonaggressive children are more likely to respond with aggressive solutions than when the attribution is one of benign intent. Thus not only do the biased perceptions of aggressive children mediate their hostile behavioral reactions to provocation, but the biased perceptions of their nonaggressive peers about them also are likely to draw aggressive youngsters into negative interchanges (Dodge & Frame, 1982).

In summary, it seems clear that aggressive children, from as early as the preschool years, are more likely to attempt to achieve some social goals by means of aggressive, hostile, or bizarre/abnormal behaviors. It seems also as if the aggressive strategies chosen to meet their social goals are mediated by a biased "reading" of the social milieu.

Data supportive of the links between information processing and aggression have been assessed mainly through the use of hypothetical-reflective interview methods. Recently, however, Rubin et al. (1991) examined observationally (during a dyadic cooperative task situation) the social goals, the means by which the goals were achieved, the relative success rates of the chosen strategies, and the subsequent responses to failure (e.g., persistence, flexibility) of third- and fourth-grade children. They found significant relations between peer-nominated aggression and children's choice of social goals, the selection of strategies to meet their goals (as measured by responses to hypothetical-reflective scenarios), the implementation of strategies (as assessed by observations of strategy usage), and social problem-solving outcome.

Beginning with social goals, Rubin et al. (1991) found that the most highly aggressive children were more likely to attempt to stop the activities of their dyadic partners or to redirect their partner's attention to themselves or to other features of the playroom. Both of these goals may be considered disruptive, especially in a situation in which the children were supposed to be completing a required task.

With regard to the selection of strategies, the data supported previous research in which aggressive children have been found to suggest more physically aggressive strategies to resolve hypothetical social dilemmas (e.g., Dodge, 1986). Furthermore, they were also more likely to suggest bargaining; this strategy often involved offering an enticement for compliance. These data are interesting for two reasons. First, they suggest that agonism is a highly salient response in the cognitive repertoire of aggressive children. That this is the case is supported by the finding that aggressive children not only were more likely to suggest aggression as a means to meet their social goals, but also by the observation that they were more likely to use aggression to meet their social goals in natural settings. Second, it is noteworthy that, for all children, the two least frequently offered solutions to the hypothetical-reflective scenarios were physical aggression and bargaining. Thus, just as it is the case that rejected children tend to select social strategies that deviate from peer group norms (Ladd & Oden, 1979), this appears to be true for aggressive children.

Finally, with regard to the outcomes of their strategic attempts, children perceived as aggressive were reinforced at high levels by their peers. These data supported earlier reports by Patterson, Littman, and Bricker (1967) that preschool aggression is highly reinforced. Thus, although agnostic strategies may not be socially acceptable, they are nevertheless relatively effective. Consequently, the strategies employed by aggressive children may be resistant to modification attempts founded on social acceptability arguments.

Patterson (1979) has suggested that aggressive behaviors are maintained by negative reinforcement, and that they function primarily to terminate the aversive behaviors of their peers. Interestingly, in Rubin *et al.*'s (1991) study, peer-assessed aggression was associated with the frequent incidence of stop-action goals; that is aggressive children often sought to terminate the activities of their peers, and they did so with much success. If the aggressive children had perceived their peers' behavior to have been underscored often by malevolent intent (as Dodge, 1986, has reported), the data would support Patterson's contention.

In summary, there is a clear relation between social problem-solving processing skills and children's aggressive behavior. Unlike withdrawn children who appear to have few information-processing difficulties but problems with enactment, aggressive children are deficient social thinkers and actors. It is this consistent finding of a relation between social information-processing deficits and aggressive behavior that has led to the development of numerous IPS skills intervention programs.

IPS and Peer Acceptance

It has long been recognized that socially skilled behavior can lead to peer acceptance and popularity, whereas unskilled behavior can lead to peer rejection and unpopularity (e.g., Hartup, 1983). These speculations have garnered a good deal of support in the literature. For example, it has been demonstrated that the strategies enacted by popular children in response to peer group entry or socially provocative situations distinguish them from their age-mates who are rejected by the peer group (see Asher & Coie, 1990, for relevant reviews). In point of fact, the ways in which rejected children think about their interpersonal dilemmas and the ways in which they are observed to behave when confronted with social problems markedly resemble the social cognitions and social behaviors of children described earlier as aggressive or as passively withdrawn. For example, rejected children are more likely than their popular counterparts to have inappropriate social goals, to misinterpret the intentions of their peers, to suggest aggressive or other unskilled strategies to deal with their interpersonal dilemmas, and to demonstrate inflexibility when confronted with initial failure (Dodge & Feldman, 1990; Ladd & Oden, 1979; Rubin & Daniels-Beirness, 1983; Rubin, Daniels-Beirness, & Hayvren, 1982).

Given that children are rejected because they deviate from acceptable forms of social behavior (e.g., aggression or passive withdrawal, Rubin *et al.*, 1990) and given that aggressive and withdrawn children deviate (albeit differently from one another) from the norms in the ways that they respond to social dilemmas, the connection between peer acceptance and IPS is hardly surprising. Thus, in the service of brevity, we refer the reader who is interested in the literature relating IPS and popularity/rejection to the review provided about aggressive and withdrawn children or to a recent review by Dodge and Feldman (1990).

TREATING IPS DEFICITS IN CHILDREN

As noted earlier, interest in deviations from the norm have been characteristic of the IPS field from the outset. During the early 1970s, correlational studies linking poor hypothetical-reflective social problem solving to behavioral maladjustment led to the development of ameliorative programs for preschool and school-aged children (e.g., Spivack & Shure, 1974). Overall, the emerging curricula focused on enhancing the child's social cognitive skills by teaching the processing steps and abilities specified in the aforementioned social problem-solving models. These programs met a receptive audience among researchers and educators for at least two reasons (Rose-Krasnor, 1991). First, there was a relatively common disillusionment with behavioristically oriented programs that typically failed to produce generalized and long-lasting results. The self-regulating and general process orientation of the social-cognitive curricula seemed more likely to be internalized by the child and thus to generalize across time and context. Second, the content of these programs was more consistent with the prevailing Piagetian zeitgeist than existing behavioral approaches and thus had ready and widespread theoretical support.

Program formats normally included 20 to 40 small-group sessions, conducted in the child's school, two or three times a week, and usually involving a variety of teaching methods (e.g., role playing, games, brainstorming, coached practice). Implementations varied as to whether they were carried out by classroom teachers or by specially trained group leaders, and in their emphasis on the use of incidental interactions to teach social problem-solving skills. A relatively small subset of interventions involved parent training in social problem solving as either primary or secondary components (Shure & Spivack, 1978; Yu, Harris, Solovitz, & Franklin, 1986).

There were two general contexts for social problem-solving training programs. One group of intervention studies had a primarily preventative focus and was directed at relatively unselected groups of middle-class (e.g., Elardo & Caldwell, 1979; Krasnor, 1981, cited in Rubin & Krasnor, 1986) or inner-city children (e.g., Spivack & Shure, 1974; Weissberg et al., 1981). Within these unselected groups, outcomes for children with relatively high levels of aggression or inhibition have been examined.

The second group of intervention studies had a more remedial function, designed for children with already identified socioemotional difficulties (e.g., Pepler, King, & Byrd, 1991; Yu et al., 1986); these difficulties were almost universally of an externalizing nature. Programs designed for aggressive children generally differed from the preventative interventions by virtue of their greater utilization of cognitive-behavioral techniques. Remedial programs, then, frequently combined a social-cognitive orientation with a behavioral one, including the training of specific target behaviors and more explicit use of reinforcement.

A series of comprehensive reviews of the social problem-solving intervention literature is now available (Denham & Almeida, 1987; Kazdin, 1987; Kendall, 1984; Pellegrini & Urbain, 1985; Urbain & Kendall, 1980; Weissberg, 1985); the reader is referred to these sources for a detailed summary. In general, the majority of reviewers have judged that social problem-solving training has been only inconsistently effective but regard the approach as promising. Recurrent questions have focused on problems in design (e.g., lack of appropriate control groups, nonblind assessments; lack of long-term follow-up) and measurement (e.g., training to task, unreliability, lack of ecological validity). Two reviewers have reached somewhat harsher conclusions. Gresham (1985) has concluded that social problem-solving "outcome" measures have poor social validity, and that social-cognitive programs have shown no greater generalizability than strictly behavioral ones. Durlak (1983) has remained unconvinced that social problem solving is important to social adjustment and has concluded that programs based on this principle have demonstrated little use in primary prevention.

A metanalysis of social problem-solving interventions has been late in coming, and recent efforts by Denham and Almeida (1987) have proven to be welcome. Their quantitative assessment of intervention efforts has yielded several clarifying conclusions. First, Denham and Almeida report that effects of social problem-solving training on outcomes of hypothetical-reflective skill reliably exist; however, effects on skilled behavior are less certain. Second, social problem-solving interventions appear to have a greater impact on "at-risk" children than on nondisordered or special-needs children, although all three groups are positively affected. In addition, the age of the child appears to be a significant boundary condition; in general, intervention has had a stronger effect on younger children. Third, the effectiveness of intervention is positively related to the experience of the investigator. Fourth, interventions lasting more than 40 sessions are more effective than shorter training programs. Finally, there was some evidence for a link between changes in social problem-solving skills and changes in behavioral adjustment. On the basis of this analysis, a conclusion of "proceed with caution" may be justified.

Interestingly, reviews of IPS interventions have typically excluded Selman's (1980) applied work, which is focused on the development of interpersonal negotiation strategies in preadolescents and adolescents with identified socioemotional difficulties. This has been somewhat surprising, because both approaches share the goal of increasing the quality and flexibility of social strategy repertoires. Selman's interventions have the specific goal of increasing the social perspective-taking level of strategies, reaching a collaborative social orientation, and showing appropriate affective control. Implementation of these programs typically occurs in classroom group discussions, with the teacher guiding discussions and modeling advanced perspective taking as needed. This approach, however, does not emphasize a step-by-step problem-solving process, nor is it characterized by the semistructured small-group lessons present in most of the social problem-solving literature.

Peer therapy, Selman's (1985; Selman & Schultz, 1990) most recent training approach, represents a further departure from the traditional approach. Therapists help adolescents to increase the level of interpersonal negotiation strategies within a developing dyadic peer relationship. Training therefore occurs within a meaningful psychological context, as the two adolescents interact repeatedly over an extended time. The peer-therapy approach is individualized and intensive, requires a highly skilled therapist, and is of unknown effectiveness. As one of the few recent innovations in social problem-solving training methods, however, it deserves note.

The popularity of IPS training seems well established in educational and research practice. Researchers designing recent IPS interventions have been responsive to many of the early reviewers' criticisms. Current studies are better designed than those of the 1970s and early 1980s and, for example, include appropriate control groups and behavioral measures (Battistich, Solomon, Watson, & Schaps, 1989; Kazdin, Esveldt-Dawson, French, & Unis, 1987; Kendall, Reber, McLeer, Epps, & Ronan, 1991; Pepler et al., 1991; Yu et al., 1986). In spite of these improvements, however, outcome results still remain inconsistent. This lack of strong positive results may reflect continuing failure to carefully specify target groups (Kazdin, 1987), adapt programs to the child's developmental level (Kendall, 1984), include methods for helping the child deal with affective interference (Rose-Krasnor, 1991), or to fully integrate the program into the school system itself (Weissberg, 1985).

SUMMARY

In this chapter, we have attempted to examine the construct of IPS not only by reviewing the literature extant but also (a) by describing conceptual models for the processing of social information and (b) by suggesting factors that may be causally associated with its development. Our overview makes it quite clear that the study of IPS and social competence is still in its infancy. For example, little is known about biological, personality, or dispositional factors that contribute to the development of interpersonal competence. Similarly, relatively little is known about the association between familial relationships, parenting behaviors, and the development of IPS. The influence of the interaction between individual characteristics and family factors is thus also unknown. Further, the significance of culture is conspicuously absent from our knowledge base, as is the importance of other factors "external" to the child and the family (e.g., the child's or family's experience of stress and unavailability of available social support).

Given that the lack of social competence is concomitantly associated with indexes of maladaptive child development such as aggression, withdrawal, and peer rejection, and given that these latter indexes are themselves predictive of negative "outcomes," there is some urgency to "fill in the blanks" of our knowledge base. Further, by filling in the blanks, we may move several steps further in creating successful, data-based prevention and intervention programs for children. As such, we would hope that, in the years to follow, any subsequent revision of this chapter will include far less conceptual "guesswork" and far more significant information that has an empirical basis.

REFERENCES

Ainsworth, M. D. S., Blehar, M., Waters, E., & Wall, S. (1978). *Patterns of attachment*, Hillsdale, NJ: Erlbaum.

Arend, R., Gove, F., & Sroufe, L. A. (1979). Continuity of individual adaptation from infancy to kindergarten: A predictive study of ego resiliency and curiosity in preschoolers. *Child Development, 50*, 950–959.

Asher, S. R., & Coie, J. D. (1990). *Peer rejection in childhood*. New York: Cambridge University Press.

Attili, G. (1989). Social Competence versus emotional security: The link between home relationships and behavior problems in preschool. In B. Schneider, G. Atilli, J. Nadel-Brulfert, & R. Weissberg (Eds.), *Social competence in developmental perspective* (pp. 293–311). Dordrecht, The Netherlands: Kluwer International Publishers.

Bandura, A. (1989). Social cognitive theory. In R. Vasta (Ed.), *Annals of child development: A research annual. Six theories of child development: Revised formulations and current issues, Vol. 6* (pp. 1–60). Greenwich, CT: TAI Press.

Barenboim, C. (1981). The development of person perception in childhood and adolescence. From behavioral comparisons to psychological constructs to psychological comparisons. *Child Development, 52*, 129–144.

Bates J., Maslin, C. A., & Frankel, K. A. (1985). Attachment security, mother-child interaction, and temperament as predictors of behavior-problem ratings at age three years. In I. Bretherton &

E. Waters (Eds.), Growing points of attachment theory and research. *Monographs of The Society for Research in Child Development*, 50, 167–193.

Battistich, V., Solomon, D., Watson, M., & Schaps, J. (1989). Effects of an elementary school program to enhance prosocial behavior vs. children's cognitive-social problem-solving skills and strategies. *Journal of Applied Developmental Psychology*, 10, 147–169.

Baumrind, D. (1967). Child care practices anteceding three patterns of preschool behavior. *Genetic Psychology Monographs*, 76, 43–88.

Belsky, J., & Nezworski, T. (1988). *Clinical implications of attachment*. Hillsdale, NJ: Erlbaum.

Berg, C. (1989). Knowledge of strategies for dealing with everyday problems. *Developmental Psychology*, 25, 607–618.

Bjorklund, D. F. (1989). *Children's thinking: Developmental function and individual differences*. Pacific Grove, CA: Brooks/Cole.

Booth, C. L., Rose-Krasnor, L., & Rubin, K. H. (1991). Relating preschoolers' social competence and their mothers' parenting behaviors to early attachment security and high risk status. *Journal of Social and Personal Relationships*, 8, 363–382.

Bowlby, J. (1973). *Attachment and loss, Vol. 2, Separation*. New York: Basic.

Brody, G. H., Stoneman, Z., & MacKinnon, C. E. (1982). Role asymmetries in interactions among school-aged children, their younger siblings, and their friends. *Child Development*, 53, 1364–1370.

Brown, J. (1989, April). *The relation between parenting styles and children's social cognitive skills*. Paper presented at the biennial meetings of the Society for Research in Child Development, Kansas City, MO.

Campbell, S. B. (1991). Longitudinal studies of active and aggressive preschoolers: Individual differences in early behavior and in outcome. In D. Cicchetti & S. Toth (Eds.), *Rochester Symposium on Developmental Psychopathology, Vol. 2. Internalizing and externalizing expressions of dysfunction* (pp. 57–90). Hillsdale, NJ: Erlbaum.

Carlson-Jones, D., Rickel, A., & Smith, R. (1980). Maternal child-rearing practices and social problem solving strategies among preschoolers. *Developmental Psychology*, 16, 241–242.

Carver, C., & Scheirer, M. (1981). *Attention and self-regulation: A control theory approach to human behavior*. New York: Springer-Verlag.

Case, R. (1987). *Intellectual development: Birth to adulthood*. New York: Academic Press.

Chandler, M. (1985). Social structures and social cognitions. In R. A Hinde, A. Perret-Clermont, & J. Stevenson-Hinde (Eds.), *Social relationships and cognitive development* (pp. 252–266). Oxford, UK: Clarendon Press.

Clark, R. A., & Delia, J. G. (1976). The development of functional persuasive skills in childhood and early adolescence. *Child Development*, 47, 1008–1014.

Clark, M. S., & Isen, A. M. (1981). Toward understanding the relationship between feeling states and social behavior. In A. H Hastorf & A. M. Isen (Eds.), *Cognitive social psychology* (pp. 73–108). New York: Elsevier.

Cooney, E. W., & Selman, R. L. (1978). Children's use of social conceptions: Towards a dynamic model of social cognition. In W. Damon (Ed.), *Social cognition: New directions for child development, Vol. 1* (pp. 23–44). San Francisco: Jossey-Bass.

Cowan, G., & Avants, S. (1988). Children's influence strategies: Structures, sex differences, and bilateral mother-child influence *Child Development*, 59, 1303–1313.

Cowan, G., Drinkard, J., & MacGavin, L. (1984). The effects of target, age and gender in the use of power strategies. *Journal of Personality and Social Psychology*, 47, 1391–1398.

Cox, D., & Waters H. (1986). Sex differences in the use of strategies: A developmental analysis. *Journal of Experimental Child Psychology*, 41, 18–37.

Crick, N. R., & Dodge, K. A. (1989, March). *Rejected children's perceptions and expectations of social interaction*. Paper presented at the annual meeting of the American Educational Research Association, San Francisco.

Crick, N. R., & Ladd, G. W. (1990). Children's perceptions of the outcomes of social strategy: Do the ends justify the means. *Developmental Psychology*, 26, 612–620.

Damon, W. (1977). *The social world of the child*. San Francisco: Jossey-Bass.

Deluty, R. (1981). Alternative thinking ability of aggressive, assertive and submissive children. *Cognitive Therapy and Research*, 5, 309–312.

Deluty, R. H. (1985). Cognitive mediators of aggression, assertive and submissive behavior in childhood. *International Journal of Behavioural Development*, 8, 355–369.

Denham, S., & Almeida, M. (1987). Children's social problem-solving skills, behavioral adjustment, and interventions: A meta-analysis evaluating theory and practice. *Journal of Applied Developmental Psychology, 8*, 391–409.

Dodge, K. A. (1980). Social cognition and children's aggressive behavior. *Child Development, 51*, 162–170.

Dodge, K. A. (1983). Behavioral antecedents of peer social status. *Child Development, 54*, 1386–1399.

Dodge, K. A. (1985). Facets of social interaction and the assessment of social competence in children. In B. Schneider, K. H. Rubin, & J. Ledingham (Eds.), *Children's peer relations: Issues in assessment and intervention* (pp. 3–22) New York: Springer-Verlag.

Dodge, K. A. (1986). A social information processing model of social competence in children. In M. Perlmutter (Ed.), *Cognitive perspectives on children's social and behavioral development. The Minnesota Symposia on Child Psychology* (Vol. 18) (pp. 77–126) Hillsdale, NJ: Erlbaum.

Dodge, K. A. (in press). Emotion and social information processing. In J. Garber & K. A. Dodge (Eds.), *The development of emotion regulation and dysregulation.* New York: Cambridge University Press.

Dodge, K. A., & Feldman, E. (1990). Issues in social cognition and sociometric status. In S. A. Asher & J. D. Coie (Eds.), *Peer rejection in childhood* (pp. 119–155). New York: Cambridge University Press.

Dodge, K. A., & Frame, C. L. (1982). Social cognitive biases and deficits in aggressive boys. *Child Development, 53*, 620–635.

Dodge, K. A., Pettit, G. S., McClaskey, C. L., & Brown, M. (1986). Social competence in children. *Monographs of the Society for Research in Child Development, 51* (Serial No. 213).

Doise, W., & Mugny, G. (1981). *Le développement social de l'intelligence.* Paris: Inter Editions.

Downey, G., & Walker, E. (1989). Social cognition and adjustment in children at risk for psychopathology. *Developmental Psychology, 25*, 835–845.

Durlak, J. A. (1983). Social problem-solving as a primary prevention strategy. In R. Felner, L. Jason, J. Maritsugu, & S. Farber (Eds.), *Preventive psychology* (pp. 31–48). New York: Pergamon Press.

Elardo, P., & Caldwell, B. (1979). The effects of an experimental social development program on children in the middle childhood period. *Psychology in the Schools, 16*, 93–100.

Elias M. J., Rothbaum, R., & Gara, M. (1986). Social-cognitive problem solving in children: Assessing the knowledge and application of skills. *Journal of Applied Developmental Psychology, 7*, 77–94.

Evans, M., & Rubin, K. H. (1979). Hand gestures as a communicative mode in school-aged children. *Journal of Genetic Psychology, 135*, 189–196.

Flavell, J. H., Bodkin, P. T., Fry, C. L., Wright, J. W., & Jarvis, P. E. (1968). *The development of role-taking and communication skills in children.* New York: Wiley.

Ford, M. E. (1982). Social cognition and social competence in adolescence. *Developmental Psychology, 18*, 323–340.

Glucksberg, S., & Krauss, R. (1967). What do people say after they have learned how to talk: Studies of the development of referential communication. *Merrill-Palmer Quarterly, 13*, 309–316.

Goetz, T., & Dweck, C. (1980). Learned helplessness in social situations. *Journal of Personality and Social Psychology, 39*, 246–255.

Goldberg, S., Lojkasek, M., Gartner, G., & Corter, C. (1989). Maternal responsiveness and social development in preterm infants. In M. H. Bornstein (Ed.), *Maternal responsiveness: Characteristics and consequences* (pp. 89–103). San Francisco: Jossey-Bass.

Goldfried, M. R., & D'Zurilla, T. J. (1969). A behavior-analytic model for assessing competence. In C. D. Spielberger (Ed.), *Current topics in clinical and community psychology* (pp. 151–198). New York: Academic Press.

Gresham, F. (1985). Utility of cognitive-behavioral procedures for social skills training with children: A critical review. *Journal of Abnormal Child Psychology, 13*, 411–423.

Guerra, N. G., & Slaby, R. G. (1989). Evaluative factors in social problem solving by aggressive boys. *Journal of Abnormal Child Psychology, 17*, 277–289.

Harter, S. (1982). The Perceived Competence Scale for Children. *Child Development, 53*, 87–97.

Harter, S. (1985). *Manual for the Self-Perception Profile for Children.* Denver: University of Denver.

Hartup, W. W. (1983). Peer relations. In E. M. Hetherington (Ed.), *Handbook of child psychology: Vol. 4. Socialization, personality and social development* (pp. 103–198). New York: Wiley.

Hartup, W. W. (1985). Relationships and their significance in cognitive development. In R. A. Hinde, A. Perret-Clermont, & J. Stevenson-Hinde (Eds.), *Social relationships and cognitive development* (pp. 66–82). Oxford, UK: Clarendon Press.

Hutt, C. (1966). Exploration and play in children. *Symposium of the Zoological Society of London, 18*, 61–81.

Hymel, S., & Franke, S. (1985). Children's peer relations: Assessing self perceptions. In B H. Schneider, K. H. Rubin, & J. E. Ledingham (Eds.), *Peer relationships and social skills in childhood: Issues in assessment and training* (pp. 251–297). New York: Springer-Verlag.

Jacquette, D. S. (1980). A case study of social-cognitive development in a naturalistic setting. In R. Selman, *The growth of interpersonal understanding: Developmental and clinical analyses* (pp. 215–242). New York: Academic Press.

Jahoda, M. (1953). The meaning of psychological health. *Social Casework, 34,* 349–354.

Kagan, J. (1989a). Temperamental contributions to social behavior. *American Psychologist, 44,* 668–674.

Kagan, J. (1989b). *Unstable ideas: Temperament, cognition, and self.* Cambridge, MA: Harvard University Press.

Kagan, J., Reznick, J. S., & Snidman, N. (1990). The temperamental qualities of inhibition and lack of inhibition. In M. Lewis & S. M. Miller (Eds.), *Handbook of developmental psychopathology* (pp. 219–226). New York: Plenum Press.

Kazdin, A. E. (1987). Treatment of antisocial behavior in children: Current status and future directions. *Psychological Bulletin, 102,* 187–203.

Kazdin, A. E., Esveldt-Dawson, K., French, N. H., & Unis, A. S. (1987). Problem-solving skills training and relationship therapy in treatment of antisocial child behavior. *Journal of Consulting Clinical Psychology, 55,* 76–85.

Keltikangas-Jävinen, L., & Kangas, P. (1988). Problem solving strategies in aggressive and nonaggressive children. *Aggressive Behavior, 14,* 255–264.

Kendall, P. C. (1984). Social cognition and problem solving: A developmental and child-clinical interface. In B. Gholson & T. Rosenthal (Eds.), *Applications of cognitive-developmental theory* (pp. 118–148). New York: Academic Press.

Kendall, P. C., Reber, M., McLeer, S., Epps, J., & Ronan, K. (1991). Cognitive behavioral treatment of conduct disordered children. In D. Pepler & K. H. Rubin (Eds.), *The developmental and treatment of childhood aggression* (pp. 341–360). Hillsdale, NJ: Erlbaum.

Krasnor, L. R. (1982). An observational study of social problem solving in young children. In K. Rubin & H. Ross (Eds.), *Peer relationship and social skills* (pp. 113–132). New York: Springer-Verlag.

Krasnor, L. R. (1985). Observational assessment of social problem solving. In B. Schneider, K. H. Rubin, & J. Ledingham (Eds.), *Children's peer relations: Issues in assessment and intervention* (pp. 57–74). New York: Springer-Verlag.

Krasnor, L. R. (1988). Social cognition. In T. Yawkey & J. Johnson (Eds.), *Integrative processes and socialization: Early to middle childhood* (pp. 79–96). Hillsdale, NJ: Erlbaum.

Krasnor, L., & Rubin, K. H. (1983). Preschool social problem solving: Attempts and outcomes in naturalistic interaction. *Child Development, 54,* 1545–1558.

Ladd, G. W., & Oden, S. L. (1979). The relationship between peer acceptance and children's ideas about helpfulness. *Child Development, 52,* 171–178.

Leadbeater, B. J., Helner, J., Allen J. P., & Aber, J. L. (1989). Assessment of interpersonal negotiation strategies in youth engaged in problem behavior. *Developmental Psychology, 25,* 465–472.

Levin, E., & Rubin, K. H. (1983). Getting others to do what you want them to do: The development of children's requestive strategies. In K. Nelson (Ed.), *Children's language* (Vol. 4). Hillsdale, NJ: Erlbaum.

McFall, R. M. (1982). A review and reformulation of the concept of social skills. *Behavioral Assessment, 4,* 1–33.

Mead, G. (1934). *Mind, self and society.* Chicago: University of Chicago Press.

Michaelson, L., & Mannarino, A. (1986). Social skills training with children: Research and clinical application. In P. Strain, M. Guralnick, & H. Walker (Eds.), *Children's social behavior* (pp 373–406). New York: Academic Press.

Miller, G., Galanter, E., & Pribram, K. (1960). *Plans and the structure of behavior.* New York: Holt, Rinehart & Winston.

Moskowitz, D. S., Schwartzman, A. E., & Ledingham, J. E. (1985). Stability and change in aggression and withdrawal in middle childhood and early adolescence. *Journal of Abnormal Psychology, 94,* 30–41.

Muus, R. (1960). Mental health implications of a preventative psychiatry program in light of research findings. *Marriage and Family Living, 22,* 150–156.

Nakamura, C., & Finck, D. (1980). Relative effectiveness of socially oriented and task oriented children and predictability of their behavior. *Monograph of the Society for Research in Child Development, 45*(3–4, Serial 185).

Newell, H., & Simon, H. (1972). *Human problem solving.* Englewood Cliffs, NJ: Prentice-Hall.

Oppenheimer, L. (1989). The nature of social action: Social competence versus social conformism. In B. Schneider, G. Atilli, J. Nadel, & R. Weissberg (Eds.), *Social competence in developmental perspective* (pp. 41–70). Dordrecht, Netherlands: Kluwer International Publishers.

Parker, J. G., & Asher, S. R. (1987). Peer acceptance and later personal adjustment: Are low-accepted children "at risk"? *Psychological Bulletin, 102,* 357–389.

Patterson, G. (1979). A performance theory for coercive family interaction. In R. Cairns (Ed.), *The analysis of social interactions* (pp. 119–161). Hillsdale, NJ: Erlbaum.

Patterson, G., Littman, R. A., & Bricker, W. (1967). Assertive behavior in children: A step toward a theory of aggression. *Monographs of the Society for Research in Child Development, 35* (No. 5).

Pellegrini, D. S., & Urbain, E. S. (1985). An evaluation of interpersonal cognitive problem solving training with children. *Journal of Child Psychology and Psychiatry, 26,* 17–41.

Pepler, D., King, G., & Byrd, W. (1991). A social cognitively based social skills training program for aggressive children. In D. Pepler & K. Rubin (Eds.), *The development and treatment of childhood aggression* (pp. 361–379). Hillsdale, NJ: Erlbaum.

Perlmutter, M. (Ed.). (1986). *Cognitive perspectives on children's social and behavioral development. The Minnesota Symposia on Child Psychology* (Vol. 18). Hillsdale, NJ: Erlbaum.

Pettit, G. S., Dodge, K. A., & Brown, M. M. (1988). Early family experience, social problem solving patterns and children's social competence. *Child Development, 54,* 107–120.

Piaget, J. (1926). *The language and thought of the child.* London: Routlege & Kegan Paul.

Piaget, J. (1970). Piaget's theory. In P. Mussen (Ed.) *Carmichael's manual of child psychology, Vol. 1.* New York: Wiley.

Piché, G., Rubin, D., & Michlin, M. (1978). Age and social class in children's use of persuasive communicative appeals. *Child Development, 49,* 773–780.

Rose-Krasnor, L. (1991). Commentary: Social cognitive treatment programs. In D. Pepler & K. Rubin (Eds.), *The development and treatment of childhood aggression* (pp. 380–386). Hillsdale, NJ: Erlbaum.

Rubin, K. H. (1982). Social and social-cognitive developmental characteristics of young isolate, normal and social children. In K. H. Rubin & H. S. Ross (Eds.), *Peer relationships and social skills in childhood* (pp. 353–374). New York: Springer-Verlag.

Rubin, K. H. (1985). Socially withdrawn children: An "at risk" population? In B. Schneider, K. H. Rubin, & J. Ledingham (Eds.), *Children's peer relations: Issues in assessment and intervention* (pp. 125–139). New York: Springer-Verlag.

Rubin, K. H., & Borwick, D. (1984). Communicative skills and sociability. In H. E. Sypher & J. L. Applegate (Eds.), *Communication by children and adults: Social cognitive and strategic processes* (pp. 152–170). Beverly Hills, CA: Sage Publications.

Rubin, K. H., Bream, L., & Rose-Krasnor, L. (1991). Social problem solving and aggression in childhood. In D. J. Pepler & K. H. Rubin (Eds.), *The development and treatment of childhood aggression* (pp. 219–248). Hillsdale, NJ: Erlbaum.

Rubin, K. H., & Clark, M. L. (1983). Preschool teachers' rating of behavioral problems Observational, sociometric, and social-cognitive correlates. *Journal of Abnormal Child Psychology, 11,* 273–285.

Rubin, K. H., & Daniels-Beirness, T. (1983). Concurrent and predictive correlates of sociometric status in kindergarten and grade one children. *Merrill-Palmer Quarterly, 29,* 337–352.

Rubin, K. H., Daniels-Beirness, T., & Bream, L. (1984). Social isolation and social problem solving: A longitudinal study. *Journal of Consulting and Clinical Psychology, 52,* 17–25.

Rubin, K. H., Daniels-Beirness, T., & Hayvren, M. (1982). Social and social cognitive correlates of sociometric status in preschool and kindergarten children. *Canadian Journal of Behavioural Science, 14,* 338–348.

Rubin, K. H., Fein, G., & Vandenberg, B. (1983). Play. In E. M. Hetherington (Ed.), *Handbook of child psychology: Socialization, personality and social development* (pp. 693–774). New York: Wiley.

Rubin, K. H., Hymel, S., Mills, R. S. L., & Rose-Krasnor, L. (1991). Pathways to and from social withdrawal in childhood: A conceptual and empirical analysis. In D. Cicchetti & M. Toth (Eds.). *Rochester Symposium on Developmental Psychopathology, Vol. 2. Internalizing and externalizing expressions of dysfunction* (pp. 91–122). Hillsdale, NJ: Erlbaum.

Rubin, K. H., & Krasnor, L. R. (1983). Age and gender differences in the development of a representative social problem solving skill. *Journal of Applied Developmental Psychology, 4,* 463–475.

Rubin, K. H., & Krasnor, L. R. (1986). Social-cognitive and social behavioral perspectives on problem solving. In M. Perlmutter (Ed.), *Cognitive perspectives on children's social and behavioral development. The Minnesota Symposia on Child Psychology* (Vol. 18; pp. 1–68). Hillsdale, NJ: Erlbaum.

Rubin, K. H., LeMare, L. J., & Lollis, S. (1990). Social withdrawal in childhood: Developmental pathways to rejection. In S. R. Asher & J. D. Coie (Eds), *Peer rejection in childhood* (pp. 217–249). New York: Cambridge University Press.

Rubin, K. H., & Lollis, S. (1988). Peer relationships, social skills and infant attachment: A continuity model. In J. Belsky (Ed.), *Clinical implications of infant attachment* (pp. 219–252). Hillsdale, NJ: Erlbaum.

Rubin, K. H., & Mills, R. S. L. (1988). The many faces of social isolation in childhood. *Journal of Consulting and Clinical Psychology, 56,* 916–924.

Rubin, K. H., & Mills, R. S. L. (1990). Maternal beliefs about adaptive and maladaptive social behaviors in normal, aggressive and withdrawn preschoolers. *Journal of Abnormal Child Psychology, 18,* 419–436.

Rubin, K. H., Mills, R. S. L., & Krasnor, L. (1989). Parental beliefs and children's social competence. In B. Schneider, G. Atilli, J. Nadel, & R. Weissberg (Eds.), *Social competence in developmental perspective* (pp. 313–331). Dordrecht, The Netherlands: Kluwer International Publishers.

Rubin, K. H., Moller, L., & Emptage, A. (1987). The Preschool Behavior Questionnaire: A useful index of behavior problems in elementary school-age children? *Canadian Journal of Behavioural Sciences, 19,* 86–100.

Rubin, K. H., Rose-Krasnor, L., & Booth, C. (1990, May). *The correlates of stable versus unstable attachment status at four years.* Paper presented at the sixth biennial meeting of the University of Waterloo Conference on Child Development, Waterloo, Ontario.

Ruble, D. N., Boggiano, A. K., Feldman, N. S., & Loebel, J. H. (1980). Developmental analyses of the role of social comparison in self-evaluation. *Developmental Psychology, 16,* 105–115.

Schank, R., & Abelson, S. (1977). *Scripts, plans, goals, and understanding.* Hillsdale, NJ: Erlbaum.

Schultz, L. H., & Selman, R. L. (1989). Bridging the gap between interpersonal thought and action in early adolescence. *Development and Psychopathology, 1* 133–152.

Selman, R. L. (1980). *The growth of interpersonal understanding: Developmental and clinical analyses.* New York: Academic Press.

Selman, R. L. (1985). The use of interpersonal negotiation strategies and communicative competences: A clinical-developmental exploration in a pair of troubled early adolescents. In R. A. Hinde, A. Perret-Clermont, & J. Stevenson-Hinde (Eds.), *Social relationships and cognitive development* (pp. 208–232). Oxford: Clarendon Press.

Selman, R. L., & Byrne, D. F. (1974). A structural developmental analysis of level of role taking in middle childhood. *Child Development, 45,* 803–806.

Selman, R. L., & Demorest, A. P. (1986). Putting thoughts and feelings into perspective: A developmental version of how children deal with interpersonal disequilibrium. In D. J. Bearison & H. Zimilies (Eds.), *Thought and emotion* (pp. 93–128). Hillsdale, NJ: LEA.

Selman, R. L., & Schultz, L. H. (1988). Interpersonal thought and action in the case of a troubled early adolescent: Toward a developmental model of the gap. In S. Shick (Ed.), *Cognitive development and child psychotherapy* (pp. 207–246). New York Plenum Press.

Selman, R. L., & Schultz, L. H. (1989). Children's strategies for interpersonal negotiation with peers: An interpretive/empirical approach to the study of social development. In T. J. Berndt & G. W. Ladd (Eds.), *Peer relationships in child development* (pp. 371–406). New York: Wiley.

Selman, R. L., & Schultz, L. H. (1990). *Making a friend in youth: Developmental theory and pair therapy.* Chicago: University of Chicago Press.

Selman, R. L., Schorin, M. Z., Stone, C. R., & Phelps, E. (1983). A naturalistic study of children's social understanding. *Developmental Psychology, 19,* 82–102.

Shantz, C. U. (1983). Social cognition. In J. H. Flavell & E. Markman (Eds.), *Handbook of child psychology: Vol. 3. Cognitive development* (pp. 495–555). New York: Wiley.

Sharp, K. (1981). Impact of interpersonal problem solving training on preschoolers' social competency. *Journal of Applied Developmental Psychology, 2,* 129–143.

Shure, M., & Spivack, G. (1978). *Problem solving techniques in childrearing,* San Francisco: Jossey-Bass.

Sigel, I. E. (1982) The relationship between parents' distancing strategies and the child's cognitive behavior. In L. M. Laosa & I. E. Sigel (Eds.), *Families as learning environments for children* (pp. 47–86). New York: Plenum.

Sigel, I., & McBane, S. (1967). Cognitive competence and level of symbolization among five-year-old children. In J. Hellmuth (Ed.), *Disadvantaged child.* New York: Brunner Mazel.

Simon, H. (1967). Motivation and emotional control of cognition. *Psychological Review, 74,* 29–39.

Spieker, S. J., & Booth, C. L. (1988). Maternal antecedents of attachment quality. In J. Belsky & T. Nezworski (Eds.), *Clinical implications of attachment* (pp. 95–136). Hillsdale, NJ: Erlbaum.

Spivack, G., Platt, J. J., & Shure, M. B. (1976). *The Problem solving approach to adjustment.* San Francisco: Jossey-Bass.

Spivack, G., & Shure, M. B. (1974). *Social adjustment of young children.* San Francisco: Jossey-Bass.

Sroufe, L. A. (1983). Infant-caregiver attachment and patterns of adaptation in preschool: Roots of maladaptation and competence. In M. Perlmutter (Ed.), *Minnesota Symposia on Child Psychology* (Vol 16). Hillsdale, NJ: Erlbaum.

Strayer, F. F. (1989). Co-adaptation within the early peer group: A psychobiological study of social competence. In B. Schneider, G. Atilli, J. Nadel, & R. Weissberg (Eds.), *Social Competence in developmental perspective* (pp. 145–174). Dordrecht, The Netherlands: Kluwer International Publishers.

Thomas, A., & Chess, S. (1977). *Temperament and development*. New York: Brunner/Mazel.

Thomas, A., Chess, S., & Birch, H. G. (1968). *Temperament and behavior disorders in children*. New York: New York University Press.

Thomas, A., Chess, S., & Korn, S. (1982). The reality of difficult temperament. *Merrill-Palmer Quarterly*, *28*, 1–20.

Urbain, E. S., & Kendall, P. C. (1980). Review of social-cognitive problem-solving interventions with children. *Psychological Bulletin*, *88*, 109–143.

Vygotsky, L. (1978). *Mind in society: The development of higher psychological processes*. Cambridge, MA: Harvard University Press.

Walters, J., & Peters, R. D. (June 1980). *Social problem solving in aggressive boys*. Paper presented at the annual meeting of the Canadian Psychological Association, Calgary.

Waters, E., & Sroufe, L. A. 91983). Social competence as a developmental construct. *Developmental Review*, *3*, 79–97.

Weissberg, R. (1985). Designing effective social problem solving for the classroom. In B. Schneider, K. Rubin, & J. Ledingham (Eds.), *Children's peer relations: Issues in assessment and intervention* (pp. 225–242). New York: Springer-Verlag.

Weissberg, R. (1989). Challenges inherent in translating theory and basic research into effective social competence promotion programs. In B. Schneider, G. Atilli, J. Nadel, & R. Weissberg (Eds.), *Social competence in developmental perspective* (pp. 313–331). Dordrecht, The Netherlands: Kluwer International Publishers.

Weissberg, R., Gesten, E., Rapkin, B., Cowan, E., Davidson, E., Flores de Apodica, R., & McKim, M. (1981). Evaluation of a social problem-solving training program for suburban and inner-city third-grade children. *Journal of Consulting Clinical Psychology*, *49*, 251–261.

Werner, H. (1948). *Comparative psychology of mental development*. New York: International Universities Press.

Wheeler, V. A., & Ladd, G. W. (1982). Assessment of children's self efficacy for social interactions with peers. *Developmental Psychology*, *18*, 795–805.

White, R. W. (1959). Motivation reconsidered: The concept of competence. *Psychological Review*, *66*, 297–333.

Yu, P., Harris, G. E., Solovitz, B., & Franklin, J. (1986). A social problem-solving intervention for children at high risk for later psychopathology. *Journal of Clinical Child Psychology*, *45*, 30–40.

Zigler, E. (1973). Project Head Start: Success or failure? *Learning*, *1*, 43–47.

13

Gender Identity and Sex Roles

Marion O'Brien

Introduction

Although infants are born with an identifiable gender, they must acquire a gender-role identity. Recent trends toward feminism, along with an increased emphasis on studying human development across the lifespan, have made it clear that an individual's gender-role identity involves more than simply recognizing oneself as male or female. Further, adoption of attitudes and behaviors that are associated with gender roles is a lifelong process, one that profoundly influences the nature of an individual's transactions with others.

The process of acquiring a gender-role identity is a crucial aspect of social development. Because gender is an enduring characteristic of an individual (unlike age or height or attractiveness), aspects of a person's childhood gender identity may influence development through adulthood. In addition, in virtually all cultures, the social world is based on gender categories. Even a very young child must be able to recognize males and females, place him- or herself in the correct category, and meet others' expectations of appropriate behavior for a girl or a boy.

Although gender roles are based on biological sex, the two are not completely overlapping. *Biological sex* refers to the morphological and physiological characteristics of males and females; these form two discrete and distinct categories. A *gender role* or *sex role* is a set of attitudes and a behavioral repertoire associated by cultural convention with being male or female. Here the categories become blurred. Attitudes and behaviors considered typical of males may also be commonly observed in females. Within a given culture, there is a set of more-or-less defining properties of male and female roles that are termed *sex-role stereotypes*. A

Marion O'Brien • Department of Human Development, University of Kansas, Lawrence, Kansas 66045.

Handbook of Social Development: A Lifespan Perspective, edited by Vincent B. Van Hasselt and Michel Hersen. Plenum Press, New York, 1992.

person's behavior is *sex typed* when it fits these stereotypes, and *cross-sex* when it fits the stereotypes for the other gender. The term *sex differences* refers to attributes and abilities that are consistently observed more often in females or in males. Finally, *gender identity* or *gender-role identity* may be defined as the extent to which an individual consciously adopts attitudes and behaviors considered typical for his or her gender.

This chapter begins with a discussion of biological sex differences and how they are reflected in cultural stereotypes and individual behavior. In the next section, theories regarding the acquisition of knowledge about gender roles and development of gender identity are reviewed. The remainder of the chapter describes the current state of knowledge concerning the development of children's gender-role identity, from the beginnings of gender-based categorization in infancy through the establishment of sexual preference in adolescence.

BIOLOGICAL AND BEHAVIORAL SEX DIFFERENCES

There is no doubt that human males and females differ. Biological gender identity is genetically determined by one pair of chromosomes: XX in females, XY in males. When the Y chromosome is present, testes develop beginning in the sixth week of gestation, and the secretion of testosterone and other androgens induces the development of male reproductive structures and external genitalia. Drawing largely from animal studies and a few human investigations, some researchers have suggested that prenatal androgens also influence brain development; however, to date, the evidence is inconclusive (see Hood, Draper, Crockett, & Petersen, 1987, for a more complete discussion of this topic).

After birth, hormonal influences on male and female development are most pronounced at puberty, with the appearance of secondary sex characteristics. Boys' voices become deeper, their beards begin to grow, and their genitals increase in size. In girls, breasts develop and hips widen. Both boys and girls grow underarm and pubic hair. Experimental manipulation of endocrine levels in animals indicate that pubertal hormonal changes are associated with increases in sexual behaviors and, for males, in aggression (Beeman, 1947; Edwards, 1969). The extent to which biological sex differences influence behavior is a key question in the study of gender identity and sex-role development. Research into the direct role of biological mechanisms on human behavior has centered on (a) studies of clinical syndromes in which biological sex and identified gender differ and (b) assessments of newborn infants.

Clinical Syndromes

Several different types of syndromes in which an individual's genetic sex, prenatal hormonal exposure, and identified gender at birth do not match have been investigated to identify the relative influence of biological and socialization factors on the development of gender-related behavior. Much of this research has been carried out at Johns Hopkins and is summarized in Money and Ehrhardt (1972).

In *adrenogenital syndrome* (AGS), genetic females are exposed to high levels of androgens prenatally, resulting in a partial masculinization of the external genitals and perhaps on the developing brain. Raised as females, AGS individuals are reported to be described as tomboys and to prefer masculine sex-typed toys and activities (Money & Ehrhardt, 1972). These findings suggest that prenatal hormones have a direct influence on behavior. However, because parents of these girls know about their condition from birth, and no observation of parental socialization practices has been carried out, the results of this investigation are ambiguous (see Eccles-Parsons, 1982, for a more extensive discussion).

Some genetic males are insensitive to androgens and therefore develop as females and are reared as girls. The girls and women with *angrogen insensitivity* described by Money and Ehrhardt (1972) were highly feminine in interests and behavior. Thus genetic sex alone appears to have little influence on the development of a consistent gender identity.

Turner's syndrome involves a chromosomal abnormality in which only one X chromosome is present, rather than a pair (XX or XY). Children with Turner's syndrome are raised as female but have neither ovaries nor testes and thus are exposed to neither androgens nor estrogen prenatally. Turner's syndrome girls are described as typical in terms of their play interest and sex-role attitudes, with perhaps a slightly more feminine orientation than a comparison group (Money & Ehrhardt, 1972).

In general, these studies of individuals with genetic or hormonal abnormalities suggest a stronger role for socialization practices than for biological factors in determining gender-role adoption. Nevertheless, the methodological difficulties, including small sample sizes and likelihood of confounds between biological and socialization factors, make it impossible to conclude that the issue is closed. As techniques for measuring hormonal levels become refined, the relative influence of different levels of prenatal androgens on the behavior and development of males and females may allow more definitive studies of the interconnections between biology and behavior.

Sex Differences in Newborn Behavior

Because boys and girls are responded to differently from the day of birth, any observation of behavioral differences that are linked directly to biology must be made in the newborn period. Few observers of newborns report sex differences. Unfortunately, investigators rarely indicate whether they have analyzed for sex effects and found no statistically significant differences or simply did not carry out the analyses. One potential problem in identifying sex differences in infancy is the instability in newborn behavior, which makes identification of a reliable and replicable statistical effect difficult.

Some newborn sex differences may be attributable to maturational effects, as girls tend to be physically more advanced than boys at birth (Garai & Scheinfeld, 1968). Probably related to this difference in maturation rate is the increased vulnerability of male infants, who are subject to higher rates of mortality and morbidity (McMilen, 1979).

A few studies have reported behavioral sex differences in newborns. In one program of research, Bell and colleagues found that girls are more sensitive to external stimuli and to pain (Bell, 1960; Bell & Costello, 1964) and that boys lift their heads higher than girls when prone (Bell, Weller, & Waldrop, 1971). Although boys are widely believed to be more active than girls (even prenatally), there is no evidence for such a difference in infants (Maccoby & Jacklin, 1974). Infant boys tend to be described as more fussy and irritable than girls (Moss, 1967) and to be less likely to maintain eye contact with a caregiver (Hittleman & Dickes, 1979). Although widely reported, none of these findings has been widely replicated, nor is there a consistent pattern of sex differences in newborns that is clearly associable with later behavioral development.

By contrast to the paucity of evidence for newborn sex differences, the behavior of adults toward newborns shows clear patterns of sex typing. Parental perceptions of infants differ depending upon the baby's sex: males are seen as more alert, better coordinated, and stronger, whereas females are described as soft, weak, and more delicate (Rubin, Provenzano, & Luria, 1974). Babies' facial expressions, too, are interpreted differently, in a direction consistent with sex-role stereotypes, depending on the perceived gender of the infant (Condry & Condry, 1976; Haviland 1977). Within the context of the family, infant boys and girls are responded to differently. Mothers talk more to girls and provide more distal stimulation to boys (Lewis, 1974; Moss, 1967); fathers cuddle girls but play actively with boys (Lamb, 1978).

The weight of evidence suggests there are few, if any, behavioral differences in infancy that occur independently of the process of socialization. It is possible that small sex-related variation in behavioral characteristics might be modified over time as children respond to and are responded to in the social environment. However, the strength of the findings for differences in adult behavior toward infants, combined with the inconsistency in findings of differences in infant behavior, suggest that biological sex has little direct influence on early behavioral development.

DEFINING PROPERTIES OF GENDER ROLES

The most obvious and pervasive aspect of the biological differences between males and females is, of course, reproductive. Females bear children; males do not. It is clear that the evolutionary heritage of humans has biologically prepared females for childbearing. What is less clear, despite the often ingenious arguments of sociobiologists, is the role of evolutionary mechanisms in determining behavioral differences between men and women.

Those who espouse an evolutionary basis for cultural sex roles cite as evidence consistencies across cultures in patterns of male and female behavior (Goldberg, 1974; Hutt, 1972a,b). For example, in almost all cultures, women are the primary nurturers of children and men the primary defenders against external threat (Rosenblatt & Cunningham, 1976). The ultimate question, for which no definitive answer is currently available, is whether or not the behavior patterns associated with these social functions arise from inherent differences in abilities and psychological traits. An alternative explanation is that gender differences arise from the consistent performance of gender-specific social roles throughout childhood and into adulthood. From another perspective, the issue is whether the similarity across cultures represents individual adaptation (genetically based and hence inevitable) or cultural adaptation (socially based and hence modifiable). (For an elegant argument against biological determinism, see Lewontin, Rose, & Karmin, 1984.)

Despite the commonalities in male and female roles across cultures, specific aspects of behavior associated with sex differences are found to vary widely across cultures. Further, men and women within a culture are typically more similar to each other than are men or women across cultures. For example, although men are considered more aggressive than women throughout most of the world, the within-culture between-sex differences are relatively small compared with the within-sex cross-cultural differences (Rohmer, 1976). In addition, cultures in which adult sex roles are similar also tend to share similar child-rearing patterns and socialization practices (Barry, Bacon, & Child, 1957), leaving open the question of causality.

Gender roles within a culture may be conceptualized as complex social conventions that are learned during childhood and adopted, to a greater or lesser degree, through the course of development. Individual differences arising from both biological and social influences will affect what is learned, the extent to which the set of attitudes and behaviors defining the social convention associated with one's gender is adhered to, and personal satisfaction with one's gender role. In the remainder of this chapter, the developmental processes involved in learning about gender roles and acquiring a behavioral repertoire that is consonant both with cultural stereotypes and individual skills and preferences will be explored.

THEORETICAL APPROACHES

The acquisition of gender identity and adoption of culturally defined sex roles are topics that have been addressed within most major developmental theories. In fact, gender issues have not infrequently served as tests of predictions arising from different theoretical perspectives. In this section, the major theoretical approaches to the development of gender identity and adoption of sex-typical attitudes and behaviors will be briefly reviewed. (For a more complete discussion of the theories of sex-role development, see Huston, 1983.)

Psychoanalytic Theory

The first comprehensive theoretical treatment of sex-role acquisition was presented by Freud (1927), who considered identification with the same-sex parent to be the primary mechanism of gender-role learning. Classical psychoanalytic theory stresses the primacy of anatomical differences that when discovered by young children, lead to penis envy in girls and castration fear in boys, and the need for all children to resolve the oedipal conflict. Within Freudian theory, the processes of sex-role learning are more clearly described for males than for females. As a consequence, more recent work from a psychoanalytic perspective has attempted to describe girls' acquisition of gender identity (e.g., Chodorow, 1978; Kleeman, 1971).

Although psychoanalytic approaches to gender have not been well supported by empirical research and have largely been subsumed into broader frameworks of modeling and imitation, the notion that the individual's psychosexual identity is at the core of a healthy personality has been a central tenet of psychological research and practice. Clinicians continue to focus on the potential consequences of early disruption of identification, especially in analyzing atypical gender-role acquisition (Green, 1974; Rekers, 1979). A recent extensive study of the development and outcomes of feminine patterns of behavior in boys suggests that factors contributing to cross-gender behavior differ in typical and atypical subjects (Roberts, Green, Williams, & Goodman, 1987). If this is true, perspectives from clinical populations may be limited in their generalizability.

Some psychoanalytic theorists have taken a view of gender-role acquisition as arising from the process of ego development, specifically with the ability to differentiate self from other (Block, 1973; Kleeman, 1971). Drawing on Loevinger's stages of ego development, Block (1973) has outlined a developmental sequence of sex-role identity acquisition, from initial self-nonself differentiation, through a period of self-assertion that brings about pressure from adults for socialization, to conformity with cultural expectations that include demands for boys to control affect and girls to control aggression. At the next level, introspection leads to moderation of stereotypical sex-role behavior and finally to the integration, within the individual, of both masculine and feminine traits. These approaches transcend the early psychoanalytic conceptions of gender identity and incorporate an awareness of the importance of cognitive development in early gender-role learning.

Cognitive Theories

COGNITIVE-DEVELOPMENTAL THEORY

The application of cognitive-developmental theory to the acquisition of gender understanding placed its emphasis entirely on the Piagetian notion of the natural unfolding of the child's processes of reasoning (Kohlberg, 1966). In Kohlberg's view, neither behavioral consequences nor socialization agents (even parents) have much to do with the acquisition of gender knowledge. According to Kohlberg, until at least the age of 6, children are incapable of grasping the unchangeable nature of gender categories, just as they are misled in their judgment of quantity by different-sized containers. Thus Kohlberg viewed the adoption of conventional gender roles as occurring *after* the acquisition of gender constancy, when a child becomes motivated to value attributes that are similar to the self and to behave in ways that are consistent with one's own gender-associated self-image. Kohlberg's theory does not describe the processes of acquisition of gender-stereotyped behavior prior to the acquisition of gender constancy.

SCHEMA THEORIES

In an effort to describe what children are acquiring during the preschool years as they observe the world and process its gender-related content, several investigators have proposed *schema* theories based on an information-processing approach to knowledge acquisition (Bem, 1981; Martin & Halverson, 1981). A gender schema is a way of representing the network of objects, attributes, and behavioral traits that are associated with gender in a given culture. These theorists see the gender schema as an organizing structure for children's selective attention to particular aspects of their environments and acquisition of information about the environment and about the self.

One prediction of gender schema theory as expressed by Martin and Halverson (1981) is that children elaborate their same-sex schema more fully than their cross-sex schema. Thus girls differentially observe and imitate same-sex models in order to learn all the varieties of appropriate female behavior in detail and devote less effort to acquiring the schema for maleness. In this manner, the schema for one's own gender serves as a filter and an attention-focusing device that facilitates the acquisition of culturally stereotyped behavior and attitudes.

Gender schemata can also be seen as accounting for individual differences in sex typing. According to the approach proposed by Bem (1984), an individual is considered more or less sex typed depending upon the degree to which that person organizes experience according to gender-linked categories. Bem sees this tendency to view the world as sex typed as a learned phenomenon, promoted by the ubiquitous nature of gender associations in many cultures, but modifiable during child rearing by consistent parental efforts to decouple gender from attributes and behaviors that are not biologically relevant to being male or female.

Social Learning Theory

Social learning theorists (Bandura, 1977; Mischel, 1966) describe two major processes of development to account for gender identity and sex-role acquisition: (a) reinforcers and punishments provided children as consequences for overt behavior that matches or conflicts with societal gender-role expectations and (b) observational learning, which leads directly to imitation. Because each culture has a set of attributes considered to define masculinity and femininity, children's behavior will be responded to differentially, depending upon its appropriateness, given the child's gender. Further, practice of same-sex-typed activities promotes competence at gender-specific tasks, which in turn provides intrinsic rewards for continued participation in those activities.

The reinforcement–punishment aspects of social learning theory have been criticized on the grounds that obvious contingencies are not readily observable in early parent–child interactions (Maccoby & Jacklin, 1974). This view discounts the potential power of subtle disparities in adults' behaviors, such as interpreting boys' and girls' facial expressions as different emotions (Condry & Condry, 1976; Haviland, 1977). Further, recent studies have made it clear that children process and respond to both positive and negative reinforcement for sex-typed behavior differentially depending upon its source, indicating that not all social reinforcement is of equal value or salience (Fagot, 1985).

Observational learning does not involve direct reinforcement but, instead, the incorporation into the child's repertoire of a large set of behaviors that can be called upon in the future as the child's skills grow. Research has shown that children may learn equally well from observing either same-sex or cross-sex models but are more likely to imitate same-sex models (Bussey & Bandura, 1984; Perry & Bussey, 1979).

According to social learning theory, children's understanding about gender and their categorization of themselves as male or female arises from their participation in sex-typical activities and the value they place on activities and attributes that are rewarding to them. Thus the environment plays a major role in children's gender-role learning, although the child brings selective perception and a learning history to the task.

Future Directions for Theory

All of the theoretical perspectives described are useful in delineating particular aspects of sex-role development. However, none alone explains the lifelong process of acquisition of core gender identity, why gender is so pervasive a factor in social organization across cultures, or what fuels change in gender-role knowledge. Too often, researchers have collected empirical data to test specific hypotheses derived from a single theoretical approach. A more complete understanding of sex-role development will require a multifaceted examination of the interaction among biological, cognitive, and social-environmental factors, and a theoretical integration that has not yet been achieved.

DEVELOPMENT OF GENDER-ROLE IDENTITY

Gender discrimination skills, self-categorization, and sex-typed behavior are apparent very early in development and undergo change over time in response to both cognitive growth and sociocultural factors. A general outline of the emergence of gender-role identity from infancy to late adolescence appears in Table 1. The major developments within each age are described in more detail in the following sections.

INFANCY: ACQUISITION OF CULTURALLY DEFINED GENDER CATEGORIES

Next to "Haven't you had that baby *yet*?", the most frequent question asked every expectant mother must be, "Do you think it is a boy or a girl?" Thus, even before birth, the salience of gender to one's core identity in others' eyes is obvious. There is a plethora of evidence to indicate that adults, and other children, treat boy and girl babies differently in a large variety of ways despite the absence of reliable evidence of differences in infant behavior (Frisch, 1977; Lewis, 1974; Moss, 1967; Rheingold & Cook, 1975; Shakin, Shakin, & Sternglanz, 1985; Snow, Jacklin, & Maccoby, 1983).

What is less clear from the empirical literature is the process by which such differential treatment influences early discrimination and acquisition of sex-typed behavior, occurring *before* children can verbally label male and female or associate toys or activities with gender categories. Clinical case studies of children whose gender was misidentified at birth suggest that basic gender-role identification is too well established by 18 months to 2 years for it to be changed (Money & Ehrhardt, 1972). It thus appears that children attach a considerable network of associations to gender categories prior to the age at which they can reliably demonstrate gender labeling.

TABLE 1. Outline of Gender-Role Acquisition Process Throughout Childhood

0–3 years	Acquisition of culturally defined gender categories
3–7 years	Stereotyped attitudes about gender, encompassing activities, clothing, social roles, personal attributes; male and female seen as opposites
7–12 years	Flexibility of gender concepts arising from separation of external characteristics and core identity
12–15 years	Reemergence of gender-role salience, especially in cross-sex relationships
15–18 years	Establishment of sexual preference; selection of adult social roles, initial career choices; for some, emergence of individual identity incorporating masculine and feminine characeristics

Although the infant–toddler period is often considered unimportant in sex-role development or dismissed as a period of undifferentiated gender roles, a closer examination indicates that children acquire an impressive set of gender-related abilities by age 3. Table 2 lists some of the milestones that have been reported in children's acquisition of gender as a category from birth to age 3. In the following sections, some of the skills involved in this acquisition are briefly described.

Discrimination

The perceptual salience of gender-related stimuli to infants is evident from research reporting clear discrimination between male and female faces (Fagan, 1972; Fagan & Singer, 1979) within the first year of life. Such discrimination does not, of course, imply that infants of 1 year or less "understand" the category of male or female in the same way that an adult or older child does. Instead, infants appear to be responding to salient visual cues such as hair length (Leinbach, 1990).

Language

Children's early words reflect the importance of gender categories in their world. The labels "mama" and "dada" appear among the first words of most children in English-speaking cultures, and they are typically used specifically to refer to Mom and Dad before the age of 18 months. The words *boy* and *girl* are also early vocabulary entries, although they are applied indiscriminately at first (Kohlberg, 1966; Leinbach & Fagot, 1986). As with most language acquisition, children's receptive recognition of gender labels applied to people or to pictures of people (at about 26 months for adults, 36 months for children) (Leinbach & Fagot, 1986; Weinraub *et al.*, 1984) precedes their expressive ability to produce the label when shown a person or a picture.

Children's early language acquisition shows more subtle effects of gender as well. In a recent analysis of children's early vocabulary development, Zima, O'Brien, and Caldera (1990) found that by 18 months of age, both girls' and boys' vocabularies contain more words with same-sex associations than with cross-sex

TABLE 2. Developmental Course of Acquisition of Gender Categories in Early Childhood

Age (months)	Ability
6	Differentiation of male/female faces; differentiation of faces of mother and father
12	Recognition of similarity across exemplars of the same gender
15	Acquisition of verbal gender labels, applied nonspecifically (receptive)
16	Acquisition of mama, dada, used specifically
18	Adoption of same-sex-typed toy and activity preferences
24	Reliable identification of picture of self
24	Acquisition of verbal labels *boy* and *girl*, applied nonspecifically
26	Reliable identification of adult male/female exemplars
30	Association of gender labels with stereotyped attributes, behaviors, and roles
30	Preference for pictures of same-sex children
31	Verbal self-categorization (gender identity)
33	Preference for same-sex playmates
36	Reliable identification of child male/female exemplars

associations. These early differences in word acquisition probably result from differential experiences of boys and girls, not from direct teaching by parents. When context is controlled, adult speech to boys and to girls is highly similar (Greif & Gleason, 1980; Masur & Gleason, 1980; O'Brien & Nagle, 1987). Across play contexts, such as trucks and dolls, however, parental speech to young children differs markedly (O'Brien & Nagle, 1987). Thus children would be expected to acquire words that describe the activities they commonly engage in, and these are highly likely to be sex typed.

Categorization of Self and Others

A crucial part of learning about gender roles is knowing how to categorize oneself. By 2 years, children can recognize themselves in pictures (Thompson, 1975), and by 2½ can reliably identify their own gender (Eaton & Von Bargen, 1981). Not surprisingly, self-categorization precedes reliable identification of others' gender. Despite the early appearance of gender knowledge, throughout most of the preschool years the identification of gender appears to be somewhat fragile, and children are easily swayed by appearances: changes of clothing, hair style, and even activity setting can lead children to change their appraisal of the gender of a pictured child (Emmerich, 1981; Marcus & Overton, 1978). The concept of gender as an unchangeable, core characteristic of a person (known as gender constancy) is achieved at about age 5, the same age as children demonstrate acquisition of other conservation principles (Marcus & Overton, 1978; Slaby & Frey, 1975).

Association of Gender with Activities and Attributes

Before the age of 3, children have adopted much of the culture's sex-typed division of activities and attributes. Two-year-olds can sort pictures of adult activities or belongings into gender categories (Thompson, 1975; Weinraub et al., 1984) and will select the stereotypically male or female figure when given information about traits (slow, mean), activities (sewing, fighting), and future roles (teacher, boss) (Kuhn, Nash, & Brucken, 1978).

Adoption of Sex-Typed Behavior

Perhaps the strongest evidence that some aspects of early gender-role acquisition are nonverbal is the pervasive finding that children prefer same-sex-typed toys and activities by the age of 18 months (Blakemore, LaRue, & Olejnik, 1979; Fagot, 1974, 1978; Fein et al., 1975; O'Brien & Huston, 1985a,b). No studies have found children of this age to be reliable in labeling the gender of their peers or sorting toys according to sex-role stereotype. Still, the majority of toddlers spend more time playing with same-sex-typed than cross-sex-typed toys.

The differential provision of toys to male and female infants and toddlers at home (O'Brien & Huston, 1985b; Rheingold & Cook, 1975) may account for at least a portion of the strong same-sex-typed play preferences observed in very young children. Because the toys they have at home are familiar and associated with play routines they know and can perform independently, toddlers may select them in laboratory or classroom situations, especially where they are expected to play without adult involvement. If children are presented with toys they have never seen or played with along with toys for which they have a well-developed play repertoire, it would not be surprising for them to choose the familiar toys, which are also likely to be same-sex-typed toys. In an observational study of toddlers and parents with a variety of masculine sex-typed, feminine sex-typed, and neutral toys, Caldera, Huston, and O'Brien (1989) found children to show higher involvement with same-sex-typed toys. Anecdotally, children appeared to have a play repertoire for same-sex-typed toys but not for cross-sex-typed toys.

EARLY CHILDHOOD: ENTRENCHMENT OF STEREOTYPES

If the first 3 years of life involve the acquisition of gender-based categories for people, activities, and attributes, the years from 3 to 6 are spent elaborating and calcifying those categories. The 3-year-old may play in a sex-stereotyped way but accepts overlap in male and female roles; the kindergartner, on the other hand, not only plays in a sex-stereotyped way with same-sex playmates but regards cross-gender behavior quite negatively. Yet this child has not yet attained a stable sense of gender as a consistent individual characteristic. In the following sections, developmental trends in children's gender-related cognition and sex-typed behavior during the preschool years are reviewed.

Knowledge of Stereotypes

During the preschool years, children's sex-role stereotypes come to match very closely those of the surrounding culture. By the time they reach kindergarten, children can clearly identify a variety of objects, activities, and attributes as gender related: toys (Perry, White, & Perry, 1984), play activities (Edelbrock & Sugawara, 1978), traits (Reis & Wright, 1982; Urberg, 1982), occupations (Katz & Boswell, 1986), and clothing (Vener & Snyder, 1966).

Preschoolers also see gender largely as a binary system in which "same as me" is viewed positively and "other than me" is viewed negatively. As a consequence, children's categorization of gender-related characteristics becomes increasingly rigid and encompasses more dimensions over the preschool years (Birnbaum & Chemelski, 1984; Marcus & Overton, 1978; Reis & Wright, 1982). Investigation of children's thinking about gender associations suggests that preschoolers view sex-typical activities and appearance as defining properties of gender (Stoddart & Turiel, 1985). Thus, to a 4- or 5-year-old, a person who wears nail polish is, by definition, a girl. The suggestion that a boy might wear nail polish violates the categorization system and is rejected by the preschool child.

The notion of the gender schema (Martin & Halverson, 1981) is a particularly useful way to conceptualize children's acquisition of gender-associated knowledge during the preschool period. By dividing the social world into male and female, children with strong gender schemata should be able to assimilate, organize, and therefore remember a considerable amount of information quite efficiently. Only a few published studies directly address the degree to which young children's tendency to organize perceptual information according to gender influences their memory for that information. Levy (1989) reported that children with a high degree of gender schematization showed better recognition memory for gender-role consistent pictures than did the less gender-schematic children but that labeling of the stimuli as gender related improved the performance of the low gender-schematic children. Further, children with a strong gender schema showed a pattern of error in which pictures depicting people engaged in cross-sex activities were transformed in memory to be gender consistent.

In a cross-sectional study of 3- to 7-year-olds, Serbin and Sprafkin (1986) found gender-based affiliation preference to be an individual difference related to degree of sex typing. Children's use of gender-based categorization, on the other hand, tended to decline over the age period as children's knowledge of cultural sex-roles increased. Young children may initially use gender as a primary basis for social classification because it is so salient a cue. As the extent of overlap in male and female behavior, attributes, and even appearance becomes evident to children, they may move beyond gender when other defining properties of stimuli are known.

Girls appear to be more advanced than boys both in learning sex-role stereotypes and in moving toward greater flexibility in defining male and female roles (Edelbrock & Sugawara, 1978; Katz & Boswell, 1986; Perry et al., 1984; Urberg, 1982). In addition, preschool-aged girls are aware of the characteristics of male as well as female roles, whereas boys learn the male stereotype earlier and more thoroughly than the female (Hartup & Zook, 1960). These early sex differences have yet to be explained and may be attributable to girls' earlier cognitive maturity, the wider range of play activities considered appropriate for girls, or the more variable socialization pressures placed on girls as compared with boys.

Play Behavior

Anyone who has observed preschoolers at play can attest to the sex-typed nature of boys' and girls' play preferences at this age and also to the overwhelming tendency of children to play in gender-segregated groups. Boys are especially likely to select masculine sex-typed toys for play, beginning before age 3 and continuing through the preschool years (Blakemore et al., 1979; O'Brien & Huston, 1985a,b; O'Brien, Huston, & Risley, 1983). Further, boys appear to actively reject stereotypically feminine toys (Lloyd, Duveen, & Smith, 1988), whereas girls' play is usually more varied. Efforts to intervene into children's play environments to reduce the level of sex-role stereotyping have shown only mixed success and often a quick return to high levels of stereotyped play once the experimental condition was removed, suggesting that gender-specific play patterns are resistant to change (see review by Katz, 1986).

The different play styles of young boys and girls may have long-term social and cognitive consequences for development. Boys' play tends to be more active, involving more rough-and-tumble activity, and toys defined as masculine often elicit manipulation and construction. Girls are provided with toys that encourage imitation of adult domestic roles and social interaction. Several studies have reported high rates of play with masculine sex-typed toys to be correlated with high scores on tests of visual-spatial skills (O'Brien, 1990; Serbin & Connor, 1979). Although the processes contributing to such differences have not been described, some have speculated that the object manipulation and eye–hand coordination required by masculine toys may contribute to the development of visual-spatial skills (Liss, 1983).

Carpenter (1983) suggested that a major difference in the play of preschool-aged boys and girls concerns the amount of "structure," or externally imposed rules or suggestions, in the play setting. Boys are more likely than girls, according to Carpenter, to create their own structure, rather than depending upon adult modeling or instructions to shape their play. It should also be noted that boys are less responsive to instructions from adults (Fagot, 1985) and so seem to actively resist adult-imposed structure in their play. Carpenter and her colleagues (Carpenter & Huston-Stein, 1980; Carpenter, Huston, & Holt, 1986) have presented data to show that these different play styles may contribute to increased peer leadership skills in boys, whose play involves ongoing negotiation, and to acquisition of academic-type cognitive skills in girls, whose play is often adult directed and learning oriented.

Recently, Eleanor Maccoby proposed that gender segregation in play throughout childhood is maintained by interaction styles that differ in males and females (Maccoby, 1988, 1990). Preschool boys' play is characterized by a rough-and-tumble style that girls find unpleasant; girls therefore seek the company of other girls, who play in a quieter, more cooperative manner. Further, according to Maccoby, girls playing in mixed-sex groups find themselves frustrated by their inability to exert any social influence over boys' behavior. The interactive styles common to boys' and girls' play groups (with boys' interactions focused on dominance and girls' on involvement and agreement) are maintained over many years and may have a pervasive influence on the development of behavioral sex differences into adulthood.

Although the peer group may take on considerable importance during the preschool years, children are also learning the rules of interaction with adults. Although it is well known that adults behave differently when playing with boys and with girls, the child's contribution to this disparity is less apparent. Fagot (1984) instructed male and female adults to respond to children's overtures and not to initiate any interaction in order to evaluate whether young children elicit differential play behavior from unfamiliar male and female adults. She found that 4-year-old children, both boys and girls, initiated playing ball significantly more often with males and asked only females for help. Boys also talked more with female adults than with males. Thus some aspects of children's interactive styles appear to be situational rather than individual variables, and from an early age are attuned to the gender of their social partner.

MIDDLE CHILDHOOD: ADDING GRADATIONS TO GENDER CATEGORIES

By the time they reach elementary school, most children in our culture have attained a sense of the constancy of gender in the face of variations in behavior and transformations in appearance. The cognitive-developmental theory proposed by Kohlberg (1966) has often been misinterpreted as predicting that sex-typed behavior should emerge and become salient only *after* a child attains gender constancy. In fact, the theory holds that understanding of gender as a stable individual characteristic should allow children to expand their view of gender categories to incorporate a wider range of behavior and greater diversity in appearance. Consistent with this prediction, during the elementary-school years, children show less rigidity in their gender-role conceptualizations, although they continue to recognize and elaborate on cultural stereotypes of masculinity and femininity. In short, children appear to be adding multiple dimensions to their previously binary view of gender categories.

Flexibility of Male and Female Roles

In middle childhood, children accept considerable overlap in what they consider acceptable for males and females in terms of behavior and appearance. In an extensive interview study of children's understanding of femininity and masculinity, Ullian (1976) found that children older than 6 or 7 years rejected appearance distinctions as defining factors in determining gender. Throughout the school years, too, children (particularly girls) view occupations as less stereotyped by gender (Alpert & Breen, 1989; Garrett, Ein, & Tremaine, 1977; Katz & Boswell, 1986).

Research showing parallels between children's broadening sex-role stereotypes and their attitudes about the rigidity of social conventions suggests that elementary-school-age children are viewing gender roles as a socially based set of rules or agreements among which individuals may choose with impugnity (Carter & Patterson, 1982; Stoddart & Turiel, 1985). Carter and Patterson (1982) asked children from kindergarten through eighth grade to identify the sex-role stereotype of a set of toys and occupations and also to describe how flexible these stereotypes were and compared these responses to children's knowledge of a rule of etiquette and a natural law. They found both children's knowledge of cultural stereotypes and their flexibility in applying stereotypes to increase with age. Similarly, the children's view of a rule of etiquette showed increasing flexibility in the older groups of children, whereas their conceptions of the natural law remained the same.

Stoddart and Turiel (1985) showed children ranging from kindergarten to eighth grade pictures of boys and girls whose appearance included an aspect appropriate to the other sex (boys wearing a barrette or nail polish; girls in a crew cut or a boy's suit) and asked the children whether they thought what the pictured children were doing was wrong. Unlike the kindergartners and eighth-graders who ranked these sex-role transgressions as very wrong, the third- and fifth-graders judged them as quite acceptable. On further questioning, the children explained their ranking by saying that what the pictured children were doing was a matter of "personal choice." Taken together, these studies suggest that during the elementary-school years, children are acquiring a rather sophisticated understanding of social conventions, including gender-related conventions, and a sense of the overlapping boundaries of the masculine and feminine categories.

Sex Differences in Behavior

During the years between 6 and 12, children's preference for same-sex playmates continues to be strong (Maccoby, 1988). Girls tend to develop a small circle of intimate friends, whereas boys increasingly play in larger groups, often organized into teams for competitive games. Although boys and girls can be observed interacting with one another when participating in adult-structured activities, their overwhelming tendency when playing without adult supervision is to segregate by gender (Hartup, 1983; Maccoby & Jacklin, 1987). Rather than being encouraged or maintained by adult socialization pressures, this separation of the sexes appears to be motivated by children's desire to avoid the appearance of either cross-sex interests (being a "tomboy" or a "sissy") or romantic involvement (Maccoby, 1988).

Within their segregated play groups, school-age children's verbal interactions take on quite different characteristics (Maltz & Borker, 1983). Girls' conversations are marked by expressions of acknowledgment and agreement and the regular exchange of speaking turns; boys interrupt each other, make demands and refuse to comply with others' demands, tell jokes or stories, and generally compete with one another for attention. These different social experiences may have long-term influences on interaction and speech styles, which are found to differ substantially in adult men and women (see Philips, Steele, & Tanz, 1987).

EARLY ADOLESCENCE: A RETURN TO RIGIDITY

Despite the obvious importance of adolescence in the development of gender-role identity and behavior, little observational research to examine these developmental processes has been carried out with children 12 and over. This is particularly unfortunate because adolescence is the point when children are making personal choices based on gender-role attitudes that have profound implications for their adult lives.

Although children entering adolescence clearly have the ability to recognize that gender-role stereotypes are social conventions open to individual preference, they tend to retreat from their position of flexibility, attained by age 11 or 12, into a conformist stance (Eccles, 1987). It is likely that as male–female relationships gain prominence, children make the "safe" choice of adapting their behavior and personality to a model of social acceptability. Alternatively, as children between ages 12 and 15 grow increasingly to look like adults, they may encounter social pressure to act in more stereotypic ways and to abandon aspects of their cross-sex behavior that may be perceived as childish. Girls may particularly move toward more traditional interests and activities as their future mothering role becomes salient.

The effects of pubertal changes taking place in early adolescence on children's cognitive and social development have recently become a topic of considerable interest to developmental psychologists (see Lerner & Foch, 1987). Few direct effects of hormone levels or timing of maturation have been described, although changes in sex hormones do appear to be related to mood shifts (Nottelman *et al.*, 1987; Susman *et al.*, 1987). Petersen (1985, 1987) has proposed that pubertal status is tied to behavior in early adolescence through mediators, particularly social norms for attractiveness and gender roles.

In a series of investigations of urban children undergoing the transition into junior high school, Blyth and colleagues (Blyth, Simmons, & Bush, 1978; Blyth, Simmons, & Carlton-Ford, 1983; Simmons, Carlton-Ford, & Blyth, 1987) have found early puberty to place seventh-grade girls at risk for low self-esteem and school problems. Boys in general appear to cope better than girls with large schools because they are able to locate a peer group that evaluates them highly, whereas girls may attempt to maintain a familiar group instead of seeking out new relationships.

Adolescence: Transcending Stereotypes

Eccles (1987) has offered a model of gender-role development in which transcendence of cultural stereotypes is seen as the mature stage of development. To Eccles and others who have written about the concept of gender-role transcendence (Block, 1973; Pleck, 1975; Ullian, 1976), an individual's ability to move past traditional concepts of male and female represents an integration of self-identity, knowledge of traditional gender roles, and principles of thought and action that go beyond prescribed roles. From the gender-schema point of view, gender-role transcendence would involve reducing one's dependence on gender-based stereotypes as a basis for decisions regarding one's own actions and beliefs and for evaluating the actions and beliefs of others. Although gender-role transcendence can be attained by adults, adolescence would appear to be a particularly important time for the development of attitudes and the selection of activities that encourage or discourage such transcendence. It is during adolescence that most boys and girls establish their sexual identity through experience with dating and its accompanying sexual experimentation (Gordon & Gilgun, 1987; Hartup, 1983). The selection as friends of same- and other-sex peers who accept and encourage behavior that goes beyond traditional gender roles may have a strong influence on an adolescent's gender identity. Early marriage or parenthood, which places an adolescent firmly into a traditional gender role, will usually be incompatible with the development of transcendence and also limits a young girl's ability to continue in school or pursue a career (Marini, 1985).

By adolescence, males and females in our culture show profound differences in social behaviors and in attitudes toward relationships with others. Gilligan (1982) has described sex differences in moral judgment criteria, with girls focusing on a morality of caring and responsiveness to others and boys on a morality of justice based on rules. In heterosexual relationships, adolescent girls (but not boys) tie sexual activity to love (Gagnon & Simon, 1973); however, both girls and boys expect males to take the lead in such relationships. Although both male and female adolescents depend to a great extent on their peers to support their developing self-esteem, male peer groups tend to be highly competitive and focused on dominance, whereas female peer groups are close knit and intimate. By adolescence, sex differences in achievement orientation are evident, with males scoring higher on measures of mastery (preference for difficult tasks) and competitiveness (desire to be better than others), and females scoring higher on work orientation (desire to work hard and do a good job) (Spence & Helmreich, 1983).

It is evident that the choices adolescents make about education, occupation, and marriage are strongly rooted in socially based perceptions of themselves as male or female. The rigidity or flexibility of the social roles inherent in these choices will, in turn, affect the further development of gender identity in adulthood. Despite the importance of adolescence in the process of gender-role development, to date little research has been directed toward describing the developmental pathways that lead to sex differences in social behavior and attitudes.

Gender is a social category around which much human interaction is organized. Learning the content of male and female stereotypes is an important developmental task for children, beginning in infancy. Similarly, children must fit themselves into a gender category in order to meet others' expectations of appropriate behavior. The task of developing a mature gender identity involves more than accepting cultural conventions, however. In later childhood and adolescence, gender-role stereotypes must be differentiated from self-identified preferences and principles if the individual is to transcend traditional gender roles and incorporate aspects of both masculine and feminine traits into an integrated adult personality.

Research into gender-role development and sex differences has become somewhat sensitive politically in recent years because of the concerns of feminists and others about unequal treatment of males and females in American society. Efforts to intervene into sex-typed behavior in early childhood, by promoting play with cross-sex toys and integrated playgroups, have indicated both the strength of early gender-based discriminations and preferences and the pervasiveness of socialization practices fostering sex differences. Interestingly, although most studies show boys to be more sex typed in their play behavior, attempts to increase cross-sex behavior in childhood are focused primarily on girls; boys who behave in feminine ways are still viewed problematically. This difference reflects our society's strong bias toward masculine traits as the standard of healthy psychological adjustment. Rather than attempting to create equality by changing either the experiences of females or society's expectations for females, it might be more productive to address adult attitudes toward social interaction patterns by placing more value on cooperation and caring and to increase the prestige (and income) afforded by female-dominated occupations.

Although gender categories have their basis in biological differences between males and females, the child-rearing practices of all cultures differ on the basis of sex. From infancy on, parents and others respond differently to boys and girls, model and reinforce gender-appropriate behavior, and hold different expectations for females than males. These pervasive cultural practices make it impossible to separate biologically based from socially based sex differences. Instead, a productive research avenue would be the analysis of the relative contributions of cognitive, social, and emotional factors, particularly in later childhood and adolescence, to the development of a mature gender-role identity.

ACKNOWLEDGMENTS   Preparation of this chapter was supported in part by NICHD grant HD18955 and by the U.S. Department of Education through the Kansas Early Childhood Research Institute. The author thanks Kathy Zima for her help.

REFERENCES

Alpert, D., & Breen, D. T. (1989). "Liberality" in children and adolescents. *Journal of Vocational Behavior,* *34,* 154–160.
Bandura, A. (1977). *Social learning theory*. Englewood Cliffs, NJ: Prentice-Hall.
Barry, H., Bacon, M. K., & Child, I. L. (1957). A cross-cultural survey of some differences in socialization. *Journal of Abnormal and Social Psychology, 55,* 327–332.

Beeman, E. A. (1947). The effect of male hormone on aggressive behavior in mice. *Psychological Zoology, 20,* 313–405.

Bell, R. Q. (1960). Relations between behavior manifestations in the human neonate. *Child Development, 31,* 463–477.

Bell, R. Q., & Costello, N. S. (1964). Three tests for sex differences in tactile sensitivity in the newborn. *Biologica Neonatorium, 7,* 335–347.

Bell, R. Q., Weller, G. M., & Waldrop, M. F. (1971). Newborn and preschooler: Organization of behavior and relations between periods. *Monographs of the Society for Research in Child Development, 46,* (Serial No. 142).

Bem, S. L. (1981). Gender schema theory: A cognitive account of sex typing. *Psychological Review, 88,* 354–364.

Bem, S. L. (1984). Androgyny and gender schema theory: A conceptual and empirical integration. In T. B. Sonderegger (Ed.), *Nebraska Symposium on Motivation* (Vol. 32, pp. 179–226). Lincoln: University of Nebraska Press.

Birnbaum, D. W., & Chemelski, B. E. (1984). Preschoolers' inferences about gender and emotion: The mediation of emotionality stereotypes. *Sex Roles, 10,* 505–511.

Blakemore, J., LaRue, A., & Olejnik, A. (1979). Sex-appropriate toy preference and the ability to conceptualize toys as sex-role related. *Developmental Psychology, 15,* 339–340.

Block, J. E. (1973). Conceptions of sex role: Some cross-cultural and longitudinal perspectives. *American Psychologist, 28,* 512–526.

Blyth, D. A., Simmons, R. G., & Bush, D. (1978). The transition into early adolescence: A longitudinal comparison of youth in two educational contexts. *Sociology of Education, 51,* 149–162.

Blyth, D. A., Simmons, R. G,. & Carlton-Ford, S. L. (1983). The adjustments of early adolescents to school transitions. *Journal of Early Adolescence, 3,* 105–120.

Bussey, K., & Bandura, A. (1984). Influence of gender constancy and social power on sex-linked modeling. *Journal of Personality and Social Psychology, 47,* 1292–1302.

Caldera, Y. M., Huston, A. C., & O'Brien, M. (1989). Social interactions and play patterns of parents and toddlers with feminine, masculine, and neutral toys. *Child Development, 60,* 70–76.

Carpenter, C. J. (1983). Activity structure and play: Implications for socialization. In M. B. Liss (Ed.), *Social and cognitive skills: Sex roles and children's play* (pp. 117–145). New York: Academic Press.

Carpenter, C. J., & Huston-Stein, A. C. (1980). Activity structure and sex-typed behavior in preschool children. *Child Development, 51,* 862–872.

Carpenter, C. J., Huston, A. C., & Holt, W. (1986). Modification of preschool sex-typed behaviors by participation in adult-structured activities. *Sex Roles, 14,* 603–615.

Carter, D. B., & Patterson, C. J (1982). Sex roles as social conventions: The development of children's conceptions of sex-role stereotypes. *Developmental Psychology, 18,* 813–824.

Chodorow, N. (1978). *The reproduction of mothering.* Berkeley: University of California Press.

Condry, J., & Condry, A. (1976). Sex differences: A study of the eye of the beholder. *Child Development, 47,* 812–819.

Cowan, G., & Hoffman, C. D. (1986). Gender stereotyping in young children: Evidence to support a concept-learning approach. *Sex Roles, 14,* 211–224.

Eaton, W. O., & Von Bargen, D. (1981). Asynchronous development of gender understanding in preschool children. *Child Development, 52,* 1020–1027.

Eccles, J. S. (1987). Adolescence: Gateway to gender-role transcendence. In D. B. Carter (Ed.), *Current conceptions of sex roles and sex typing: Theory and research* (pp. 225–241). New York: Praeger.

Eccles-Parsons, J. (1982). Biology, experience, and sex dimorphic behaviors. In W. Gove & G. R. Carpenter (Eds.), *The fundamental connection between nature and nurture: A review of the evidence.* Lexington, MA: Lexington Books.

Edelbrock, C., & Sugawara, A. I. (1978). Acquisition of sex-typed preferences in preschool-aged children. *Developmental Psychology, 14,* 614–623.

Edwards, D. A. (1969). Early androgen stimulation and aggressive behavior in male and female mice. *Physiology and Behavior, 4,* 335–338.

Emmerich, W. (1981). Non-monotonic developmental trends in social cognition: The case of gender constancy. In S. Strauss (Ed.), *U-shaped behavioral growth* (pp. 249–269). New York: Academic Press.

Fagan, J. F. (1972). Infants' recognition memory for faces. *Journal of Experimental Child Psychology, 14,* 453–476.

Fagan, J. F., & Singer, L. T. (1979). The role of smile feature differences in infant recognition of faces. *Infant Behavior and Development, 2,* 39–46.

Fagot, B. I. (1974). Sex differences in toddlers' behavior and parental reaction. *Developmental Psychology*, 10, 554–558.

Fagot, B. I. (1978). The influence of sex of child on parental reactions to toddler children. *Child Development*, 49, 459–465.

Fagot, B. I. (1984). The child's expectations of differences in adult male and female interactions. *Sex Roles*, 11, 593–600.

Fagot, B. I. (1985). Beyond the reinforcement principle: Another step toward understanding sex role development. *Developmental Psychology*, 21, 1097–1104.

Fein, G., Johnson, D., Kosson, N., Stork, L., & Wasserman, L. (1975). Sex stereotypes and preferences in the toy choices of 20-month-old boys and girls. *Developmental Psychology*, 11, 527–528.

Freud, S. (1927). Some psychological consequences of the anatomical distinction between the sexes. *International Journal of Psychoanalysis*, 8, 133–142.

Frisch, H. L. (1977). Sex stereotypes in adult-infant play. *Child Development*, 48, 1671–1675.

Gagnon, J. H., & Simon, W. (1973). *Sexual conduct*. New York: Aldine.

Garai, J. E., & Scheinfeld, A. (1968). Sex differences in mental and behavioral traits. *Genetic Psychology Monographs*, 77, 169–299.

Garrett, C. S., Ein, P. L., & Tremaine, L. (1977). The development of gender stereotyping of adult occupations in elementary school children. *Child Development*, 48, 507–512.

Gilligan, C. (1982). *In a different voice*. Cambridge: Harvard University Press.

Goldberg, S. (1974). *The inevitability of patriarchy*. New York: Morrow.

Gordon, S., & Gilgun, J. F. (1987). Adolescent sexuality. In V. B. Van Hasselt & M. Herson (Eds.), *Handbook of adolescent psychology* (pp. 147–167). New York: Pergamon Press.

Green, R. (1974). *Sexual identity conflict in children and adults*. New York: Basic Books.

Greif, E. B., & Gleason, J. B. (1980). Hi, thanks, and goodbye: More routine information. *Language in Society*, 9, 159–166.

Hartup, W. W. (1983). Peer relations. In P. H. Mussen (Series Ed.) and E. M. Hetherington (Vol. Ed.), *Handbook of child psychology* (4th ed.): *Vol. 4. Socialization, personality, and social development* (pp. 103–196). New York: Wiley.

Hartup, W. W., & Zook, E. A. (1960). Sex-role preferences in three- and four-year-old children. *Journal of Consulting Psychology*, 24, 420–426.

Haviland, J. M. (1977). Sex-related pragmatics in infants. *Journal of Communication*, 27, 80–84.

Hittleman, J. H., & Dickes, R. (1979). Sex differences in neonatal eye contact time. *Merrill-Palmer Quarterly*, 25, 171–184.

Hood, K. E., Draper, P., Crockett, L. J., & Petersen, A. C. (1987). The ontogeny and phylogeny of sex differences in development: A biopsychosocial synthesis. In D. B. Carter (Ed.), *Current conceptions of sex roles and sex typing* (pp. 49–77). New York: Praeger.

Huston, A. C. (1983). Sex typing. In P. H. Mussen (Series Ed.), and E. M. Hetherington (Vol. Ed.), *Handbook of Child Psychology* (4th ed.): *Vol. 4. Socialization, personality and social development* (pp. 387–457). New York: Wiley.

Hutt, C. (1972a). Sex differences in human development. *Human Development*, 15, 153–170.

Hutt, C. (1972b). *Males and females*. Harmondsworth, UK: Penguin Books.

Katz, P. A. (1986). Modification of children's gender-stereotyped behavior: General issues and research considerations. *Sex Roles*, 14, 591–602.

Katz, P. A., & Boswell, S. (1986). Flexibility and traditionality in children's gender roles. *Genetic, Social, and General Psychology Monographs*, 112, 105–145.

Kleeman, J. A. (1971). The establishment of core gender identity in normal girls. *Archives of Sexual Behavior*, 1, 103–116.

Kohlberg, L. (1966). A cognitive-developmental analysis of children's sex-role concepts and attitudes. In E. Maccoby (Ed.), *Development of sex differences* (pp. 81–173). Stanford: Stanford University Press.

Kuhn, D., Nash, S. C., & Brucken, L. (1978). Sex role concepts of two- and three-year-olds. *Child Development*, 49, 445–451.

Lamb, M. E. (Ed.). (1978). *Social and personality development*. New York: Holt, Rinehart & Winston.

Leinbach, M. D. (1990, April). *Infants' use of hair and clothing cues to discriminate pictures of men and women*. Paper presented at the International Conference on Infant Studies, Montreal.

Leinbach, M. D., & Fagot, B. I. (1986). Acquisition of gender labels: A test for toddlers. *Sex Roles*, 15, 655–666.

Lerner, R. M., & Foch, T. T. (1987). *Biological-psychosocial interactions in early adolescence*. Hillsdale, NJ: Erlbaum.

Levy, G. D. (1989). Developmental and individual differences in preschoolers' recognition memories: The influences of gender schematization and verbal labeling of information. *Sex Roles, 21,* 305–423.

Lewis, M. (1974). State as an infant-environment interaction: An analysis of mother-infant interactions as a function of sex. *Merrill-Palmer Quarterly, 20,* 195–204.

Lewontin, R. C., Rose, S., & Karmin, L. (1984). *Not in our genes: Biology, ideology, and human nature.* New York: Pantheon.

Liss, M. B. (1983). Learning gender-related skills through play. In M. B. Liss (Ed.), *Social and cognitive skills: Sex roles and children's play* (pp. 147–166). New York: Academic Press.

Lloyd, B., Duveen, G., & Smith, C. (1988). Social representations of gender and young children's play: A replication. *British Journal of Developmental Psychology, 6,* 83–88.

Maccoby, E. E. (1988). Gender as a social category. *Developmental Psychology, 24,* 755–765.

Maccoby, E. E. (1990). Gender and relationships: A developmental account. *American Psychologist, 45,* 513–520.

Maccoby, E. E., & Jacklin, C. N. (1974). *The psychology of sex differences.* Stanford: Stanford University Press.

Maccoby, E. E., & Jacklin, C. N. (1987). Gender segregation in childhood. In E. H. Reese (Ed.), *Advances in child development and behavior* (Vol. 20, pp. 239–287). New York: Academic Press.

Maltz, D. N., & Borker, R. A. (1983). A cultural approach to male-female miscommunication. In J. A. Gumperz (Ed.), *Language and social identity* (pp. 195–216). New York: Cambridge University Press.

Marcus, D. E., & Overton, W. F. (1978). The development of cognitive gender constancy and sex role preferences. *Child Development, 49,* 434–444.

Marini, M. M. (1985). Determinants of adult role entry. *Social Science Research, 14,* 309–350.

Martin, C. L., & Halverson, C. F. (1981). A schematic processing model of sex typing and stereotyping in children. *Child Development, 52,* 1119–1134.

Masur, E. F., & Gleason, J. B. (1980). Parent-child interaction and the acquisition of lexical information during play. *Developmental Psychology, 16(5),* 404–409.

McMilen, M. M. (1979). Differential mortality by sex in fetal and neonatal deaths. *Science, 204,* 89–91.

Mischel, W. (1966). A social learning view of sex differences in behavior. In E. Maccoby (Ed.), *Development of sex differences* (pp. 56–81). Stanford: Stanford University Press.

Money, J., & Ehrhardt, A. A. (1972). *Man and woman, boy and girl: Differentiation and dimorphism of gender identity from conception to maturity.* Baltimore: Johns Hopkins University Press.

Moss, H. A. (1967). Sex, age, and state as determinants of mother-infant interaction. *Merrill-Palmer Quarterly, 13,* 19–36.

Nottelmann, E. D., Susman, E. J., Blue, J. H., Inoff-Germain, G., Dorn, L. R., Loriaux, D. L., Cutler, G. B., & Chrousos, G. P. (1987). Gonadal and adrenal hormone correlates of adjustment in early adolescence. In R. M. Lerner & T. T. Foch (Eds.), *Biological-psychosocial interactions in early adolescence* (pp. 303–324). Hillsdale, NJ: Erlbaum.

O'Brien, M. (1990). *Stability of sex-typed toy preferences and relation to spatial abilities in young children.* Unpublished manuscript, University of Kansas, Lawrence, Kansas.

O'Brien, M., & Huston, A. C. (1985a). Activity level and sex stereotyped toy choice in toddler boys and girls. *Journal of Genetic Psychology, 146,* 527–534.

O'Brien, M., & Huston, A. C. (1985b). Development of sex-typed play behaviors in toddlers. *Developmental Psychology, 21,* 866–871.

O'Brien, M., Huston, A. C., & Risley, T. R. (1983). Sex-typed play of toddlers in a day care center. *Journal of Applied Developmental Psychology, 4,* 1–9.

O'Brien, M., & Nagle, K. J. (1987). Parents' speech to toddlers: The effect of play context. *Journal of Child Language, 14,* 269–279.

Perry, D. G. & Bussey, K. (1979). The social learning theory of sex differences: Imitation is alive and well. *Journal of Personality and Social Psychology, 37,* 1699–1712.

Perry, D. G., White, A. J., & Perry, L. C. (1984). Does early sex typing result from children's attempts to match their behavior to sex role stereotypes? *Child Development, 55,* 2114–2121.

Petersen, A. C. (1985). Pubertal development as a cause of disturbance: Myths, realities, and unanswered questions. *Genetic, Social, and General Psychology Monographs, 111,* 205–232.

Petersen, A. C. (1987). The nature of biological-psychosocial interactions: The sample case of early adolescence. In R. M. Lerner & T. T. Foch (Eds.), *Biological-psychosocial interactions in early adolescence* (pp. 35–61). Hillsdale, NJ: Erlbaum.

Philips, S. U., Steele, S., & Tanz, C. (Eds.). (1987). *Language, gender, and sex in comparative perspective.* Cambridge: Cambridge University Press.

Pleck, J. H. (1975). Masculinity-feminity: Current and alternative paradigms. *Sex Roles, 1,* 161–178.

Reis, H. T., & Wright, S. (1982). Knowledge of sex-role stereotypes in children aged 3 to 5. *Sex Roles, 8*, 1049–1056.

Rekers, G. A. (1979). Psychosexual and gender problems. In E. Mach & L. Terdal (Eds.), *Behavioral assessment of childhood disorders* (pp. 483–526). New York: Guilford Press.

Rheingold, H. L., & Cook, K. V. (1975). The content of boys' and girls' rooms as an index of parent behavior. *Child Development, 46*, 459–463.

Roberts, C. W., Green, R., Williams, K., & Goodman, M. (1987). Boyhood gender identity development: A statistical contrast of two family groups. *Developmental Psychology, 4*, 544–557.

Rohmer, R. P. (1976). Sex differences in aggression: Phylogenetic and enculturation perspectives. *Ethos, 4*, 57–72.

Rosenblatt, P. C., & Cunningham, M. R. (1976). Sex differences in cross-cultural perspective. In B. Lloyd & J. Archer (Eds.), *Exploring sex differences* (pp. 71–94). London: Academic Press.

Rubin, J. Z., Provenzano, F. J., & Luria, Z. (1974). The eye of the beholder: Parents' views on sex of newborns. *American Journal of Orthopsychiatry, 44*, 512–519.

Serbin, L. A., & Connor, J. M. (1979). Sex-typing of children's play preferences and patterns of cognitive performance. *Journal of Genetic Psychology, 134*, 315–316.

Serbin, L. A., & Sprafkin, C. (1986). The salience of gender and the process of sex typing in three- to seven-year-old children. *Child Development, 57*, 1188–1199.

Shakin, M., Shakin, D., & Sternglanz, S. H. (1985). Infant clothing: Sex labeling for strangers. *Sex Roles, 12*, 955–963.

Simmons, R. G., Carlton-Ford, S. L., & Blyth, D. A. (1987). Predicting how a child will cope with the transition to junior high school. In R. M. Lerner & T. T. Foch (Eds.), *Biological-psychosocial interactions in early adolescence*, (pp. 325–375). Hillsdale, NJ: Erlbaum.

Slaby, R. G., & Frey, K. S. (1975). Development of gender constancy and selective attention to same-sex models. *Child Development, 46*, 849–856.

Snow, M. E., Jacklin, D. N., & Maccoby, E. E. (1983). Sex-of-child differences in father-child interaction at one year of age. *Child Development, 54*, 227–232.

Spence, J. T., & Helmreich, R. L. (1983). Achievement-related motives and behaviors. In J. T. Spence (Ed.), *Achievement and achievement motives: Psychological and sociological approaches* (pp. 7–74). San Francisco: W. H. Freeman.

Stoddart, T., & Turiel, D. (1985). Children's concepts of cross-gender activities. *Child Development, 56*, 1241–1252.

Susman, E. J., Inoff-Germain, G., Loriaux, D. L., Cutler, G. B. & Chrousos, G. P. (1987). Hormones, emotional dispositions, and aggressive attributes in young adolescents. *Child Development, 58*, 1114–1134.

Thompson, S. K. (1975). Gender labels and early sex role development. *Child Development, 46*, 339–347.

Ullian, D. Z. (1976). The development of conceptions of masculinity and femininity. In B. Lloyd and J. Archer (Eds.) *Exploring sex differences*. London: Academic Press.

Urberg, K. A. (1982). The development of the concepts of masculinity and femininity in young children. *Sex Roles, 8*, 659–668.

Vener, A., & Snyder, C. A. (1966). The preschool child's awareness and anticipation of adult sex-roles. *Sociometry, 29*, 159–168.

Weinraub, M., Clemens, L. P., Sockloff, A., Ethridge, T., Gracely, E., & Myers, B. (1984). The development of sex role stereotypes in the third year: Relationships to gender labeling, gender identity, sex-typed toy preference, and family characteristics. *Child Development, 55*, 1493–1503.

Zima, K., O'Brien, M., & Caldera, Y. M. (1990). *Gender differences in early vocabulary acquisition.* Unpublished manuscript. University of Kansas, Lawrence, Kansas.

14

Adolescence and Family Interaction

Susan B. Silverberg, Daniel L. Tennenbaum, and Theodore Jacob

Introduction

Since the early 1980s, the area of adolescence and the family has become one of the most rapidly growing fields in social science research. Although interest in, and conclusions about, family relations at this point in the lifespan find strong origins in the psychoanalytic writings and clinical work of the 1950s (e.g., A. Freud, 1958), they have undergone major transformations since that time—especially over the past 15 years. The psychoanalytic model painted a picture of inevitable stress, tension, and hostility in family relations at adolescence. And, indeed, this negative image, also apparent in early sociological writings (e.g., Davis, 1940), has shaped our popular stereotypes about adolescence and is still maintained by many parents and clinicians today (Offer, Ostrov, & Howard, 1981). Systematic empirical research conducted since the early 1970s has tempered this storm-and-stress portrayal considerably. In place of the earlier emphasis on conflict and detachment between parents and adolescents, there is growing agreement among scholars regarding the significance of family ties at adolescence and the reciprocal influence between adolescents and their families (Powers, Hauser, & Kilner, 1989). Current research suggests that parent–child relations do not change in *dramatic* ways at adolescence; rather the transition from childhood to adolescence marks a time of important, if subtle, realignments in parent–child relations (see reviews by Collins, 1990 and Steinberg, 1990).

Susan B. Silverberg and Theodore Jacob • Division of Family Studies, University of Arizona, Tucson, Arizona 85721.   Daniel L. Tennenbaum • Department of Psychology, Kent State University, Kent, Ohio 44242.

Handbook of Social Development: A Lifespan Perspective, edited by Vincent B. Van Hasselt and Michel Hersen. Plenum Press, New York, 1992.

John Hill (1982), an influential scholar of adolescence and the family, wrote that "early adolescence brings with it the onset of the most rapid and dramatic changes in the human organism since infancy" (p. 1410). These changes range from the physical aspects of pubertal development, to the psychological issues associated with autonomy and identity development, to the social changes linked with peer group membership and dating. To researchers who maintain a contextual approach to the study of human development, a focus on the family as a critical context of adolescent development would seem to go without question (Bronfenbrenner, 1986). Somewhat surprisingly, however, family studies of adolescence were relatively limited until the early 1980s. The wealth of new research is welcome but increases the challenge of summarizing the work in one short chapter.

We have organized our review of the literature around three main themes. In the first section, we briefly trace the field from its storm-and-stress roots of the psychoanalytic tradition to its more recent conceptual and empirical bases that have a more balanced, less dramatic flavor. Part of this section includes discussion of the extent and role of conflict and closeness in parent–child relations at adolescence. Our second theme concerns adolescent development as a stimulus for family change. Here, we review research that has attempted to answer the question, How does a child's development at adolescence serve to influence the nature and quality of his or her family relations? How do the changes experienced by the adolescent reverberate throughout the family system? We devote special attention to pubertal and cognitive changes as catalysts for transformations in parent–child relations. In our third section we review the growing body of literature concerning the influence of family interaction patterns and parenting styles on adolescent competence and psychosocial development. We touch upon selected research regarding the role of family factors in the development and maintenance of behavioral and psychiatric problems among adolescents; however, a full review of this literature is beyond the scope of the present chapter (see Halweg & Goldstein, 1987; Jacob, 1987; Loeber & Stouthamer-Loeber, 1986). Throughout these sections, we briefly highlight areas that warrant additional study. We conclude the chapter with some thoughts on directions for future research.

CHANGING PERSPECTIVES ON ADOLESCENCE AND THE FAMILY

Prevailing views of what constitutes normal and healthy parent–child relationships during adolescence have swung somewhat like a pendulum over the last 30 years. At one extreme, one finds the orthodox psychoanalytic perspective wherein explosive family conflict, adolescent rebellion, and emotional detachment from parents describes the normative and healthy scenario for youngsters in this age group. The largely clinically based work of Anna Freud (1958) was especially influential in promoting this storm-and-stress view of adolescence and the family. According to A. Freud, the physiological changes of puberty bring a resurgence of sexual impulses that disrupt the relative calm of latency; intrapsychic conflicts repressed since early childhood (unconscious attraction toward the opposite-sex parent and ambivalent feelings toward the parent of the same sex) are suddenly reawakened. The resurgence of these sexual impulses leads inevitably to severe intrapsychic turmoil and anxiety for the young adolescent and makes continued emotional attachment to parents extremely difficult. This inner emotional upheaval is not dealt with by the adolescent consciously but gets expressed in rebelliousness toward parents, severe arguments in the home, and emotional detachment from parents. Most important, A. Freud considered these hostile and distant parent–adolescent relationships to be normative and desirable because they act to stimulate the development of greater autonomy from parents and the development of mature extrafamilial attachments and sexual relationships in later adolescence and early adulthood. Interestingly, A. Freud interpreted the continued presence of close, harmonious parent–child relations at adolescence as indicative of a delay in normal development and a symptom of immaturity deserving serious attention.

The disturbing storm and stress view of adolescence and the family prompted a number of researchers in the mid-1960s and early 1970s to conduct much-needed empirical investigations on samples of adolescents more representative of the general population (e.g., Douvan & Adelson, 1966; Offer, 1969; Rutter, Graham, Chadwick, & Yule, 1976). These now classic accounts of parent–child relations at adolescence discounted the long-held belief of the inevitability of stormy and stressful family relations, rebelliousness, and adolescents' feelings of emotional detachment vis-à-vis their parents. Instead, they suggested that the vast majority of adolescents feel close to and respect their parents. Rutter *et al.* (1976), for example, suggested that most adolescents did not see their parents as adversaries but considered their parents as supportive and guiding influences. This new stream of research also revealed that the relatively small group (perhaps 15% to 20%) of young people who seem to have poor relationships with their parents at adolescence most often evidenced poor relationships with their parents during childhood as well; sudden deterioration of the parent–child relationship seemed to be a relatively rare exception. Thus, although adolescence is a period of change, the weight of the empirical evidence from these studies greatly modified the tumultuous image of adolescents and their family relations. That is, most nonclinical scholars in the field concluded that the quality of parent–child relations remains largely continuous from childhood through adolescence and that most families show signs of continued closeness (Dornbusch, 1989). The pendulum had swung to its other extreme.

As revealing as this empirical work on adolescence and the family was, the resulting continuity perspective seemed to downplay changes that one would expect to find in parent–child relations from childhood through adolescence (Grotevant & Cooper, 1986). Parent–child relationships of 10- and 11-year-olds seem to differ from those of 16- and 17-year-olds to a greater extent than these studies suggested. Part of the reason for the discrepancy between intuitive predictions and early research findings may be attributable to the methodological and conceptual shortcomings of the research conducted in the 1960s and early 1970s. For example, "virtually all studies were questionnaire or interview based, and relied on global assessments of closeness, independence, or intergenerational tension" (Steinberg, 1987c, p. 193). Without more detailed questions to both youngsters and parents and without assessments of actual interactions and daily life, many questions regarding the nature of family interaction and the changing quality of family relations during adolescence remained unexplored.

In response to the limitations of the earlier empirical literature, recent research efforts have become more methodologically sophisticated, often including combinations of questionnaire/interview, standardized instrument, and observational approaches (Hill, 1987). Moreover, researchers have devoted increasing attention to the processes of change in family relations at adolescence. Although the issue of conflict continues to be studied, it is no longer based on adolescents' global descriptions of parent–child relations. Investigations using a wide variety of self-report techniques, including detailed questionnaires (Steinberg, 1987b), time sampling with electronic beepers (Csikszentmihalyi & Larson, 1984), and periodic, randomly timed phone interviews concerning the previous day's interactions (Montemayor, 1983) reveal (as did earlier studies) that serious parent–child conflict and family turmoil are not inevitable features of family relations at adolescence for most families. These more recent studies also indicate that the conflicts that do occur are best characterized as occasional bickering and squabbling over day-to-day topics, such as chores, personal appearance, curfew, and the like, rather than over major values (Hill & Holmbeck, 1986). Many disagreements also concern issues of consideration and accommodation to the needs of others, issues that may be as likely to cause conflict at other times of life (Montemayor & Hanson, 1985). Interestingly, the rather mundane topics of parent–adolescent conflict have remained quite similar over the past 60 years. For example, in Lynd and Lynd's (1929) study of Middletown, "hours and home duties were most often subject to disagreement, and club and society memberships and religious observance were least often subject to disagreement" (Hill, 1987, p. 15). Montemayor's (1986) review of the literature suggests a good deal of between-family differences in the frequency and intensity of parent–adolescent conflict; nevertheless, most adolescents and parents report quarreling on a regular basis.

Other research suggests that although the early psychoanalytic predictions severely exaggerated the extent of normative parent–adolescent conflict, our current picture of parent–adolescent relationships may underestimate conflict levels (Gecas & Seff, 1990). For example, Hill and Holmbeck (1987) remind us that research on parent–adolescent conflict resolution shows that over half of specific conflicts do not reach the point of parent–adolescent verbal interchange leading toward resolution (Montemayor & Hanson, 1985). That is, instead of heatedly talking through or negotiating the area of disagreement, family members often "solve" conflicts through withdrawal—by one or both members walking away. Hill and Holmbeck (1987) suggest that data collection methods that consider conflict to have occurred *only* if an actual parent–child interchange was involved, may yield underestimations. And it is, perhaps, the more sensitive topics that are most likely to involve withdrawal.

Although few studies have permitted longitudinal comparisons of conflict before and during adolescence, research to date indicates that no dramatic increases in family conflict occur from childhood to adolescence in most families. Nonetheless, *early adolescence* does seem to be a time of temporary "perturbations" in parent-child interactions (Hill, 1988), as well as a stressful time for many parents (Ballenski & Cook, 1982; Pasley & Gecas, 1984; Silverberg & Steinberg, 1987; Small, Eastman, & Cornelius, 1988). Youngsters become somewhat more assertive and influential in family interactions, especially at the expense of their mothers (Steinberg, 1990). (We discuss the important realignments in parent–child relations at early adolescence in a section to follow.)

Moreover, although the orthodox psychoanalytic conception of emotional detachment does not provide an accurate description of parent–child relations at early adolescence (i.e., emotional bonds are not threatened), researchers have noted that early adolescence is a time of diminished positive interactions between children and parents. For example, a recent study of parent–child interaction indicates that as youngsters mature physically during early adolescence, both parents and adolescents express less positive affect toward one another (Flannery, 1991). Compared with their interactions during childhood and later adolescence, parents and young teenagers are less likely to say positive things to each other and are less apt to engage in pleasant activities with each other (Montemayor, 1986). Relatedly, neo-analytic theorists have suggested that a gradual process of individuation (i.e., a gradual relinquishing of childish dependencies on parents in favor of a more mature, realistic, and responsible relationship) begins during early adolescence (Blos, 1962). Part of this process, according to Blos (1962), involves the gradual deidealization of one's parents. And indeed, in their questionnaire study of 10- to 15-years-olds, Steinberg and Silverberg (1986) found increases in youngsters' deidealization of parents (e.g., "My parents sometimes make mistakes") over the age range studied.

Similarly, Smollar and Youniss's (1989) interviews with adolescents suggest that by middle adolescence most youngsters have moved away from an idealized image of their parents as "all-knowing" and "all-powerful." For example, when asked to describe changes in their relationships with their parents over the past 5 years, one 15-year-old said about his father, "I used to listen to everything. I thought he was always right. Now I have my own opinions. They may be wrong, but they're mine and I like to say them" (Smollar & Youniss, 1989, p. 77). In this context, however, most youngsters continue to identify with and be influenced by their parents during adolescence. For example, when it comes to long-term questions concerning educational or occupational plans, or questions of values, adolescents seem to follow parental advice even over peer advice (Brittain, 1963; Young & Ferguson, 1979).*

In summary, even in families with positive, close relationships, some bickering and squabbling is present during adolescence (Hill & Holmbeck, 1986; Montemayor, 1986). Although parent–child relationships appear to change over the transition from childhood to adolescence, this change is rather gradual and is not marked by feelings of detachment. Young adolescents, although not rejecting parental values, begin to form a less idealized image of their parents. Research suggests, however, that it may not be until late adolescence or young adulthood that individuals begin to perceive their parents in a fully realistic way, that is, as individuals beyond their role as parents (Smollar & Youniss, 1989; Steinberg & Silverberg, 1986; White, Speisman, & Costos, 1983).

Interestingly, recent investigations have reintroduced the idea that parent–adolescent conflict may serve a positive, functional purpose for adolescents. Hill (1988), for example, suggests that although severe conflict is rare in most families, it would be premature to regard the conflicts that occur in the majority of families as insignificant and of little adaptive importance (Hill & Holmbeck, 1986). In this vein, both Hill (1988) and Cooper (1988) have proposed that conflict that occurs within a hostile, defensive context is a sign of problematic parent–adolescent relations and is detrimental to youngsters' development, whereas low-level parent–adolescent conflict, *if* worked out in an otherwise supportive relational environment, may be beneficial to youngsters and help transform parent–child relations in a favorable direction. The proposal, briefly stated, is that "conflict can function constructively when it co-occurs with the subjective conditions of trust and

---

*See, however, Sebald (1986) for a discussion of shifts in parent and peer orientation over the past three decades.

closeness and their behavioral expressions" (Cooper, 1988, p. 183). Disagreements worked out under these conditions may help youngsters develop a more realistic appraisal of their parents, safely test-out their own ideas, and loosen childish dependence on parents (Steinberg, 1990). Although few researchers have conducted studies to examine this hypothesis directly, Cooper and Grotevant's studies of structured family interaction indicate that expressions of individuality (self-assertions and disagreements) in the context of interpersonal connectedness (agreement, acknowledgments, and compromise) are associated with adaptive identity and relational skills among older adolescents (Cooper, Grotevant, & Condon, 1983; Grotevant & Cooper, 1985). (We will elaborate on this, and related research, in a later section.)

One assumption of the view just described is that the adaptive value of conflict will prevail only if a tolerant and open verbal give-and-take between parent and child accompanies the disagreement. In light of research indicating that more than half of parent–adolescent disagreements are ended by means of withdrawing from the scene and that relatively few disagreements involve true negotiation and discussion (Montemayor & Hanson, 1985), Steinberg (1990) suggests that most parents may be missing an opportunity to facilitate their adolescent's development.

Adolescent Development as a Stimulus for Family Change

A growing number of researchers studying the adolescent years have devoted attention to the issue of how youngsters' development during the transition to adolescence might serve as a potential catalyst for change in family relations and perceptions of family functioning (Kidwell, Fischer, Dunham, & Baranowski, 1983). This relatively new avenue of research corresponds well with one of the most significant changes in the study of human development and family relations—the shift away from models that focus exclusively on *parents'* influence on their children, toward an examination of the *child's* influence on the family, in general, and on parenting, in particular (Bell, 1968; Maccoby & Martin, 1983). The existing body of research on "child effects" during adolescence began with studies that compared family interaction patterns of preadolescent youngsters with those of adolescents (Alexander, 1973a,b; Jacob, 1974). Chronological age (the independent variable in these studies) served merely as a proxy for more specific aspects of youngsters' development (e.g., maturing physical appearance, expanding social relations, more sophisticated cognitive skills, and increasing demands for greater autonomy). And, there are reasons to believe that it is the more specific aspects of youngsters' development that influence family relationships (Powers *et al.*, 1989). We know, moreover, that there is a fair degree of variability *between* youngsters of the same chronological age on these more specific aspects of development. Therefore, to group youngsters according to chronological age alone may blur important differences among youngsters and, in turn, among families exhibiting changes over time. Nevertheless, these initial, age-focused studies set the stage for later research on the impact of youngsters' pubertal and cognitive development on family relations.*

---

*The complexity of predictions regarding family change as a function of child development multiplies when we consider families with multiple children of different ages. The existing research, as well as our discussion, assumes a one-child family as a prototype.

Jacob (1974) was among the first researchers to examine the nature of familial realignment over the transition to adolescence. In his cross-sectional study, he compared mother–father–son patterns of interaction (with a focus on indices of dominance and influence) in families of 11-year-old boys with those in families of 16-year-old boys. After making independent choices on a series of emotionally charged topics, mother, father, and son were asked to reach consensus—to arrive at a family decision on the topics. Analyses of the taped triadic discussions revealed "definite shifts in family power structure as a function of child age" (p. 9). The nature of the shifts differed, however, for middle- versus working-class families. The power structure of middle-class families with a younger son reflected relative equality between mothers and fathers in their influence over family final decisions, and both mothers and fathers appeared more influential than their son (father = mother > son). With an adolescent son in middle-class families, an influence shift appeared in which the sons become more influential at the expense of mothers, whereas fathers maintained their relative power status (father > son > mother). Although sons gained influence in working-class families as well, this shift in influence was not only at the expense of mothers but also at the expense of many fathers. Jacob proposed that the shift in working-class families tends to move from a father = mother > son structure to a (rather unstable) father = mother = son structure.

Overall, this laboratory research suggests that a specific pattern of realignment in family relations occurs across the transition from preadolescence to middle adolescence, at least among families with boys. These transformations may play a critical role in the maintenance of healthy development of youngsters.* In fact, other research indicates that families that resist making adaptations during adolescence—by discouraging greater symmetry in the parent–child relationship and developing hostility around old patterns of interaction—are more likely to include a delinquent adolescent (Alexander, 1973b).

Changes in Family Relations as a Function of Pubertal Development

The realignments and adaptations in family relations from preadolescence to middle adolescence may progress, however, not so much as a function of youngsters' age *per se* but as a function of their pubertal, cognitive, and social development (Kidwell *et al.*, 1983). Pubertal development is characterized by well-documented changes in the physical characteristics of the child (Tanner, 1962). Accompanying internal endocrinological changes are easily observable changes in height, facial features, body proportions, and voice. As youngsters mature, they move from a prepubertal status when they show no signs of pubertal development, to their apex of pubertal growth, to full pubertal maturation. To date, researchers interested in family adaptation to youngsters' development at adolescence have focused primarily on the impact of these overt signs of pubertal maturation on family relations. Many of the studies that include families of girls have used menarcheal status as an alternative means of tracking pubertal status.

---

*As we discuss in a later section, the process of transforming parent–child relationships may, however, be less favorable when one considers the well-being of mothers.

Laurence Steinberg and John Hill have conducted some of the most influential research on family adaptation to adolescent pubertal development. For example, in a longitudinal follow-up of their initial cross-sectional work (Steinberg & Hill, 1978), Steinberg (1981) examined whether family interaction patterns seem to shift as boys progress across the phases of pubertal development. Steinberg assessed pubertal status and collected family interaction data at 6-month intervals, three times over the course of 1 year among a small sample of middle- and upper middle-class 11- to 14-year-old boys and their mothers and fathers (all boys were firstborns). Family interaction patterns were assessed via a method similar to Jacob's (1974) already described. The taped family interactions were coded with respect to indexes of conflict, power, and deference (in the form of interruptions, lack of explanations, yielding to interruptions, and influence on family final decisions). When the interaction data were examined as a function of sons' chronological age, no clear or consistent pattern emerged. However, when they were examined as a function of sons' pubertal maturation, systematic transformations in family inter-action, and especially in the mother–adolescent relationship, were apparent.

Specifically, as the boys approached the pubertal apex, both mothers and sons interrupted each other more frequently and offered fewer explanations for their assertions. Not only did sons interrupt their mothers with increasing frequency, they less often yielded to their mothers' interruptions. In brief, a somewhat more vigorous and conflictual-like pattern of interaction emerged between mothers and their sons near the midpoint of the pubertal cycle. This conflictual-like pattern seemed to subside as sons moved from the midpoint of pubertal development toward full pubertal maturation. Interestingly, this was not due to a decrease in sons' assertiveness toward their mothers; rather, it was due to mothers "backing off" (i.e., to a decrease in mothers' interruptive behaviors toward their sons and an increase in mothers' yielding to their sons' interruptions). As the boys passed the pubertal apex, they also became more influential in the family decisions. Like Jacob's (1974) findings for middle-class families, this increase in sons' influence comes at the expense of mothers. In summary, following strained mother–son interactions at the pubertal apex, sons appeared to gain influence, whereas their mothers showed a complementary pattern of giving in to their sons more and commanding less influence in decisions. In high contrast to this pattern, Steinberg (1981) found that fathers tended to become more dominant and sons more deferent to them across the pubertal cycle, at least as revealed in father–son patterns of interruptions and yields to interruptions. Moreover, fathers continued to be the most influential family member even as their sons matured. Here again, the pattern is quite consistent with Jacob's (1974) findings for middle-class families.

In an independent program of research, Hill and his colleagues later at-tempted to examine whether Steinberg's (1981) findings would be confirmed using self-report rather than observational methods and whether similar findings would emerge for families of boys and families of girls (Hill, Holmbeck, Marlow, Green, & Lynch, 1985a,b). These researchers focused on perceptions of parent–child rela-tionships in samples of firstborn, seventh-grade youngsters who ranged from prepubescent to postpubescent. Like Steinberg (1981), Hill *et al.* (1985b) found that "there appear to be perturbations in mother-son relations in the apex pubertal group" relative to the pre- and post-pubertal groups (p. 40). For example, mothers' reports of sons' oppositionalism peaked in the apex pubertal group, whereas mothers' reports of sons' involvement in family activities and maternal satisfaction were at their lowest levels in the apex group. This curvilinear pattern of strained parent–child relations was not apparent in father–son relationships. Although the magnitude of Hill *et al.*'s (1985b) findings suggests that the degree of change in mother–son relations is not dramatic, the findings' consistency with those of observational studies (Steinberg, 1981; Steinberg & Hill, 1978) supports the view that family interaction patterns tend to shift at the peak of the pubertal cycle.

Hill *et al.*'s (1985a) study of seventh-grade girls also supports the idea of temporary perturbations in parent–child relations; in this case, the strain appears among families whose daughters have just recently experienced menarche (0–6 months ago). Relative to premenarcheal girls and to girls who experienced menarche 7 to 12 months ago, girls who recently experienced menarche were more likely to perceive their parents as controlling and were more apt to have disagreements over rules. Moreover, these girls were less apt to seek guidance from their parents, less likely to be involved in family activities, and less likely to perceive their mothers as accepting. Thus, Hill *et al.* (1985a) conclude that "if not out-right storm, there certainly does appear to be a period of stress and strain in mother-daughter relations shortly after menarche" (p. 315). However, because their data also indicate strain in mother–daughter relations for the seventh-grade girls who were greater than 12 months postmenarche, Hill and colleagues suggest that whereas a *temporary* period of perturbations follows menarche when the event is "on time," early maturing girls may be at risk for distance and dissatisfaction in their relations with parents well beyond the months just past menarche (Hill & Holmbeck, 1987). Future, longitudinal-based research is needed to test this intriguing hypothesis. It is also noteworthy that although sons and most daughters experience a temporary period of strained parent–child interactions as they mature physically, observational research reveals that unlike boys, girls do not appear to gain in influence in family decision making with advanced pubertal development (Hill, 1988).

On the whole, the results of these initial research endeavors began to suggest that puberty may be linked to a form of distancing in the parent–child relationship. And indeed, more recent studies, including those using longitudinal designs, indicate that pubertal maturation is associated with somewhat diminished parent–child closeness, increased feelings of emotional autonomy on the part of youngsters (Steinberg, 1987b, 1988), as well as decreased expression of youngsters' and parents' positive affect toward each other (Flannery, 1991). Other studies also suggest that mothers perceive some loss of control over their adolescent's behavior with increased maturation (Papini & Sebby, 1987).

In summary, puberty seems to serve as a catalyst for transformations in the parent–child relationship including modest increases in parent–child distance and notable shifts at the apex of pubertal development (Steinberg, 1990). Mother–child relations seem to undergo greater change than father–child relations as youngsters mature; this entails mothers bearing some of the less favorable aspects of familial change, such as parent–child bickering. It is important to keep in mind, however, that although findings are consistent across various studies, pubertal status alone accounts for a relatively small proportion of the variation in adolescent–parent relations (Steinberg, 1988). Moreover, the "perturbations" in parent–child relations tend to occur (in most families) within a context of generally positive feelings and not with feelings of detachment and hostility. The transformations in no way imply that emotional ties between parent and child have been severed. They do, however, suggest that puberty plays a role in the gradual process of adolescent individuation (see Steinberg, 1989, for an evolution-based discussion of puberty and parent–adolescent distance).*†

In an interesting extension of this research area, Anderson, Hetherington, and Clingempeel (1989) investigated whether the patterns of transformation found among intact, two-parent families hold for divorced, single-parent families as well. In brief, their analyses suggest that unlike the pattern found in intact families, there does not seem to be any systematic increase in mother–child conflict or decrease in maternal warmth as a function of child's pubertal status among single-mother families. (Single mothers did, however, become less effective monitors of their daughters' behavior as girls matured.) To make sense of this curious difference between their intact and single-mother families, Anderson *et al.* speculated that, at least for families of boys, conflict around issues of independence and autonomy may have already peaked when the single-parent families were in the initial process of adjustment to divorce—a period prior to the study. This interpretation suggests that strain and eventual realignment of mother–child relations can be prompted prior to puberty as a result of a dramatic intrafamilial event. Although Anderson *et al.*'s (1989) study revealed no increase in conflict between single-mothers and daughters as a function of pubertal status in girls, single-mothers of daughters (relative to other mothers) expressed negative expectations when asked to describe how they felt about their child's becoming a "teenager."

We know from a number of studies that adolescent detachment (Ryan & Lynch, 1989) and familial conflict (Montemayor, 1986) tend to be greater in single-parent homes than in intact, two-parent homes. In light of Anderson *et al.*'s (1989) findings, we can tentatively conclude that for families of boys this difference in level of conflict and distance is not due to greater difficulty in adapting to puberty on the part of single mothers and sons; instead, it may be due to adaptation to a single-parent household. On the other hand, the adaptation of single-parent mothers to their daughter's pubertal development, and in particular *early* pubertal development, may have its special difficulties and warrants further study (Hetherington, 1988). Indeed, the vast majority of research in the area of family adaptation to pubertal development has been confined to samples of white, middle-class, two-parent intact families. Whether patterns of family realignment are similar in other families remains to be seen. Future research efforts should pay special attention to stepfamilies at the transition to adolescence given other research which suggests that early adolescents may be particularly vulnerable and less able to adapt to the remarriage of their custodial parent (Hetherington, Stanley-Hagan, & Anderson, 1989) and investigations which point to the stepparent–adolescent relationship as one at risk for the occurrence of maltreatment (Garbarino, Sebes, & Schellenbach, 1984).

---

*Interestingly, in a test of the potential reciprocal relation between parent–child distance and pubertal maturation, Steinberg (1988) found that distance in the mother–child relationship—in the form of more frequent arguments and fewer calm discussions—seems to accelerate pubertal maturation in girls.
†Studies of the effects of pubertal *timing* on family relations yield less consistent patterns (Hauser, *et al.*, 1985; Savin-Williams & Small, 1986; see Steinberg, 1987*b* for a review).

Although pubertal changes may be the most visible and dramatic aspect of the transition from childhood to adolescence, this period is also marked by changes in youngsters' ways of thinking about themselves, others, and the day-to-day events in their lives. Each of these changes presents a potential challenge to existing patterns of interaction between parents and children (Laursen, 1988; Robin, Koepke, & Nayor, 1986). For example, the emergence of the ability to think and reason in more sophisticated ways may permit youngsters to present more rational and convincing arguments to their parents (Clark & Delia, 1976). Similarly, newly developing abilities to think in terms of possibilities, alternatives, and principles may provide youngsters with the cognitive means to take a new perspective on their family's situation, rules, and regulations (Hill & Holmbeck, 1986).

Only very recently have researchers begun to investigate empirically the link between social-cognitive changes of adolescence and changing family relations during this period, and Smetana's work (1988b, 1989) is of particular interest in this area. She argues that cognitive changes in adolescents influence their view of legitimate parental authority such that areas previously considered to be under parental jurisdiction come to be viewed as under their own personal jurisdiction. Parents, on the other hand, may continue to view many of these areas as subject to their authority. Smetana (1988b) proposes that this potential discrepancy may help to account for conflicts during the adolescent years. And, indeed, based on extensive interviews with parents and their fifth- through twelfth-graders, Smetana (1988a) has demonstrated that compared to pre-adolescents, older youngsters increasingly view issues that arise at home (e.g., how clean their room is, manner of dress) as matters of personal choice or taste rather than as matters of convention. Whereas adolescents seem to view more and more issues as rightly under their own jurisdiction, parents (especially mothers) continue to perceive most issues as subject to rules and legitimately under their authority, to some degree. This divergence in definition or conceptualization of issues increases the likelihood of parent–child conflict. Smetana's (1988a) results do not, however, coincide with the prediction that parent–child conceptions of parental authority are maximally disjunctive at early adolescence. Instead, they appear to be disjunctive throughout adolescence. The typical decrease in parent–adolescent conflict by middle or late adolescence, then, may be attributable either to parents gradually conceding to their youngsters in actual interactions or to youngsters' increasing ability, at least, to understand their parents' point of view.

Parent–child relations may also be affected by youngsters' changing self-conceptions from childhood through adolescence (Laursen, 1988). Damon and Hart (1982) note that as children mature, their conceptions of self change toward greater reliance on social and psychological aspects of self and lesser reliance on physical and active aspects. Self-conceptions at early adolescence tend to focus on how the self appears to others; there is a concern with obtaining the approval of others and integrating the self into social networks (Level 3 in Damon and Hart's terminology). This dependency on the views of others diminishes for most youngsters by late adolescence, when a more abstract, unified conception of self forms that coordinates seemingly inconsistent characteristics (Level 4). Unfortunately, researchers have not as yet explored the implications of these developmental changes in youngsters' self-conceptions upon parent–child relations. Laursen (1988) suggests, however, that "the potential for conflict between peer and parent norms and resulting tensions within the family seem greatest during the Level 3 period as the adolescent strives to conform to both groups" (pp. 10–11).

In summary, although researchers who have assessed youngsters' cognitive development in terms of *formal operational* thinking skills have not found significant associations with patterns of parent–child interaction (Steinberg & Hill, 1978; Walters & Norrell, 1987), there is evidence that indexes of *social-cognitive* development are linked with changes in parent–child relations. In accord with Smetana's (1988a) view, Powers *et al.* (1989) suggest that

> basic realignments in family relationships and new views of parental authority and of family roles and rules may be necessary to permit continued growth of the adolescent and the family, rather than an impasse resulting from sustained opposition by the adolescent or parents' reluctance or inability to appreciate new perspectives from their changing son or daughter. (p. 204)

What the current body of research now requires are longitudinal studies that closely monitor the independent *and* combined effects of pubertal and social-cognitive development on parent–child relations, perceptions of familial relations, and behavioral interactions during the transition into and through adolescence. Of great value would be studies initiated at a pretransition point such that researchers could discern how preexisting characteristics of the family and the child moderate the effects of puberty and social-cognitive development on family relations.

In addition, the question of whether and how these changes in family relations, in turn, affect parents' well-being is just beginning to receive empirical attention. Studies, to date, have found that reports of parental stress are highest among parents of early adolescents and are associated with youngsters' demands for greater say in decision making (Small *et al.*, 1988). Moreover, distance between parents and children at early adolescence may provoke life/self-reappraisal and reevaluation among parents, especially among parents with adolescents of the same sex (Silverberg & Steinberg, 1987). The strength of the link between development at adolescence and parental well-being appears to be moderated by characteristics of the parent, however, including the parent's orientation toward his or her paid work role (Silverberg & Steinberg, 1990). Silverberg and Steinberg's (1990) study, for example, indicates that among parents with a weak orientation toward work, signs of their child's transition to adolescence are negatively associated with well-being. However, among parents with a relatively strong orientation toward work, well-being may be favorably affected by development during this transitional period. Of interest in future research is whether the families of these two groups of parents differ in their ability to adapt to the new challenges of the adolescent years, and whether other characteristics of parents (e.g., their belief system regarding the period of adolescence) also moderate the effects of youngsters' development on parental mental health.

FAMILY INFLUENCES ON ADOLESCENT PSYCHOSOCIAL DEVELOPMENT

A long-standing and dominant trend in research on child development casts parenting practices and the general family environment as major contexts for development (Collins, 1984). How parenting styles and family interaction patterns differ across families and what consequences these differences may have for children's healthy development have been central questions in this field of research. Although most research on parenting practices and developmental outcomes focuses on the early-and middle-childhood years (Maccoby & Martin, 1983), researchers have recently extended their efforts toward adolescence.

Connectedness, Individuality, and Adolescent Development

A number of active research teams have focused on the link between patterns of family interaction and key developmental tasks of adolescence: identity exploration, ego development, and formation of interpersonal perspective-taking skills (Cooper *et al.*, 1983, Grotevant & Cooper, 1985, 1986; Hauser *et al.*, 1984; Powers, Hauser, Schwartz, Noam, & Jacobson, 1983). Much of this work has been guided by the hypothesis that encouragement of adolescent individuality (permitting disagreement and the expression of alternative views) within a context of family affective support and connectedness provides an optimal environment for adolescent psychosocial development. (This suggestion is closely tied to the idea, discussed previously, that moderate parent–child conflict may serve a facilitating role if expressed within an otherwise supportive social environment.)

Hauser, Powers, and their colleagues (Hauser *et al.*, 1984; Powers *et al.*, 1983), for example have attempted to specify the role that family interactions play in facilitating (enabling) or inhibiting (constraining) adolescent ego development.* Their work is generally based on the premise that in order to stimulate youngsters' development, parent–child interactions must combine cognitive-enabling behavior (communication of different viewpoints, challenging of views, focusing, problem solving) with affective support (acceptance, empathy, encouragement of discussion). Inhibiting interactions, according to these researchers, include those in which parents actively resist their child's differentiation (through devaluing, distortion, and avoidance), especially in the context of affective conflict.

Hauser and Powers's empirical work provides support for these hypotheses. For example, in a structured interactional study of 14- to 15-year-old adolescents and their parents, Powers *et al.* (1983) found that adolescent ego development was most advanced when families exhibited a high amount of noncompetitive sharing of perspectives or challenging behavior within a context of high affective support and low affective conflict. Somewhat less advanced youngsters experienced sharing of perspectives in their family interactions as well. However, this was combined with high amounts of avoidance (perhaps indicating that family members felt uneasy about openly dealing with differences of opinion). Families whose youngsters were least advanced in ego development were most likely to exhibit high amounts of task rejection and distortion within a context of affective conflict. These findings, as well as those of Hauser *et al.* (1984) point to strong links between parents' affective responsiveness and adolescent ego development.

*In Loevinger's (1976) theory, ego development follows a hierarchically ordered, invariant sequence of stages where "the lower stages of ego development are characterized by impulsive, exploitative, and dependent orientations; the middle levels are typified by conformist thinking; and the higher stages are distinguished by cognitive complexity, autonomy, and respect for individual differences" (White *et al.*, 1983).

Additional analyses on this cross-sectional data set (Powers, Beardslee, Jacobson, & Noam, 1987) and its 4-year longitudinal follow-up (Leaper et al., 1989), however, point to possible differences in facilitative family interactions for males and females during adolescence. Unfortunately, these two reports yielded somewhat conflicting results regarding the relative beneficial effects of the encouragement of individuality and overt affective support for the two sexes. On the one hand, by means of a quantitative and qualitative examination of the data, Powers and her colleagues (1987) found that a combination of sharing alternative perspectives and overt affective support was associated with high functioning among girls; overt expression of support appeared to be less important among boys. On the other hand, Leaper et al.'s (1989) coding and analyses of the Hauser data indicated that for girls, progression in ego development toward a postconformist stage is associated with patterns suggestive of greater separation; for boys such progression is associated with family discussions marked by greater warmth and support. Perhaps slight variations in coding systems, somewhat disparate outcomes variables, and/or differences in the age of the target adolescents may be able to account for the conflicting results of Powers et al. (1987) and Leaper et al. (1989). Leaper et al.'s findings, however, are in keeping with Steinberg's view that:

> Healthy psychosocial development among young women may require more of a concerted effort to establish autonomy in family relations, among young men, however, the same goal may require maintaining more connectedness in the family. Because girls in our society may be oversocialized toward dependence, and boys toward independence, it may be necessary for individuals to depart from traditional sex roles in late adolescence in order to be able to strike a balance between agency and communion in their intimate relations with peers. (Steinberg, 1987c, pp. 194–195)

Additional research that focuses on potential differences in facilitative family interaction for males and females is clearly warranted.

Aside from this unresolved issue, the recent longitudinal data begin to reveal the full import of Hauser and Powers's earlier cross-sectional results (Hauser, Powers, Noam, & Bowlds, 1987). By assessing stage of adolescent ego development annually over 4 years (beginning at age 14), Hauser et al. (1987) were able to trace ego development *trajectories* (early arrested, consistent, precociously advanced, and progressive) and the antecedent family interaction patterns that appear to contribute to these various developmental paths. Parents proved to be least enabling toward those adolescents who showed early arrested ego development.

> There were few instances of connectedness. . . . Instead, there were many moments of disengagement, turning away, or indifference between parent and child. . . . Rather than being permeable in their responses to one another, they express opaqueness, rejecting and devaluing ideas and feelings from one another. (Hauser et al., 1987, p. 267)

In contrast, parents expressed a good deal of cognitive and affective enabling toward adolescents who subsequently showed trajectories of progressive ego development. Parents in these families appear to permit, encourage, and accept the expression of multiple perspectives or points of view. In summary, family discussion patterns during middle adolescence can predict whether adolescents will exhibit arrested, consistent, or progressive paths of development in the years to follow (Powers et al., 1989).

In a related program of research, Grotevant and Cooper (1986) outline a model of adolescent development that highlights the facilitative role of individuation in family dyadic relationships. According to this model, an individuated relationship is one that displays a balance between individuality and connectedness (Cooper *et al.*, 1983). Using this model as a framework, Grotevant and Cooper developed a four-part system for assessing family communication patterns, where individuality is reflected by *separateness* (expressing differentness of self from others) and *self-assertion* (expressing one's own point of view clearly); connectedness is reflected by *mutuality* (expressing sensitivity to and respect for others' ideas) and *permeability* (expressing openness and responsiveness to others' views).*

The results from Grotevant and Cooper's (1985) observational study of high-school seniors and their families provide some support for the view that an effective combination of cohesion and separation in family relationships is associated with adolescent identity exploration and perspective-taking skills (Cooper *et al.*, 1983). In general, "adolescents rated highest in both identity exploration and role-taking skill were found to have participated with at least one parent in an individuated relationship . . . examining their differences, but within the context of connectedness" (Grotevant & Cooper, 1986, p. 92). The specific results, however, were complicated enough to underscore the importance of examining individuation at the level of specific dyads within the family (including the marital dyad) and of considering differences in relationship qualities that are associated with male and female competence. For example, Grotevant and Cooper (1985) found that in families with boys, only father–son communication style was related to identity exploration. Boys rated high on exploration were more likely to express disagreements and suggestions directly with their father, and fathers complemented these behaviors with relatively high levels of mutuality. For girls, the strongest associations were between father–mother communication and daughter's identity-exploration level. Daughters who showed high identity exploration were likely to come from families where husbands exhibited more separateness, and lower mutuality and permeability in relating to their wives, and where wives expressed their opinions directly but also seemed more responsible for coordinating the discussion, as seen in their higher mutuality scores toward their husbands. As with other initial efforts, the need for replication and longitudinal extension of this research is clear.†

An assumption that underlies the work of Hauser, Powers, Grotevant, and Cooper is that parent–child relationship patterns that encourage genuine individu-

---

*Factor loadings reported in their work appear to be lower than optimal, however.

†Most descriptions of the family during adolescence are based on the study of *individuals'* behavior occurring during family, or dyadic, interactions. Reiss argues, however, that family members have a *shared* subjective experience of the world around them (a family paradigm) and that this way of experiencing the world may have important implications for adolescent behavior and psychosocial competence (Reiss, Oliveri, & Curd, 1983). According to this model, a family paradigm involves three components: (a) whether the family perceives the world as a masterable place, governed by understandable rules; (b) the family's sense of itself as a unit—whether they perceive actions by one family member as reflecting on all family members in the eyes of the community; and (c) how comfortable a family is in seeking out information before deciding on a solution to a family problem. Reiss's work is unique in its theoretical contribution to the field. Thus far, however, empirical applications of the model indicate surprisingly similar family paradigms in families with high-empathy adolescent males (Reiss *et al.*, 1983), with conduct-disordered adolescents (Reiss, 1971), and with alcoholic fathers (Davis, Stern, Jorgenson, & Steier, 1980).

ality on the part of the adolescent while maintaining positive emotional ties, provide a firm foundation from which youngsters can develop a healthy sense of self and autonomy. Interestingly, theorists from both family systems and psychodynamic perspectives have hypothesized that family patterns that hinder the path to autonomy and to consolidation of individual identity can give rise to the development of eating disorders during the adolescent years (Humphrey, 1989; Minuchin, Rosman, & Baker, 1978). In fact, although still a relatively small empirical literature, existing evidence suggests that families with an eating-disordered adolescent differ in their patterns of relationships from nondistressed families and that specific subtypes of eating disorders (e.g., anorexia, bulimia) appear to be associated with different family interactional styles (see reviews by Humphrey, 1989, and Strober & Humphrey, 1987). Humphrey (1989), for example, used a complex system to code mother–father–daughter interaction during a 10-minute discussion concerning separation. She found that:

> Parents of anorexics communicated a double message of nurturant affection combined with neglect of their daughters' needs to express themselves and their feelings. Anorexic daughters, in turn, were ambivalent about disclosing their feelings versus submitting to their parents. In contrast, bulimics and their parents were hostilely enmeshed and, for them, this appeared to undermine the daughter's separation and self-assertion. (p. 206)

Humphrey's results, especially for families of bulimics, are reminiscent of the family behaviors identified by Hauser *et al.* (1984) as constraining ego development because they involve more negative and affectively conflictual interaction and, at the same time, discourage the expression of the adolescent's independent thought. Although nonfamilial factors may be implicated in the etiology of eating disorders, these initial studies suggest that specific familial strategies may play a role by hindering the process of healthy individuation among adolescent girls. However, whether difficulties in adolescents' age-appropriate attempts at individuation are causally related to the development of eating disorders or are the result of the disorder or a third factor is unclear. Moreover, even if the current hypothesis is confirmed, how and why adolescent girls' problems with individuation result in *eating* disorders rather than in other behavioral or emotional disturbances is certainly not well understood. Without replications and longitudinal extensions of these findings, strong conclusions cannot be drawn; however, the success researchers have had in observing theoretically meaningful distinctions in family process across these families should encourage further investigations.

Variations in Parenting Styles and Adolescent Development

A conceptually related stream of research focuses explicitly on parental rearing practices, or styles, and their links with youngsters' psychosocial competence, on the one hand, and problem behavior, on the other. One of the most consistent findings in this literature on socialization is the favorable association between an authoritative parenting style and psychosocial competence among preschoolers, school-age children, and adolescents alike. The notion of authoritative parenting derives from the seminal work of Diana Baumrind (1978), who sought to identify a cluster of parental practices that promotes healthy child development. Based on her writings and those of other researchers in the field (e.g., Lamborn, Mounts, & Steinberg, 1990), one can conceptualize parenting styles under a fourfold classification scheme: authoritative, authoritarian, indulgent, and indifferent (see Maccoby & Martin, 1983).

Authoritative parents seem to strike an effective balance in their parenting practices. They encourage warm parent–child relationships, permit their children to take part in decision making and express their opinions and individuality, and at the same time, set age-appropriate rules, standards, and limits for their youngsters' behavior. These parents provide rational explanations for family rules and engage in verbal give-and-take with their children especially around issues of discipline. In short, authoritative parents combine high levels of warmth, demandingness (behavioral control and monitoring), and psychological autonomy (Steinberg, 1990). Recent, large-scale questionnaire studies on parenting styles and adolescent development indicate that adolescents raised in authoritative homes tend to score higher than other adolescents on indexes of self-reliance, positive work attitudes, school performance, and mental health (Dornbusch, Ritter, Leiderman, Roberts, & Fraleigh, 1987; Lamborn *et al.*, 1990; Steinberg, Elmen, & Mounts, 1989). These adolescents are less likely than their peers to experience psychological problems or to exhibit externalizing problems such as drug and alcohol use, delinquency, and school misconduct.* Longitudinal research suggests that the positive impact of authoritative parenting on academic success is mediated, in part, through its favorable influence on attitudes toward effort and work (Steinberg *et al.*, 1989).

Authoritarian parents also set limits and rules for their youngsters' behavior, that is, engage in a high degree of demandingness and behavioral control. However, they tend to be lower on warmth and acceptance and to restrict their youngsters' autonomy, self-expression, and involvement in decision making. Their underlying belief is that children should accept, without question or explanation, rules and standards set by parents. Adolescents raised in authoritarian households show a mixture of positive and negative outcomes (Lamborn *et al.*, 1990). Although they appear to score reasonably well on indexes of work orientation and school performance and are less likely than peers raised in indulgent or indifferent households to engage in deviant activities, they are more depressed and somatically distressed than their peers and have a poorer self-image. In summary, these youngsters seem to be obedient but suffer from internalizing problems and a lack of self-confidence (Lamborn *et al.*, 1990).

Indulgent parents are warm and supportive of their youngsters' behavior but are rather passive when it comes to matters of rules, limits, and discipline. They make relatively few demands on their children for mature behavior and take a rather tolerant, even accepting attitude toward their youngsters' impulses (Steinberg, 1987a). Their permissiveness is often based in an ideological commitment to the idea that parental control is an infringement on children's freedom and may interfere with healthy development. Lamborn *et al.*'s (1990) work suggests that, like youngsters raised in authoritarian homes, adolescents from indulgent households fair reasonably well in terms of school performance and work orientation (though not as well as their authoritatively raised counterparts). Unlike youngsters raised in

---

*See, however, Dornbusch's discussion of the differential effectiveness of authoritative and authoritarian parenting practices across ethnic groups (1989; Dornbusch *et al.*, 1987).

authoritarian homes, adolescents from indulgent households score well on indexes of self-confidence and show no particular signs of psychological distress. However, indulgently raised adolescents are more susceptible to peer pressure (Steinberg, 1987a) and are more likely to engage in drug and alcohol use and school misconduct (e.g., cheating, copying homework, and lateness). Lamborn *et al.* (1990) point out that these particular "deviant" behaviors are rather peer oriented in nature and in some groups of adolescents, "normative." They note

> the fact that this group does not score higher on other measures of delinquency [e.g., carrying a weapon, theft, trouble with the police], and does score among the highest on the measure of social competence, suggests a picture of youngsters who are especially oriented toward their peers, and toward the social activities valued by adolescents—including some activities not especially valued by adults. (p. 15)

Thus the potential negative effects of warm, but permissive parenting seem to manifest themselves in youngsters' more impulsive and peer-oriented, problem behavior during adolescence.

For some parents, permissiveness may entail reduced parental monitoring: low-level awareness of their child's whereabouts, friends, and activities. This becomes a critical issue in light of studies that have found that deficiency in parental monitoring is a good predictor of adolescent susceptibility to, and actual, problem-related behavior (Patterson & Stouthamer-Loeber, 1984; Steinberg, 1986). For example, Patterson and Stouthamer-Loeber (1984) studied the relation between delinquency and several family management practices including parental monitoring, discipline consistency, problem solving, and positive reinforcement. Of all the variables studied, delinquency was most strongly related to a lack of parental monitoring. It is worth noting in this context that youngsters living in single-parent households are more involved in problem-related behavior than are those living in two-parent intact families (Dornbusch *et al.*, 1985). Research is beginning to suggest that differences in level of parental monitoring across family structures may be one critical explanatory factor. For example, a recent comparative study indicated that single parents engage in the least amount of parental monitoring, whereas parents in intact families engage in the most; parents in stepfamilies are intermediate in their degree of monitoring (Silverberg & Small, 1991). Moreover, analyses suggested that this variation in monitoring across family structures can account for part of the variation observed in adolescent engagement in problem-related behaviors. Dornbusch (1989) suggests that the higher rate of delinquency among adolescents from single-parent families may also be due to single parents' tendency to permit their youngsters earlier control over their own behavior, that is, to be more permissive in their parenting.

Whereas permissiveness within a context of warm parent–child relations may contribute to an increased probability of engagement in certain problem behaviors, permissiveness within a context of distant, uninvolved, and aloof parenting appears to have more detrimental consequences. Maccoby and Martin (1983) label parents who minimize their commitment to parenting, *indifferent-uninvolved*. Indifferent parents know little about their youngster's activities and whereabouts, do not establish rules or guidelines that might benefit their child, rarely converse with their child, and structure their lives around their own needs with little, if any, consideration to the needs and opinions of their child. In its extreme form, indifferent parenting is neglectful. Lamborn *et al.*'s (1990) study indicates that adolescents from indifferent households are at risk for problems across the board, be they attitude- or school-related, psychological in nature, or behavioral. These youngsters score lowest on measures of work orientation and school performance and highest on indexes of delinquency, including behaviors such as carrying a weapon, theft, and getting in trouble with the police. Like youngsters raised in authoritarian homes, adolescents from indifferent homes are more likely than other teens to experience internalizing problems and problems with self-confidence. And like those from indulgent homes, adolescents raised in indifferent households are more likely than other teens to use drugs and alcohol and engage in school misconduct. Consistent with these findings is Loeber and Stouthamer-Loeber's (1986) conclusion that the strongest predictors of delinquency are related to socialization practices including lack of parental supervision, parental rejection, and parent–child uninvolvement. Indeed, those adolescents who exhibit enduring, recurrent, and serious problem behavior are likely to have had problems during childhood and to have experienced disrupted parent–child relations from an early age (Steinberg, 1987a).

If parenting practices indeed play a causal role in youngster's development (and are not merely a response to child characteristics), the research reviewed suggests that parental acceptance and warmth may be a primary contributor to healthy emotional development and positive self-conceptions. On the other hand, firm behavioral control, including appropriate levels of parental monitoring and limit setting, may help to deter or delay the development of problem behaviors among adolescents (Lamborn *et al.*, 1990; Steinberg, 1990). Further, longitudinal studies that examine these tentative conclusions in samples of varied ethnic background and socioeconomic status would both strengthen our knowledge base and better inform programs aimed at enhancing parental effectiveness.

SUMMARY

Throughout this review, we have pointed to gaps in the literature on adolescence and the family and some promising directions for future research. We repeatedly highlighted the genuine need for longitudinal research as well as for studies that examine samples that vary with respect to ethnic background, family structure, and socioeconomic status. We also called for careful analysis of the potential differences in facilitative family interaction for male and female adolescents. In addition, we indicated the need to examine factors that could help to account for individual differences in family functioning and adaptation over the course of adolescence. Likely candidates exist not only within the family system itself (e.g., openness of communication, parental personality characteristics) but also outside the boundaries of the family *per se* (e.g., at the work–family interface). Investigations initiated prior to the transition to adolescence would be especially helpful. To date, students of adolescence and the family have relied heavily on the detailed investigations of a few, well-designed, but small-sample observational studies. A valuable addition to the field would be a series of replications of these studies.

With respect to observational research, there is also a need to clarify the relationship between behaviors identified by various coding systems (Jacob &

Tennenbaum, 1988). Although teams of researchers observe families for relatively similar reasons, they employ a variety of coding systems that makes comparison and integration of their results, at all but a global level, rather difficult. We would encourage greater use of well-documented coding systems across multiple research projects. Another important issue related to coding systems is the extent to which affective expression is adequately captured (Tennenbaum & Jacob, 1989). Although researchers, including Hauser and Powers, discuss the importance of the affective dimension of family interactions they apply their coding systems to transcripts of audiotaped discussions. The importance of nonverbal expressions in the coding of affect should serve as a stimulus for greater use of videotaped interaction data. And, finally in this vein, researchers have begun to question whether interruptive behavior is always an indicator of conflict or power assertion, an assumption of many coding systems. Alternatively, interruptions may be indicative of high excitement, the ability to anticipate what a family member will say, or even greater flexibility (Hill, 1988). The simultaneous coding of affect and interruptive behavior will enable researchers to discriminate between interruptions indicative of negative escalation or power attempts and those reflecting mutual spontaneity and anticipation.

Bronfenbrenner (1986) has called on researchers to move beyond the microsystem of the family toward systematic study of how *multiple* microsystems may interact to have an effect on youngsters' development. A good example of recent research on adolescent development that has moved in this direction examined the complex ways that peers and parents together influence school achievement and educational aspirations among a group of ethnically diverse high-schoolers (Brown, Steinberg, Mounts, & Philipp, 1990). The field of adolescent development would surely benefit from future research that maintains this multicontextual approach.

Finally, although we have a growing body of literature that confirms the beneficial effects of authoritative parenting (parenting that combines parental acceptance, firm control, and democratic parent–child interaction), we know very little about the determinants of effective parenting practices themselves or about the nature of stability and change in parenting practices during the transition into and through adolescence. Answers to these questions will inevitably move our research agenda toward more systematic study of both intraindividual processes (e.g., parents' cognitions, attributions, and expectations about adolescence and adolescents' behavior) and sociocultural and family factors (e.g., ethnicity, place of residence, family structure) that are likely to influence parent–adolescent relations.

REFERENCES

Alexander, J. F. (1973a). Defensive and supportive communications in family systems. *Journal of Marriage and the Family, 35*, 613–617.

Alexander, J. F. (1973b). Defensive and supportive communications in normal and deviant families. *Journal of Consulting and Clinical Psychology, 40*, 223–231.

Anderson, E. R., Hetherington, E. M., & Clingempeel, W. G. (1989). Transformations in family relations at puberty. *Journal of Early Adolescence, 9*, 310–334.

Ballenski, C., & Cook, A. (1982). Mother's perceptions of their competence in managing selected parenting tasks. *Family Relations, 31*, 489–494.

Baumrind, D. (1978). Parental disciplinary patterns and social competence in children. *Youth and Society*, 9, 239–276.

Bell, R. Q. (1968). A reinterpretation of the direction of effects in studies of socialization. *Psychological Review*, 75, 81–95.

Blos, P. (1962). The second individuation process. *Psychoanalytic Study of the Child*, 22, 162–186.

Brittain C. V. (1963). Adolescent choices and parent/peer cross-pressures. *American Sociological Review*, 28, 385–391.

Bronfenbrenner, U. (1986). Ecology of the family as a context for human development. *Developmental Psychology*, 22, 723–742.

Brown, B. B., Steinberg, L., Mounts, N., & Philipp, M. (1990, March). *The comparative influence of peers and parents on high school achievement: Ethnic differences*. Biennial Meeting of the Society for Research on Adolescence, Atlanta.

Clark, R., & Delia, J. (1976). The development of functional persuasive skills in childhood and early adolescence. *Child Development*, 47, 1008–1014.

Collins, W. A. (1984). Commentary: Interaction and child development. In M. Perlmutter (Ed.), *Parent-child interaction and parent-child relations in child development: The Minnesota Symposium on Child Psychology* (Vol. 17, pp. 167–175). Hillsdale, NJ: Erlbaum.

Collins, W. A. (1990). Parent-child relationships in the transition to adolescence: Continuity and change in interaction, affect, and cognition. In R. Montemayor, G. R. Adams, & T. P. Gullotta (Eds.), *From childhood to adolescence: A transitional period?* (pp. 85–106). Newbury Park, CA: Sage.

Cooper, C. R. (1988). Commentary: The role of conflict in adolescent-parent relationships. In M. G. Gunnar & W. A. Collins (Eds.), *Development during the transition to adolescence: Minnesota Symposium on Child Development* (Vol. 21; pp. 181–187). Hillsdale, NJ: Erlbaum.

Cooper, C. R., Grotevant, H. D., & Condon, S. M. (1983). Individuality and connectedness in the family as a context for adolescent identity formation and role-taking skill. In H. D. Grotevant & C. R. Cooper (Eds.), *Adolescent development in the family: New directions for child development* (pp. 43–59). San Francisco: Jossey-Bass.

Csikszentmihalyi, M., & Larson, R. (1984). *Being adolescent*. New York: Basic Books.

Damon, W., & Hart, D. (1982). The development of self-understanding from infancy through adolescence. *Child Development*, 53, 841–864.

Davis, K. (1940). The sociology of parent-youth conflict. *American Sociological Review*, 5, 523–535.

Davis, P., Stern, D., Jorgenson, J., & Steier, F. (1980). *Typologies of the alcoholic family: An integrated systems perspective*. Philadelphia: University of Pennsylvania, Wharton Applied Research Center.

Dornbusch, S. M. (1989). The sociology of adolescence. *Annual Review of Sociology*, 15, 233–259.

Dornbusch, S., Carlsmith, J., Bushwall, S., Ritter, P., Leiderman, P., Hastorf, A., & Gross, R. (1985). Single parents, extended households, and the control of adolescents. *Child Development*, 56, 326–341.

Dornbusch, S., Ritter, P., Leiderman, P., Roberts, D., & Fraleigh, M. (1987). The relation of parenting style to adolescent school performance. *Child Development*, 58, 1244–1257.

Douvan, E., & Adelson, J. (1966). *The adolescent experience*. New York: Wiley.

Flannery, D. J. (1991). *The impact of puberty on parent-adolescent relations: An observational study of the relationship between affect and engagement in interactions, parent-adolescent conflict, and adolescent problem behavior*. Unpublished doctoral dissertation, Ohio State University, Columbus.

Freud, A. (1958). Adolescence. *Psychoanalytic Study of the Child*, 13, 255–278.

Garbarino, J., Sebes, J., & Schellenbach, C. (1984). Families at risk for destructive parent-child relations at adolescence. *Child Development*, 55, 174–183.

Gecas, V., & Seff, M. (1990). Families and adolescents: A review of the 1980s. *Journal of Marriage and the Family*, 52, 941–958.

Grotevant, H. D., & Cooper, C. R. (1985). Patterns of interaction in family relationships and the development of identity exploration in adolescence. *Child Development*, 56, 415–428.

Grotevant, H. D., & Cooper, C. R. (1986). Individuation in family relationships: A perspective on individual differences in the development of identity and role-taking skill in adolescence. *Human Development*, 29, 82–100.

Halweg, K., & Goldstein, M. J. (Eds.). (1987). *Understanding major mental disorder: The contribution of family interaction research*. New York: Family Process Press.

Hauser, S. T., Liebman, W., Houlihan, J., Powers, S. I., Jacobson, A. M., Noam, G. C., Weiss, B., & Follansbee, D. J. (1985). Family contexts of pubertal timing. *Journal of Youth and Adolescence*, 14, 317–337.

Hauser, S. T., Powers, S. I., Noam, G., & Bowlds, M. K. (1987). Family interiors of adolescent ego development trajectories. *Family Perspective, 21,* 263–282.

Hauser, S. T., Powers, S. I., Noam, G. C., Jacobson, A. J., Weiss, B., & Follansbee, D. J. (1984). Familial contexts of adolescent development. *Child Development, 55,* 195–213.

Hetherington, E. M. (1988). Parents, children, and siblings: Six years after divorce. In R. A. Hinde & J. Stevenson-Hinde (Eds.), *Relationships within families: Mutual influences* (pp. 311–331). Oxford: Clarendon Press.

Hetherington, E. M., Stanley-Hagan, M., & Anderson, E. R. (1989). Marital transitions: A child's perspective. *American Psychologist, 44,* 303–312.

Hill, J. P. (1982). Guest editorial. *Child Development, 53,* 1409–1412.

Hill, J. P. (1987). Research on adolescents and their families: Past and prospect. In C. E. Irwin (Ed.), *Adolescent social behavior and health: New directions for child development* (pp. 13–31). San Francisco: Jossey-Bass.

Hill, J. P. (1988). Adapting to menarche: Familial control and conflict. In M. G. Gunnar & W. A. Collins (Eds.), *Development during the transition to adolescence: Minnesota Symposium on Child Development* (Vol. 21, pp. 43–77). Hillsdale, NJ: Erlbaum.

Hill, J. P., & Holmbeck, G. N. (1986). Attachment and autonomy during adolescence. In G. Whitehurst (Ed.), *Annals of child development* (Vol. 3, pp. 145–189). Greenwich, CT: JAI.

Hill, J. P., & Holmbeck, G. N. (1987). Familial adaptation to biological change during adolescence. In R. M. Lerner & T. T. Foch (Eds.), *Biological-psychosocial interactions in early adolescence* (pp. 207–223). Hillsdale, NJ: Erlbaum.

Hill, J. P., Holmbeck, G. N., Marlow, L., Green, T. M., & Lynch, M. E. (1985a). Menarcheal status and parent-child relations in families of seventh-grade girls. *Journal of Youth and Adolescence, 14,* 301–316.

Hill, J. P., Holmbeck, G. N., Marlow, L., Green, T. M., & Lynch, M. E. (1985b). Pubertal status and parent-child relations in families of seventh-grade boys. *Journal of Early Adolescence, 5,* 31–44.

Humphrey, L. L. (1989). Observed family interactions among subtypes of eating disorders using structural analysis of social behavior. *Journal of Consulting and Clinical Psychology, 57,* 206–214.

Jacob, T. (1974). Patterns of family conflict and dominance as a function of child age and social class. *Developmental Psychology, 10,* 1–12.

Jacob, T. (Ed.). (1987). *Family interaction and psychopathology: Theories, methods, and findings.* New York: Plenum Press.

Jacob, T., & Tennenbaum, D. L. (1988). *Family assessment: Rationale, methods and future directions.* New York: Plenum Press.

Kidwell, J., Fischer, J. L., Dunham, R. M., & Baranowski, M. (1983). Parents and adolescents: Push and pull of change. In H. I. McCubbin & C. R. Figley (Eds.), *Stress in the family: Coping with normative transitions* (pp. 74–89). New York: Bruner/Mazel.

Lamborn, S., Mounts, N., & Steinberg, L. (1990). *Patterns of competence and adjustment among adolescents from authoritative, authoritarian, indulgent, and neglectful families.* Manuscript submitted for publication.

Laursen, B. (1988, March). *Cognitive changes during adolescence and effects upon parent-child relationships.* Paper presented at the biennial meetings of the Society for Research on Adolescence, Alexandria, VA.

Leaper, C., Hauser, S. T., Kremen, A., Powers, S. I., Jacobson, A. M., Noam, G. C., Weiss-Perry, G., & Follansbee, D. (1989). Adolescent-parent interactions in relation to adolescents' gender and ego development pathway: A longitudinal study. *Journal of Early Adolescence, 9,* 335–361.

Loeber, R., & Stouthamer-Loeber, M. (1986). Family factors as correlates and predictors of juvenile conduct problems and delinquency. In M. Tonry & N. Morris (Eds.), *Crime and justice* (Vol. 7, pp. 29–149). Chicago: University of Chicago Press.

Loevinger, J. (1976). *Ego development: Conceptions and theories.* San Francisco: Jossey-Bass.

Lynd, R. S., & Lynd, H. M. (1929). *Middletown.* New York: Harcourt Brace.

Maccoby, E., & Martin, J. (1983). Socialization in the context of the family: Parent-child interaction. In E. M. Hetherington (Ed.), *Handbook of child psychology: Vol. 4, Socialization, personality, and social development* (pp. 1–101). New York: Wiley.

Minuchin, S., Rosman, B. L., & Baker, L. (1978). *Psychosomatic families: Anorexia nervosa in context.* Cambridge, MA: Harvard University Press.

Montemayor, R. (1983). Parents and adolescents in conflict: All of the families some of the time and some families most of the time. *Journal of Early Adolescence, 3,* 83–103.

Montemayor, R. (1986). Family variation in storm and stress. *Journal of Adolescent Research, 1,* 15–31.

Montemayor, R., & Hanson, E. (1985). A naturalistic view of conflict between adolescents and their parents and siblings. *Journal of Early Adolescence, 5*, 23–30.

Offer, D. (1969). *The psychological world of the teenager*. New York: Basic Books.

Offer, D., Ostrov, E., & Howard, K. (1981). The mental health professional's concept of the normal adolescent. *Archives of General Psychiatry, 38*, 149–152.

Papini, D. R., & Sebby, R. (1987). Adolescent pubertal status and affective family relationships: A multivariate assessment. *Journal of Youth and Adolescence, 16*, 1–15.

Pasley, K., & Gecas, V. (1984). Stresses and satisfactions in the parental role. *Personnel and Guidance Journal, 2*, 400–404.

Patterson, G., & Stouthamer-Loeber, M. (1984). The correlations of family management practice and delinquency. *Child Development, 55*, 1299–1307.

Powers, S. I., Beardslee, W., Jacobson, A. M., & Noam, G. G. (1987, April). *Family influences on the development of adolescent coping processes*. Paper presented at the biennial meeting of the Society for Research in Child Development, Baltimore.

Powers, S. I., Hauser, S. T., & Kilner, L. (1989). Adolescent mental health. *American Psychologist, 44*, 200–208.

Powers, S. I., Hauser, S. T., Schwartz, J. M., Noam, G. C., & Jacobson, A. M. (1983). Adolescent ego development and family interaction: A structural-developmental perspective. In H. D. Grotevant & C. R. Cooper (Eds.), *Adolescent development in the family: New directions for child development* (pp. 5–24). San Francisco: Jossey-Bass.

Reiss, D., (1971). Varieties of consensual experience: 1. A theory for relating family interaction to individual thinking. *Family Process, 10*, 1–28.

Reiss, D., Oliveri, M. E., & Curd, K. (1983). Family paradigm and adolescent social behavior. In H. D. Grotevant & C. R. Cooper (Eds.), *Adolescent development in the family: New directions for child development* (pp. 77–92). San Francisco: Jossey-Bass.

Robin, A. L., Koepke, T., & Nayor, M. (1986). Conceptualizing, assessing, and treating parent-adolescent conflict. In B. B. Lahey & A. E. Kazdin (Eds.), *Advances in clinical child psychology* (Vol. 9, pp. 87–121). New York: Plenum Press.

Rutter, M., Graham, M, Chadwick, O., & Yule, W. (1976). Adolescent turmoil: Fact or fiction? *Journal of Child Psychology and Psychiatry, 17*, 35–56.

Ryan, R. M., & Lynch, J. H. (1989). Emotional autonomy versus detachment: Revisiting the vicissitudes of adolescence and young adulthood. *Child Development, 60*, 340–356.

Savin-Williams, R., & Small, S. (1986). The timing of puberty and its relationship to adolescent and parent perceptions of family interaction. *Developmental Psychology, 22*, 322–347.

Sebald, H. (1986). Adolescents' shifting orientations toward parents and peers: A curvilinear trend over recent decades. *Journal of Marriage and the Family, 48*, 5–13.

Silverberg, S. B., & Small, S. A. (1991, April). *Parental monitoring, family structure, and adolescent problem-related behavior*. Paper presented at the biennial meetings of the Society for Research in Child Development, Seattle.

Silverberg, S. B., & Steinberg, L. (1987). Adolescent autonomy, parent adolescent conflict, and parental well-being. *Journal of Youth and Adolescence, 16*, 293–312.

Silverberg, S. B., & Steinberg, L. (1990). Psychological well-being of parents with early adolescent children. *Developmental Psychology, 26*, 658–666.

Small, S. A., Eastman, G., & Cornelius, S. (1988). Adolescent autonomy and parental stress. *Journal of Youth and Adolescence, 17*, 377–391.

Smetana, J. G. (1988a). Adolescents' and parents' conceptions of parental authority. *Child Development, 59*, 321–335.

Smetana, J. G. (1988b). Concepts of self and social convention: Adolescents' and parents' reasoning about hypothetical and actual family conflicts. In M. G. Gunnar & W. A. Collins (Eds.), *Development during the transition to adolescence: Minnesota Symposium on Child Development* (Vol. 21, pp. 79–122). Hillsdale, NJ: Erlbaum.

Smetana, J. G. (1989). Adolescents' and parents' reasoning about actual family conflict. *Child Development, 60*, 1052–1067.

Smollar, J., & Youniss, J. (1989). Transformations in adolescents' perceptions of parents. *International Journal of Behavioural Development, 12*, 71–84.

Steinberg, L. (1981). Transformations in family relations at puberty. *Developmental Psychology, 17*, 833–840.

Steinberg, L. (1986). Latchkey children and susceptibility to peer pressure: An ecological analysis. *Developmental Psychology, 22*, 433–439.

Steinberg, L. (1987a). Familial factors in delinquency: A developmental perspective. *Journal of Adolescent Research, 2,* 255–268.

Steinberg, L. (1987b). Impact of puberty on family relations: Effects of pubertal status and pubertal timing. *Developmental Psychology, 23,* 451–460.

Steinberg, L. (1987c). Recent research on the family at adolescence: The extent and nature of sex differences. *Journal of Youth and Adolescence, 3,* 191–197.

Steinberg, L. (1988). Reciprocal relation between parent-child distance and pubertal maturation. *Developmental Psychology, 24,* 122–128.

Steinberg, L. (1989). Pubertal maturation and parent-adolescent distance: An evolutionary perspective. In G. R. Adams, R. Montemayor, & T. P. Gullotta (Eds.), *Biology of adolescent behavior and development* (pp. 71–97). Newbury Park, CA: Sage.

Steinberg, L. (1990). Autonomy, conflict, and harmony in the family relationship. In S. Feldman & G. Elliot (Eds.) *At the threshold: The developing adolescent* (pp. 255–276). Cambridge, MA: Harvard University Press.

Steinberg, L., Elmen, J., & Mounts, N. (1989). Authoritative parenting, psychosocial maturity, and academic success among adolescents. *Child Development, 60,* 1424–1436.

Steinberg, L., & Hill, J. P. (1978). Patterns of family interaction as a function of age, the onset of puberty, and formal thinking. *Developmental Psychology, 14,* 683–684.

Steinberg, L., & Silverberg, S. B. (1986). The vicissitudes of autonomy in early adolescence. *Child Development, 57,* 841–851.

Strober, M., & Humphrey, L. L. (1987). Familial contributions to etiology and course of anorexia nervosa and bulimia. *Journal of Consulting and Clinical Psychology, 55,* 654–659.

Tanner, J. M. (1962). *Growth at adolescence* (2nd Ed.). Oxford: Basil Blackwell.

Tennenbaum, D. L., & Jacob, T. (1989). Observational methods for assessing psychological state. In N. Schneiderman, S. M. Weiss, & P. G. Kaufman (Eds.), *Handbook of research methods in cardiovascular behavioral medicine* (pp. 543–552). New York: Plenum Press.

Walters, L. H., & Norrell, E. (1987). Pubertal status, cognitive development, and parent/adolescent relationships. *Family Perspective, 21,* 355–368.

White, K. M., Speisman, J. C., & Costos, D. (1983). Young adults and their parents: Individuation to mutuality. In H. D. Grotevant & C. R. Cooper (Eds.), *Adolescent development in the family: New directions for child development* (pp. 61–76). San Francisco: Jossey-Bass.

Young, H., & Ferguson, L. (1979). Developmental changes through adolescence in the spontaneous nomination of reference groups as a function of decision context. *Journal of Youth and Adolescence, 8,* 239–252.

15

Adolescent Heterosocial Interactions and Dating

DAVID J. HANSEN, JEANETTE SMITH CHRISTOPHER, AND DOUGLAS W. NANGLE

INTRODUCTION

The transitional period of adolescence is characterized by a number of changes and challenges that occur both within and outside the individual (Petersen & Hamburg, 1986). One of the most significant developmental changes is the emergence of new social interaction patterns (Kelly & Hansen, 1987). Social interactions and relationships become increasingly complicated and adultlike, and more independence and responsibility are required. The peer group becomes larger and more complex, more time is spent with peers, and interactions with opposite-sex peers increase. For example, Csikszentmihalyi and Larson (1984) found that high-school freshman spent 44% of their time in same-sex groups and 4% in opposite-sex dyads, whereas seniors spent 21% of their time in same-sex groups and 24% in opposite-sex dyads. Most adolescents begin dating between the ages of 13 and 15 years (Spreadbury, 1982).

Social interactions and relationships with same- and opposite-sex peers are necessary for social development and thus may be related to adjustment and coping with the challenges of adolescence (cf. Kelly & Hansen, 1987; Petersen & Hamburg, 1986). Social interactions may be critical for an adolescent's adjustment in a number of ways, such as (a) establishing support systems for emotional and

DAVID J. HANSEN • Department of Psychology, University of Nebraska, Lincoln, Nebraska 68588. JEANETTE SMITH CHRISTOPHER AND DOUGLAS W. NANGLE • Department of Psychology, West Virginia University, Morgantown, West Virginia 26506-6040.

Handbook of Social Development: A Lifespan Perspective, edited by Vincent B. Van Hasselt and Michel Hersen. Plenum Press, New York, 1992.

social needs; (b) developing sexual attitudes, interests, and sex-role behaviors; (c) developing moral judgment and social values; and (d) improving or maintaining self-esteem (Kelly & Hansen, 1987). Dating and heterosocial interactions also serve a variety of additional functions, including (a) promotion of interpersonal competence and adultlike social behavior; (b) recreation, entertainment, and sexual stimulation; (c) enhancement of status within the peer group; (d) development of independence assertion to aid in separation from the family; (e) experimentation, particularly with sex-role behaviors and sexual activity; and (f) courtship and mate selection (Damon, 1983; Kelly & Hansen, 1987).

The purpose of this chapter is to examine developmental and clinical issues related to adolescent heterosocial interactions and dating. The full range of adolescent development is discussed, from young adolescents (e.g., age 12) to adolescents in college. First, a variety of issues associated with normal development of heterosocial interaction and dating will be examined, including the developmental context, components of heterosocial skills, influences on heterosocial interactions, and sexual activity. Next, problems in the development of heterosocial interactions and assessment and intervention approaches are discussed. Finally, future directions for examining heterosocial interaction and dating among adolescents are proposed.

DEVELOPMENTAL ISSUES

Developmental Context

A brief examination of the developmental context in which adolescent heterosocial interaction and dating occurs is warranted. For a more thorough review of the changes associated with puberty, see Berger (1986), Brookman (1990), or Kimmel and Weiner (1985).

PHYSICAL DEVELOPMENT

The average onset of male puberty is 11 to 12 years (range 9 to 14 years); the average for females is 10 to 11 years (range 8 to 13 years) (Brookman, 1990). With the onset of puberty, differences between males and females become more readily apparent (Berger, 1986). Females gain a more rounded appearance with fat depositing in the pelvis, breast, upper back, and backs of upper arms. Males tend to lose the subcutaneous fat of childhood. Their shoulders become broader and their legs become relatively long compared with their trunk length. Other obvious changes for males include the growth of facial hair and voice change. Males also experience growth of their penis and testes and their first ejaculation of semen. Female internal sex organs increase in weight and size, and the onset of menarche occurs. Both sexes experience an increase in muscle growth and in the size and capacity of the heart and lungs. Their faces become longer, the jaw becomes more prominent, and the nose projects more. Axillary and pubic hair also develop with puberty. The growth spurt in height occurs approximately 2 years earlier for females than it does for males. Early-maturing girls and late-maturing boys are more likely to be distressed by their physical development (or their lack of it) (Berger, 1986). The problem may be temporary for most girls, but the effects on the self-confidence of boys may persist into adulthood.

COGNITIVE DEVELOPMENT

373

ADOLESCENT
HETEROSOCIAL
INTERACTIONS
AND DATING

Adolescents' cognitive abilities differ from those of children in many ways (Berger, 1986; Kimmel & Weiner, 1985). They are able to think in abstract terms, develop hypotheses, ponder about their own thoughts, and plan ahead. Adolescents are able to look beyond the obvious surface characteristics of another person's behavior and make inferences about the causes and meaning of behavior. Because adolescents are able to think about abstract possibilities, they are able to consider the possible causes and effects of another person's behavior. They also see consistencies in other people's behavior that lead them to make overall judgments of their personal characteristics. Adolescents know that other people have perspectives different from their own.

Although adolescents are able to think about relationships and sexuality in the abstract, their egocentric styles may create difficulties in thinking objectively (Berger, 1986; Kimmel & Weiner, 1985). Adolescents may believe that they lead a special, unique existence. For example, adolescents may believe that other people get pregnant or contract AIDS but that they will not. Fortunately, cognitive abilities appear to improve with age. As such, the older adolescent may be better able to consider the consequences of sexual intercourse and take precautions to prevent an unwanted pregnancy or sexual disease (Kimmel & Weiner, 1985).

Components of Heterosocial Skills

The social competencies that bring about contact with opposite-sex persons are generally termed "date-initiation" or "heterosocial" skills (Kelly, 1982). Date initiation is the behavior of asking another person to join in some prearranged social dating activity. Dating, subsequent to date initiation, can be defined as "a dyadic interaction that focuses on participation in mutually rewarding activities that may increase the likelihood of future interaction, emotional commitment, and/ or sexual intimacy" (Pirog-Good & Stets, 1989, p. 5). Heterosocial skills are the behaviors necessary for initiating, maintaining, and terminating social and/or sexual relationships with persons of the opposite sex (Barlow, Abel, Blanchard, Bristow, & Young, 1977; Galassi & Galassi, 1979). Because the skills needed for competent performance may be different in the various stages of a relationship, a global definition or description of heterosocial skills is not meaningful (Galassi & Galassi, 1979). In general, the literature has focused on a narrow range of heterosocial skills (e.g., getting dates) and excluded other types, such as heterosexual skills and heterosocial friendships.

The extent of the similarity between skills needed for social and heterosocial interactions and between same- and opposite-sex peer relations is unclear but commonly assumed to be significant (Kelly, 1982). Same- and opposite-sex interactions and popularity appear to be more strongly related for males than females (Himadi, Arkowitz, Hinton, & Perl, 1980; Miller, 1990).

Most of the specific behaviors that have been proposed as components of heterosocial competence or date initiation are the same as those that have been proposed to comprise conversational competence (Kelly, 1982). Global skills necessary for normal adolescent heterosocial interactions, as well as interactions with the same-sex persons, are varied and include knowing how to initiate and maintain conversation, interpret and understand the affective state of others, assess peer norms and values, monitor the social impact of behavior, and match social behaviors to the demands of the situation (Conger & Conger, 1982; Kelly, 1982). Specific behaviors that have been related to skill in date-initiation or heterosocial interactions include eye contact or gaze, affect (including smiles, voice quality, facial expressions), head nods, gestures, appropriate laughter, duration of speech, conversational questions, self-disclosing statements, complimentary comments, follow-up or acknowledgment statements, and requesting a date (Conger & Conger, 1982; Kelly, 1982; Kolko & Milan, 1985; Kupke, Hobbs, & Cheney, 1979). A number of behaviors have also been associated with unskilled or anxious performance, including silences of 5 to 10 seconds, negative-opinion statements, speech dysfluencies (e.g., "uh," "ah"), and long or delayed response latencies (Kelly, 1982).

Although investigators are beginning to look at skills exhibited by males (e.g., Kupke *et al.*, 1979) or females (e.g., Kolko & Milan, 1985), further research is needed to delineate specific gender differences in heterosocial competence. Heterosocial skills identified for females include eye contact, response latency, talk time, interest, initiation, and attractiveness (Galassi & Galassi, 1979). In a specific examination of female heterosocial skills, Muehlenhard, Koralewski, Andrews, and Burdick (1986) identified several verbal cues (initiates conversation, compliments, asks questions, provides phone number if asked) and nonverbal cues (eye contact, smiling, animated speech, touching while laughing) that convey interest in dating.

Influences on Heterosocial Interactions and Dating

SOCIAL LEARNING MECHANISMS

A variety of mechanisms may facilitate the development of social and heterosocial skills during adolescence. These are (a) exposure to appropriate social skill models; (b) the consequences (e.g., reinforcement, punishment, extinction) associated with an adolescent's social behavior; (c) exposure to, and participation in, peer social activities; and (d) "cognitive" factors such as self-statements and attributional processes (Kelly, 1982; Kelly & Hansen, 1987).

Adolescents are highly influenced by and likely to imitate peers (Berger, 1986). Hairstyles, clothing style, musical interests, vocabulary and slang, activities and interests, and values are some of the many characteristics that teenagers learn, in part by exposure to peer models (Kelly & Hansen, 1987). Adolescents also learn methods of handling social relationships by observing and imitating peers. For example, the double dating and group dating common in early and middle adolescence permit teenagers to learn heterosocial skills by modeling from peers (Kelly & Hansen, 1987). Even physical affection may often be a semipublic affair (Berger, 1986).

Individuals who are heterosocially competent have a repertoire of social strategies or skills that produce reinforcing interpersonal outcomes (Kelly, 1982). An adolescent will be more likely to initiate conversations, assert views or opinions, initiate a date, and engage in other social interactions if the youth has a history of reinforcement (as opposed to punishment or extinction) for such behaviors (Kelly & Hansen, 1987). The consequences associated with social behavior provide "feedback" to the individual regarding the appropriateness and impact of the behavior. Research is needed to identify the social behaviors that will be reinforced in adolescence. For example, research suggests that adolescents find certain conversational topics more reinforcing than others, such as discussing family and friends, television, movies, music, sports, school activities, recreation and hobbies, and appearance (e.g., clothes and hair) (Hansen, St. Lawrence, & Christoff, 1988).

Because adolescents can gain skills through observation and from receiving reinforcement and feedback in social situations, participation in peer activities is a necessary precursor for naturalistic skill learning to occur (Kelly & Hansen, 1987). Adolescents who engage in few peer activities have reduced opportunities to observe and interact with competent models, as well as fewer opportunities to practice social behaviors and learn which skills will be reinforced in which situations.

Self-evaluation and attributional factors that may influence social and heterosocial adjustment include (a) acceptance of physical change and maturation, as well as physical attractiveness; (b) success at separation and independence from the parents; (c) acceptance of and by a peer social group; and (d) the development of adaptive self-appraisals of performance in social situations (Kelly & Hansen, 1987). Feedback from others concerning characteristics such as attractiveness and social acceptability, whether accurate or not, may foster either social anxiety or confidence.

PARENTAL AND RELIGIOUS INFLUENCES

A variety of parent and family characteristics may be related to adolescent heterosocial interactions and dating. Parents who raise their children with traditional masculine and feminine sex roles may be more likely to raise males who have a sexual orientation toward dating and females who have an affectional orientation toward dating (McCabe, 1984). Children who are raised with an androgynous orientation may be more likely to have both a sexual and affectional orientation toward dating (McCabe, 1984). In terms of family structure, Coleman, Ganong, and Ellis (1985) found no differences between adolescents from intact versus nonintact families with regard to total dating partners or number of steady involvements. Adolescents from nonintact households, however, began dating at younger ages. Children from families of higher socioeconomic status also reportedly start dating earlier (McCabe, 1984).

The education level of the mother and the adolescent may be associated with sexual behavior. Mothers who had higher educational levels were less likely to have sexually active 15- to 19-year-old adolescents (Leigh, Weddle, & Loewen, 1988; Scott-Jones & White, 1990). With an older, college-student population, however, parental education had little or no effect on sexual behavior and attitudes (Roche, 1986). Adolescents with higher educational expectations for themselves are less likely to be sexually active. Scott-Jones and White (1990) found that 50% of those adolescents who did not plan to go to college were sexually active, whereas only 13% of the adolescents who planned to attend graduate school were sexually active.

Leslie, Huston, and Johnson (1986) found that parents of college students were more likely to support relationships in which their offspring were highly involved. Approving behaviors most frequently engaged in by parents included relaying phone messages from partner, asking how partner is doing, being pleasant to partner, and letting offspring and partner be alone. Disapproving behaviors included talking about other people the offspring could date, telling offspring to wait until he/she has finished school before getting serious, cautioning offspring about getting involved with partner, and "nicknaming" the partner something strange.

Religious affiliation and church activity may also play a role in adolescent dating behavior (McCabe, 1984). Female college students who attend church regularly and/or for whom religion is very important are more conservative in their sexual behavior and attitudes (Roche, 1986). These results were also found for black females who reported being members of churches holding more conservative sexual mores (Leigh *et al.*, 1988). Roman Catholics were found to be more sexually conservative than Protestants in the more involved stages of dating (i.e., dating one person only and being in love, or being engaged), although there were no differences in the earlier stages of dating (Roche, 1986).

OTHER INFLUENCES

Peer group factors may also play a large role in determining the age of the first date and the frequency and intensity of dates (Coleman *et al.*, 1985). Because of the increased independence of adolescents and the hesitancy to discuss sex and dating with their parents, adolescents often discuss these issues with peers (Roscoe, Kennedy, & Pope, 1987). Treboux and Busch-Rossnagel (1990) found that both social networks and discussion with parents were related to sexual attitudes and behavior for high-school students.

Adolescents may often seek dates because of the impact that dating has on their peer status and self-esteem (Damon, 1983). Elkind (1983) believes that teenagers often seek dates more for the sake of their "audience" than for the sake of the dating activity itself. Dating provides many opportunities for "strategic interactions" to maintain or enhance self-esteem (Elkind, 1983). Every aspect of dating, from asking someone for a date to sexual activity, entails a number of potential rewards and risks from a strategic point of view. Getting a date and refusing date offers from others can represent attractiveness, popularity, and social status, and thus contribute to an adolescent's self esteem. Sexual intercourse is a status-gaining behavior not only for males but also increasingly for females (McCabe, 1984).

In general, social expectations and age may have a greater effect on dating than does sexual maturation (Miller, McCoy, & Olson, 1986). As such, younger adolescents have different reasons for dating than do older adolescents (Roscoe, Diana, & Brooks, 1987). Younger adolescents weigh a potential dating partner's superficial features (e.g., fashionable clothing) and approval by others more heavily than do older adolescents, whereas older adolescents weigh their partner's future plans most heavily (Roscoe *et al.*, 1987). Additionally, older adolescents may feel pressure to begin dating because of their age and the frequency of dating among same-age peers.

The influence of physical attractiveness on dating activity is not entirely clear. Stelzer, Desmond, and Price (1987) found that attractiveness was not related to the age at which females began dating but that it was positively related to sexual activity. Bailey and Kelly (1984) found that daters in the early phases of a dating relationship, compared to steady and engaged daters, appeared insecure about their own and their partner's physical attractiveness. Steady male daters perceived their partner as corresponding to their idealized physical image of a female.

Sexual Activity

There is popular belief that adolescent sexual activity has changed dramatically in recent decades, especially since the "sexual revolution" of the 1960s. Although there have been some gradual changes in the ages at which youth initiate sexual activity, the changes have been taking place since early in this century, with the largest increase occurring shortly after World War I (Damon, 1983). There has also been a trend over several decades toward valuing premarital sexual intercourse. Yet, the majority of adolescents still seek stability and commitment in their sexual relationships (Damon, 1983). Although males traditionally have higher rates of sexual intercourse, the gap between sexually active males and females has narrowed (Brooks-Gunn & Furstenberg, 1989). This is primarily due to changes in the behavior of female youth (McAnarney & Hendee, 1989; Sherwin & Corbett, 1985). More than half of American adolescents have had intercourse by the time they are 17 or 18 (Brookman, 1990; Jemmott & Jemmott, 1990). MacDonald *et al.* (1990) found that 74.3% of the college males and 68.9% of college females were coitally active.

Adolescent sexual involvement has been related to the age at first date. Adolescents who began dating at an earlier age (e.g., age 12) are more likely to have experienced intercourse than those adolescents who begin dating later (e.g., age 17) (Miller *et al.*, 1986; Scott-Jones & White, 1990). As expected, the degree of sexual involvement has also been strongly related to the degree of dating involvement (Christopher & Cate, 1988; Miller *et al.*, 1986; Roche, 1986). Adolescents who are in a more involved relationship are more likely to have experienced intercourse than those adolescents who are not in an involved dating relationship (Miller *et al.*, 1986; Scott-Jones & White, 1990).

Stelzer *et al.* (1987) found that attractive females were significantly more likely to engage in sexual intercourse and oral sex than were unattractive- or average-rated females. Additionally, attractive and unattractive women had a significantly greater number of sexual partners than the average rated females. Attractiveness was not related to the age of first sexual intercourse.

Black adolescents are generally younger at first coitus (Jemmott & Jemmott, 1990) and may have significantly higher rates of intercourse than white females (Brooks-Gunn & Furstenberg, 1989; McAnarney & Hendee, 1989). These figures may be partially explained by the association between early sexual intercourse and either living in a lower income home and/or single-parent home; black children are three times as likely as white children to live below the poverty line and to live in a single-parent household (Leigh *et al.*, 1988). Therefore, it is not surprising that they may have higher rates of intercourse than white females.

Christopher and Cate (1988) investigated the relational correlates of sexual involvement at four stages of dating: first date, casually dating, considering becoming a couple, and being a couple. In the early stages, conflict (e.g., arguing, expressing negative feelings) was the best predictor of sexual involvement. Love and conflict were the best and second-best predictors, respectively, of sexual involvement when considering becoming a couple. Females are more likely than males to believe that love and commitment between partners is important before becoming sexually intimate (Christopher & Cate, 1988; Miller et al., 1986; Roche, 1986).

Roche (1986) examined sexual attitudes and behavior of college students by five dating stages: dating with no particular affection (Stage 1), dating with affection but not love (Stage 2), dating and being in love (Stage 3), dating one person only and being in love (Stage 4), and engaged (Stage 5). During the early stages, males and females have very different views regarding what is proper behavior and also in their reported behavior. For example, for Stage 1, 17% of males and 1% of females felt that light petting was proper behavior, and 25% of males and 8% of females reported engaging in the behavior. For Stage 5, 93% of males and 90% of females felt that light petting was proper behavior, and 94% of males and 94% of females reported engaging in the behavior. The percentage of males who engaged in intercourse during the increasing stages of involvement was 15%, 18%, 49%, 63%, and 74%. The percentages for females were 4%, 11%, 32%, 68%, and 81%. In general, adolescents are most restrictive in what they believe is proper sexual behavior, less restrictive in their reported actual behavior, and most permissive in their perceptions of what others are doing (Roche, 1986).

PROBLEMS IN THE DEVELOPMENT OF HETEROSOCIAL INTERACTIONS AND DATING

Many heterosocial difficulties experienced by adolescents may be transitory, the result of normal awkwardness that is likely to occur in new social roles during maturational-developmental change (Kelly & Hansen, 1987). Yet, for some adolescents, problems may signal a more long-standing pattern of heterosocial maladjustment that may persist into adulthood.

The bulk of existing research on heterosocial problems has focused on the early stages of dating by college students. Klaus, Hersen, and Bellack (1977) found that the most difficult stages of dating for both sexes have been reported to be finding possible dates, initiating contact with prospective dates, initiating sexual activity, avoiding or curtailing sex, and ending a date. Knox and Wilson (1983), in a survey of 227 female and 107 male college students, found that the most frequently identified dating problems for the female students were (a) unwanted pressure to engage in sexual behavior (23%); (b) places to go (22%); (c) communication with date (20%); (d) sexual misunderstandings (e.g., "accidentally leading a guy on") (13%); and (e) money (e.g., "who pays") (9%). The most frequently identified problems for male students were (a) communication with date (35%); (b) places to go (23%); (c) shyness (20%); (d) money (17%); and (e) honesty/openness (8%).

Heterosocial problems have been defined from a variety of perspectives including skill deficits, frequency of dates, and anxiety (Curran, 1977; Galassi & Galassi, 1979). A variety of terms have been used to describe persons with heterosocial problems, including *heterosocially incompetent*, *shy*, *socially anxious*, *low-frequency* or *minimal dater*, and *unskilled dater* (Galassi & Galassi, 1979). Differences in terminology result from the variety of ways that the problem has been conceptualized and from a tendency to focus on the individual rather than on the behaviors being exhibited (Galassi & Galassi, 1979). Although much of the previous literature has focused on "heterosocial skill deficits" or "heterosocial anxiety," a more integrative term, used in this chapter, is to focus on *heterosocial dysfunction*. The following sections review causal models and common problems of heterosocial dysfunction and assessment and treatment approaches for identifying and remediating heterosocial problems.

Causal Models of Heterosocial Dysfunction

Four models have been commonly proposed to account for heterosocial dysfunction, including social skill deficits, conditioned anxiety, negative cognitive self-evaluations, and personal unattractiveness (Arkowitz, Hinton, Perl, & Himadi, 1978; Curran, 1977; Galassi & Galassi, 1979; Kelly, 1982). It is likely, however, that difficulties during heterosocial or dating situations are multidetermined (Curran, 1977; Kelly, 1982). In fact, a general problem with the four-model approach as commonly discussed is that interactive influences of the various mechanisms are generally ignored. For example, the influence of skill and anxiety on attractiveness, or the influence of skill and attractiveness on anxiety, are not adequately understood.

Anxiety

Difficulty with dating and heterosocial interactions appears to be a relatively frequent problem. Arkowitz *et al.* (1978) reported that 31% of 3,800 college students (37% of the males and 25% of the females) evaluated themselves as "somewhat" to "very" anxious about dating. Borkovec, Stone, O'Brien, and Kaloupek (1974) found that 15.5% of the males and 11.5% of the females in introductory psychology classes reported at least some fear of being with the opposite sex. The greater incidence in males may be due to their more common role as initiators of heterosocial dating (Kelly, 1982).

Although survey research indicates that social-interaction problems are a concern of many adolescents, little is known about the severity and duration of these difficulties, and the ability of the adolescent to overcome social anxiety or inhibition through increased exposure to naturally occurring social interactions (Kelly & Hansen, 1987). Unfortunately, it is not generally clear from the survey research whether adolescent's responses represent normal, transient social self-consciousness or more long-standing, serious relationship deficits (Kelly & Hansen, 1987).

Anxiety is frequently associated with date-initiation behavior, even among clients who can effectively handle everyday conversations that are not in the context of dating (Kelly, 1982). Anxiety associated with dating appears to occur for a variety of reasons, such as (a) the desire to establish heterosocial relationships; (b) the social importance and status associated with dating; (c) the fact that dating is a social skill that emerges relatively late in development and, therefore, is not based on an extensive set of personal learning experiences; and (d) the relationship between dating and heterosexual involvement, with the latter also being a common source of anxiety (Kelly, 1982).

There is significant disagreement and controversy over current theories for children's fears and anxieties (Barrios & O'Dell, 1989). The respondent-conditioning model postulates that heterosocial anxiety develops as a result of the classical conditioning of fear or anxiety with date-related situations, in a manner analogous to phobic responses (Arkowitz et al., 1978; Kelly, 1982). Two-factor theory suggests that subsequent avoidance of feared situations may also be negatively reinforced by the removal of an aversive stimulus (Barrios & O'Dell, 1989). Such models have not adequately addressed heterosocial anxiety. Further research is needed regarding possible mechanisms by which social and heterosocial anxiety originate and are maintained.

Heterosocial anxiety may be associated with a variety of problems. Dodge, Heimberg, Nyman, and O'Brien (1987) found that high-anxious students participated in fewer heterosocial interactions over a 2-week period and reported higher anxiety, poorer social performance, and less satisfaction with their performance than low-anxious students. Himadi et al. (1980) found that socially anxious, low-dating men, but not low-dating women, exhibited general adjustment problems and difficulties in same-sex friendship interactions. In addition to interfering with the development of relationships (Arkowitz et al., 1978), social anxiety and avoidance may be related to problems such as depression, alcoholism, and sexual dysfunction (Arkowitz, 1977; Dodge et al., 1987).

SKILL DEFICITS

The social skills deficit model assumes that an individual lacks the interpersonal behaviors needed to perform effectively in heterosocial interactions (Kelly, 1982). Anxiety may also be present, possibly as a result of previous unsuccessful interactions, and it may prevent successful exhibition of skilled behaviors. As described previously, research has documented a variety of behaviors or "skills" that discriminate heterosocially successful from unsuccessful youth (cf. Curran, 1977; Kupke et al., 1979; Twentyman & McFall, 1975). Unfortunately, relatively little research has been conducted specifically with females, and the similarity of behaviors needed for same- and opposite-sex interactions is unclear.

COGNITIVE INFLUENCES

Cognitive models emphasize the causal relationship between negative self-evaluations and subsequent anxiety. The cause of negative self-evaluations may include high performance standards, anxiety-related self-statements, and selective recall of unsuccessful past experiences (Arkowitz, 1977; Kelly, 1982). Compared to low-anxious persons, high-anxious individuals are more likely to attend to negative experiences, interpret experiences less favorably, expect more negative evaluations, reward themselves less, and make less frequent use of problem-solving and other self-control procedures (Galassi & Galassi, 1979).

PHYSICAL ATTRACTIVENESS

The role of physical attractiveness on dating is also suggested (Galassi & Galassi, 1979; Kelly, 1982). Physical attractiveness, however, has received little attention in theoretical formulations or in the development of treatment programs.

Analog research as well as research involving actual interactions has reported that physically attractive individuals date more frequently, are rated as more likable and more popular, and are stereotyped as having more pleasant personalities than less attractive persons (Galassi & Galassi, 1979; Kelly, 1982). Attractiveness may be particularly influential for younger daters (Bailey & Kelly, 1984) and in the initial stages of heterosocial interaction because it may be the only readily available information. The relationship between attractiveness and dating may be stronger for females than males (Galassi & Galassi, 1979).

Problems Related to Sexual Activity

The sexual behavior of adolescents may lead to serious problems that are a concern and cost not only for individuals and their families but for society as well. Over 50% of 15- to 19-year-olds are sexually active; by age 19, over 70% of teenagers have been sexually active (Select Committee on Children, Youth, and Families, 1988).

Adolescents seldom complain about sexual dysfunction, possibly due to embarrassment, fear of adult reactions, or lack of knowledge about normal human sexual responses (Brookman, 1990). Problems may include premature ejaculation or lack of erection for males, and painful intercourse or lack of orgasm for females. Hasty intercourse, which may be associated with fear of discovery, increases the chance of performance difficulties.

Little is known about the psychological consequences of early sexual activity and intercourse, separate from the consequences of adolescent pregnancy. The literature suggests that the psychological problems associated with early intercourse include self-devaluation, unsatisfactory sexual experiences, substitution of intercourse for intimacy, anorgasmia, and promiscuity (see Alexander, 1990). More is known about the potential physical consequences, reviewed in the following sections.

SEXUALLY TRANSMITTED DISEASES (STDs)

It is estimated that 2.5 million teenagers are affected by STDs each year (Select Committee on Children, Youth, and Families, 1988). MacDonald *et al.* (1990) found that approximately 70% of college students were sexually active, and of these, 5.5% reported a previous STD. Prevalence data on gonorrhea, syphilis, chlamydia, and pelvic inflammatory disease reveal that higher rates occur among adolescents more than any other age group (DiClemente, 1990; Jemmott & Jemmott, 1990; Select Committee on Children, Youth, and Families, 1988). There is an association between ethnicity and STDs in adolescents, with blacks having significantly higher rates than whites (Select Committee on Children, Youth, and Families, 1988).

Acquired Immune Deficiency Syndrome (AIDS) is currently uncommon among adolescents. Only approximately 1% of all AIDS cases has occurred in persons under age 20, most of whom were infected by transfusion or perinatal transmission (Select Committee on Children, Youth, and Families, 1988). There is, however, growing awareness of the threat that HIV infection poses for adolescents (DiClemente, 1990). Burke *et al.* (1987) studied seroprevalence rates of HIV infections among applicants for U.S. military service. The mean prevalence of the sample comprised mostly of teens and young adults was 1.5 per 1,000. Demographic factors that were positive, independent predictors of a positive HIV-antibody test were increasing age, black race, male sex, residence in a densely populated county, and residence in a metropolitan area with a high incidence of AIDS.

Unfortunately, evidence suggests that increased knowledge of AIDS does not significantly influence AIDS-preventive behaviors among adolescents (DiClemente, 1990). Roscoe and Kruger (1990) surveyed 296 college juniors and seniors in 1987 and found that late adolescents were quite knowledgeable regarding AIDS and its transmission; however, only 33% of the females and 37% of the males reported that they had made some change in their sexual behavior as a result of fear of AIDS. The most common changes included being more selective about partners (18.1% of females, 19.1% of males) and use of condoms (6.6% of females, 10.1% of males).

PREGNANCY

Another serious, widespread consequence of adolescent sexual activity is pregnancy. Approximately 1 million teenagers in the United States become pregnant each year. Almost one-half of all teenage girls become pregnant at least once before age 20 (Select Committee on Children, Youth, and Families, 1988). Koenig and Zelnick (1982) found that within the first 2 years of intercourse, as many as 35.9% of sexually active teenage girls become pregnant (33.2% of unmarried white teenagers and 43.3 percent of unmarried black teenagers). Approximately 10% of adolescent pregnancies are spontaneously aborted, and about 40% are aborted by induction (Berger, 1986; McAnarney & Hendee, 1989).

A major problem associated with adolescent pregnancy is higher risk of neonatal problems, such as low birth weight, increased mortality, and increased behavioral and developmental problems as children (McAnarney & Hendee, 1989). The social, economic, and psychological consequences of pregnancy can be very disruptive to the development and adjustment of the teenage mother. The absence of a supportive father is only one of the many reasons that adolescent pregnancy may result in lower self-esteem, less education, reduced lifetime income for the young mother, repeated pregnancy, and a higher incidence of birth complications and problems throughout childhood for the offspring (Berger, 1986; McAnarney & Hendee, 1989).

INADEQUATE CONTRACEPTIVE BEHAVIOR

It is not surprising that recent data indicate that inadequate contraceptive behavior is widely prevalent among adolescents. MacDonald *et al.* (1990) found that only 24.8% of the college males and 15.6% of the college females always used a condom during sexual intercourse. For the 21.3% of males and 8.6% of females with 10 or more partners, regular condom use was reported in only 21% and 7.5%, respectively. In a telephone survey of 1,773 16- to 19-year-olds, Hingson, Strunin, Berlin, and Heeren (1990) found that although 61% were sexually active, only 31% of those reported always using condoms.

A variety of factors have been associated with inadequate contraceptive behavior. Among sexually active young adolescents, whites are more likely than blacks to use contraception regularly and to use effective methods (Scott-Jones & White, 1990). In a large sample of sexually active black males between the ages of 11 and 19, only 46% said they would avoid intercourse if neither they nor their partner were using contraception (Clark, Zabin, & Hardy, 1984). Approximately 25% of those who claimed to use contraception were actually using withdrawal as their only form of birth control. In a survey of 200 black male inner-city junior and senior high-school students, Jemmott and Jemmott (1990) found that 96.7% reported having coitus at least once, with 78.3% reporting no contraception use during initial coitus, and 53.9% reporting no contraception use during their most recent coitus.

Lack of information about STDs and contraception and lack of appreciation of the personal significance of the consequences of sexual behavior are believed to be common problems (Select Committee on Children, Youth, and Families, 1988). Recent research has shown that factors associated with not using a condom are number of sexual partners, embarrassment about condom purchase, difficulty discussing condom use with a partner, use of oral contraceptives, insufficient knowledge of STDs, and belief that condoms interfere with pleasure (MacDonald *et al.*, 1990). Behavior problems and juvenile delinquency may also be related to inadequate contraceptive behavior (Melchert & Burnett, 1990). Other factors have not been found to be related, such as physical attractiveness for college females (Stelzer *et al.*, 1987) or general self-esteem of college students (Burger & Inderbitzen, 1985).

Use of contraceptives requires a variety of skills, including (a) identifying oneself as sexually active; (b) accepting erotic feelings and sexuality itself; (c) overcoming expectations of negative reactions in purchasing contraceptives; (d) overcoming expectations that one will be perceived as "easy" or "experienced" because of preparation for intercourse; and (e) interrupting the spontaneity of intercourse (Select Committee on Children, Youth, and Families, 1988). Factors related positively to use of condoms may be (a) the belief that condoms are effective in preventing HIV transmission; (b) concern about getting AIDS; (c) carrying condoms; (d) discussing AIDS with a physician; (e) belief that condoms do not reduce sexual pleasure; (f) lack of embarrassment using condoms; (g) lack of alcohol and drug use; and (h) general and sexual communication with one's partner (Burger & Inderbitzen, 1985; Byrne, 1983; Hingson *et al.*, 1990).

Discussion with parents was found to have a positive direct influence on sexual behavior for virgin males and on contraceptive use for nonvirgin males, suggesting that parents are accepting of sexuality in their adolescent sons (Treboux & Busch-Rossnagel, 1990). However, for females, discussion with parents provided a negative indirect influence on sexual behavior for virgin females and did not influence either sexual behavior or contraceptive use among nonvirgin females. A double standard is apparent; the message conveyed to daughters may be "Don't— and if you do, we don't want to know about it" (Treboux & Busch-Rossnagel, 1990, p. 185).

In recent years, anxiety has been an increasingly investigated factor in contraceptive behavior (Bruch & Hynes, 1987; Byrne, 1983; Leary & Dobbins, 1983). Bruch and Hynes (1987) found that for a woman's first intercourse experience, general heterosocial anxiety was inversely correlated with discussion of birth control, male partner's communication effectiveness, and use of more effective contraceptive methods. For recent intercourse experiences, general heterosocial anxiety was inversely correlated with discussion about birth control and male partner's communication effectiveness, whereas contraceptive task anxiety was inversely correlated with use of more effective contraceptive methods.

Problems that have been increasingly recognized in heterosocial relationships are dating violence and date rape. Estimates of involvement in dating violence (either expressing or sustaining violence) range from approximately 9% to 65%, with females more likely to report that they have ever been a victim of or have expressed violence in a dating relationship (Sugarman & Hotaling, 1989).

Much of the research on dating violence has been with college students. O'Keeffe, Brocropp, & Chew (1986) surveyed 256 high-school students and found that 35.5% had experienced some form of violence and/or threats in their dating relationships (victim and/or perpetrator). Almost 27% of the sample had experienced actual violence (7.8% were victims only, 7.4% were perpetrators only; 11.7% were both). The most common type of violence was slapping (45.5%), followed by pushing or shoving (34.8%), and object throwing (19.7%). Alcohol was associated with violence approximately 40% of the time. There was no significant relationship with social demographic variables such as race, economic status, and parent's marital status.

Estimates of the incidence of date rape are also alarmingly high. Aizenman and Kelley (1988), in a survey of 204 female and 140 male undergraduates, found that 22% of females and 6% of males reported being involved in an acquaintance rape, and 43% of females and 17% of males were pressed into unwanted, noncoital sexual contact. In a survey of 380 female and 368 male undergraduates, Muehlenhard and Linton (1987) found that 14.7% of the females and 7.1% of the males had been involved in unwanted sexual intercourse. Factors associated with increased risk were (a) the male partner's initiating the date, driving, and paying all of the expenses; (b) miscommunication about sex; (c) heavy alcohol or drug use; (d) "parking," and (e) male acceptance of traditional sex roles, interpersonal violence, adversarial attitudes about relationships, and rape myths (Muehlenhard & Linton, 1987). The length of time that the individuals had known each other was not a risk factor.

Lundberg-Love and Geffner (1989) proposed a "precondition model" of date rape. According to this model, the potential offender (a) needs to have some type of motivation to abuse sexually (power and control needs, miscommunication about sex, sexual arousal, emotional incongruence, imbalance in power); (b) has to overcome internal inhibitions against acting on that motivation (attitudes such as traditional sex roles, acceptance of violence, endorsement of rape myths, adversarial relationships; prior abusive acts); (c) has to overcome external impediments to acting on that motivation (date location, mode of transportation, date activity, alcohol or substance use); and (d) has to encounter some other factor(s) that undermines or overcomes the potential victim's resistance to sexual abuse (passivity, poor self-defense abilities, history of sexual abuse, traditional attitudes, poor sexual knowledge).

Additional Problems

SPECIAL POPULATIONS

Given the extent of heterosocial problems among adolescents, it seems likely that special populations of youth may also experience significant problems. For example, although sexual development may parallel that of nonhandicapped individuals, mentally and physically handicapped individuals have increased vulnerability for problems related to dating and sex and may benefit from interventions to improve heterosocial interactions (Mueser, Valenti-Hein, & Yarnold, 1987; Van Hasselt, 1983). Social skills training has frequently been used to improve the interpersonal functioning of handicapped persons, yet there is little research specifically targeting heterosocial skills (Mueser *et al.*, 1987; Van Hasselt, 1983).

Behavior-disordered and emotionally disturbed youth may also have heterosocial problems (e.g., Swanson, 1985). For example, in a study of adolescents involved in the juvenile justice system, Melchert and Burnett (1990) found that 92% were nonvirgins, 27% had been involved in a pregnancy, 59% reported that they never or seldom used birth control.

JEALOUSY AND INFIDELITY

Jealousy and infidelity in adolescent relationships are beginning to receive attention. Hansen (1985) found that college females were more jealous than males over situations involving the partner spending time on a hobby or with family members, but other situations showed no sex differences. Beginning in the early stages of a relationship, many expect dating partners to give up close personal friendships with members of the opposite sex, and most begin to expect sexual exclusiveness. Roscoe, Cavanaugh, and Kennedy (1988) surveyed undergraduates about infidelity, which may range from flirting and kissing to coitus or may consist solely of emotional involvement. Reasons for unfaithfulness strongly paralleled those found in extramarital relationships, including dissatisfaction, revenge or jealousy, variety or experimentation, and sexual incompatibility. In general, females were more likely to focus on emotional components such as dissatisfaction with the relationship, whereas males focus on physical components such as sexual attraction or incompatibility.

Assessment Procedures

In this section, a discussion of the major issues in the assessment of heterosocial dysfunction precedes a brief review of the more frequently used assessment procedures. The review is selective, as an exhaustive review is beyond the scope of this chapter (see Galassi & Galassi, 1979, or Hersen & Bellack, 1977, for a more complete review). Although there is a considerable research on the assessment of heterosocial interaction and dysfunction, the research has been conducted almost exclusively with college students.

A major assessment issue is the general lack of psychometric considerations in the development and validation of instruments (Galassi & Galassi, 1979; Hersen & Bellack, 1977). The focus of most of the assessment research has been on the evaluation of treatment effects or the discrimination of high- and low-competent groups, and not on instrument development.

Most assessment instruments are based on either face validity or known-groups research. The known-groups research that compares heterosocially competent and incompetent individuals has been criticized methodologically (e.g., same measures used to divide samples are used as dependent measure) (Conger & Conger, 1982). Further, there is an implicit assumption in this approach that all heterosocially incompetent individuals have similar deficits across all situations.

Given the many personal and situational variables possible, this assumption is highly questionable.

The assessment of heterosocial dysfunction has been dominated by self-report measures and global ratings of role-play performances. High- and low-competent groups are generally formed on the basis of self-report measures and then compared behaviorally using global ratings of role-play performances (e.g., Kolko, 1985; Twentyman & McFall, 1975). Unfortunately, many studies do not compare self-reports of anxiety with physiological and/or behavioral indexes or they fail to compare global ratings with objective behavioral observation using frequency and duration measures (Conger & Conger, 1982).

SELF-REPORT INVENTORIES

Self-report measures have been used in research primarily for subject selection and treatment evaluation. Clinically, self-report measures can be helpful for conceptualizing heterosocial difficulties, indirectly assessing fears, anxiety, and dating frequency, and as dependent measures (Kelly, 1982). They do not, however, provide the clinician with the kind of detailed behavioral information needed to design an intervention.

Self-report instruments typically have respondents rate their expected degree of anxiety or competence in various heterosocial situations. The most frequently employed instruments are (a) the Social Anxiety and Distress Scale (SAD) (Watson & Friend, 1969), (b) the Situation Questionnaire (SQ) (Rehm & Marston, 1968), (c) the Survey of Heterosocial Interactions (SHI) (Twentyman & McFall, 1975), (d) the Survey of Heterosocial Interactions for Females (SHI-F) (Williams & Ciminero, 1978), (e) the Social Activity Questionnaire (SAQ) (Christensen & Arkowitz, 1974), and (f) the Dating and Assertion Questionnaire (DAQ) (Levensen & Gottman, 1978). The Heterosocial Assessment Inventory for Women (HAI-W) (Kolko, 1985) is a promising, recently developed measure that evaluates five dimensions (likelihood of initiation, anxiety, skillfulness, expectation of outcome, and influence of attractiveness) that may influence performance in a variety of heterosocial situations from three categories of difficulty (finding dates, making conversation, and initiating physical or sexual activity). Another recent measure is the Dating Anxiety Survey (DAS) (Calvert, Moore, & Jensen, 1987), which assesses anxiety related to passive contact, active intentions for dating, and dating interactions. Behaviors addressed range from meeting someone to kissing goodnight at the end of a date.

Despite the tremendous influence of self-report measures in heterosocial research, their psychometric integrity is generally unclear. For example, in a study comparing the psychometric properties of four major self-report instruments (i.e., the SAD, SQ, SHI, SAQ), Wallander, Conger, Mariotto, Curran, and Farrell (1980) concluded that the intercorrelations between the instruments were generally low, the battery of variables assessed were multidimensional, and that the instruments selected independent groups of subjects.

ANALOG PERFORMANCE TESTS

Sampling of behavior in analog heterosocial situations is a frequently used assessment procedure. It allows for the direct observation of performance without the ethical and pragmatic limitations of conducting such observations in the natural environment. Analog procedures are generally used to determine which behaviors discriminate between high- and low-competent groups, to validate other assessment procedures, and as dependent measures in treatment studies.

Typically, analog procedures consist of role-play tests using either audiotaped stimuli or live confederates. The Situation Test (ST) (Rehm & Marston, 1968) is an example of a role-play test using audiotaped stimuli. Subjects respond to 10 situations that are described by a male narrator and followed by a line of dialogue from a female confederate. Measures of performance include self-ratings of anxiety, global ratings by others of anxiety, latency of responding, and number of words per response. Another procedure that uses audiotaped stimuli is the Heterosocial Adequacy Test (HAT) (Perri & Richards, 1979).

The Heterosocial Skills Behavior Checklist (Barlow *et al.*, 1977) requires the subject to interact for 5 minutes with a female confederate whose behavior is standardized and to behave toward the confederate as if he wants a date. Interactions are videotaped and responses are coded using an empirically derived checklist that includes the following categories: (a) voice (loudness, pitch, inflection), (b) form of conversation (initiation, follow-up, flow, interest), and (c) affect (facial expression, eye contact, laughter).

The Heterosocial Skill Observational Rating System (HESORS) (Kolko & Milan, 1985) is a role-play observational rating system for women that has been found to have acceptable reliability, internal structure, and discriminant and criterion validity. Four situations related to heterosocial conversation are role-played with a male confederate for 4 minutes each, and 16 component behaviors are assessed: loudness, tone, inflection, active time, follow-up latency, follow-up answers to questions, topic transition, reinforcing feedback, personal attention, topic development, positive statements, smiles, gaze, eye contact in listener role, eye contact in speaker role, and self-manipulation. Other examples of "live" role plays are the Behaviorally Referenced Rating System for Heterosocial Skills (BRISS) (Wallander, Conger, & Conger, 1985) and the Forced Interaction Test (FIT) (Twentyman & McFall, 1975).

Despite their use as validation measures, there are concerns over the internal and external validity of role-play measures. Although the measures often discriminate between high- and low-competent groups on the basis of global ratings, consistent specific behavioral differences have not been found (Hersen & Bellack, 1977). The major concern about role-play procedures is the degree to which behavior in these assessments corresponds to behavior in natural settings. Research investigating the ecological validity of heterosocial role-play measures is rare and inconclusive (e.g., Kupke *et al.*, 1979; Twentyman & McFall, 1975). Kern, Miller, and Eggers (1983), in a comparison of role-play methodologies, observed male undergraduates in an "unobtrusive criterion situation" talking with a female confederate, and then assessed subjects 3 weeks later with one of three role-play procedures. The 'typical' role play required examinees to simulate their behavior in a situation described by the examiner. The "replication" and "specification" role plays required examinees to replicate their behavior from the prior criterion situation. On the specification role play, examinees were also told of specific dependent measures that were important to simulate accurately. The specification method was superior to the other methods, and the replication method was a more valid measure than the typical role play. The results suggest that the most commonly used role-play methods may not be the most valid.

Other assessment measures used in heterosocial skills research include self-monitoring, self-ratings of anxiety or skill, and peer-assessment in the natural environment (cf. Arkowitz, 1977; Galassi & Galassi, 1979). In general, self-monitoring and self-ratings suffer from low reliability and reactivity, whereas the reliability of heterosocial peer assessments is unknown.

Treatment Approaches

The major approaches to the treatment of heterosocial dysfunction are reviewed briefly in this section (see reviews by Arkowitz, 1977; Curran, 1977; Galassi & Galassi, 1979). Similar to the assessment research, the treatment investigations have been conducted almost exclusively with college students.

ANXIETY-REDUCTION PROCEDURES

Systematic desensitization and practice dating are commonly discussed anxiety-reduction techniques (Arkowitz, 1977; Galassi & Galassi, 1979). Using systematic desensitization, heterosocial fears are treated like any other phobia. A hierarchy of feared heterosocial situations is constructed and systematically paired with relaxation (e.g., Curran & Gilbert, 1975).

It should be noted that many techniques traditionally labeled *anxiety reduction* may also function to improve skill deficits through information/education, practice, and feedback components. For example, practice dating, which involves repeated exposure, is generally considered an anxiety-reduction procedure (Arkowitz, 1977; Galassi & Galassi, 1979). In general, volunteers are paired and told to arrange weekly practice dates. Christensen and Arkowitz (1974) used practice dating to treat 14 males and 14 females who volunteered in response to an advertisement for a program designed to increase dating comfort, skill, and frequency. The treatment lasted 6 weeks and consisted of having matched opposite-sex subjects go out on a practice date once a week. After the date, each subject completed a feedback form for his or her partner, which was returned to the experimenter. The treatment resulted in significant decreases in self-reported anxiety, increases in dating frequency, and improved skills. This approach is economical, can be applied to many clients simultaneously, and can enhance generalization by utilizing the natural setting (Galassi & Galassi, 1979). Unfortunately, the current prevalence of dating aggression and rape, STDs, and adolescent pregnancy may discourage use of such a procedure.

SKILLS-TRAINING APPROACHES

Skills-training approaches generally use a combination of behavioral techniques, such as instruction, modeling, rehearsal, and feedback, to treat heterosocial dysfunction (cf. Curran, 1977; Kelly, 1982). The purpose of these strategies is to improve the heterosocial skill repertoire, which should result in more positive heterosocial interactions and lowered anxiety (e.g., Curran & Gilbert, 1975; Kupke *et al.*, 1979; Twentyman & McFall, 1975).

In an often-cited investigation, Twentyman and McFall (1975) used a skills-training approach to treat 15 college males selected on the basis of their scores on the Survey of Heterosocial Interactions, which was developed for use in the study. After an extensive pretreatment assessment, subjects in the skills-training group received instruction that focused on several different heterosocial situations (e.g., telephoning for a date). Training sessions consisted of listening to a modeling tape, instructions, coaching, behavioral rehearsal with a female confederate, and self-critique of performance with the option of repeating it if not pleased. Compared to a no-treatment control group, the skills-training group was rated as less anxious and more skilled in the posttraining assessments. They also showed increased heterosocial activity in the natural environment and improved SHI scores.

ADDITIONAL INTERVENTIONS

Alternative approaches to treating heterosocial dysfunction have also shown positive effects. "Cognitive modification" procedures (Arkowitz, 1977; Galassi & Galassi, 1979) have included self-evaluation and self-reinforcement (Rehm & Marston, 1968) and modification of negative self-statements and self-appraisals (Glass, Gottman, & Shmurak, 1976). A group contingency token system has been shown to be more effective than an individual contingency at increasing rates of heterosocial and same-sex interaction (Swanson, 1985).

Interventions for heterosocial difficulties have generally focused on the reduction of anxiety and the remediation of skills deficits. Identifying additional targets for intervention seems appropriate, as the problems related to adolescent heterosocial interactions are wide ranging. For example, one relatively uninvestigated area is the treatment of heterosexual problems. Sex education is popular but is generally considered an issue for the schools and parents (see review by Otto, 1977). The lack of psychological intervention research on heterosexual difficulties is disappointing, given the fact that it seems to be a highly problematic aspect of heterosocial relationships (e.g., Knox & Wilson, 1983; Muehlenhard & Linton, 1987).

Potentially helpful heterosexual interventions for adolescents might be assertion training and social problem-solving training (Hynes & Bruch, 1985). It seems important to not only teach adolescents about safe sex, but to teach assertion or problem-solving skills so that they may apply that knowledge in their own relationships (MacDonald et al., 1990). Such interventions could be carried out in a typical social-skills training format, using instruction, modeling, rehearsal, and feedback. These skills could be helpful in preventing unwanted pregnancies, AIDS and other STDs, and date rape and violence.

Another possible area for intervention is the parent–adolescent relationship because parents may influence adolescent sexual activity (McCabe, 1984) and issues surrounding heterosexual relationships may be a significant source of friction between parents and adolescents (Forgatch & Patterson, 1989). The addition of assertion, problem solving, and/or parent–adolescent communication interventions may prove to be very beneficial for improving adolescent heterosocial difficulties.

TREATMENT EFFECTIVENESS

There is ample research on the effectiveness of anxiety-reduction and skills-training treatments (see reviews by Curran, 1977; Galassi & Galassi, 1979). In general, systematic desensitization and practice dating are effective in reducing heterosocial anxiety. Skills training not only reduces anxiety but also results in improvements on global ratings of heterosocial skills.

Research comparing the effectiveness of various treatment approaches can be misleading, however, because heterosocial dysfunction is often multidetermined, with anxiety, skill, cognitive, and social factors all influencing performance. It is highly unlikely that any one treatment would prove to be the most effective for all individuals. For example, some individuals might have the requisite skills and still experience anxiety in heterosocial interactions, whereas others might lack skill and do not experience anxiety.

An idiographic approach to assessment is needed to determine what approach is the most effective for which specific problems and which clients (Galassi & Galassi, 1979). And, consistent with the general literature on social-skills training, much more information is needed on the generalization and social validity of the treatment procedures (Hansen, Watson-Perczel, and Christopher, 1989).

SUMMARY

In the 1970s and early 1980s, there was a significant amount of attention directed to heterosocial interactions and dysfunction. This was due in part to dissatisfaction with target behaviors chosen for previous therapy studies (e.g., small-animal phobias) (cf. Curran, 1977; Galassi & Galassi, 1979). Heterosocial anxiety was found to be more pervasive and complicated, with an abundance of available research subjects. Unfortunately, research activity on adolescent heterosocial interactions appears to have declined in recent years. This is especially disappointing given the extent and seriousness of the problem and the variety of questions to be addressed.

Based on the literature discussed in this chapter, a variety of directions for research and practice are evident. One needed direction is expansion of the populations studied, such as (a) more research with adolescents who are not college students (i.e., younger adolescents and noncollege populations); (b) more attention to gender differences; (c) more research on the heterosocial interaction and dating of handicapped and behavior-disordered adolescents; and (d) increased investigation of racial and cultural differences in heterosocial interactions and dating.

Research is needed regarding the causes of heterosocial dysfunction, especially the interrelationships among the models proposed for heterosocial problems (i.e., anxiety, skill deficits, cognitions, attractiveness) and the role of physical appearance, including style of dress as well as physical attributes. Assessment and treatment research that considers the multiple causes of heterosocial dysfunction and avoids taking a single, limited perspective is also needed.

Additional areas in need of further investigation include (a) the various stages of dating and their impact on measures and procedures; (b) the situational specificity of the occurrence of heterosocial behaviors (and avoidance of simplistic, traitlike labels such as "high-anxious subjects"); (c) further identification of which behaviors are required for socially competent performance (and in which situations with which individuals); and (d) examination of heterosocial interactions in situations for which the goal is not dating or sexual activity (i.e., when adolescent males and females are interacting as friends and how these may be different from interactions with same-sex persons).

Research needed in the area of intervention, in addition to these suggestions, includes (a) development and identification of measures for evaluating intervention effectiveness; (b) development of procedures for assessing and programming generalization; (c) evaluation of the social validity of treatment goals, procedures, and effects (e.g., actual increases in dating frequency and satisfaction); and (d) application of assertion, social problem solving, and parent–adolescent communication training to heterosexual problems.

It is hoped that researchers and practitioners will address these important issues. There is clearly a need for increased understanding of the heterosocial development and dysfunction of adolescents.

References

Aizenman, M., & Kelley, G. (1988). The incidence of violence and acquaintance rape in dating relationships among college men and women. *Journal of College Student Development, 29*, 305–311.

Alexander, B. (1990). Teenage sex risks. *Medical Aspects of Human Sexuality, 24*, 55–56.

Arkowitz, H. (1977). Measurement and modification of minimal dating behavior. In M. Hersen, R. Eisler, & P. Miller (Eds.), *Progress in behavior modification* (Vol. 5, pp. 1–61). New York: Academic Press.

Arkowitz, H., Hinton, R., Perl, J., & Himadi, W. (1978). Treatment strategies for dating anxiety in college men based on real-life practice. *Counseling Psychologist, 7*, 41–46.

Bailey, R. C., & Kelly, M. (1984). Perceived physical attractiveness in early, steady, and engaged daters: Distinguishing intimate from nonintimate relationships. *The Journal of Psychology, 116*, 39–43.

Barlow, D. H., Abel, G. G., Blanchard, E. B., Bristow, A. R., & Young, L. D. (1977). A heterosocial skills behavior checklist for males. *Behavior Therapy, 2*, 229–239.

Barrios, B., & O'Dell, S. L. (1989). Fears and anxieties. In E. J. Mash & R. A. Barkley (Eds.), *Treatment of childhood disorders* (pp. 167–221). New York: Guilford.

Berger, K. S. (1986). *The developing person through childhood and adolescence* (2nd ed.). New York: Worth.

Borkovec, T. D., Stone, N. M., O'Brien, G. T., Kaloupek, D. G. (1974). Evaluation of a clinically relevant target behavior for analogue outcome research. *Behavior Therapy, 5*, 503–511.

Brookman, R. R. (1990). Adolescent sexual behavior. *Sexually transmitted diseases* (2nd ed., pp. 77–84). New York: McGraw-Hill.

Brooks-Gunn, J., & Furstenberg, F. F. (1989). Adolescent sexual behavior. *American Psychologist, 44*, 249–257.

Bruch, M. A., & Hynes, M. J. (1987). Heterosocial anxiety and contraceptive behavior. *Journal of Research in Personality, 21*, 343–360.

Burger, J. M., & Inderbitzen, H. M. (1985). Predicting contraceptive behavior among college students: The role of communication, knowledge, sexual anxiety, and self-esteem. *Archives of Sexual Behavior, 14*, 343–350.

Burke, D. S., Brundage, J. F., Herbold, J. R., Berner, W., Gardner, L. I., Gunzenhauser, J. D., Voskovitch, J., & Redfield, R. R. (1987). *New England Journal of Medicine, 317*, 131–136.

Byrne, D. (1983). Sex without contraception. In D. Byrne & W. A. Fisher (Eds.), *Adolescents, sex, and contraception* (pp. 3–31). Hillsdale, NJ: Erlbaum.

Calvert, J. D., Moore, D., & Jensen, B. J. (1987). Psychometric evaluation of the dating anxiety survey: A self-report questionnaire for the assessment of dating anxiety in males and females. *Journal of Psychopathology and Behavioral Assessment, 9*, 341–350.

Christensen, A., & Arkowitz, H. (1974). Preliminary report on practice and feedback as treatment for college dating problems. *Journal of Counseling Psychology, 21* 92–95.

Christopher, F. S., & Cate, R. M. (1988). Premarital sexual involvement: A developmental investigation of relational correlates. *Adolescence, 22*, 793–803.

Clark, S. D., Zabin, L. S., & Hardy, J. B. (1984). Sex, contraception and parenthood: Experiences and attitudes among urban black young men. *Family Planning Perspectives, 16*, 77–82.

Coleman, M., Ganong, L. H., & Ellis, P. (1985). Family structure and dating behavior of adolescents. *Adolescence, 20,* 537–543.

Conger, J. C., & Conger, A. J. (1982). Components of heterosocial competence. In J. P. Curran & P. M. Monti (Eds.), *Social skills training: A practical handbook for assessment and treatment* (pp. 313–347). New York: Guilford.

Csikszentmihalyi, M., & Larson, R. (1984). *Being adolescent: Conflict and growth in the teenage years.* New York: Basic Books.

Curran, J. P. (1977). Skills training as an approach to the treatment of heterosexual-social anxiety: A review. *Psychological Bulletin, 84,* 140–157.

Curran, J. P., & Gilbert, F. S. (1975). A test of the relative effectiveness of a systematic desensitization program and an interpersonal skills training program with date anxious subjects. *Behavior Therapy, 6,* 510–521.

Damon, W. (1983). *Social and personality development.* New York: Norton.

DiClemente, R. J. (1990). The emergence of adolescents as a risk group for human immunodeficiency virus infection. *Journal of Adolescent Research, 5,* 7–17.

Dodge, C. S., Heimberg, R. G., Nyman, D., & O'Brien, G. T. (1987). Daily heterosocial interactions of high and low socially anxious college students: A diary study. *Behavior Therapy, 18,* 90–96.

Elkind, D. (1983). Strategic interactions in early adolescence. In W. Damon (Ed.), *Social and personality development: Essays on the growth of the child* (pp. 434–444). New York: Norton.

Forgatch, M. S., & Patterson, G. R. (1989). *Parents and adolescents living together—Part 2: Family problem solving.* Eugene, OR: Castalia.

Galassi, J. P., & Galassi, M. D. (1979). Modification of heterosocial skills deficits. In A. S. Bellack & M. Hersen (Eds.), *Research and practice in social skill training* pp. 131–187). New York: Plenum Press.

Glass, C. R., Gottman, J. M., & Shmurak, S. H. (1976). Response-acquisition and cognitive self-statement modification approaches to dating-skills training. *Journal of Counseling Psychology, 23,* 520–526.

Hansen, D. J., St. Lawrence, J. S., & Christoff, K. A. (1988). Conversational skills of inpatient conduct-disordered youth: Social validation of component behaviors and implications for skills training. *Behavior Modification, 12,* 424–444.

Hansen, D. J., Watson-Perczel, M., & Christopher, J. S. (1989). Clinical issues in social-skills training with adolescents. *Clinical Psychology Review, 9,* 365–391.

Hansen, G. L. (1985). Dating jealousy among college students. *Sex Roles, 12,* 713–721.

Hersen, M., & Bellack, A. J. (1977). Assessment of social skills. In A. R. Ciminero, K. R. Calhoun, & H. E. Adams (Eds.), *Handbook of behavioral assessment* (pp. 509–554). New York: Wiley.

Himadi, W. G., Arkowitz, H., Hinton, R., & Perl, J. (1980). Minimal dating and its relationship to other social problems and general adjustment. *Behavior Therapy, 11,* 345–352.

Hingson, R. W., Strunin, L., Berlin, B. M., & Heeren, T. (1990). beliefs about AIDS, use of alcohol and drugs, and unprotected sex among Massachusetts adolescents. *American Journal of Public Health, 80,* 295–299.

Hynes, M. J., & Bruch, M. A. (1985). Social skills and responses in simulated contraceptive problem situations. *Journal of Sex Research, 21,* 422–436.

Jemmott, L. S., & Jemmott, J. B. (1990). Sexual knowledge, attitudes, and risky sexual behavior among inner-city black male adolescents. *Journal of Adolescent Research, 5,* 346–369.

Kelly, J. A. (1982). *Social-skills training: A practical guide for interventions.* New York: Springer.

Kelly, J. A., & Hansen, D. J. (1987). Social interactions and adjustment. In V. B. Van Hasselt & M. Hersen (Eds.), *Handbook of adolescent psychology* (pp. 131–146). New York: Pergamon.

Kern, J. M., Miller, C., & Eggers, J. (1983). Enhancing the validity of role-play tests: A comparison of three role-play methodologies. *Behavior Therapy, 14,* 482–492.

Kimmel, D. C., & Weiner, I. B. (1985). *Adolescence: A developmental transition.* Hillsdale, NJ: Erlbaum.

Klaus, D., Hersen, M., & Bellack, A. S. (1977). Survey of dating habits of male and female college students: A necessary precursor to measurement and modification. *Journal of Clinical Psychology, 33,* 369–375.

Knox, D., & Wilson, K. (1983). Dating problems of university students. *College Student Journal, 17,* 225–228.

Koenig, M. A., & Zelnik, M. (1982). The risk of premarital first pregnancy among metropolitan-area teenagers: 1976 and 1979. *Family Planning Perspectives, 14,* 239–247.

Kolko, D. J. (1985). The heterosocial assessment inventory for women: A psychometric and behavioral evaluation. *Journal of Psychopathology and Behavioral Assessment, 7,* 49–64.

Kolko, D. J., & Milan, M. A. (1985). A women's heterosocial skill observational rating system: Behavior-analytic development and validation. *Behavior Modification, 9*, 165–192.

Kupke, T. E., Hobbs, S. A., & Cheney, T. H. (1979). Selection of heterosocial skills. I. Criterion-related validity. *Behavior Therapy, 10*, 327–335.

Leary, M. R., & Dobbins, S. E. (1983). Social anxiety, sexual behavior, and contraceptive use. *Journal of Personality and Social Psychology, 45*, 1347–1354.

Leigh, G. K., Weddle, K. D., & Loewen, I. R. (1988). Analysis of the timing of transition to sexual intercourse for Black adolescent females. *Journal of Adolescent Research, 3*, 333–344.

Leslie, L. A., Huston, T. L., & Johnson, M. P. (1986). Parental reactions to dating relationships: Do they make a difference? *Journal of Marriage and the Family, 48*, 57–66.

Levenson, R. W., & Gottman, J. M. (1978). Toward the assessment of social competence. *Journal of Consulting and Clinical Psychology, 8*, 453–462.

Lundberg-Love, P., & Geffner, R. (1989). Date rape: Prevalence, risk factors, and a proposed model. In M. A. Pirog-Good & J. E. Stets (Eds.), *Violence in dating relationships: Emerging social issues* (pp. 169–184). New York: Praeger.

MacDonald, N. E., Wells, G. A., Fisher, W. A., Warren, W. K., King, M. A., Doherty, J. A., & Bowie, W. R. (1990). High-risk STD/HIV behavior among college students. *Journal of the American Medical Association, 263*, 3155–3159.

McAnarney, E. R., & Hendee, W. R. (1989). Adolescent pregnancy and its consequences. *Journal of the American Medical Association, 262*, 74–77.

McCabe, M. P. (1984). Toward a theory of adolescent dating. *Adolescence, 19*, 159–170.

Melchert, T., & Burnett, K. F. (1990). Attitudes, knowledge, and sexual behavior of high-risk adolescents: Implications for counseling and sexuality education. *Journal of Counseling and Development, 68*, 293–298.

Miller, B. C., McCoy, J. K., & Olson, T. D. (1986). Dating age and stage as correlates of adolescent sexual attitudes and behavior. *Journal of Adolescent Research, 1*, 361–377.

Miller, K. E. (1990). Adolescents' same-sex and opposite-sex peer relations: Sex differences in popularity, perceived social competence, and social cognitive skills. *Journal of Adolescent Research, 5*, 222–241.

Muehlenhard, C. L., Koralewski, M. A., Andrews, S. L., & Burdick, C. A. (1986). Verbal and nonverbal cues that convey interest in dating: Two studies. *Behavior Therapy, 17*, 404–419.

Muehlenhard, C. L., & Liton, M. A. (1987). Date rape and sexual aggression in dating situations: Incidence and risk factors. *Journal of Counseling Psychology, 34*, 186–196.

Mueser, K. T., Valenti-Hein, D., & Yarnold, P. R. (1987). Dating-skills groups for the developmentally disabled: Social skills and problem-solving versus relaxation training. *Behavior Modification, 11*, 200–228.

O'Keeffe, N. K., Brockopp, K., & Chew, E. (1986). Teen dating violence. *Social Work, 31*, 465–468.

Otto, H. (Ed.). (1977). *The new sex education: The sex educator's resource book.* New York: Association Press.

Perri, M. G., & Richards, C. S. (1979). Assessment of heterosocial skills in male college students: Empirical development of a behavioral role-playing test. *Behavior Modification, 3*, 337–354.

Petersen, A. C., & Hamburg, B. A. (1986). Adolescence: A developmental approach to problems and psychopathology. *Behavior Therapy, 17*, 480–499.

Pirog-Good, M. A., & Stets, J. E. (Eds.). (1989). *Violence in dating relationships: Emerging social issues.* New York: Praeger.

Rehm, L. P., & Marston, A. R. (1968). Reduction of social anxiety through modification of self-reinforcement: An instigation therapy technique. *Journal of Consulting and Clinical Psychology, 32*, 565–574.

Roche, J. P. (1986). Premarital sex: Attitudes and behavior by dating stage. *Adolescence, 21*, 107–121.

Roscoe, B., Cavanaugh, L. E., & Kennedy, D. R. (1988). Dating infidelity: Behaviors, reasons and consequences. *Adolescence, 23*, 35–43.

Roscoe, B., Diana, M. S., & Brooks, R. H. (1987). Early, middle, and late adolescents' views on dating and factors influencing partner selection. *Adolescence, 22*, 59–68.

Roscoe, B., Kennedy, D., & Pope, T. (1987). Adolescents' views of intimacy: Distinguishing intimate from nonintimate relationships. *Adolescence, 22*, 511–516.

Roscoe, B., & Kruger, T. L. (1990). AIDS: Late adolescent' knowledge and its influence on sexual behavior. *Adolescence, 25*, 39–48.

Scott-Jones, D., & White, A. B. (1990). Correlates of sexual activity in early adolescence. *Journal of Early Adolescence, 10*, 221–238.

Select Committee on Children, Youth, and Families, U.S. House of Representatives. (1988). *AIDS and teenagers: Emerging issues.* Washington, DC: U.S. Government Printing Office.

Sherwin, R., & Corbett, S. (1985). Campus sexual norms and dating relationships: A trend analysis. *Journal of Sex Research, 21,* 258–274.

Spreadbury, C. L. (1982). First date. *Journal of Early Adolescence, 2,* 83–89.

Stelzer, C., Desmond, S. M., & Price, J. H. (1987). Physical attractiveness and sexual activity of college students. *Psychological Reports, 60,* 567–573.

Sugarman, D. B., & Hotaling, G. T. (1989). Dating violence: Prevalence, context, and risk markers. In M. A. Pirog-Good & J. E. Stets (Eds.), *Violence in dating relationships: Emerging social issues* (pp. 4–32). New York: Praeger.

Swanson, H. L. (1985). Improving same-sex and heterosocial interactions of emotionally-disturbed adolescents. *Journal of School Psychology, 23,* 365–374.

Treboux, D., & Busch-Rossnagel, N. A. (1990). Social network influences on adolescent sexual attitudes and behaviors. *Journal of Adolescent Research, 5,* 175–189.

Twentyman, C. T., & McFall, R. M. (1975). Behavioral training of social skills in shy males. *Journal of Consulting and Clinical Psychology, 43,* 384–395.

Van Hasselt, V. B. (1983). Social adaptation in the blind. *Clinical Psychology Review, 3,* 87–102.

Wallander, J. L., Conger, A. J., & Conger, J. D. (1985). Development and evaluation of a behaviorally referenced rating system for heterosocial skills. *Behavioral Assessment, 7,* 137–153.

Wallander, J. L., Conger, A. J., Mariotto, M. J., Curran, J. P., & Farrell, A. D. (1980). Comparability of selection instruments in studies of heterosexual-social problem behaviors. *Behavior Therapy, 11,* 548–560.

Watson, D., & Friend, R. (1969). Measurement of social-evaluative anxiety. *Journal of Consulting and Clinical Psychology, 33,* 448–457.

Williams, C. L., & Ciminero, A. R. (1978). Development and validation of a heterosocial skills inventory: The Survey of Heterosexual Interactions for Females. *Journal of Consulting and Clinical Psychology, 46,* 1547–1548.

IV

Adults

In looking at one's social development in adulthood the preeminent factors to be considered are marriage and work. Indeed, when interviewing successful adults who are devoid of major psychopathology, it would seem that satisfaction with their mates (or other loved ones) and their occupation are most often emphasized. However, as will be apparent in the three chapters that comprise this part, neither the relationship nor one's chosen profession remains static throughout one's adult years. Indeed, the combination of biological and maturational changes in concert with the vicissitudes of life interweave and can result in difficulties. Especially difficult for some men is the so-called "midlife" period when a critical reevaluation of one's life often takes place. This tends to happen as a function of aging, increased concern about death or variance between past aspirations and present accomplishments, and role changes that have taken place over times.

Gary R. Birchler (Chapter 16) examines marriage and its implications from a number of perspectives. In so doing he divides marriage into five development stages: (1) the new couple, (2) the transition to parenthood, (3) midlife adolescence, (4) the postparental stage, and (5) culmination. At different stages the couple will enjoy differing degrees of marital satisfaction. The author notes that by conceptualizing such stages it enables one to understand better when a marital relationship is functional. Lynda J. Katz and Ray Feroz (Chapter 17) describe work activity as central to human existence. Over centuries the meaning and function of work have changed and are strongly affected by cultural values, individual values, race, ethnicity, gender, age, education, and aptitude. The authors examine in detail the measurement of the meaning of work and the future of work. External factors that impact on work, such as economics, environmental concerns, resources available, regulatory influences, and politics, are outlined. Richard M. Eisler and Kim Ragsdale (Chapter 18) evaluate masculine gender role and midlife transition in men. The major thesis of this chapter is that men who adhere to the dictates of the supermasculine role are those who will experience the greatest distress in the midlife period. It is argued that American males have been taught to associate masculinity with (1) diminished expressiveness in intimate relationships, (2) superachievement in work roles, (3) power and control, and (4) maintenance of physical strength and sexual potency. Apparently, less reliance in the masculine gender role will result in a smoother transition during the midlife period.

16

Marriage

GARY R. BIRCHLER

INTRODUCTION

The lifespan perspective of marriage becomes broader and more complicated each year. First, the "normal" family household unit in America, popularly idealized to be the traditional nuclear family composed of working father, housekeeping mother, and the children is fast becoming a myth. Today the majority of household units in our country is headed by single adults and single parents (Norton, 1983). When husband and wife *are* living together, in approximately half the cases, both husbands and wives work (Locksley, 1980). Second, increased longevity has expanded dramatically the postparental and the old age stages of marital life into new lifespan phenomena. Third, the changing role of women has had a powerful impact on marriage over the past two decades. Fourth, the empirical support for relationships between marital satisfaction and life cycle stages lags far behind the theoretical descriptions of these relationships.

The organization and scope of this chapter are constrained by several factors. First, although it should be obvious that the life cycles of the individual, the marriage, and the family are intertwined, in this review an emphasis will be placed on the *marital life cycle*. Other chapters in this book will elaborate upon individual and family issues more appropriately. Second, most of the existing literature on the development of marriage over the lifespan describes first-marriage nuclear families in white, middle-class America. Therefore, this group shall perforce form the basis for our current understanding of change in marriage over the lifespan. Third, the literature on marriage and the life cycle is derived primarily from broad demographic cross-sectional studies in the field of family sociology and from family-

GARY R. BIRCHLER • Veterans Affairs Medical Center, San Diego, California 92161 and University of California School of Medicine, San Diego, California 92093.

Handbook of Social Development: A Lifespan Perspective, edited by Vincent B. Van Hasselt and Michel Hersen. Plenum Press, New York, 1992.

systems-oriented clinicians. Sorely missing are well-controlled longitudinal studies of the development of marriage and marital dysfunction. Contemporary marital researchers most likely to design empirical studies, the social-learning-oriented, behavioral marriage therapists, have rarely (Markman, 1979, 1981) and only recently (Gottman & Krokoff, 1989; Markman, Floyd, Stanley, & Storaasli, 1988) employed longitudinal, developmental approaches.

The present chapter will review the existing sociological, family systems, and related clinical/research literatures as they describe our present understanding of marriage over the lifespan. The development of marriage can only be understood in the context of the *family life cycle*. Consequently, several renditions of marital/family life cycle stages (and their associated tasks and issues) will be considered. After progression through the five marital life cycle stages arbitrarily chosen for this exposition, aspects of the rapidly changing family life cycle will be discussed, followed by therapeutic and research considerations.

ORIGINS AND PROPOSITIONS OF THE DEVELOPMENTAL PERSPECTIVE

The Family and Marital Life Cycles

The most frequent reference to the family life cycle is Duvall (1967). She based her eight developmental stages on the ages and the presence or absence of children in the family and from the beginning of marriage to the death of one or both parents (see Table 1). Duvall suggested that families grow through transitional stages of development that are predictable and that have associated tasks. The successful accomplishment of these tasks leads to happiness and to easier transition through future stages of development. In contrast, failure to accomplish these personal and relationship tasks leads to unhappiness and increased difficulty with later transitions. The work of Duvall (1967) played an important early role in influencing later theorists (e.g., Berman & Lief, 1975; Solomon, 1973) to further develop and integrate individual, marital, and family life cycle concepts. Solomon (1973) described five stages of development (Table 1) and suggested, as have others (e.g., Carter & McGoldrick, 1980; Hoffman, 1988), that the transitions between family life cycle stages represent crises for the family and its members. The outcomes of struggling with these transitions can be either healthy transformations or the development of psychopathological symptoms (Haley, 1973).

Berman and Lief (1975) were perhaps the first to outline an elaborate conceptual matrix that invited comparison and integration of individual and marital aspects of development across seven age-based stages. Dimensions of marital conflict, intimacy, power, and marital boundaries were introduced in this outline. Since the formative work of Duvall, Solomon, and Berman and Lief, many others have proposed various renditions of marital (Campbell, 1980; Kovacs, 1988; Monte, 1989; Nadelson, Polonsky, & Mathews, 1984; Nichols, 1988; Rock, 1986) and family (Carter & McGoldrick, 1988a) developmental stages (Table 1). However, before proceeding to a consideration of specific developmental stages, we will examine some assumptions underlying the developmental approach.

General Assumptions Underlying the Developmental Perspective

Arguably, the edited books by Carter and McGoldrick (1980, 1988b) have presented the most comprehensive concentration of writings about the family life

TABLE 1. Stages of Marital and Family Life Cycles

Duvall, 1967	*Solomon, 1973*
I. Beginning families	I. The marriage
II. Childbearing famlies	II. The birth of the first child and subsequent childbearing
III. Families with preschool children	III. Individuation of family members
IV. Families with school-age children	IV. The actual departure of children
V. Families with teenagers	V. The integration of loss
VI. Families as launching center	
VII. Family in the middle years	
VIII. Aging families	

Campbell, 1980[a]	*Nadelson et al., 1984[a]*
I. Romance	I. Idealization
II. Power struggle	II. Disappointment, disillusionment, disenchantment
III. Stability	III. Productivity, parenting
IV. Commitment	IV. Career resolution
V. Co-creation	V. Redefinition, child launching
	VI. Reintegration, postparenting

Carter & McGoldrick, 1988[a]	*Kovacs, 1988[a]*
I. Leaving home: single young adults	I. Honeymoon
II. The joint of families through marriage: the new couple	II. Early marriage-dependence
III. Families with young children	III. Growing divergence
IV. Families with adolescents	IV. Independence (7-year itch)
V. Launching children and moving on	V. Working through
VI. Families in later life	VI. Interdependence-mutuality

Nichols, 1988[a]	*Monte, 1989[a]*
I. Mating and marriage	I. Starting up
II. Expansion: parental beginnings and subsequent years	II. Settling in
III. Contraction: individuation and eventual separation of youth	III. Decision time
IV. Postparental	IV. Moving on/latency age
	V. Midlife adolescence
	VI. Launching
	VII. Older age and death

[a]Denotes *marital* as opposed to *family* life cycle.

cycle and family therapy. The notion that the family is a complex system moving through time is axiomatic. To quote Carter and McGoldrick (1988a):

> In our view family stress is often greatest at transition points from one stage to another of the family developmental process, and symptoms are most likely to appear when there is an interruption or dislocation in the unfolding family life cycle. (p. 4)

Particular difficulty in health development may occur in families when transgenerational, historical, developmental, and contemporary stressors converge and intersect (Carter & McGoldrick, 1988a).

Kovacs (1982, 1988) suggests that marital development has an orderly progression but that disruptions are common. These "crises" associated with stage transitions are considered normal and represent opportunities for growth or failure. The lifelong marital process includes complex, polarized struggles for independence/dependence, closeness/distance and autonomy/belongingness. Marital relationship boundaries expand and contract over time to accommodate additions and losses.

Contemporary theorists concur that there are three major sources of development and influence on marriage: (1) individual factors (e.g., genetic, personality, and behavioral predispositions); (2) interactional factors; and (3) extramarital factors (e.g., influences from previous generations, extended family, society, and natural occurrences [Martin, 1987; Monte, 1989; Nichols, 1988]). In a perfect marriage, these three sources of influence are synthesized in harmony. In reality, there are progressions, disruptions, and constant changes that lead to a very few high-quality, long-term, intimate relationships and to possibly a majority of failed marriages.

Another important concept, which is endorsed by most family therapists, sociologists, and life cycle advocates, is the phenomenon of *epigenesis of relational systems*. With regard to the epigenetic principle, Wynne (1984) stated that "the interchanges or transactions of each developmental phase build upon the outcomes of earlier transactions" (p. 298). The success (satisfaction, health) or failure (dissatisfaction, psychopathology) associated with each sequential stage of individual, marital, or family life cycles is dependent upon the outcomes of previous tasks, transitions, and stages. Wynne (1984) presents an interesting model of four major processes in the epigenesis of enduring relational systems: attachments/caregiving, communicating, joint problem solving, and mutuality. The epigenetic nature of intimate relationships is a fundamental premise of all contemporary developmental models of marriage (Bader & Pearson, 1988; Campbell, 1980; Kovacs, 1988; Monte, 1989; Nadelson *et al.*, 1984; Nichols, 1988).

COMPARATIVE STAGES OF THE FAMILY AND MARITAL LIFE CYCLE

Over the past three decades, the family life cycle has been separated into as many as 24 stages (Rodgers, 1960) and into as few as 3 (Flori, 1989). Rodgers's systems accounted for the progression of multiple children through family life; Flori considered periods of family *establishment*, *expansion*, and *culmination*. Table 1 presents an additional 8 models, ranging in number of developmental stages from 5 to 8. The models developed by Duvall (1967), Carter and McGoldrick (1988a), and ᶜᴐlomon (1973) represent the basic *family* life cycle; schema by Campbell (1980), Kovacs (1988), Monte (1989), Nadelson *et al.* (1984), and Nichols (1988) represent the *marital* life cycle. Note that although somewhat different names, stages, and developmental markers are used by various authors, there is a considerable degree of overlap in these stages (e.g., presence or absence of children, length of marriage, epigenetic relationship processes).

For purposes of this chapter, a five-stage model has been adopted, utilizing some of the stage names of existing models and incorporating many of the stages described in the literature: (a) Stage I: the new couple; (b) Stage II: the transition to parenthood; (c) Stage III: midlife adolescence; (d) Stage IV: postparental; and (e) Stage V: culmination.

Stage I: The New Couple

Taking note of the changing family life cycle, one might conclude that young people are shying away from the traditional marriage. The number of lifelong single people and the number of co-habiting pairs are increasing. Given greater access to contraception and economic support, young women are pursuing careers more frequently. Couples are having sex earlier but getting married significantly later (Glick, 1984). As the divorce rate has skyrocketed over the past generation, the offspring from these broken families are appropriately reluctant to perpetuate the process (see Mueller & Pope, 1977). Nevertheless, by age 40, the marriage rate is as high as ever; well over 90% of our single adults eventually do marry (Glick, 1975).

Another interesting phenomenon is that of all the stages of the marital life cycle, the new couple stage is undoubtedly the most adventurous, exciting, and results in the highest level of marital satisfaction for the greatest numbers of people (Nadelson *et al.*, 1984). Yet the first 2 years of marriage also result in the highest divorce rate of all the marital stages (Carter & McGoldrick, 1988a; Nadelson *et al.*, 1984). How do we account for this phenomenon? The selection process and the development of the relationship from acquaintanceship through the first few years of marriage seem to be the problem.

Regarding mate selection, marital success is relatively more assured to the extent that partners are similar in background and status on the following variables: education, socioeconomic status, race, religion, age, culture, physique, physical attraction, and values (Meyer & Pepper, 1977; Murstein, 1976). Although similarities and differences in personality variables have received inconsistent support for decades, there is some evidence that a couple's effectiveness in basic communication skills predicts later marital satisfaction (Markman, 1979, 1981).

Individuals also seem to get married for the wrong reasons, at the wrong time, and in the wrong circumstances. Too frequently people marry (a) to escape unpleasant aspects of their family of origin (Carter & McGoldrick, 1988a; Martin, 1987); (b) to resolve unfinished business with family members by displacing the conflict onto their mate (Nadelson *et al.*, 1984); (c) to cure severe psychological deficits (Nadelson *et al.*, 1984); or (d) to meet the expectations of peers, family, or community (Ryder, Kafka, & Olson, 1971). Carter and McGoldrick (1988a) also determined from the literature that adjustment problems may arise if couples meet or marry after one mate has sustained a significant loss (e.g., death in the family), marry before age 20, marry after being acquainted for less than 6 months or for more than 3 years, get pregnant before marriage or within the first year of marriage, become dependent on families of origin for financial or housing support, or live either too close to or too far away from extended families (Carter & McGoldrick, 1988a). In summary, there seems to be an overwhelming number of reasons and circumstances why *not* to marry. Unfortunately, soon after marriage, if not before, blind love must be reconciled with practical reality.

Experts on marriage reach fair consensus on the adjustment problems of the new couple. Nadelson *et al.* (1984) discuss the stage of idealization, in which each partner expects the other to fulfill all of one's needs; negative or incompatible traits in the opposite partner are denied. In their model (Table 1), idealization is followed by disappointment, disillusion, and disenchantment, where the reality of living together soon confronts and dispels the romantic high. Formerly overlooked personality, behavioral habit, lifestyle, and value differences emerge abruptly. Basically, in the ideal progression, one's identity must mature from an adolescent, to a single young-adult independent of family, to an integral, even exclusive partner of a new couple entity, and once again to a more differentiated individual in a marriage. One who has matured to the latter stage can maintain a healthy balance of meeting personal and relationship needs. To the extent that the newly married partners cannot support, tolerate, and adapt to one another through these early complex changes, the new couple is threatened.

Finally, there are the practical aspects of role adoption and dealing with the various content areas of making a life together. Women are balking increasingly at the sex roles assigned on the basis of the traditional marriage (see McGoldrick, 1988). Although it is clear that men and women still have somewhat different expectations placed upon them and somewhat different tasks to perform, rigid divisions of labor are evolving to a more negotiated and equitable transaction. Typical responsibilities and adjustments for the new couple include (a) finding job(s) and establishing a foundation of economic security (often still more expected of the male); (b) establishing a home and comfortable living space (often still expected of the female); (c) working through revisions of the relationships with premarital friends and family; (d) establishing a satisfying sexual relationship; (e) accommodating to one another's personal habits, tastes, and activity preferences; and (f) developing an initial pattern of communication, decision making, and conflict resolution. Many marital therapists believe that the acquisition of effective communication and problem-solving processes is required in order to establish (Nichols, 1988), maintain (Markman, 1984; Wynne, 1984), and remediate distress associated with long-term intimate relationships (e.g., Birchler & Gershwin, 1991).

Using PREPARE, a 125-item inventory designed to identify relationship strengths and weaknesses in 11 relationship areas, Olson, Fournier and Druckman (1987) completed two longitudinal studies that sought to predict later marital satisfaction and dissolution of large groups of engaged couples (Fowers & Olson, 1986; Larson & Olson, 1989). Variables that significantly predicted happiness or divorce after 3 years were a couple's realistic expectations, personality issues, communication, conflict resolution, leisure activities, family and friends, equalitarian roles, and religious orientation. Longitudinal studies of engaged couples are important in that they (a) provide empirical support for long-held theoretical constructs of successful marital interaction in the new couple and (b) may help define high-risk couples who can benefit from premarital counseling. On the presumption that the new couple survives the first few years of marriage, let us now consider the second stage of our five-stage model.

Stage II: The Transition to Parenthood

In the present five-stage model, the transition to parenthood stage lasts basically from the birth of the first child until the first child reaches adolescence. For the majority of married couples in our society, typically after a couple years of marriage and in the couples' early to middle 20s, there are several important options and tasks that can affect marital satisfaction significantly: (a) whether or not to have children, (b) commitment to career and work inside or outside of the home, and (c) working through the inevitable power struggles that result from identity and role changes associated with family, career, and individual versus marital development over this period of time. Much of the following discussion comes from resources identified in Table 1.

COMMITMENT

New and renewed commitments are a dominant theme of this stage of marital development. Following recovery from the idealization and disillusionment of early marriage, surviving couples reach a more realistic appraisal of the prospects for gratification in the marriage. Either the decision to join the majority who have children or the minority who do not constitutes a form of renewed commitment to live together (Monte, 1989). Commitment is also required to maintain secure employment or to establish a career (Nadelson *et al.*, 1984). For mothers, commitment to being either a full-time homemaker or a dual-role working mother is required. Associated with changes in role definition and identity differentiation and as a result of generalized erosion of spousal emotional attachment, significant adjustment problems occur for many couples during this stage of marriage.

CHILDBEARING

In previous research over the past two decades, there have been two main propositions regarding the advent of parenthood: (a) the transition from couple to family causes a "crisis," and (b) children cause a decrease in marital satisfaction. There still exists some debate as to whether the transition to parenthood constitutes a kind of family life cycle crisis, with unpredictable course and outcome (e.g., Berman & Lief, 1975; Carter & McGoldrick, 1988a; Combrinck-Graham, 1985; Hoffman, 1988). Alternatively, family structure may evolve both predictably and unpredictably, depending on the introduction of unplanned influences, such as a death in the family, loss of a job, seriously ill child, and so forth (Kovacs, 1988; Wynne, 1984). The divergence of opinion (and some data) on this issue may be accounted for by the fact that "crises" and unpredictability are characteristic of clinical populations, whereas relatively minor adjustments and predictable stages of transition are associated with nonclinical (so-called "normal") families (Lewis, 1988b).

Some recent findings relevant to the crisis-in-transition issue are found in the well-described longitudinal study of 40 prenatal couples who were in the second trimester of their first pregnancies (Lewis, 1988a, b; Lewis, Owen, & Cox, 1988). A rather sophisticated measure of *marital competence* was obtained on four occasions based on personal interviews, home observations of marital and family interaction, and paper-and-pencil inventories. The families were assessed during the second trimester, at birth, at 3 months, and 1 year postpartum. Results indicated that at 1 year postpartum, 58% of the couples remained at the same levels of marital competence demonstrated prenatally. However, 37% showed deterioration, whereas two couples (5%) improved. Highly competent couples were the most likely to remain unchanged by the introduction of the child, and relative to the more dysfunctional couples, they were also more apt to show interest, warmth, and sensitivity while interacting with their children. This study lends important support to Wynne's (1984) notion of epigenesis; that is, successful completion of a given stage of family development is related to the completion of tasks in the prior stage. The results also challenge the view that most families experience unpredictable crises related to this transition. Developmental predictability during this particular transition may depend on the couple's levels of personal adjustment and marital competence before the birth of the child (Lewis, 1988a, b).

The second and related issue in this area concerns the relationship between the presence or absence of children and level of marital satisfaction. Most recent longitudinal research, though not conclusive, and usually conducted on nonclinical samples, strongly suggests that most couples experience a decline in marital satisfaction soon after the 1- to 3-month period of excitement associated with the birth (Belsky, Spanier, & Rovine, 1983; Cox, 1985; Lewis, 1988b). Based on these studies, it also appears that any major difficulties during this time impact greatest on the wife/mother (Belsky *et al.*, 1983; Gove & Peterson, 1980; Grossman, Eichler, & Winickoff, 1980). However, if the wife experiences happiness and support in her marriage, she appears to be extremely adaptable to stressors associated with the transition to parenthood.

Additional information that bears on children and marital satisfaction comes from the few studies that compare adjustment levels of childless versus child-rearing couples. Early in the marriage at least, childless couples score somewhat higher on general marital satisfaction measures (Glenn & McLanahan, 1982; Houseknecht, 1979). Also, childless couples are more likely to have stimulating conversations and to engage in outside interests together (Houseknecht, 1979). In contrast, young parents are more likely to be dissatisfied with finances and with the division of labor (White, Booth, & Edwards, 1986). The group differences found in these investigations appear to increase as each additional child is brought into the family. Interestingly, Gove and Peterson (1980) review this literature and suggest that certain adjustment differences found early on which favor childless over child-rearing couples seem to be reversed after about 7 years of marriage.

WORKING WIVES AND MOTHERS

The period between the transition to parenthood and the midlife adolescence stages of the marital life cycle presents the option, and increasingly the necessity, for wives and mothers to work. Potential benefits of working include diversified sources of self-esteem, independence, money, and decision-making power relative to the husband. The costs are that women will be paid, trained, and promoted less frequently. Also, women may be burdened by the dual roles of employee and homemaker or criticized by their husbands for working (Gove & Peterson, 1980; Hoffman, 1974a; Romer, 1981). The impact on the marriage and family of working mothers is variable. Trying to determine the motivations of women who work and those who do not severely complicates this area of research. In decades past, it was believed that most women who worked did so to increase family income (Gove & Peterson, 1980; Romer, 1981). More recently, with greater access to employment, many more women also are working for personal (i.e., nonfinancial) reasons and are pursuing career objectives (McGoldrick, 1988).

Overall, full-time housewives seem to be more prone to poor self-esteem, feelings of incompetence, alcohol and drug abuse, and marital dissatisfaction than working wives (Romer, 1981). However, full-time housewives who do not want to work seem better adjusted than working wives, who seem better adjusted than housewives who want to work but cannot (Gove & Peterson, 1980). Within the group of working mothers, those with preschool children have a more difficult challenge and generally experience lower marital satisfaction than those with children in school or out of the home. However, if working mothers want to work, obtain satisfaction from their jobs, do not regret leaving the children, receive emotional and administrative support from their husbands, and can make satisfactory child care arrangements, then they *and the children* seem to adjust fairly well (Gove & Peterson, 1980; Hoffman, 1974b; Romer, 1981).

In summary, children do affect level of marital satisfaction in a fairly predictable way. However, the effect is relatively minor for couples who function well before the birth of the child and seems fairly limited to the preschool years. The burden of child rearing is felt most by the mother (and especially the working mother); yet, emotional support from the husband is a critical variable in her and the family's overall adjustment. Having children and making work commitments serve to distance and differentiate husband and wife relative to the idealistic new couple stage. How these formative adjustments are made constitute a classic struggle during this time of marriage.

POWER STRUGGLES

Several developments contribute to the notorious "7-year itch," a time in marriage when the divorce rate is second only to the first 2 years (Kovacs, 1988). Marital problems are reported to be at their peak (Levinson, 1977); early child-rearing responsibilities (White *et al.*, 1986) and males' requirement and devotion to work tend to exacerbate the inequalities associated with traditional sex roles. Mothers who work tend to exercise their independence and assertiveness in decision making (Gove & Peterson, 1980), whether they resent the burden of multiple role responsibilities (Carter & McGoldrick, 1988a). Family boundaries must expand, not only to incorporate the child, but also to reintroduce the new grandparents into a more active (sometimes intrusive) role. In addition, the age of 30 transition for the individual is known to be one of high energy, perceived power and control, and heightened desire for self-expression and independence. There-fore, there is a significant potential for power struggles between partners (Berman & Lief, 1975; Campbell, 1980; Kovacs, 1988; Levinson, 1977).

Couples who meet this developmental challenge most effectively must work continually toward commitment, caring, communication, conflict resolution, and intimacy (Nichols, 1988; Wynne, 1984). They have to confront together the tasks of starting a family and making commitments to work and homelife. Divisions of labor have to be identified and negotiated. Marital satisfaction will probably decline somewhat, and marital boundaries have to be expanded as the relationship is reorganized to include children, grandparents, and to accommodate differentiat-ing personal growth.

Couples who fail during the transition to parenthood stage seem to take one of two paths: They struggle overtly and aggressively to determine who is in charge; they may not be able to resolve individual differences well enough to maintain the marriage (Nichols, 1988). Alternatively, many partners begin to drift apart gradu-ally over the years, covertly developing in their disparate ways (Monte, 1989; Nichols, 1988). Family members who break up at this stage constitute the increas-ing numbers of remarried adults and stepparented or single-parented children in our country. Couples who persevere in an unsatisfactory marriage, perhaps "for the sake of the children," join the many relatively satisfied and fewer very satisfied couples who enter the midlife adolescence stage of the marital life cycle.

Stage III: Midlife Adolescence

The third stage of the marital life cycle is called midlife adolescence, taken after Monte's (1989) fifth stage (Table 1). Although the word *adolescence* suggests appropriately that the nuclear family is coping with adolescents, in Monte's model the term actually refers to the adults' level of development. The midlife adolescence stage is the period between when the first child reaches adolescence and the last child leaves home. Obviously this is a highly variable period for individual families. However, the majority of couples are between their mid-30s and early 50s, having been married between 15 to 30 years. As appropriate, the various titles of the life cycle stages in Table 1 suggest the nature of the challenges and tasks during this time frame. Ironically, the classic struggles of the adolescent are rather stressfully revisited by the midlife couple as well, for example, trying to find one's identity, trying to fully differentiate from, but not destroy parental relationships, trying to define one's sexuality, and trying to determine and pursue one's life work.

MIDLIFE IDENTITY CRISIS

Somewhere in the early 40s, men are likely to encounter a "midlife crisis" (Berman & Lief, 1975; Levinson, 1977, 1986). It is as though mortality dawns on them (Nadelson *et al.*, 1984). Perhaps working for over two decades has gotten them nowhere (Romer, 1981); the better part of life is behind them; there is more uncertainty ahead than optimism. At best their marriage and sex life are all too familiar; at worst they are boring or conflict-ridden (Kovacs, 1988; Monte, 1989; Nichols, 1988). Men's minds and bodies are growing perceptively older, slower, and less capable of the performance they expect (Monte, 1989). In a family context where the adolescents are rebelling against authority, acting out behaviorally, and preparing to leave, many men do the same, and sometimes they leave rather impulsively. In the *early* part of this stage some men are more unhappy and confused than ever before in their lives.

For women, the *early* part of this stage also can be very stressful. Mothers, perhaps dangerously, have established overly strong ties of intimacy with the children instead of or to compensate for, a gradually deteriorating relationship with the husband (Carter & McGoldrick, 1988a). This arrangement is doomed to failure if the husband is neglectful of, or otherwise withdraws from the marriage because the children, during adolescence, make it their business to distance themselves from even the most loving parents. This is the most difficult stage in parenting (Nichols, 1988). Any failure of the marital pair to maintain the marital bond and to cooperate and communicate fully about raising the adolescents will tend to be magnified as a burden on the wife and mother. She, too, may be forced to reevaluate the meaning of her life. In distressed relationships, this distancing process between husband and wife may have been going on for years, or it may be a relatively new cause for open conflict and resentment. During this stage, talk of separation and divorce tends to increase (Kovacs, 1988). In the wake of relating to distant husbands and exiting adolescents, women confront an identity crisis that must be resolved.

REDEFINITION, REORGANIZATION, AND STABILITY

As suggested, most of this time period is characterized by self-examination, attempting to maximize personal goals in the context of diverging marital and family relationships, and to be sure, dealing with the collision of children's adolescence and parents' midlife adolescence (Monte, 1989). The goals of this stage include (a) achieving a sufficient degree of personal separateness and independence and *simultaneously* reconnecting with one's mate, (b) managing the challenges of rearing adolescent children and making personal midlife adjustments, using effective communication, negotiation, and conflict resolution skills, and (c) consciously choosing the marital relationship as a way of life (Kovacs, 1988; Monte, 1989; Nichols, 1988).

One very interesting reorganizational phenomenon associated with the latter part of the midlife adolescence stage is the role reversals that many husbands and wives first begin to experience. Grunebaum (1979) and Romer (1981) found that middle-aged men begin to shift their focus from work and instrumental effectiveness to affiliation needs (i.e., closer ties with wife, children, extended family, friends, and coworkers). In contrast, middle-aged women, relatively free of child rearing demands, often shift focus from affiliation and nurturance to rejoining the workforce and to experiencing a more independent, assertive, task-oriented side of their personalities. A similar role reversal is known to occur in the sexuality arena (Romer, 1981). Women may become more interested in sex; men may express relatively less interest in sex. Once again, the onus is on open and effective marital communication to identify and resolve these relative shifts in personalities and sexual desires.

At some point in the midlife adolescence stage, couples who survive intact reach accommodation to these changing goals and interests. Campbell (1980) calls this the stage of *stability*; Kovacs (1988) calls it *working through* (Table 1). In Campbell's model, stability is characterized by spouses having progressed through the romance and power struggle stages to a point of finally *accepting* the relationship with all its benefits and drawbacks. Conflict patterns become more familiar, more predictable, more comfortable, less threatening, and less catastrophic. Individuals have seemingly progressed through the midlife transitions of a reevaluation of self and marriage, a redefinition of relationship boundaries, goals, and realistic expectations, and a mutual couple reorganization of central issues and priorities. The foundation is now laid for the newest stage of the marital life cycle.

Stage IV: The Postparental Stage

The postparental stage begins when the last child leaves home and ends when wife and/or husband retires. If the couple has children late in life (or a belated exit of adult children), this stage may last as little as a few months. More typically, the postparental stage can last for 15 to 20 years, which is a relatively new phenomenon of the last half of the twentieth century (Deutscher, 1964; Nichols, 1988). As the reader may have come to suspect, the literature also suggests some confusion concerning what really happens to couples who survive to reach this stage of development.

THE EMPTY NEST SYNDROME

Earlier literature and considerable folklore suggest that the so-called *empty nest* transition causes severe strain on couples (cf. Deutscher, 1964; Kerckhoff, 1976). Difficulties may be caused by (a) women and many men (Duvall, 1985) going through the climacteric, (b) many men still encountering their midlife crisis (between the ages of 40–65), (c) mothers having overly invested in children to the detriment of the marital bond, (d) a physiological and psychological loss of sexual interest and performance (in men especially), (e) many couples having developed such rigid personalities and sex-role structures that they cannot negotiate diverging interests and role changes (Monte, 1989; Nadelson *et al.*, 1984; Sinnott, 1977), and (f) the inattention to and gradual deterioration in marital competence and quality over the years such that the relationship becomes totally "devitalized" (Cuber & Haroff, 1965). Such reasons for postparental adjustment problems seem powerful, indeed.

However, most studies (Duvall, 1985) have failed to support either greater personal or marital dissatisfaction in menopausal versus premenopausal women (Neugarten, 1970) or in postparental versus parental couples of the same age (Glenn, 1975; Kerckhoff, 1976; Le Shan, 1973, Neugarten, 1970). On the contrary, there is strong if not conclusive evidence that marital satisfaction follows a curvilinear trend over the marital life cycle, with the highest level occurring in the new couple stage, lower levels in Stages II and III, and a rebound to the second highest level overall in the postparental stage (Miller, 1976; Rollins & Cannon, 1974; Spanier, Lewis, & Cole, 1975). Thus it does not appear that the empty nest transition has any lasting negative impact.

Several investigators describe the positive potential of the postparental stage as one of renewed and deepened commitment. Spouses finally understand and accept their differences, and devote their energies to companionship and caring (Campbell, 1980; Kovacs, 1988; Monte, 1989; Neugarten, 1970). There are significant losses experienced during this period: of children leaving the home; of dying parents, relations, and friends; and of one's former mental and physical prowess. Such losses serve to close the marital boundary so that spouses, who now have become the "oldest generation," have increased appreciation of and reliance on one another (Monte, 1989; Nichols, 1988).

A number of developmental tasks confront couples who desire to achieve and maintain personal and marital satisfaction. Examples of wives' tasks include adjust to the drastically changed role of mother (Duvall, 1985), prepare for the loss of husband (Kovacs, 1988; Neugarten, 1970), coordinate or provide care for any remaining aged parents (Duvall, 1985), and maintain or develop an avocational or vocational outlet for time diverted from motherhood (Duvall, 1985; Nadelson *et al.*, 1984; Neugarten, 1970). For men, one possible unique task is to adjust to a relative plateau in career achievements, satisfaction, and remuneration (Duvall, 1985; Kerckhoff, 1976; McCullough & Rutenberg, 1988; Neugarten, 1970). Tasks for both partners include maintaining emotional well-being and physical health in the face of general mental and physiological decline (Duvall, 1985; Neugarten, 1970), developing new personal and couple leisure activities (Duvall, 1985), planning for financial security in anticipation of retirement (Duvall, 1985; Kovacs, 1988; Monte, 1989), and developing adult and grandparental relationships with grown children and their families (McCullough & Rutenberg, 1988). Most couples manage to accomplish these tasks adequately, with fair satisfaction (Deutscher, 1964; Duvall, 1985; Monte, 1989; Nadelson *et al.*, 1984).

SEX-ROLE REVERSAL

As discussed previously, the later life phenomenon of sex-role reversal may begin in the midlife adolescence stage; typically, however, the phenomenon becomes more pronounced in the postparental stage. It is an accepted proposition that women are predisposed biologically and culturally to take on the socioemotional, nurturing, affectionate, and domestic roles in marriage and family. In contrast, men are expected to take on the instrumental roles of provider, problem solver, and protector from the outside world. Curiously, as people grow older, particularly after the children leave home, and again after retirement, there is a distinct tendency for these traditional sex roles to shift. As McGoldrick (1988) points out, men and women seem to be moving in opposite directions psychologically. Women often make the most abrupt change, jolted into awareness by children's leaving, that after years of nurturing they now can venture out of the home for personal gratification of unmet needs. Although some women struggle with this transition (Hesse-Biber & Williamson, 1984), most find the new opportunities for work, avocation, and outside friends energizing, exciting, and confidence building (McGoldrick, 1988). Many of these wives become more assertive, sexually active, and from their husbands' perspectives, even domineering in their decision-making preferences (Dressler, 1973; Hesse-Biber & Williamson, 1984). At the same time, after over three decades of investment in the working world and prompted by the loss of their children from the home (Duvall, 1985; McGoldrick, 1988), men turn inward to focus on the family. Older men tend to become less aggressive, less sexual, less ambitious, and more interested in interpersonal relationships (Duvall, 1985; McGoldrick, 1988; Nadelson et al., 1984).

For most couples, these various personality changes and lifestyle adjustments are accepted or tolerated and may even be a source of renewal and mutual sharing. However, for some couples these changes can be quite troublesome. They have not prepared well enough for this stage of development by acquiring adequate communication, problem-solving, and relationship-nurturing skills (Kovacs, 1988; Nichols, 1988; Wynne, 1984). For a variety of reasons, many spouses also exhibit personality or character structures, or conditioned marital interaction patterns that are so rigid that they cannot make the necessary changes to accommodate the required age-related and stage-related adjustments (Kerckhoff, 1976; Monte, 1989; Nadelson et al., 1984). In fact, there is increasing evidence that older couples who are more cooperative and flexible in daily tasks and who manifest *convergent* as opposed to *traditional* sex-role attitudes and behaviors are more likely to be personally and maritally satisfied (Baucom & Aiken, 1984; Romer, 1981; Sinnott, 1977).

In summary, most recent research indicates that the postparental stage is relatively positive for most couples. Marital satisfaction improves relative to the previous two stages. The departure of children, though difficult for some overly invested parents, is greeted by women especially as liberating—ushering in opportunities for personal growth and marital enrichment. At the same time, physiological and psychological changes associated with aging are cause for sobering reflection and active planning for the culmination of one's life.

Stage V: Culmination

Fortunately, most couples who reach the final stage of the marital life cycle have learned to be rather good partners. The culmination stage is defined as that period of marriage between retirement and the death of one spouse. It may last a few weeks, months, or from 10 to 15 years and more. According to norms for our average, white, middle-class, married couple, (Romer, 1981), the husband typically lives for a few years after retirement (age 69); his wife typically lives for over a decade after retirement (age 76.5). They will have been married 40 to 50 years.

The culmination stage is at the same time a relatively new and the least studied stage of the marital life cycle (Flori, 1989). Earlier research on marital satisfaction suggested a gradual decline over the entire marital life cycle (e.g., Blood & Wolfe, 1960; Luckey, 1966). More recently, the majority of studies suggest an increase in marital satisfaction following the child-rearing years. Focusing on three later life age groups, Gilford (1984) studied marital satisfaction among these age groups: 55–62, 63–69, and 70–90. Social, personal, and marital adjustment measures were obtained on 318 married individuals. The results indicated that marital satisfaction was highest in the group of 63- to 69-year-old subjects and significantly lower in the two adjacent age groups. Gilford (1984) attributed these differences to the significant adjustments required of couples and families in the midlife child-rearing years (see Stage III), to the relative stability and new opportunities of the postparental and immediately postretirement years (Stage IV), and to the typical decline of health, resources, and vitality of the latest years (Stage V). Thus for many couples who live to a "ripe old age" together, marital satisfaction may decline slightly relative to the early postretirement years (Gilford, 1984). This important study needs to be replicated. Nevertheless, most couples who reach the culmination stage generally experience a solid companionship, an increased interdependence and need for mutual support, and a relative contentment with one another (Dressler, 1973; Lee, 1988; Monte, 1989; Nadelson et al., 1984; Romer, 1981; Walsh, 1988).

The major tasks of this stage concern adjusting to retirement and preparing for the loss of one's spouse. Retirement brings on major adjustments in both the practical and psychological aspects of the relationship. Daily living is a central focus (Monte, 1989), and each day may become savored or resented depending on two key factors: health and relationship quality. In fact, health and vigor may be better determinants of personal satisfaction than chronological age (Romer, 1981; Streib & Beck, 1980). Most couples also must adjust to a drastic reduction in income (Kovacs, 1988; Romer, 1981), and many choose relocation into another home and community (Duvall, 1985; Walsh, 1988). Men may have the most difficult task in dealing with retirement because they typically are giving up their primary occupation and important relationships in which they invested many years (Romer, 1981; Walsh, 1988).

On the other hand, retirement also can be stressful for the woman. A major transition is the successful incorporation of the husband into the household (Dressler, 1973; Duvall, 1985; Romer, 1981; Walsh, 1988). This task presents a problem when a couple has established a rigid traditional sex-role marriage: working husband and housekeeper/mother (or the formerly working wife has retired). When the husband retires, having lost his occupation as a major source of power, control, and self-esteem, he may take over wife's domestic tasks. In deference, when she withdraws and becomes depressed, he takes over even more to "relieve her burden," and she (her role) is rejected even more. Should she assert herself, he becomes resentful and withdraws because now he has no productive role. Suicide and depression rates increase for males during this stage (Romer, 1981). Therefore, as discussed relative to the postparental stage, couples who do not communicate and negotiate well and who cannot be flexible in sex-role assignments (especially after retirement) do poorly in personal and marital adjustment (Duvall, 1985; Nadelson et al., 1984; Romer, 1981; Walsh, 1988).

Retirement is one of the most significant changes for a couple during the entire course of the marriage. If couples have developed effective communication, decision-making, and problem-solving skills and have worked through such issues as finances, sexual preferences, relating to children, family, inlaws, and household tasks, then retirement will be pleasurable. If they have not, retirement can turn into a despairing disaster quickly. Fears of desertion, loneliness, poor health, sexual failure, survival, and death can stir up issues of control and dominance (Berman & Lief, 1975). Some elderly spouses complain that their partners become more rigid, resentful, hostile, and angry with age (Duvall, 1985; Monte, 1989; Nadelson *et al.*, 1984). Surprisingly, other golden anniversary couples remain very flexible and adaptive to changes within and around them (Neugarten, 1975).

In summary, the years of culmination from retirement to death of a spouse are relatively satisfactory and compatible for most couples. Although far too many couples face poverty, isolation, chronic illness, and psychological distress, married individuals do relatively better than their separated, divorced, and widowed counterparts (Carter & McGoldrick, 1988a). Couples who make it this far are certainly a rare and understudied minority. However, there are some wonderful vigorous elderly couples in our country who should be models of the best that marriage has to offer: lifelong, intimate friendship (Neugarten, 1975).

The Changing Family Life Cycle

Of considerable import, the five stages of the marital life cycle described apply to many of us, but *conceivably*, many aspects of these developmental stages do not apply to most family units in society today. Having occurred within one generation, some rather dramatic changes must be highlighted as we look to the future of marriage. World economics, political developments, social movements, and medical/technical advancements—all these forces have contributed to recent development of the American family. For example, our inability to compete as well with other industrialized nations has meant a rapid drop in Americans' standard of living (Thurow, 1987). In an attempt to maintain a middle-class standard of living, most wives and mothers have joined the workforce. The women's movement has been effective in pursuing social and economic equality of the sexes. However, thus far the major gains have been made in the consciousness raising, psychological sphere. Women's increased pursuit of equality has, in the short run, had a disruptive impact on contemporary marriage (Gurman & Klein, 1980; McGoldrick, 1988). Women who are better educated, employed, or career-oriented are most apt to never marry or to remain single once divorced (Glick & Lin, 1986; Norton & Moorman, 1987). Finally, given birth control advancements and societal health improvements, women have been able to remain childless or limit birthrate and to outlive the child-rearing period long enough to embark on independent careers. Therefore, to the extent that companionship and marital happiness become the primary criteria for remaining in a relationship, the divorce rate is likely to remain as distressingly high as it is.

Given that the majority of first *and second* marriages end in divorce, the changing family life cycle must account for the projection that by 1990, 50% of the children in our country are expected to live with a stepparent and/or single parent for some time before age 18 (Brown, 1988). The investigation of remarried or blended families is relatively new to the field. Several writers have begun to describe the similar and unique interaction processes and developmental tasks of remarried families (e.g., Glick & Lin, 1986; Kleinman, Rosenberg, & Whiteside, 1979; McGoldrick & Carter, 1988; Peek, Bell, Waldren, & Sorell, 1988; Whiteside, 1982). For families in which divorce occurs, 35% of the women do not remarry (Brown, 1988), and this event adds one phase to the "normal" life cycle (divorce and restabilization). Sixty-five percent of women remarry and two additional family life cycle stages have been proposed: divorce and remarriage (McGoldrick & Carter, 1988). Needless to say, these adjustments are very difficult for all concerned. However, there is no indication that our worldwide high divorce and remarriage rates will change anytime soon (Glick & Lin, 1986). Although the future of marriage as an institution seems assured, the number of marriages per adult and the complex adjustments and transitions required of families and society are less predictable.

THERAPEUTIC CONSIDERATIONS

During the past decade, in particular, more attention has been directed to integrating the broad-scale family sociology and the family systems clinical literatures (see Carter & McGoldrick, 1980, 1988b). In addition, more attention has been paid to the investigation of the normal functional family (e.g., Glick & Kessler, 1980; L'Abate, 1985) in order to gain a better perspective on the well-studied dysfunctional family.

Therapeutic considerations relevant to the marital life cycle are important. Marital therapists must not overlook clients' stage-related tasks and potential individual and couple stressors. One could always pursue a development-oriented answer to the question, "Why now?" is this couple seeking therapy. Why are they in the office now rather than 5 years ago or 5 years from now? Often, the answer is related to a life cycle transition or stressor (Barnhill & Longs, 1978; Berman & Lief, 1975; Birchler & Gershwin, 1991; Glick & Kessler, 1980; Hoffman, 1988).

Marital and family therapists have proposed a number of important variables to account for the development and maintenance of a satisfactory marriage. For example, Weiss (1980), Jacobson and Margolin (1979), and Birchler (1983) have stressed the importance of communication and problem-solving skills. Wynne (1984) underscores the importance of attachment/caregiving, communicating, joint problem solving, and mutuality. Nichols (1988) espouses commitment, caring, communication, and conflict/compromise. Berman and Lief (1975) emphasize the resolution of power, intimacy, and inclusion–exclusion issues. Monte (1989) stresses the importance of identity, differentiation, commitment, trust, power, and competence. Kovacs (1988) highlights the paradoxical dynamics of autonomy/belongingness, separateness/connectedness, dependence/independence, and closeness/distance/privacy. Lewis (1986) stresses the importance of commitment, allocation of power, and the balance of separateness and attachment. Obviously, there are many other related tasks and processes (e.g., decision making, sex-role assignments, patterns of affection and sexuality, cohesion, parenting roles). The point is, maritally distressed couples will be better served if therapists carefully assess these areas of interaction and development.

Another important therapeutic consideration is the gender issue. As Hare-Mustin (1987) points out, gender bias in family therapy is often an unintended, subtle process influenced by the larger values in society and by values incorporated into certain therapeutic orientations. Bernard (1972) is often credited with raising the consciousness of many by documenting a number of reasons why the *traditional marriage*, at least, is good for men and bad for women. Since then, a fairly extensive literature has developed, substantiating that, although men have their own problems and adjustments to make throughout life, the institution of marriage serves them fairly well (e.g., Schafer & Keith, 1981). In contrast, for women, many aspects of the traditional marriage appear to be depressive and detrimental, if not oppressive (Gurman & Klein, 1980; Hesse-Biber & Williamson, 1984; McGoldrick, 1988; Whisman & Jacobson, 1989). Equality and egalitarian therapeutic principles are laudable concepts. However, effectively assuring that women and men have equal opportunities for work, education, decision making, self-expression, activities apart from children and away from home, and sharing the burdens of work, parenting, and household tasks, and the like is a major challenge for couples and an important responsibility for therapists (Hare-Mustin, 1987; McGoldrick, 1988).

RESEARCH CONSIDERATIONS

Current Problems

Despite the existence of a rather rich clinical literature based on the marital and family life cycle schema, there has been considerable difficulty establishing empirical support for these models. There is continuing debate concerning their utility (Hudson & Murphy, 1980; Spanier, Sauer, & Larzelere, 1979). Briefly, the problems with research in this area have included (a) the number of, and definitions of, the life cycle stages of development; (b) the relevance of these stages to contemporary family units; (c) the validity, reliability, and comparability of the dependent variables (e.g., measures of marital satisfaction, marital quality); (d) the frequently negligible or small amount of variance associated with dependent variables and life cycle stages; and (e) the inherent methodological dilemma associated with sampling methods used to investigate marital phenomena that span a 50-year period of time.

First, as implied in Table 1, the comparability, starting, and stopping points of given stages are nearly impossible to determine. For example, even limited to one model, determination of when the last child leaves home is very difficult. These days some adult children return to live at home several times before the final break (Berger & Berger, 1985).

Second, the "goodness of fit" problem of the traditional marital or family life cycle schema has already been mentioned. Nuclear families no longer comprise the majority of family units in this country. Thus findings from even the best studies of the "normal" marital or family life cycle do not generalize well to family households headed by single parents, divorced, remarried, and widowed adults.

Third, the definitions of marital satisfaction, marital happiness, marital adjustment, and marital stability have long been problematic in this field (Barry, 1970; Hicks & Platt, 1970). During the 1970s, the concept of *marital quality* gained prominence, in recognition of the fact that the quality of marriage involves multidimensional phenomena: adjustment, communication, happiness, integration, and satisfaction (Spanier & Lewis, 1980). However, even this more comprehensive measure has been criticized as being dependent on *subjective* evaluations by *individuals* in the marriage (Anderson, Russell, & Schumm, 1983).

Fourth, most investigations have failed to attribute much variance in marital satisfaction or marital quality measures specifically to life cycle stages. Moreover, in a number of empirical studies, it has been demonstrated that such variables as length of marriage, the presence or absence of children, and subjects' age account for certain findings as well as or better than stage of family life cycle (Gilford & Bengtson, 1977; Miller, 1976; Nock, 1979; Spanier *et al.*, 1979). Related to these problems and the basic inadequacy of statistical analyses, Hudson and Murphy (1980) went so far as to conclude that the family life cycle concept has little utility for future research. Subsequent research has retained the family life cycle stage stratification scheme. However, these efforts have yet to account for more than 8% to 9% of the variance in marital satisfaction as a function of family life cycle categories (Anderson *et al.*, 1983; Schumm & Bugaighis, 1986).

Finally, there is no single method of studying marital satisfaction over the life cycle that does not have an inherent problem. Retrospective surveys of older married people are vulnerable to inaccurate recollections of the respondents. Longitudinal studies, though preferred but few in number, confound life cycle stages with the age of the subjects, the effects of aging *per se*, and changes in society over time. Cross-sectional studies, the most prevalent, confound the results with length of marriage, age, and cohort membership. Because there is no perfect method, investigators should work toward standardizing their instruments, independent and dependent variables, and employ a variety of methods to gather converging data on the important questions.

Future Directions

Research on the marital life cycle is in its own early developmental stages. As suggested by Spanier and Lewis (1980), some improvements in research methodology are evident. More studies have included men, and more importantly, husbands and wives in the same relationship. More attention has been given to psychometric properties of various measures of marital quality. Sample sizes have increased, and multivariate statistics and sophisticated research designs have been employed more frequently. More attention has been directed to nontraditional family structures and to gender issues. However, research in this area is very complex and much remains to be done.

Perhaps the best strategy for the future would be to accumulate multiple studies and employ transition period longitudinal, multimethod, multivariate designs that span known transitions in the marital life cycle. The transition to parenthood research project discussed earlier is a good example (Lewis, 1988a,b; Lewis *et al.*, 1988). Another example of a transition period longitudinal approach to marital life cycle research is the innovative work of Markman (1979, 1981, 1984). The basic objectives were to identify developmental, interaction-based, modifiable, behavioral, or cognitive antecedents of future marital dysfunction. Accordingly, 26 engaged couples completed a marital satisfaction inventory and participated in several laboratory interactions designed to assess positive and negative communication patterns. Laboratory observational measures were repeated at 1 year and 2.5 years; marital satisfaction and relationship status also were assessed at 5.5 years follow-up. Outcome measures were marital satisfaction (if still together) and relationship status (never got married, still married, divorced). Results indicated that certain negative communication behaviors that preceded marriage significantly predicted relationship satisfaction 2.5 and 5.5 years later. Interestingly, the best predictor of relationship stability (5.5 years later) was the couple's confidence that they would get married. An interactional measure of give-and-take in the laboratory discussion was the second best predictor.

Results from Markman's earlier work and related studies have now been incorporated into a premarital intervention program designed to teach engaged couples effective communication and problem-solving skills (Markman et al., 1988). Compared to a nonintervention control group, at 3 years follow-up, the treated couples had higher levels of marital and sexual satisfaction and lower levels of problem intensity. Moreover, the dissolution rate was 24% for the control couples, compared to 5% for the treated couples. As an example of quality research methods applied to the marital life cycle, this study suggests that premarital intervention using a cognitive-behavioral treatment program can serve to prevent the decline in marital satisfaction that has been observed in early marriage (Spanier et al., 1975).

Finally, Markman (1984) and others (Carter & McGoldrick, 1988a) emphasize the significant impact on couples and families of external variables and the need for more and better research to understand their influence. These powerful variables have tremendous importance in determining the quality of individual, marital, and family life: separation, divorce, and remarriage; chronic illness, death of spouse or other family members; mental illness, drug and alcohol problems; ethnic and cultural factors; and other social factors such as sex-role changes, employment patterns of women, changing economy, and war. These variables must be accounted for in both clinical and research endeavors if the concepts of the marital and family life cycles are to be useful and fully understood.

SUMMARY

For approximately two-thirds of men's lives and three-fifths of women's lives, the quality of one's marital relationship is a critical factor in one's satisfaction with life. Determinants of marital satisfaction are complex and difficult to specify, but no doubt include (a) our expectations of marriage based on what we learned in our families of origin; (b) our individual biological and learned predispositions for thinking, feeling, and behaving; (c) our choice of mates; (d) our efforts to realize expectations for marriage in interaction with our mates; (e) our experiences with extramarital society via work, outside relationships, extended family, and various social and economic factors; (f) our relative acquisition of communication and problem-solving skills to maintain and improve interpersonal relationships, and (g) our abilities to cope with stresses, strains, illnesses, and various transitions and losses associated with the marital and family life cycles.

Five stages of the marital life cycle were discussed, including somewhat different tasks and struggles typical for each stage. Each stage has the potential for mature growth, development, and certain relationship satisfactions. At the same time, each stage is vulnerable to individual, marital, and societal developments that lead many couples to dissolve their marriages. Marital satisfaction is believed to be at its highest level in the new couple stage; however, the divorce rate is also highest during this period. With the advent of children, and during the following decade or so of child rearing, marital satisfaction is believed to decline. There may or may not be a gradual rise in marital satisfaction during children's teenage years, depending upon some dangerous transitions to be made in the midlife-adolescence stage. The level of marital satisfaction then reaches its second highest level during the postparental stage and early retirement years, with a possible slight decline for elderly couples in their 70s and 80s.

There exists a relatively rich theoretical and descriptive literature on the marital life cycle, complemented by years of sociological and family investigations. However, much of the research has been flawed by various methodological problems; there are few well-controlled empirical studies of the marital life cycle. In addition, the rapidly changing nature of the family life cycle and the composition of household units in our country have made the study of the traditional American nuclear family an increasingly narrow focus.

Despite these issues, it is believed that the marital life cycle schema have merit. Conceptualizing stages and transitions in marital development helps us to organize our thinking and understanding of functional marriages. Important reference points also are established for understanding developmental aspects of dysfunctional marriages. In the future, the use of appropriate research methodologies can lead us to better understand the increasingly complex and often distressed marital life cycle through which over 90% of us will progress. Multivariate, multimethod, longitudinal studies designed to span important developmental transition points in marriage can help to point the way toward better prevention and remediation programs.

REFERENCES

Anderson, S. A., Russell, C. S., & Schumm, W. R. (1983). Perceived marital quality and family life-cycle categories: A further analysis. *Journal of Marriage and the Family, 45*, 127–139.

Bader, E., & Pearson, P. T. (1988). *In quest of the mythical mate*. New York: Brunner/Mazel.

Barnhill, L. R., & Longo, D. (1978). Fixation and regression in the family life cycle. *Family Process, 17*, 469–478.

Barry, W. A. (1970). Marriage research and conflict: An integrative review. *Psychological Bulletin, 73*, 41–54.

Baucom, D. H., & Aiken, P. A. (1984). Sex role identity, marital satisfaction, and response to behavioral marital therapy. *Journal of Consulting and Clinical Psychology, 52*, 132–142.

Belsky, J., Spanier, G. B., & Rovine, M. (1983). Stability and change in marriage across the transition to parenthood. *Journal of Marriage and the Family, 45*(3), 567–578.

Berger, M., & Berger, S. D. (1985). Individual and family life-span development. In L. L'Abate (Ed.), *The handbook of family psychology and therapy*, (Vol. I, pp. 143–176). Homewood: IL: Dorsey Press.

Berman, E. M., & Lief, H. I. (1975). Marital therapy from a psychiatric perspective: An overview. *American Journal of Psychiatry, 132*, 583–592.

Bernard, J. (1972). *The future of marriage*. New York: Bantam.

Birchler, G. R. (1983). Marital dysfunction. In M. Hersen (Ed.), *Practice of outpatient behavior therapy: A clinician's handbook* (pp. 229–271). New York: Grune & Stratton.

Birchler, G. R., & Gershwin, M. (1991). Marital dysfunction. In M. Thase, B. Edelstein, & M. Hersen (Eds.), *Handbook of outpatient treatment of adults* (pp. 463–488). New York: Plenum Press.

Blood, R. O., & Wolfe, D. M. (1960). *Husbands and wives: The dynamics of married living*. Glencoe, IL: Free Press.

Brown, F. H. (1988). The postdivorce family. In B. Carter & M. McGoldrick (Eds.), *The changing family life cycle* (2nd ed., pp. 371–401). New York: Gardner Press.

Campbell, S. (1980). *The couple's journey: Intimacy as a path to wholeness.* San Luis Obispo, CA: Impact Publishers.

Carter, B., & McGoldrick, M. (Eds.). (1980). *The family life cycle.* New York: Gardner Press.

Carter, B., & McGoldrick, M. (1988a). Overview: The changing family life cycle. In B. Carter & M. McGoldrick (Eds.), *The changing family life cycle* (2nd ed., pp. 3–28). New York: Gardner Press.

Carter, B., & McGoldrick, M. (1988b). *The changing family life cycle* (2nd ed.). New York: Gardner Press.

Combrinck-Graham, L. A. (1985). Developmental model for family systems. *Family Process, 24,* 139–150.

Cox, M. (1985). Progress and continued challenges in understanding transition to parenthood. *Journal of Family Issues, 6,* 395–408.

Cuber, J. F., & Haroff, P. B. (1965). *The significant Americans: A study of sexual behavior among the affluent.* New York: Appleton-Century-Croft.

Deutscher, I. (1964). The quality of post-parental life. *Journal of Marriage and the Family, 26,* 52–60.

Dressler, D. M. (1973). Life adjustment of retired couples. *International Journal of Aging and Human Development, 4*(4), 335–349.

Duvall, E. M. (1967). *Marriage & family development,* (3rd ed.). Philadelphia: Lippincott.

Duvall, E. M. (1985). *Marriage and family development* (6th ed.). Philadelphia: Lippincott.

Flori, D. E. (1989). The prevalance of later life family concerns in the marriage and family therapy journal literature (1976–1985): A content analysis. *Journal of Marital and Family Therapy, 15,* 289–297.

Fowers, B. J., & Olson, D. H. (1986). Predicting marital success with PREPARE: A predictive validity study. *Journal of Marital and Family Therapy, 12,* 403–413.

Gilford, R. (1984). Contrasts in marital satisfaction throughout old age: An exchange theory analysis. *Journal of Gerontology, 39,* 325–333.

Gilford, R., & Bengtson, V. (1979). Measuring marital satisfaction in three generations: Positive and negative dimensions. *Journal of Marriage and the Family, 41,* 387–398.

Glenn, N. D. (1975). Psychological well-being in the post-parental stage: Some evidence from national surveys. *Journal of Marriage and the Family, 37,* 105–110.

Glenn, N. D., & McLanahan, S. (1982). Children and marital happiness: A further specification of the relationship. *Journal of Marriage and the Family, 44,* 63–72.

Glick, P. A. (1975). A demographer looks at American families. *Journal of Marriage and the Family, 37*(1), 15–26.

Glick, P. (1984). How American families are changing. *American Demographics,* January, pp. 21–25.

Glick, I. D., & Kessler, D. R. (1980). *Marital and family therapy.* New York: Grune & Stratton.

Glick, P. C., & Lin, S. L. (1986). Recent changes in divorce and remarriage. *Journal of Marriage and the Family, 48*(4), 737–747.

Gottman, J. M., & Krokoff, L. J. (1989). Marital interaction and satisfaction: A longitudinal view. *Journal of Consulting and Clinical Psychology, 57*(1), 47–52.

Gove, W. R., & Peterson, C. (1980). An update of the literature on personal and marital adjustment: The effect of children and the employment of wives. *Marriage and Family Review, 3*(3/4), 63–96.

Grossman, F. K., Eichler, L. S., & Winickoff, S. A. (1980). *Pregnancy, birth, & parenthood.* San Francisco: Jossey-Bass.

Grunebaum, H. (1979). Middle age and marriage: Affiliative men and assertive women. *American Journal of Family Therapy, 7*(3), 46–50.

Gurman, A. S., & Klein, M. H. (1980). Marital and family conflicts. In A. M. Brodsky & R. T. Hare-Mustin (Eds.), *Women and psychotherapy: An assessment of research and practice* (pp. 159–188). New York: Guilford Press.

Haley, J. (1973). *Uncommon therapy: The psychiatric techniques of Milton H. Erickson.* New York: Norton.

Hare-Mustin, R. T. (1987). The problem of gender in family therapy. *Family Process, 26*(1), 15–27.

Hesse-Biber, S., & Williamson, J. (1984). Resource theory and power in families: Life cycle considerations. *Family Process, 23*(2), 261–278.

Hicks, M., & Platt, M. (1970). Marital happiness and stability: A review of the research in the 60s. *Journal of Marriage and the Family, 32,* 553–574.

Hoffman, L. (1988). The family life cycle and discontinuous change. In B. Carter & M. McGoldrick (Eds.), *The changing family life cycle* (2nd ed., pp. 91–106). New York: Gardner Press.

Hoffman, L. W. (1974a). Psychological factors. In L. W. Hoffman & F. I. Nye (eds.), *Working mothers.* San Francisco: Jossey-Bass.

Hoffman, L. W. (1974b). Effects on child. In L. W. Hoffman & F. I. Nye (Eds.), *Working mothers.* San Francisco: Jossey-Bass.

Hoffman, L. W. (1977). Changes in family roles, socialization, and sex differences. *American Psychologist, 32*, 644–657.

Houseknecht, S. K. (1979). Childlessness and marital adjustment. *Journal of Marriage and the Family, 41*, 259–265.

Hudson, W. W., & Murphy, G. J. (1980). The non-linear relationship between marital satisfaction and stages of the family life cycle: An artifact of Type I errors? *Journal of Marriage and the Family, 42*, 263–267.

Jacobson, N. S., & Margolin, G. (1979). *Marital therapy: Strategies based on social learning and behavior exchange principles.* New York: Brunner/Mazel.

Kerckhoff, R. K. (1976). Marriage and middle age. *The Family Coordinator, 25*, 5–11.

Kleinman, J., Rosenberg, E., & Whiteside, M. (1982). Common developmental tasks in forming reconstituted families. *Journal of Marital and Family Therapy, 5*, 79–86.

Kovacs, L. (1982). Development of the marital relationship (dissertation). Ann Arbor, MI: University Microfilms International.

Kovacs, L. (1988). Couple therapy: An integrated developmental and family system model. *Family Therapy, 15*, 133–155.

L'Abate, L. (Ed.). (1985). *The handbook of family psychology and theory, Vol. I.* Homeward, IL: Dorsey Press.

Larson, A. S., & Olson, D. H. (1989). Predicting marital satisfaction using PREPARE: A replication study. *Journal of Marital and Family Therapy, 15*(3), 311–322.

Lee, G. R. (1988). Marital satisfaction in later life: The effects of nonmarital roles. *Journal of Marriage and the Family, 50*, 775–783.

Le Shan, E. J. (1973). *The wonderful crisis of middle age.* New York: David McKay Company.

Levinson, D. J. (1977). The mid-life transition: A period of adult psychological development. *Psychiatry, 40*, 99–112.

Levinson, D. J. (1986). A conception of adult development. *American Psychologist, 41*, 3–13.

Lewis, J. M. (1986). Family structure and stress. *Family Process, 25*, 235–247.

Lewis, J. M. (1988a). The transition to parenthood: I. The rating of prenatal marital competence. *Family Process, 27*, 149–165.

Lewis, J. M. (1988b). The transition to parenthood: II. Stability and change in marital structure. *Family Process, 27*, 273–283.

Lewis, J. M., Owen, M. T., & Cox, M. J. (1988). The transition to parenthood: III. Incorporation of the child into the family. *Family Process, 27*, 411–421.

Locksley, A. (1980). On the effects of wives' employment on marital adjustment and companionship. *Journal of Marriage and the Family, 42*, 337–346.

Luckey, E. B. (1966). Number of years married as related to personality perception and marital satisfaction. *Journal of Marriage and the Family, 28*, 44–48.

Markman, H. J. (1979). The application of a behavioral model of marriage in predicting relationship satisfaction of couples planning marriage. *Journal of Consulting and Clinical Psychology, 4*, 743–749.

Markman, H. J. (1981). Prediction of marital distress: A 5-year follow-up. *Journal of Consulting and Clinical Psychology, 49*(5), 760–762.

Markman, H. J. (1984). The longitudinal study of couples' interactions. In K. Hahlweg & N. S. Jacobson (Eds.), *Marital interaction: Analysis and modification* (pp. 253–284). New York: Guilford Press.

Markman, H. J., Floyd, F. J., Stanley, S. M., & Storasli, R. D. (1988). Prevention of marital distress: A longitudinal investigation. *Journal of Consulting and Clinical Psychology, 56*(2), 210–217.

Martin, B. (1987). Developmental perspectives on family theory and psychotherapy. In T. Jacob (Ed.), *Family interaction and psychopathology* (pp. 163–202). New York: Plenum Press.

McCullough, P. G., & Rutenberg, S. K. (1988). Launching children and moving on. In B. Carter & M. McGoldrick (Eds.), *The changing family life cycle* (2nd ed., pp. 285–309). New York: Gardner Press.

McGoldrick, M. (1988). Women and the family life cycle. In B. Carter & M. McGoldrick (Eds.), *The changing family life cycle* (2nd ed., pp. 29–68). New York: Gardner Press.

McGoldrick, M., & Carter, B. (1988). Forming a remarried family. In B. Carter & M. McGoldrick (Eds.), *The changing family life cycle* (2nd ed., pp. 402–432). New York: Gardner Press.

Meyer, J. P., & Pepper, S. (1977). Need compatibility and marital adjustment in young married couples. *Journal of Personality and Social Psychology, 35*(5), 331–342.

Miller, B. C. (1976). A multivariate developmental model of marital satisfaction. *Journal of Marriage and the Family, 38*, 643–657.

Monte, E. P. (1989). The relationship life-cycle. In G. R. Weeks (Ed.), *Treating couples* (pp. 287–316). New York: Brunner/Mazel.

Mueller, C. W., & Pope, H. (1977). Marital instability: A study of its transmission between generations. *Journal of Marriage and the Family, 39*, 83–92.

Murstein, B. I. (1976). *Who will marry whom?* New York: Springer.

Nadelson, C., Polonsky, D. C., & Mathews, M. A. (1984). Marriage as a developmental process. In C. Nadelson & D. C. Polonsky (Eds.), *Marriage and divorce: A contemporary perspective* (pp. 127–141). New York: Guilford Press.

Neugarten, B. (1970). Dynamics of transition of middle to old age: Adaptation and the life cycle. *Journal of Geriatric Psychiatry, 4*, 71–87.

Neugarten, B. (1975). The future and the young old. *Gerontologist, 15*, 4–9.

Nichols, W. C. (1988). *Marital therapy.* New York: Guilford Press.

Nock, S. L. (1979). The family life cycle: Empirical or conceptual tool? *Journal of Marriage and the Family, 41*, 15–26.

Norton, A. J. (1983). Family life cycle: 1980. *Journal of Marriage and the Family, 45*(2), 267–275.

Norton, A. J., & Moorman, J. E. (1987). Current trends in marriage and divorce among American women. *Journal of Marriage and the Family, 49*(1), 3–14.

Olson, D. H., Fournier, D. G., & Druckman, J. M. (1987). *Counselor's manual for PREPARE/ENRICH* (rev. ed.). Minneapolis, PREPARE/ENRICH.

Peek, C. W., Bell, N. J., Waldren, T., & Sorell, G. T. (1988). Patterns of functioning in families of remarried and first-married couples. *Journal of Marriage and the Family, 50*, 699–708.

Rock, M. (1986). *The marriage map: Understanding and surviving the stages of marriage.* Atlanta: Peachtree Publishers.

Rodgers, R. (1960). *Proposed modifications of Duvall's family life cycle stages.* Paper presented at American Sociological Association, New York.

Rollins, B. C., & Cannon, K. L. (1974). Marital satisfaction over the family life cycle: A reevaluation. *Journal of Marriage and the Family, 36*, 271–282.

Romer, N. (1981). *The sex-role cycle: Socialization from infancy to old age.* New York: McGraw-Hill.

Ryder, R., Kafka, J., & Olson, D. H. (1971). Separating and joining. *American Journal of Orthopsychiatry, 2*, 450–464.

Schafer, R. B., & Keith, P. M. (1981). Equity in marital roles across the family life cycle. *Journal of Marriage and the Family, 43*(2), 359–367.

Schumm, W. R., & Bugaighis, M. A. (1986). Marital quality over the marital career: Alternative explanations. *Journal of Marriage and the Family, 48*, 165–168.

Sinnott, J. D. (1977). Sex-role inconstancy, biology, and successful aging: A dialectical model. *Gerontologist, 17*, 459–463.

Solomon, M. A. (1973). A developmental, conceptual premise for family therapy. *Family Process, 12*, 179–188.

Spanier, G. B., & Lewis, R. A. (1980). Marital quality: A review of the seventies. *Journal of Marriage and the Family, 42*, 825–839.

Spanier, G. B., Lewis, R. A., & Cole, C. L. (1975). Marital adjustment over the family life cycle: The issues of curvilinearity. *Journal of Marriage and the Family, 37*, 263–275.

Spanier, G. B., Sauer, W., & Larzelere, R. (1979). An empirical evaluation of the family life cycle. *Journal of Marriage and the Family, 41*, 27–38.

Streib, G., & Beck, R. (1980). Older families: A decade review. *Journal of Marriage and the Family, 42*, 937–956.

Thurow, L. (1987). The surge in inequality. *Scientific American, 256*(5), 30–37.

Walsh, F. (1988). Family in later life. In B. Carter & M. McGoldrick (Eds.), *The changing family life cycle* (2nd ed., pp. 311–334). New York: Gardner Press.

Weiss, R. L. (1980). Strategic behavioral marital therapy: Toward a model for assessment and intervention. In J. P. Vincent (Ed.), *Advances in family intervention, assessment and theory* (Vol. 1, pp. 229–271). Greenwich, CT: JAI Press.

Whisman, M. A., & Jacobson, N. S. (1989). Depression, marital satisfaction, and marital and personality measures of sex roles. *Journal of Marital and Family Therapy, 15*(2), 177–186.

White, L. K., Booth, A., & Edwards, J. N. (1986). Children and marital happiness: Why the negative correlation? *Journal of Family Issues, 7*, 131–147.

Whiteside, M. (1982). Remarriage: A family developmental process. *Journal of Marital and Family Therapy, 8*(2), 59–68.

Wynne, L. C. (1984). The epigenesis of relational systems: A model for understanding family development. *Family Process, 23*, 297–318.

17

Work

Lynda J. Katz and Ray Feroz

Introduction

Work plays a central role in human existence, inextricably intertwined into the fabric of society and circumscribing the individual lives of its members. The initiation and involvement of individuals in the workforce are related to dominant cultural values and the overall economic development of nations. According to Moore (1969), "the character of social organization in the contemporary world . . . assures that work will be the principal normal link between consuming families and the system of economic production" (p. 861).

In general, in more primitive (i.e., agrarian) economies, greater amounts of time are expended in work, and there is an earlier onset of the work role for the individual. In more advanced industrialized nations, children and adolescents can more easily postpone the requirement to work for pay in order to attend school, which leads to a more desirable, exalted, and/or less physically demanding job in the future. Indeed, in advanced societies, there are often proscriptions pertaining to child labor that would be incomprehensible in more primitive societies.

A formal definition of work is not easily developed. Traditional definitions are vocationally oriented, involving physical or mental activity leading to some outcome. In exchange for this activity (i.e., labor), the worker/employee receives pay in the form of currency, barter, or share of production yield. Newer definitions tend to be broader, undoubtedly related to the expanding relationship of work vis-à-vis self-esteem and personal fulfillment, which are themselves tied closely to changing social values, advanced economics, and occupational specialization. Indeed,

Lynda J. Katz • University of Pittsburgh School of Medicine, Western Psychiatric Institute and Clinic, Pittsburgh, Pennsylvania 15213.   Ray Feroz • Clarion University of Pennsylvania, Clarion, Pennsylvania 16214.

Handbook of Social Development: A Lifespan Perspective, edited by Vincent B. Van Hasselt and Michel Hersen. Plenum Press, New York, 1992.

LYNDA J. KATZ and
RAY FEROZ

the perception of work in the United States has broadened to the point that it has been defined as "any human activity undertaken in a quest for extrinsic rewards" (Rettig, 1982, p. 22). This is in contrast to activity undertaken for purposes of intrinsic rewards, defined as "nonwork" by Rettig (1982). Of special interest is the area in the continuum between these two poles, where the employee finds the activity intrinsically satisfying, but with potential or actual extrinsic payoffs. This is precisely where concepts of "job enrichment" (building intrinsic rewards into jobs) are rooted.

The Individual Need to Work

Work fulfills a variety of needs for the individual; among these are subsistence, personal fulfillment, independence, social support, structuring of time, and establishing identity. In fact, "in a society that values work, not to have work is a stigma and a loss of purpose and of meaning" (Super, 1984, p. 75). This is supported by the fact that in the United States, unemployment has been frequently associated with psychopathology (Brenner, 1976; Droughton, 1975; Sayers, 1988). Paradoxically, as Moore (1969) has observed, "Work is ambiguous for modern man" (p. 862). Work can be (and often is) a necessity to sustain life, but it can also be an internally satisfying commitment to a "calling." Moreover, these outlooks can exist simultaneously in the same person.

In addition to internal regards, work provides the individual with an occupational role or position by which to identify herself or himself. This work-role identity is embedded in society and connected to reciprocal roles and obligations that give further meaning to life and status to the holder (Merton, 1957). In a society that places high value on work, not to be engaged in an occupation can lead to personal devaluation. This is evident in the way America treats mothers who prefer to stay home with small children rather than return to the workplace (Brazelton, 1989), in the way we treat persons who are incapable of work because of severe cognitive deficiencies, and in the way retirees drop in social status when compared with those who remain actively engaged in the workplace.

Conversely, Lefkowitz (1979) has observed that a growing number of Americans are choosing not to work rather than be engaged in jobs perceived to be irrelevant and/or unsatisfying. Given the affluence of our society and the availability of government support for the "unemployed," the "nonwork" option has become viable for many Americans:

> Look around . . . and what do you see? Those that are still working count the days until they stop. And those who have stopped are not despised. They are envied. Things have changed. (p. 117)

Suffice it to say, however, that in general work satisfies needs for both the individual and the larger society. And as the essence and nature of work evolve, the entire society will be transformed.

The Changing Nature of Work

Social, legal, and technological changes obviously have an impact upon the world of work. For example, technical progress in robotics, while resulting in the elimination of many mundane assembly-line jobs, has, nonetheless, created the need for skilled technicians with specialized expertise to design, manufacture, program, and service high-tech equipment. Political changes in the European Common Market will result in prolific opportunity for business and legal experts with foreign language expertise. Aging baby-boomers will increasingly require health and nursing services. Old jobs die out and new specialties are born with the inevitable progression of economic, social, and technological change. The impact of these changes and projections and their effect on the future will be addressed at a later point.

Implications

As Calvin Coolidge observed in 1925, "The business of America is business." Sociologists determine one's social class by occupation, that of self for adults or father's occupation for children. Business and work and social validation go hand in hand in America. Work, together with family, plays a central role in defining one's identity (Moore, 1969). We cannot escape from the conclusion that work exerts a critical influence on adult development. This is especially true in American society with its unabashed valuing of business, consumption, and personal status. All of these are directly rooted in the concept we call *work*. Thus the character of work in contemporary American society to a large extent defines who we are. It makes us feel good or not good about ourselves. It allows us to live the "good life" in terms of consumption and status. It puts us into contact with persons with whom we spend more time than the very members of our own families. In this chapter we will discuss the meaning, dimensions, and future of work, with special focus on the adult in postindustrial American society.

MEASURING THE MEANING OF WORK

The meaning of work for modern Western culture took on its current reality from the era of the Protestant Reformation, initially as a result of the efforts of Martin Luther. Luther's preaching was to alter the value of life's work from that espoused by the "other worldliness" philosophy of the monastics of the time to a belief in fulfilling one's worldly duties as a way to live acceptably to God (Robertson, 1985). The Calvinists further solidified the value of worldly vocations, with the added dictum to improve one's station in life rather than remaining with Luther's idea of a vocational calling as a fixed station in life. Because the individual was now to improve his or her station in life, the notion of how this improvement was to be measured was the next aspect of the Protestant work ethic to emerge. Factors such as time, monetary wealth, and work as a necessary endeavor in order to fulfill one's duty to God came to be valued and as such have served as measuring sticks over time for the development of the traditional work ethic. Quantitative values, money and time, individualism, and impersonal work environments were reflective of how the meaning of work would be actualized for centuries to follow.

The Protestant work ethic, however, was to be modified in time by virtue of the heterogeneous societies in which work was to have meaning. Thus, measuring the meaning of work is heavily influenced by individual and cultural work values, racial and ethnic factors, the educational level of workers themselves, and their innate ability levels, gender, and age. It is these dimensions of work, which help to measure its meaning in contemporary society, that we will now address. And although each dimension is discussed as a singular entity, it will become clear that overlaps exist and lines blur as we attempt to define and operationalize the meaning of work.

Cultural and Individual Work Values

The concept of values has generally been defined as an individual's belief about modes of conduct (instrumental values) and end states of existence (terminal values) (Rokeach, 1968). How individual values are shaped including work values is profoundly influenced by the economic and social system of which an individual is a part, the implicit and explicit conceptions of that society that the individual holds, and by his or her status and role within that society. Numerous writers have addressed those specific sociological, cultural, economic, and historical factors that have influenced work values in particular (Pine & Innis, 1987). Thus it would appear that an understanding of cultural values and the dynamic nature of societies that give rise to and nourish personal values would be necessary in order to understand the value of work for the individual and his or her culture.

Schnall (1981) traced the development of value shifts over a 50-year period in the United States, beginning with the 1930s. She posited four stages that had an impact upon the development of values. Stage 1 incorporated the depressing 30s, the patriotic 40s, and the square 50s, where the major value focus was on denial of self and compliance with others. Stage 2 was composed of the revolutionary 60s, where self-indulgence and rejection of others were major values, commitment and discipline were dissolved, and keeping one's options open and instant gratification were prized. The overall value orientation concerned itself with the here-and-now. In Stage 3, the selfish 70s, values were reflective of self-reliance and a distrust of others. Stage 4, the concerned 80s, saw values revolve around the fulfillment of the self, balanced by a concern for others. It can be hypothesized that a Stage 5 may now be envisioned (which we shall call the unpredictable 90s), where values will be highly influenced by the speed of information processing, the shrinking of the globe, and the overwhelming complexities, fostered by a technological revolution, that must be absorbed into the value-driven decision making of individuals in society. In this context, Rosenberg's (1987) comments on individual occupational choice as a function of values is most appropriate.

> When an individual chooses an occupation, he [sic] thinks there is something good about it, and this conception of the "good" is part of an internalized mental structure which establishes priorities regarding what he wants out of life. To ask what an individual wants out of his work is to a large extent to ask what he wants out of life. It is, therefore, indispensable to an adequate understanding of the occupational decision making process to consider what people want or consider good or desirable, for these are the essential criteria by which choices are made. (Rosenberg, 1987, p. 6)

What individuals "want or consider good or desirable," personal values as it were, cannot be separated from the cultural context within which these values arise (Hofstede, 1984). Therefore, if we are to evaluate the quality of an individual's work life, the quality of his or her total life must be considered. "At the level of culture, work and life cannot and should not be separated" (Hofstede, 1984, p. 389). In his work on the cultural relativity of the quality of life concept, Hofstede validated four dimensions of cultural work values that had been derived factorially in an earlier study. These four dimensions were power distance, individualism, masculinity, and uncertainty avoidance. Power distance as a cultural characteristic defines the extent to which a less powerful person in society accepts inequality in power and considers it to be the norm. Individualism in a culture depicts the extent to which individuals are concerned primarily with their own interests and those of their immediate families. Masculinity is a measure of a culture's use of the two sexes to define different social roles for men and women. Feminine cultures, on the other hand, define relatively overlapping roles for the sexes. Uncertainty avoidance is a measure of the extent to which individuals within a culture are made "nervous by situations that they consider to be unstructured, unclear, or unpredictable" (Hofstede, p. 390). The United States is an example of a country where cultural work values involve small power distance, high individualism, weak uncertainty avoidance, and masculinity. In Japan, on the other hand, cultural work values include large power distance, low individualism, strong uncertainty avoidance, and masculine values.

Further, in his validation study of these work-related value patterns in 53 countries and regions, Hofstede demonstrated that the traditionally accepted hierarchies of human needs, such as those proposed by Maslow (1954) and McClelland (1961), are ethnocentric and do not recognize cultural differences. In this context, Hofstede illustrates the difference between the North American and the North European school of improving the quality of work life, humanization of work, and job restructuring:

> In North America, the dominant objective is to make individual jobs more interesting by providing workers with an increased challenge. This grew out of the earlier "job enlargement" and "job enrichment" movements. In countries such as Sweden and Norway, the dominant objective is to make group work more rewarding by allowing groups to function as self-contained social units (semiautonomous groups) and by fostering cooperation among group members. Humanization of work means "masculinization" in North America, but "feminization" in Sweden. (Hofstede, 1980, p. 397)

Finally, Hofstede points out that to the extent that he was able to measure, shifts over time in the masculinity–femininity and uncertainty avoidance dimensions were relatively small and inconsistent. "There was no sign of convergency among countries, rather there was an indication of increasing divergence" (p. 397), a finding he had also reported earlier (Hofstede, 1980).

Occupational Roles

Measuring the meaning of work, its role in the life of workers in specific occupational groups, and its impact upon these groups have also been discussed extensively in the literature (Mottaz, 1985, 1988; O'Reilly & Caldwell, 1980; Porter, Crampom, & Smith, 1976; Quinn & Cobb, 1971; Rabinowitz & Hall, 1977; Tausky, 1960; Vroom, 1962; Yankelovich, 1979). As part of a larger study conducted by an international team of researchers in eight countries engaged in a comparative study of the major pattern of meanings attached to work (MOW International Research Team, 1981), Harpaz (1985) found three major "meaning of work" profiles among his sample population of Israeli workers. The sample surveyed consisted of 896 individuals (501 males, 395 females): students in their final year at vocational-technical high school, temporary workers, self-employed businessmen, chemical engineers, teachers, tool and die makers, white-collar workers, textile workers, individuals who were unemployed, and those who were retired. Forty percent of the population under study fit a profile characterized by high levels of work centrality and high intrinsic work orientation. The domain of work centrality was assessed in absolute terms, "How important and significant is working in your life" and in relative terms: work's importance in relation to leisure, community, religion, and family. A measure of intrinsic work orientation was obtained based upon responses to a job satisfaction questionnaire that assessed 11 work goals: opportunity to learn, interpersonal relations, promotional opportunities, convenient work hours, variety, interesting work, job security, match between job requirements and abilities, pay, working conditions, and autonomy. The intrinsic rating was based upon specific responses to variety, autonomy, and work is interesting and satisfying, an item taken from a valued work outcome domain that was assessed as well.

Those occupational groups whose members concentrated around the cluster profile characterized by high levels of work centrality and high intrinsic work orientation were chemical engineers, tool and die makers, the self-employed, and teachers. These occupations were considered to have relatively higher prestige, status, pay, and professionalism as compared with the total sample. The second most dominant profile resembled the major one in terms of the emphasis placed upon work centrality. The difference was in these workers' association with an extrinsic orientation. Dominating this profile were textile workers, white-collar workers, and some tool and die makers. The common denominator for these groups was their status as manual workers and/or their situation in low-level positions within their respective organizations.

Similar results have been reported by Mottaz (1988) based on data obtained from 1,385 workers drawn from five occupational groups: professional (university faculty, nurses, elementary-school teachers); managerial, including police, educational administrators, and factory supervisors; clerical (secretaries); service (police officers); and blue-collar workers. In this study, aimed at identifying determinants of organizational commitment, it was found that work rewards (intrinsic and extrinsic) have a stronger positive effect on organizational commitment than do work values (what the worker wants, desires or seeks to attain from work). Also, organizational commitment, when given the same level of intrinsic and extrinsic rewards, tends to be lower among workers with high work values, that is, task autonomy, significance, and involvement. That is, if workers have high work values, it may be very difficult for an organization to provide levels of work rewards sufficient to meet these high work standards. Thus "the more one's experiences in the organization are congruent with one's values, the more likely the individual will be committed to the organization" (Mottaz, 1988, p. 479).

Age

The factor of age intersects with the other dimensions that are being considered (ethnicity, culture, gender) as we attempt to measure the meaning of work, and in addition, makes a unique contribution to the measurement process. For simplicity's sake, workers will be categorized as young, adult, and older workers as we examine the dimension of age.

THE YOUNG WORKER

In general, much of life constitutes socialization for work for young persons. In preindustrial America, families typically owned the agricultural or craft enterprises in which children worked alongside adults. Career choice was not an issue for most children because they grew up doing the same kind of work their parents did. Industrialization, which removed work to enterprises not owned by employees, left parents without any direct way to teach their children how to make a living.

Children in contemporary industrialized societies, therefore, are faced with the developmental task of preparing themselves for adult work without being able to rely on direct instruction by parents or other adults to whom parents delegate specific authority (as in traditional apprenticeship arrangements where parents could "bind out" children to another household for a period of time). In preindustrial times, only children who were very privileged, very poor, or unusual in some other way had to face this problem. Now, however, most children cannot rely on their parents to teach them, in any detail, what work to do when they mature (Stern & Eichorn, 1989).

Adolescence is the time of life when this question becomes salient. Indeed, getting ready to do some kind of adult work is said to be the main problem for contemporary adolescents. Erik Erikson (1963), whose writings on adolescent identity formation have a had a strong influence on clinical and developmental psychology, observed that "in most instances . . . it is inability to settle on an occupational identity which disturbs individual young people" (p. 262). Because adolescence has emerged historically as the period in industrual societies when individuals must make the transition from childhood dependence to economically independent adulthood, the search for occupational identity can be considered a defining characteristic of contemporary adolescence (Stern and Eichorn, 1989).

Although the official labor force in the United States is defined in terms of persons 16 years of age and older who are paid full- or part-time workers (Hall, 1986), many more youth are in school until the age of 18 than are in the labor force, and many younger than 16 have part-time jobs while in school or during the summer. The kinds of work that young people do is differentiated in terms of setting and most importantly in terms of quality of work experience. Among a sample of middle-class suburban teenagers surveyed by Greenberger and Steinberg (1986), approximately one-half of those employed worked as store clerks or food service workers. The results of their survey led them to conclude that the poor quality of many contemporary teenage jobs threaten to make young workers "economically rich . . . but psychologically poor" (p. 238).

Data from the National Longitudinal Survey (NLS) of Youth Labor Market Experience (Stein & Nakata, 1989), based on a representative sample of 12,686 youth ages 14 to 22 in 1979, demonstrated that overall, the amount of time spent in paid jobs during high school was positively associated with labor market success in the first 3 years after graduation. However, these data also validated Greenberger and Steinberg's earlier conclusion. Specifically there was greater initial success in the labor market among recent graduates whose high-school jobs gave them more of a chance to use and develop skills. Stein and Nakata concluded that "skill use and development in teenagers' jobs also stands for opportunity to develop the capacity for learning on the job, and students who experience more of it in high school do better in the labor market after they graduate" (p. 205). This finding substantiates the work of the National Academy of Sciences Panel, Secondary School Education for the Changing Workplace (1984), whose chairperson, Richard Heckert of Dupont, had written earlier:

> The major asset required by employers of high school graduates . . . is the ability to learn and to adapt to change in the workplace. The continual evolution of work functions will require that workers master new knowledge and new skills throughout their lives. The ability to learn will be the essential hallmark of the successful employee. (p. xi)

In contrast, other kinds of "synthetic" work experiences (Dement, 1982) have been created for low-income, unemployed teenagers. Evaluation of these programs has found disappointing results (Burtless, 1984; Dement, 1982; Manpower Demonstration Research Corporation, 1980; Taggart 1981). In fact, they may create a negative credentialing effect, "if would-be employers assume that participants in these programs are *ipso facto* undesirable as employees" (Stein & Nakata, 1989, p. 192). It is well documented that the dominant characteristic of young workers is their high rate of unemployment, with a striking differential between African-American and white youth. And although it would appear that at least in terms of white youth there is no overall decline in psychological well-being associated with leaving school and becoming unemployed (Gurney, 1980; Winefield & Tiggemann, 1985), unemployed young persons compare unfavorably with their employed counterparts in terms of self-esteem and depressive affect. Longitudinal studies suggest that these differences are due more to an improvement in both dimensions shown by those working rather than a decline in these characteristics by those who are unemployed (Winefield & Tiggermann, 1985).

However, although unemployment is somewhat voluntary among school leavers who are engaged in a job search, it has become increasingly clear that job loss and/or prolonged unemployment in the young can lead to potentially damaging longer term consequences. In the last three decades the problem of unemployment for youths has received increasing attention from both policymakers and researchers in the United States and other industrialized countries (Ogbu, 1989). In 1984 youth unemployment rose to approximately 25%, more than double that of the adult working force. And although it is high for all young people in this country, it is significantly higher for minority teenagers—American Indian, African-American, and Hispanic youth. In 1984, the unemployment rate for African-American youth was 43%; in 1987 it was 35%, in contrast to 14% for white youth.

> A study by the Education Commission of the States (1985) concluded: The number of young people who are disconnected from school and work and the benefits they confer is on the rise. The entry-level labor pool, then, contains more and more of the kinds of teenagers employers have been able to overlook in the past: poorly motivated, lacking fundamental literacy skills and unacquainted with the responsibilities and demands of the work world. (p. 5)

In trying to explain the source of this large and widening differential between African-American and white teenagers, it has been argued that minorities, on the average, are less qualified (Osterman, 1989). Evidence for this argument comes from higher dropout rates that lead to lesser educational attainment. According to the Carnegie Foundation in 1980, 78% of white 19-year-olds in the United States were high-school graduates (Sum, 1983). In the same year, 61% of African-American and 56% of Hispanic 19-year-olds held high-school diplomas; "while 13% of all 17 year-old youth are functionally illiterate, this percentage rises to 44% for African-American youth and 56% for Hispanics" (Osterman, p. 240).

Although there is no agreement among researchers as to whether the problem is a result of the supply side or the demand side of the labor market, Ogbu (1974) argues rather that a reciprocal relationship exists between the two sides of these labor market forces: (1) minority youths' employment opportunities on the one hand and (2) preparation for the labor market on the other. He espouses a cultural-ecological framework in which he examines the issues of social opportunities and efforts expended by individuals or groups to pursue the educational credentials necessary for labor force participation and remuneration. Ogbu (1989) argues that the existence of a "job ceiling," the practice of requiring additional qualification from African-Americans, and the development in minorities of an institutionalized discrimination perspective contribute to a folk theory of getting ahead (members of a society tend to share a theory of getting ahead based on their past and present experiences) for black members of society including its youth that differs from the folk theory of success of the dominant culture.

Finally, much has been written about the "transition" from young worker or student to adult worker. Miller and Form (1964) have provided a useful conceptualization of how this transition process forms part of the individual's overall career path. In the *preparatory* stage, relevant work behavior and attitudes are developed in the home and at school. The *initial* phase involves the young person's engagement in part-time or full-time work while still a student, and jobs are viewed as temporary. During the *trial* phase, the individual may change jobs several times as expectations and career goals are shaped. The final stages are *stable* work and then *retirement*.

The trial phase is considered to be the *transition* stage and can vary widely in terms of its duration and the degree of flux experienced. Ginzberg (1981) has suggested several patterns for this transition stage.

> *The Straight Pattern.* Those who make the transition with little or no difficulty because they have the qualifications that employers seek and have family support to draw on.
> *The Interrupted Pattern.* Those who are unable or unwilling to move directly from school to work because they have not acquired the necessary credentials, because they are undergoing emotional turmoil, or because they are confused about their aims and goals. They need time to sort out their feelings, conflicts, and goals.
> *The Disturbed Pattern.* Those who, because of poor preparation, alienation, minority status, or police records, are not acceptable to most employers and who find getting and holding a job unrewarding and frustrating. As an alternative this group often drifts into illicit activities. (p. 72)

The relationship between age and work appears obvious—young people do not work because they are in school, and older people do not work because they are retired. Fortunately and unfortunately, the matter is not that simple. Although young people may not be working, what they are doing has a crucial impact on

LYNDA J. KATZ and
RAY FEROZ

their future work lives. People who are retired are vitally affected by the kind of work they did in terms of their economic situations after retiring, their outlook on life, and their social relationships. In addition, many older people continue to work.

The transition stage is considered to be a major turning point in the life of the individual because it typically contains certain other major life events—the end of schooling, the first real job, marriage. Thus, based on the previous discussion, it is not surprising that the successful completion of this transition stage (the timing, spacing, and sequencing of events) is directly related to the dimension of age and the interconnections between age and ethnicity, occupational status, cultural diversity and gender (which has yet to be discussed).

THE OLDER WORKER

Although the transition from adult worker to older worker can also occur over a wide span of years, it is otherwise characteristically very different from the transition of young worker to adult worker. These differences stem from societal views of older persons in general, specific corporate and governmental policies regarding mandatory retirement and support for older retired persons, and negative stereotypes about the older worker (Hall, 1986).

Giving rise to these negative stereotypes was the rapid industrialization and labor-intensive employment expansion that took place in the United States between 1920 and 1940. Scientific management principles, first espoused and practiced with religious ferocity in industry during this period, were based on the theory that a worker's lifetime individual capacity was relatively fixed and therefore would decline over time until it was exhausted. The requirement for speed was seen to increase stress and thereby decrease productive capacity with age. And although there has never been empirically derived support for the relationship between age and declining capacities (Baltes, Reese & Lipsitt, 1980; Schaie, 1974), these negative beliefs (ageism in the workplace) have persisted over time along with negative assumptions regarding reduced learning capacity, skills obsolescence, resistance to change, and slower decision making with aging (Morrison, 1986).

More recently, however, societal values and expectations about older persons and their roles in society have changed to a large degree in response to a number of demographic, economic, political, and sociocultural circumstances. By the year 2000, 20% of the population of the United States will be age 65 or older. The declining birth rate and aging of the baby boom generation have contributed to this dramatic shift in the age distribution of the U.S. population (Cahill & Salomone, 1987). This phenomenon as manifest in employment settings has been dubbed the "graying of the workforce" (Work in America Institute, 1980). Moreover, a variety of factors—(a) developments in the economy such as the spiraling rate of inflation; (b) certain proposed changes in the Social Security system; (c) the experience of extended longevity in spite of impaired health; and (d) the 1978 Amendment to the Age Discrimination in Employment Act, which enables older workers to remain on their job until the age of 70—have contributed to a reversal in the previous trend toward early retirement (Shkop, 1982). In a Harris survey (Harris, 1979), 75% of the then-current working population expressed a desire to continue working beyond the typical retirement age.

One measure of the value of work across the life span, because the work role is particularly important to an individual's sense of identity, is job satisfaction. The study of age differences in job satisfaction focuses on how age combines with work and self-and family concepts to produce differences in work rate outcome over the life cycle (Kalleberg & Loscocco, 1983). The most consistent research finding on age differences in job satisfaction is that older workers are more satisfied with their jobs than are younger workers (Janson & Martin, 1982; Kalleberg, 1977; Quinn *et al.*, 1974; Wright & Hamilton, 1978).

In attempting to systematically explore the form and determinants of the age–job satisfaction relationship, Kalleberg and Loscocco (1983) concluded that (a) chronological age differences in job satisfaction are substantial compared to the effects of other variables (education, sex, race, work structures, family life cycle, job rewards and work-related values; (b) perceived job rewards and work values account for the effects of work structure and family life cycle positions on job satisfaction; but (c) job rewards and work values do not completely account for the total age differences in job satisfaction. "Chronological age is significantly related to job satisfaction independently of all of our variables" (p. 84). The authors argue that this effect reflects processes of adaptation to the work alone. This conclusion was further supported by the fact that only among workers for whom work is a highly salient role was this effect observed.

Another measure of the meaning of work as a reflection of age is its relationship to perceived health, life satisfaction, and activity among the older population. Continued employment into old age has been associated with higher morale, happiness, adjustment and longevity (Palmore & Stone, 1973). However, establishing a causal relationship between work and these factors has been difficult because most studies have not controlled adequately for self-selection among ill versus healthy workers in opting for retirement. Because poor health is one of the main causes of voluntary and early retirement, the independent effects of retirement on health are difficult to estimate (Soumerai & Avorn, 1983). On the other hand, mandatory retirement as a significant life event with possible negative consequence on health and moral has been researched (Fox, 1976; Sheldon *et al.*, 1975; Thompson, 1973).

In an effort to evaluate the impact of flexible employment programs on the status of older persons, Soumerai and Avorn (1983) conducted a study involving a random selection of elderly applicants in a demonstration employment program for retirees. Results from this controlled, randomized study documented the positive effects of part-time employment on the life satisfaction and perceived health on this sample of urban, community-dwelling retirees. The investigators postulated that a major factor influencing these results was that the experimental group was given an opportunity to "exert meaningful control over their [*sic*] environment and to satisfy the need to engage in useful, valued activity" (p. 360).

Although the data demonstrated that some elderly persons are eager and able to undertake demanding jobs quite different from the ones from which they retired, certain caveats were noted concerning the translation of work-in-retirement research into policy. First, older workers are prime candidates for salary exploitation; and second, placing part-time elderly workers in jobs to displace currently employed full-time workers as a cost containment measure could intensify intergenerational economic rivalry. In addition, the investigators cautioned that "although the opportunity to work far into advanced age may be a right owed to every citizen, such a right could easily be distorted into an obligation at a time when publicly supported pension systems are under increasing economic pressure" (Soumerai & Avorn, 1983, p. 362).

As a final note, organizations in the United States and abroad are experimenting with flexible retirement policies and with the alteration of an older employees' work situation (i.e., transfer to another job, modifications in the current job structure and/or time schedule) (Morrison, 1979; Jacobson, 1980; Rosenblum & Sheppard, 1977). Such alterations may alleviate the pressures that often force a person to retire and, at the same time, allow the organization to capitalize on that employee's particular skills (Sheppard, 1978; Walker & Lazer, 1978). In addition, job transfers may result in openings that would allow promotion of younger employees. The success of a plan of job modification appears to be highly dependent, however, on the nature of the job and the job holder (Shkop, 1982). Alternatives such as (a) use of annuitant pools (employment of a company's own retirees for temporary full- or part-time assignments); (b) contract work (employment of older persons as independent contractors on fee-for-service basis); (c) retraining (where recruitment of trained personnel is difficult and costly); (d) multiple flexible work arrangements and job redesign (when experienced employees have long-standing clients and the firm values older workers); and (e) part-time employment could enable older workers to develop second careers, participate in phased retirement programs, receive additional training and education, and obtain flexible work schedules. Morrison (1986) wrote:

> In addition to the work options that are being provided for older "retired" persons today, it is also possible to foresee another approach for older employees who might remain in the work force instead of retiring early. This would require employers and workers to accept a different view of work life, including such policies as horizontal job mobility without increased pay, reduced responsibility and income, and gradual diminution of responsibility and reward. In a society that values and requires the productive participation of greater numbers of older persons, these types of human-resource policy adjustments may become increasingly necessary. But they will be feasible only if the social values that now emphasize progressively upward mobility and increasing reward can be modified to reflect a continuum of work life, encompassing upward, horizontal, and downward mobility. (p. 287)

Race and Ethnicity

As will become evident in the following discussion, although race and ethnicity interact with the dimensions of gender and educational level, over the years a variety of stereotypic linkages have been made between work, race, and ethnicity. And although at times these stereotypes can be both accurate and mean-spirited, they "inadvertently represent the racial and ethnic dimension of work in that members of various racial and ethnic groups are over- and underrepresented across the spectrum of work" (Hall, 1986, p. 251). The reasons for this are rooted in historical and economic traditions.

Agricultural work has been the point of entry into the world of work for many immigrants into the United States over the years. Slavery was agricultural work, as was the work found by northern and western European immigrants who came to the United States in the early 1800s. The majority of Scandinavian and German immigrants, for example, moved to the rich farmlands of the Midwest, settling in rural areas. Many, however, while entering the labor force as agricultural workers, saw this only as a stepping stone on their way to an urban area. Such was the case with Jamaican migrant farm workers (Foner & Napolic, 1978) and Mexicans who migrated to South Texas (Jones, 1984). These and other later migrants from southern, central, and eastern Europe (post-1880) settled in large cities where industrial jobs were located. However, neither these later migrants nor African-Americans found particularly desirable jobs. The European migrants found employment in the manufacturing sector, whereas African-Americans found work primarily in service jobs (Lieberson, 1980).

In one of the few studies concerned with Hispanic workers, Arbona (1989) looked at the representation of Hispanics in the workplace utilizing Holland's work typology and its corresponding levels of educational prerequisites. Earlier work by Gottfredson and Gaiger (1977) had analyzed occupation of men and women, utilizing data from the 1970 census, according to educational level and the Holland work typology, a well-researched classification of career interest (Holland, 1985). Gottfredson (1978) extended these earlier studies by examining race and gender composition within these work types reaching the following conclusion: (a) Some types of work are more scarce than others; (b) various types of work are distributed unevenly across various educational and prestige levels; (c) the different types of work are not equally available to men and women; and (d) African-Americans are underrepresented in some types of work and substantially overrepresented in others, particularly low-prestige positions.

Using 1980 census data, Arbona (1989) extended a similar analysis to the Hispanic population. Hispanics are the fastest growing minority group in the United States as well as the youngest subpopulation. Although Hispanics comprised 7.2% of the U.S. population in 1985, it is expected that their numbers will rise to nearly 10% in the year 2000. Arbona's work looked at where Hispanic men and women have found employment in the past and where they may find the greatest opportunities in the future. Results from Arbona's study were several. Three types of work (social, enterprising, and conventional) accounted for over 50% of all jobs available to Hispanics, and within these, 40% were in the realistic as opposed to investigative or artistic categories. With respect to educational level, at the high-school GED level, 41% of the jobs held were realistic, 27% were conventional, and 10% social. Among African-Americans, who represented 5% of the employed labor force in 1980, there was an overrepresentation in low- and moderate-level realistic jobs and a dramatic underrepresentation in all other categories. Finally, for Hispanic men who represented 3% of the labor force and Hispanic women who represented 2%, the same job characteristics as found with African-American workers held true. But, Hispanic women, like African-American women, appeared to be somewhat better represented in the various job types as well as in the higher GED-level jobs than were their male counterparts. In both instances, women were overrepresented in social and conventional work.

However, according to Silvestri and Lukasiewicz (1985), employment projections for 1995 are that the predominant sources of employment for Hispanics—realistic work (construction, mechanics, repairers, production occupations, and transportation) and conventional work (office clerical work)—are expected to grow slightly or decline in number. When this projection is coupled with the fact that a lower percentage of Hispanics than African-Americans complete high school or college, the situation becomes even more negative. In the words of Arbona (1989):

> These findings suggest that the interplay of specific school factors may result in decreased educational and, possibly, decreased occupational opportunities for Hispanics. The relationship between these school factors and the occupational segregation of Hispanics in the U.S. economy needs to be examined further. (p. 266)

In a study using national data, Fligstein and Fernandez (1985) found that both Hispanic and white students who attended schools having a high percentage of Hispanics were more likely to have experienced grade delay and to drop out of school. Other studies have shown that Hispanic students are very often "tracked" in high-school general or vocational programs and are rarely placed in college preparatory programs (Amato, 1980; Orum, 1986). Often the students in these vocational programs do not meet admissions requirements for 4-year colleges. Furthermore, Ballesteros (1986) found that, in general, both white and Hispanic students placed in college preparatory programs scored higher on aptitude tests, made better grades in high school and college, and aspired to higher degrees than did students placed in vocational or general education curriculums.

Central to the discussion of race and ethnicity as dimensions of work is the phenomenon of discrimination in the workplace. Discrimination has been defined by Cain (1984) as long-lasting inequality in economic well-being among individuals based on their color, gender, or ethnic ties and as differences in pay or wage rates for equally productive groups. Kaufman (1983) found that minorities are differentially distributed in labor market sectors. In addition, competition for limited jobs tends to breed racial prejudice. In their study of changes in socioeconomic opportunity Hauser and Featherman (1977) wrote:

> If black men in the labor force have experienced greater increases in educational attainment, occupational status, and income than white men of the same age over the past decade, these gains have not been great enough to offset the discriminatory obstacles faced by black men. (p. 134)

Cain (1984) reported similar trends. The African-American/white earnings ratio for men shifted from .45 in 1939 to .73 in 1982, with a nearly identical earnings ratio for Hispanic men. In addition, a dramatic shift in the earnings ratio for women has occurred. In 1939 the African-American/white earnings ratio for women was .38; in 1982 it was .94. This near parity is offset, however, by the fact that white women only earn 59% of the income earned by men; thus the African-American women's gain has only caught them up with white women. The ratio for Hispanic women was .86. According to Cain, these figures mean that equally productive men and women are discriminated against in terms of their pay (Hall, 1986).

A number of factors appear to contribute to racial and ethnic discrimination in the workplace. In the search for cheap labor pools, racial and ethnic minorities who have few other alternatives will work for lower wages. Craft unions still appear to discriminate against African-American workers, whereas industrial unions do not (Leigh, 1978). Over the years, geographic distribution appears to have played a significant role in job entry for many immigrants resulting in their need to find "niches" in particular occupation groups (Lieberson, 1980, p. 379). Lieberson cited statistics gathered in 1950 that indicated that, for example, Greek immigrant men ran eating and drinking establishments 29 times more frequently than the national average for other nationality groups. Irish men became policemen or firemen at a rate three times greater than for all other caucasian males. Russian immigrant males became tailors or furriers at a rate 17 times greater than all other caucasians. Lieberson's findings are significant when one recognizes that the migration experience from the South to the North for African-Americans in such sizable numbers served to reduce the negative, discriminatory practices that were experienced by these new European groups overall.

The experience of Asians in the workplace presents some contrasting discriminatory practices. Except in the West, where the responses to Asians were at times severe and violent, Asian immigrants have not been perceived historically to pose economic threats to whites. However, although educational levels for Asians have been equal to that of whites or at times better, they almost always have entered the labor force at the bottom, even if they arrived with financial resources and credentials (Hall, 1986).

Generally speaking, although there has been a growing interest in the experience and problems of minority groups in the workplace, their vocational aspirations and ultimate career choices, there is a paucity of research specifically addressing Asian-American individuals. Although several explanations have been posited to account for this seeming neglect (Minatoya & Sedlacek, 1981; Sue & Sue, 1972; Sue, Sue, & Sue, 1975; Sue & Wagner, 1973; Hsia, 1980), it is clear that a combination of factors have most probably interacted to contribute to this state of affairs. Issues such as segregation of occupational choice and interest; occupational values that reflect Asian-American culture; the process of acculturation and assimilation; societal and cultural barriers to occupational aspirations; and personality traits such as external locus of control, social anxiety, and intolerance for ambiguity have been identified as significant and relevant variables in the career development of Asian-American persons. In the words of Leong (1985), in addressing the issue of career counseling specifically:

> Although the majority of Asian Americans do become engineers, mathematicians, and computer scientists, counselors need to be cautious not to overgeneralize from this pattern of occupational segregation to individual cases. To do so would be similar to encouraging female clients to seek careers in traditional fields (e.g., elementary school teaching) because many other women have chosen those fields. At the same time, counselors need to be aware that Asian-American students may have certain personality traits, such as social anxiety and low tolerance of ambiguity, that may influence their career choices. The degree to which these personality traits are important in an Asian-American student's career choice may be moderated by his or her level of acculturation, which would have to be assessed by the counselor. Differences in Asian Americans' occupational values would also need to be taken into consideration. These implications are quite tentative, in need of empirical validation, and should be implemented cautiously. (p. 544)

Finally, more recent researchers have argued in support of Wilson's (1978) contention that race has become a less significant issue than is social class in the employment pattern of African-Americans. However, the same trend does not appear to be the case when one focuses on the issue of ethnic group membership.

Portes (1984) and Wilson and Portes (1980) reported, for example, that among Cuban workers in Miami who traditionally had lived in enclaves, the opportunity to create their own labor markets resulted in the establishment of a somewhat insulated position for them with respect to competition with the dominant labor market. Such ethnic enclaves have been described elsewhere, that is, Jewish people in Manhattan, Japanese on the West Coast, Koreans in Los Angeles, with essentially "positive" outcomes in terms of work opportunities and other quality-of-life measures for these disparate ethnic groups (Alba & Chamblin, 1983).

Education

The impact of education on the workplace and on the worker has received considerable attention in sociological and industrial psychology literature since World War II. A number of competing forces have had a direct bearing on the importance of educational attainment levels as one measure of work's meaning in modern Western society. What does it mean to be overeducated and/or underemployed? Are they necessarily related? Why the recent focus on the crisis in workplace literacy? How does level of education influence the worker's commitment to his or her organization? And finally, how does education influence work satisfaction as a major work value?

On the one hand, until 1970, rapid growth in fields and professions requiring highly educated labor saw a dramatic rise in the educational attainment of young persons from a particularly small birth cohort resulting in occupational opportunities available to them that were unprecedented. In response to the demand from the marketplace to a large extent from 1950 until 1980, the number of high-school graduates in the United States increased from 59% to 80%, and the number of college graduates rose from 14.8% to over 25% during this same time period (U.S. Bureau of the Census, 1981). This trend in educational attainment paralleled the market demand for more highly educated and trained workers until the period from 1970–1982 when employment growth tapered off to a significant degree particularly for men. It was during this time period that Freeman among others wrote treatises whose titles included "Overinvestment in College Training" (1975), *The Overeducated American* (1976), "The Decline in Economic Rewards to College Education" (1977), and "The Facts about the Declining Economic Value of College" (1980).

Giving rise to Freeman's arguments is the fact that between 1970 and 1975, the proportion of both male and female college graduates who were able to obtain high-paying entry-level jobs declined noticeably in relation to the rate between 1950 and 1970 as did the quality of entry-level jobs for males with 1 to 3 years of college education (Smith, 1986). However, even as the rate of increase in professional and managerial jobs waned, the proportions of college graduates grew. It has been hypothesized that what will ultimately deter young people from enrolling in college will not be occupational mismatch *per se* but rather declining returns to investment in higher education (Smith, 1986). In the words of the economists Galper and Dunn (1969), "Individuals are . . . assumed to invest in higher education until the marginal rate of return from additional education is equal to some market rate of return" (p. 766). In other words, "A college education will seem a worthwhile investment as long as college graduates earn sufficiently more than high school graduates—i.e., enough to offset the expense of college plus the delay in entering the labor force "(Smith, 1986, p. 91). This hypothesis has been borne out in the recent press that has accompanied the decline in applications to and enrollment in medical schools in this country today, for example.

On the other hand, the idea that college graduates could be overeducated but still not suffer any loss of relative income has been argued by several authors (Rumberger, 1980; Smith, 1986). Relying on Thurow's (1974) job competition model, Rumberger concluded that education indicates to employers which potential employees are most qualified or easiest to train for a given job. In the words of Smith (1986):

> Education is a comparative marker, not an absolute marker. As more people become educated, the best-educated still get the best jobs and wages. Inevitably, however, as the stock of educated labor increases, more and more college graduates will get, say, clerical and sales jobs. (p. 95)

And, although we may be concerned with the prospects of college graduates, prospects for those persons without college degrees may be even more dismal. Clogg and Shockey (in Smith, 1986) conducted an exhaustive study of occupational mismatch that demonstrated that although college graduates were squeezing high-school graduates out of their traditional jobs, high-school graduates were squeezing those without high-school degrees out of theirs and so on. According to Smith,

> A college education was once sufficient for the attainment of a good job. It is clearly no longer sufficient, but at the same time, it is all the more necessary. Data from the 1980 Detroit Area Study show that the public has acknowledged this state of affairs. Two thirds of all adult respondents believed that a college education was not worth what it was thirty years ago. Included in this group were 65 percent of the college graduates in the study and 69 percent of the parents with a child aged 5 to 17 in the house. Yet 75 percent of these same parents said that they intended to send their oldest child to college. (p. 95)

However, it has become increasingly clear that individuals seek a college education for reasons other than its economic value. Dresch (1975) addressed this phenomenon in particular when he described the "marginal" college student, whose diminished abilities may not be compatible with a reasonable return on investment in a college education. He concluded that these marginal students may have come to the realization "that a college education confers no specific set of opportunities" (Smith, 1986, p. 97). Instead, for some, the nonmonetary rewards of a college education may be as important as the monetary ones (i.e., social status, prestige, at least for the short run).

At the other extreme is the fact that 45 million adults holding jobs in the United States at the present time are functionally or marginally illiterate. The U.S. Department of Education has produced statistics that estimate that persons who are functionally illiterate account for 30% of the unskilled work force, 29% of all semiskilled workers, and 11% of all managers, professionals, and technicians (Goddard, 1987). At the same time the down trend in employment opportunities prevalent in the 1979s has undergone a major transformation in the 1980s, particularly in the latter third of the decade. Some regions of the country report twice as many new jobs created in 1988 than in the period from 1985 to 1987 (The Face of Change, 1989). This "new economy" will be faced with a potential workforce among whose members 25% will be high school-dropouts while 95% of the new jobs will pay $6.00 per hour or more and will require a high school diploma. In general, occupation trends across the United States reflect rapid growth in service and health jobs, an increase in white collar jobs, and emergence of an elite "gold collar" worker, the highly educated generalist who can integrate information from several factors and use advanced software to meet increased needs for information (The Face of Change, 1989).

Thus, although the forecasted expanding economy will require a more highly trained workforce, a significant portion of the future workforce are and will be ill prepared for workforce demands. In the city of Pittsburgh, Pennsylvania, for example, one out of four students drops out of school before graduation, whereas one-fourth of white public-school students and one-half of African-American students score below the national average in reading. In the state of Georgia, 45% of the current high-school population of students never receive a high-school diploma. Illiteracy as a social, economic, and political dilemma affects a variety of disadvantaged groups, most seriously of all displaced industrial workers, poor urban youth, and ethnic and racial minorities. According to Goddard (1987):

> Rather than criticize the schools, parents, immigration, poverty and others outside our domain, it's time to examine the marketplace itself. Recently several social, demographic and economic events have conspired to produce our present predicament. The labor pool has contracted and educational standards have declined; both have forced corporate America to lower its employment requirements to fill available openings. Affirmative action and equal employment guidelines have further complicated the search for excellence.
>
> The automation and computer revolutions have eliminated many low-literacy-level industrial and clerical jobs and replaced them with jobs requiring a high order of workplace literacy. There has been and will continue to be an increasing demand for knowledge workers who are skilled in the use of advanced technologies . . . and possess good writing, reading, listening, memory, computation, and comprehension skills. (p. 75)

This state of affairs has led to the development in large corporations of programs for remedial education. According to the Center for Public Resources, 75% of the country's largest corporations now offer some kind of basic skills training (Goddard, 1987). Presently, one-third of corporate training expenditures are invested in remedial education and fundamental job skills. Examples of programs aimed at eradicating illiteracy in the workplace are as follow:

- American Telephone and Telegraph currently spends $6 million yearly on remedial courses for its employees.
- General Motors Corp. and International Business Machines spend a total of $700 million annually on adult education.
- Ford Motor Co. offers basic reading courses at 25 plants.
- In 1981, Pratt and Whitney instituted an in-house general education program to enable employees to obtain high-school equivalency diplomas.
- Texas Instruments reimburses tuition costs for 4,000–5,000 employees per semester, some of whom take very basic learning classes.
- New York Telephone funds a large-scale program to boost the education of barely literate employees to ninth- and tenth-grade levels.
- Aetna Life and Casualty and United Technologies have employees tutor coworkers on a one-to-one basis.

- Standard Oil Co. in Indiana hired a former schoolteacher to conduct classes in grammar and spelling to newly hired secretaries.
- Nabisco Brands offers 4 hours of elementary-school courses each week, on company time, to employees at its Virginia factory.
- Polaroid targets 500 to 750 employees annually for remedial programs, which also include teaching English to immigrants.

The issue is squarely one of economics for all interested parties. The direct cost to American business for illiterate employees is at least

> 20 billion a year in lost profits, lowered productivity, reduced international competitiveness, reduced promotability, and increased remedial training. Moreover, as machinery increases in sophistication and as technical manuals become essential reading for industrial technicians, labor unions, as well, are including training, and in particular literacy training, in their negotiable collective bargaining agendas. (Goddard, 1987)

The final two issues to be discussed within the domain of education are studies that have addressed the relationship between level of education, organizational commitment, and worker satisfaction. As has been previously noted, a major factor that influenced the trend toward rising educational levels in the workforce in the 1970s was the belief that the more formal education people have, the more likely they are to obtain rewarding and satisfying jobs. In like manner, one of the alleged consequences of underemployment has been viewed as work dissatisfaction (Blumberg & Murtha, 1977; O'Toole, 1977; Westley & Westley, 1971). This argument is based on the notion that education tends to increase work expectations that cannot be met by low-level jobs and therefore contributes to dissatisfaction with work (Glenn & Weaver, 1982a,b). Thus it appears that education may have either a positive or negative effect on work satisfaction (Gruneberg, 1980; Glenn & Weaver, 1982a,b; King, Murry & Atkinson, 1982; Quinn & Mandilovitch, 1975).

In an effort to elucidate highly complex and inconsistently reported relationships between education and overall work satisfaction, Mottaz (1984) looked at data on 1,385 workers representing a variety of occupational groups from a midwestern metropolitan area (previously described in this chapter). Questionnaires were distributed on which these workers were to respond to questions concerning work satisfaction, intrinsic task factors (task autonomy, task significance, and task involvement), extrinsic social and policy factors (supervisory and coworker assistance, adequate working conditions, pay equity, promotional opportunity, and adequate fringe benefits), work values, and demographic characteristics. Results from a 74% response rate were analyzed and led to the following conclusion: (1) For both sexes, the more educated worker tends to assign greater weight to task significance and task involvement than does the less educated worker, (2) For workers in upper- and lower-level occupations, impact of education on work-related values is much greater in the former (upper-level occupations) than in the latter, (3) The effect of education on work rewards is considerably stronger and more pervasive in upper-level than in lower-level occupations, (4) Intrinsic work rewards are by far the most powerful predictors of overall work satisfaction. That is, it is primarily the nature of the task itself that determines one's attitude toward work, (5) Education may thus increase work satisfaction by increasing the availability of intrinsic work rewards, (6) However, level of education seems to have little effect on extrinsic returns. These findings led Mottaz to conclude tentatively that "education which does not lead to intrinsic rewards may diminish work satisfaction through its effect of increasing the value assigned to these rewards. Thus, for workers who report equal levels of intrinsic rewards, work satisfaction tends to be considerably lower among the better (educated) workers" (p. 1,001).

As a final note, in a later publication that reported the results of a parallel study to examine the relationship between level of education and organizational commitment, Mottaz (1986) wrote:

> Taken together, the data suggest that in both upper and lower level occupational categories the positive effect of education on organizational commitment is, for the most part, indirect through intrinsic work rewards. The apparent reason for this finding is that education tends to significantly increase intrinsic rewards and intrinsic rewards are the major determinants of organizational commitment. The data additionally indicate that the effect of education on commitment becomes negative only when intrinsic rewards are held constant. (p. 224)

Gender

Although it is recognized that there are indeed two sexes, this discussion will purposely have as its focus the meaning of work as measured by its impact upon women. The reasons for this are several. First, by the year 2000, 90% of the national work force will be comprised of women and minorities; women will represent 47% of the labor force. Second, at the present time, 55.9% of all women in the United States are in the civilian labor force, and of those women with infants less than 1 year old, nearly half are employed (Green & Epstein, 1988). Third, an analysis of women's employment by multinationals involved in manufacturing for export in the Third World has established that women constitute an overwhelming proportion of those employed in the unskilled and manual labor positions. These unskilled labor jobs represent 90% of the total employment generated by such Third World industrial investments (Pineda-Ofreneo, 1984). Reasons for this differential preference for women as "cheap labor" when there is a surplus labor pool of both sexes are complex. According to Person (1988), the factors of lower wages and higher productivity levels appear to contribute to the employment of women in both traditional and new technology industries in spite of the unequivocal existence of unemployed male labor in the Third World.

Austin (1984) has argued that basic work motivation is the same for men and women but that they make different choices because their early socialization experiences and structural opportunities are different. Before examining evidence to support this premise, it is first necessary to briefly review the historical context in which society's view of women has served to diminish an understanding of the meaning of work and its impact upon the lives of women.

The reader is referred to an excellent review by Scott (1987) on women workers in the discourse of French political economy, 1840–1860. In this work Scott contrasts the writing of Jules Simon, a political economist who wrote the book *L'Ouvriere* in 1860 and the writings of Julie-Victoire Daubie whose book was published in 1866 under the title, *La Femme Pauvre au XIXe siecle*. The economist and the feminist, while writing, ostensibly about women's manual labor, were also dealing with questions of order and justice. Scott (1987) wrote:

In effect, Simon and Daubie simply reversed the emphasis of earlier constructions, making explicit what had before been implicit (that modest women and
good mothers were the antitheses of prostitutes, that discipline and domestic
order were the opposite of misery). The effect on representations of women
workers was striking: they were now portrayed more often as victims torn by
economic necessity (misery) from their "natural" labour as mothers and wives,
or from the work and workplaces appropriate to their sex. . . . The differences of
argument and intention between them were crucial, but the similarities were
also revealing. In both cases discussions of women workers converged on the
question of motherhood, viewed as the defining quality or characteristic of
femininity. (pp. 133–134)

In the words of Simon, "The woman who becomes a worker is no longer a
woman. . . . All material improvements will be welcome, but if you want to
improve the condition of women workers and at the same time guarantee order . . .
do not separate children from their mothers" (Scott, 1987, pp. 134, 136). At stake
was the essence of femininity; wage earning was not harmful as long as it did not
detract women from their "natural vocation." The social values of women did not
derive from their roles as wage earners but rather from their duty to exemplify and
enforce family morality.

On the other hand, Daubie addressed as separate issues what for Simon and
others had been inherently contradictory concepts: wage labor and motherhood.
According to Daubie, the problem of women's poverty was due to the monopoly by
men of previously all-female trades or of trades suitable for women and the
selfishness of men. Scott quotes Daubie:

I have searched in vain for man's duty in social organizations; I have found only
his right to the unlimited liberty to oppress. That, if I am not mistaken, is the
node of all questions of work and political economy. (p. 139)

Equality for women in the workplace for Daubie would not eradicate sexual
differences but would allow women to protect themselves. She advocated equal
access to jobs to break the unjustified male monopolies, equal pay to enable
women to support themselves without depending upon men and thus be sexually
vulnerable to them, and legal rights for women to enable them to force seducers to
acknowledge paternity and recalcitrant husbands to recognize their financial
obligations to their families (Scott, 1987).

Thus it can be seen that early on the meaning of work for women, at least in
Western civilization, has been historically tied to the institutions of the family and
of education. For it is in these institutions that the early socialization process occurs
and also in these arenas that the structure of opportunity or lack thereof is
reinforced.

After an extensive review of the literature on the subject of socialization, Fox
and Hesse-Biber (1984) concluded that:

Of all the groups that socialize the sexes for different roles, two of the most
important institutions are the family and the school. Almost immediately after
birth, parents sex-type their children and respond differently to boys and girls.
They regard daughters as softer, quieter, and more delicate, and sons as
stronger, bolder, and more active. This brings us then to the long-debated
argument over origin of sex differences as a function of: (1) nature or biology, or

(2) nurture or experience. From our examination of these major perspectives, we conclude that biological differences between the sexes are just a starting point in the development of sex-role differences and their occupational consequences. Biology may influence certain tendencies, but these differences are strengthened by the social environment of the child. In addition, the "cognitive perspective" on development stresses that the children themselves play an active part in their development by selecting, organizing, and acting on the messages they receive about sex-appropriate and sex-inappropriate behavior and occupational roles.

The family is the earliest socializing experience. But the schools join in and, in certain ways, intensify the process of socializing males and females and influencing their occupational outcomes. The schools influence the destinies of females compared to males through a variety of social arrangements and processes, including:

1. The segregation, tracking, and funneling of boys and girls into different groups, activities, classes, and courses.
2. The imagery of books, texts, and readers depicting boys and men as the doers, goers, and makers of ideas, places, and things, and women and girls as spiritless observers.
3. The schools' structure of power and authority in which children see males in superordinate and females in subordinate positions.
4. The teachers' preference for male students in spite of girls' good behavior; and teachers' more active interaction with boys, not just in reprimands, but also in instruction, careful listening, and opportunities for response.
5. The guidance staff's covert and overt reinforcement of traditional cultural definitions of masculinity and femininity.

Each of these educational processes and arrangements operate toward the following final outcomes. First, they lower women's esteem and depress confidence so that as they progress through school, girls become less confident about their accomplishments and the adequacy of their whole gender group. Second, they form self-defeating attributions of success and failure. Third, they inhibit the development of growth and potential so that between adolescence and adulthood, when men's I.Q.'s are still rising, women are making few gains. Fourth, they restrict development, particularly, of the mathematical, technical, and scientific skills on which are based 75 percent of the majors in higher education, and 75 percent of all well-paying jobs. (pp. 67–68)

To further substantiate Fox and Hesse-Biber's findings, Fitzgerald and Betz (1983), in presenting a rationale for the study of women's career development, pointed out that clear sex differences exist that are relevant to vocational choices and patterns exhibited by women. Among these differences are the relatively restricted range of occupations pursued by women in contrast to the range pursued by men, the continuance of stereotypic career aspirations in young women (Matthews & Rodin, 1989), and the fact that women's intellectual capacities and talents are not reflected in their educational and occupational achievements in comparison to their male peer group. Fitzgerald and Betz (1983) cite Terman and Oden's 1959 follow-up study of gifted California children.

The follow-up study of the gifted group at midlife indicated that, as expected, the great majority of men had achieved prominence in professional and managerial occupations. They had, by their mid-40's, been exceptionally productive scientists, made literary and artistic contributions, and become prominent lawyers, physicians, and psychologists. In contrast to the men, the women were primarily housewives or were employed in the traditionally female occupations. About 50% of the women, in their mid-40s, were full-time housewives. Of those who were working full time, 21% were teachers in elementary or secondary school, 8% were social workers, 20% were secretaries, and 8% were either librarians or nurses. Only 7% of those working were academicians, 5% were physicians, lawyers, or psychologists, 8% were executives, and 9% were writers, artists or musicians. As children, these women had been as intellectually gifted as their male counterparts, but their achievements in adulthood were clearly in contrast to their early intellectual promise. Their sex was a better predictor of their occupational pursuits in adulthood than were their capabilities as individuals. (p. 87)

Fitzgerald and Betz (1983) concluded: "In terms of vocational theory, then, sex has been a far more powerful predictor of vocational role choices in women than have the other individual factors postulated as important in vocational theories focusing . . . on male career development" (p. 87).

Finally, relying on Austin's (1984) model, early socialization is not the only force that shapes work expectations in women. Indeed, in recent years accelerations in trends connected with the family, education, and work have occurred that have modified the structure of opportunities available to women. These environmental trends include (a) increased longevity and the need to plan for meaningful life activity over a longer timespan; (b) a declining birthrate, with the proportion of childless married women increasing from 24% to 41% between 1960 and 1974; (c) an increasing divorce rate wherein women can no longer afford to believe they will have their survival needs satisfied by someone else; (d) the proliferation of nontraditional lifestyles allowing for a multiplicity of social roles for both men and women that will of necessity transcend gender-differentiated occupational boundaries; (e) medical advances and reproductive technology giving women more control of their lives and bodies and the freedom to plan and prepare for their life's work; (f) the codification of women's rights helping to assure greater equality of opportunity for women in the workplace; and (g) changes in the nation's economy that have necessitated dual-income families and redistribution in some cases of the traditional "breadwinner" role.

In the words of Austin (1984):

> In summary, then, recent sociostructural trends have reduced the barriers that women faced in trying to pursue careers (in the form of paid employment) and have increased the career options available to them. Thus, changes in the structure of opportunity have led to modifications in the work expectations of women that were initially shaped by their socialization experiences and early perceptions of the opportunity structure. (p. 124)

In conclusion, although many women today work primarily because the family needs the money and secondarily for their own personal actualization (Scarr, Philips, & McCartney, 1989), it is also true that most women would not leave their paid employment even if the family did not need the money (DeChick, 1988). The preponderance of married women with children in the workplace has led to numerous studies concerned with marital relationships and child development. National concerns about the possible ill-effects of maternal employment on the development of children are extremely reminiscent of the writings in nineteenth century France of Jules Simon rather than Julie Daubie. However, it is the words of a twentieth-century female researcher that appear to be most appropriate as we conclude this discussion on the meaning of work in the context of gender.

> All in all, the question of what effects (if any) maternal employment has on children is not a productive one because it ignores the many contextual features of family life that moderate the effects of maternal employment (Grossman, Pollack, and Golding, 1988). We do know that the straighforward results of bad emotional, social, and intellectual outcomes for children of working mothers were not found, but no research can rule out yet unstudied subtleties. All we know is that the school achievement, IQ test scores, and emotional and social development of working mothers' children are every bit as good as that of children whose mothers do not work." (Scarr, 1984, p. 25)

THE FUTURE OF WORK

> The world has not just "turned upside down." It is turning every which way at an accelerating pace. (Peters, 1987, p. 45)

In times of turbulence, future projections can be risky; this is especially true when a multitude of variables are involved. Economics, changing social values, technological innovation, and regulatory influences interact reciprocally at local, national, and global levels to influence the future of work. In this section, the future of work from both micro- and macroperspectives will be addressed, exploring specific projections for employment growth into the next century, as well as broader, more ambitious scenarios that envision dramatic transformations of the character of work in the postindustrial age.

Maccoby (1988) argues that changes spurred by global competition, advances in information and telecommunication technology, and deregulation require business to change from traditional bureaucratic-industrial heirarchies to a "technoservice" game, defined as

> **technoservice** n. (fr. *techno*, a combining form from from the Greek *techne* meaning *art, skill, craft*, and the modern *technology*, industrial science or systematic knowledge of the industrial arts, and *service*, fr. OF *servise*, service, fr. L. *servitium* meaning labor for the benefit of another)
>
> 1. The use of systematic knowledge and information-communications technology for the benefit of customers and clients.
> 2. The most advanced way of working at the end of the twentieth century, brought about by international competition, and information and communications technology. Technoservice is characterized by customizing products and services for customers and clients both internal and external to the organization. Technoservice organization is characterized by networks and teams; flexible work roles with authority based on competence and knowledge; flat hierarchy, front-line freedom and responsibility to make decisions to satisfy customers and adapt to different conditions; work measurements based on customer satisfaction and profitability; management as strategic planning; and leadership that develops a motivating corporate culture which supports teamwork. Ant: standardized work, mass production, industrial bureaucracy. (p. 21)

According to *US News and World Report*, "The 1990s will offer . . . less job security, but they will distinctly enrich . . . job possibilities" ("Best Jobs," 1989, p. 60). Five major trends are delineated that are predicted to shape the future of work:

1. Small Start Ups—Small business (i.e., 100 or less employees) will continue to create more new jobs than big corporations. Females will launch more than half of the new small businesses.
2. Aging Population—With the "graying of the workforce" (Work in America Institute, 1980) it is projected that there will be growth in many industries, such as travel, recreation, health care, personal services, retailing, food services, and law. Indeed, by the year 2010, a deluge of new retirees from the baby boom generation will cause elder care to surpass child care as a national priority and potential career market ("Best Jobs," 1989, p. 61).
3. Advancing Technology—Since 1980, automation has eliminated two thirds of all assembly line jobs in the United States but the development of new jobs is projected to outpace the elimination of old ones as new employment opportunities are created to keep pace with technological advances (Cetron & Davies, 1989; Cyert & Mowery, 1989).
4. Foreign Competition—Peters (1987) has strongly recommended that American business go international or risk decline. The globe continues to shrink as a result of technology and communication. This translates into opportunity for knowledgeable people fluent in foreign language and culture, as overseas offices expand. The economic unification of the European continent, scheduled to occur in 1992, will have particular effect on American business ("Suddenly, High Tech," 1990).
5. Skills Gap—Purely as a function of population demographics, there is already a shortage of young people entering the workforce. This should increase entry level wages for less desirable jobs, but compensation will likely not meet requirements necessary to support a family. It has also been projected that the need for many new and expanding jobs will outstrip the number of qualified persons to fill them ("Best Jobs," 1989). The result will be that many middle-level technical jobs will go unfilled—partly as a function of demographics, and partly due to the presence of unemployable persons who have chosen a "nonwork" lifestyle (Lefkowitz, 1979) or who have been simply left behind due to lack of education, illiteracy, or significant impairment which renders them unemployable (e.g., drug habit, prison record, poor health, or in combination).

Of the 20 occupations projected by U.S. Department of Labor (1990) to have the greatest percentage increase in the next 10 years, every one is in the service sector. Examples of occupations with the greatest projected growth rates are paralegal, 75%; medical assistant, 70%; home health aide, 68%; radiology technician, 66%; computer technician, 61%; medical records technician, 60%; and medical secretary, 58%. The decline in manufacturing jobs has been dramatic. Seventy-five percent of Americans are now presently employed in the service sector of the American economy (Peters, 1987).

Various business writers have advocated a "smaller is better" philosophy, which, they argue, facilitates customer responsiveness, innovation, employee empowerment, and improved managerial leadership, not to mention the enhance-ment of quality and productivity (Emery, 1985; Peters, 1987; Zemke & Schaaf, 1989). Even within large corporations, breaking down large workforces into smaller, relatively autonomous "teams" seems to be the trend of the future. Technical progress has eroded "economy of scale" advantages that previously forced masses of workers into mammoth factories (Kolodny & Stjernberg, 1986). Moreover, business forecasters project that the greatest employment growth will continue to be generated in small (i.e., less than 100 employees) businesses.

Thus it is fair to project that the future will not be characterized by bigger business and larger factories, but in smaller, tighter businesses and/or industrial enclaves, which allow individual employees to have greater autonomy and control over their employment situation. But greater responsibility will mean the need for greater skills on the part of each individual employee. Employees will need to be more self-reliant, resourceful, better trained/educated, and more tolerant of ambi-guity (Mohrman & Mitroff, 1987). They will need to build teams, develop support, and create adaptive alliances in order to compete (Maccoby, 1988). Thus predictions that the workforce of the future will need to be more highly educated and resilient would certainly appear to be true.

Broader Scenarios

A most ambitious discussion of the future of work has been compiled by Robertson (1985) who described three differing views of work in the "postindus-trial society." They are "Business As Usual," "Hyper-Expansionist" (HE), and "Sane, Humane, Ecological" (SHE). "Business As Usual" assumes that there will be no real differences from the current industrial society of today. That is, full employment is pursued; housework, child raising, volunteer work, and the like are considered to be lesser status activities. Also, there are sharp value distinctions drawn between work and leisure (work is more desirable), social status depends upon occupation, and those who do not work are devalued.

HE and SHE represent contrasting visions of a postindustrial society. Both recognize that full employment will never be restored. HE is described as "super-industrial . . . based on big science, big technology and expert know-how" (Robert-son, 1985, p. 4). HE features the presence of a technocratic elite who will have access to state-of-the-art technology and the advanced skills required to generate the bulk of required work. The remainder of the population will be involved primarily in consumption and leisure activities. The skilled working elite would be highly paid, with others receiving a reasonable, but unspecified, subsistence stipend from the government.

SHE represents a more desirable, albeit utopian, change in direction, charac-terized by psychological and social breakthroughs. Under the SHE vision, work would be essentially redefined to include all forms of contribution to the common good, whether paid or unpaid. Individuals would exercise choice in engaging in activities of relatively equal perceived value. "Ownwork" would not be limited to specific locations or ages or hours. Finally, some sort of guaranteed basic income (GBI) would be provided to all, and those who do not need it because of other earnings would have it taxed back.

Robertson (1985, p. 5) delineates contrasting values and tendencies characteris-tic of the HE and SHE visions:

HE	SHE
Quantitative values and goals	Qualitative values and goals
Economic growth	Human development
Organizational values and goals	Personal and interpersonal values and goals
Money values	Real needs and aspirations
Contractual relationships	Mutual exchange relationships
Intellectual, rational, detached	Intuitive, experiential, empathetic
Masculine priorities	Feminine priorities
Specialization/helplessness	All-round competence
Technocracy/dependence	Self-reliance
Centralizing	Local
Urban	Countrywide
European	Planetary
Anthropocentric	Ecological

Related to this, Lefkowitz (1979) suggests that there has been a profound shift in American work values, to the point that not working (i.e., "nonwork") has become acceptable and even desirable in the minds of many Americans. Lefkowitz (1979) interviewed 100 individuals, who had chosen not to work, from different social classes, backgrounds, and work histories. He concluded that the American work ethic has been significantly eroded, observing that people do not have to choose between work and the poorhouse. "Now they only have to decide whether or not working is worth a modest reduction in consumption" (p. 37). Unemployment is seen as "an opportunity to escape (p. 42) from tension, trivia, and boredom. "In an age of affluence, a person need not work to survive" (p. 48). According to Lefkowitz (1979):

> The details of economic survival vary from person to person. When husbands stop working, some wives start. College-age children are asked to go to work to help pay for tuition; or they are transferred to low-tuition public universities. Life insurance policies are cashed in. People barter services and material goods. They move to less expensive apartments or sell their houses and buy cheaper ones. They share their living quarters or live collectively. They may take temporary jobs when bills are due, or they may raise money in other more ingenious ways. (p. 160)

Similarly, Sherman (1986) describes "a quiet revolution" (p. 120) occurring in the workplace. He cites increases in part-time employment, job splitting, job sharing, flextime, shorter work weeks, short-term/fixed-term employment contracts, increased use of subcontracts, earlier retirement, expansion of holidays, and home work "telecommuting" to support his contention that the "changes have been sweeping" (p. 120). He also notes that such changes are not without cost and that flexibility on the part of both employers and employees will be increasingly important. Finally, he suggests that these changes require "statesmen and stateswomen of firm purpose and wide vision" (p. 141) to guide nations along this turbulent path.

A sample of legislation codifying this kind of change was the Family and Marital Leave Act that President Bush vetoed in June 1990. Note, however that

> many medium and large sized companies already have policies and half the states require them in limited form. Those firms that can afford the investment

often find it pays in the long run because it lead to happier more productive workers. ("Despite Bush, parental leave policies are here to stay," 1990, p. 19)

With or without formal/legal sanction, inevitable change will evolve along a contorted path, making Robertson's (1985) HE and SHE scenarios all the more plausible.

SUMMARY

The meaning of work cuts through and significantly defines the meaning of adult life in most of Western civilization. The values and behaviors associated with work are interwoven with the very fiber of individuals, cultures, and nations. Change, whether by evolution or revolution, that has an impact upon any one of these areas can profoundly affect the nature, role, and meaning of work, Historically, the meaning and character of work has been one of dynamic change determined, for each individual, to a great extent by a variety of interacting factors. These factors include internal variables, such as cultural and individual values, race, ethnicity, gender, age, education, and ability level. They also include external factors (e.g., economics, environmental concerns, resources available, regulatory influences, and politics). Thus work now and in the future in all societies will continue to reflect this complex dynamic interaction. However, some societal, political, and economic trends have become well established and will continue as dominant forces well into the twenty-first century, particularly for individuals who are members of Western society.

It is a relatively safe prediction to contend that there will be continued growth in health and service jobs well into the next several decades; that higher education and advanced skill levels will be directly correlated to higher pay; that openness to continuing education will be more important than ever for those already employed; that employers will become more involved in employee training and education; and that the number of women and minorities in the workforce will grow. In addition, it would appear that employers, in an effort to retain individuals from an ever-shrinking labor pool, will make increased efforts to provide employment settings in which employees find their work more satisfying and fulfilling. There is some evidence that society will extend greater tolerance and acceptance to persons who do not fill standard work roles (i.e., "nonworkers"). On the other hand, there is some reason to believe that the definition of work will continue to broaden and that government financial entitlements for those who do not hold "traditional" jobs will continue and expand.

Finally, there is sufficient evidence to support the contention that work, however narrowly or broadly defined, will continue its dominant role in the life of adults in Western society. Although beyond the limits of this discussion, one can surmise that as the globe continues to shrink, the impact of Western civilization, insofar as work is concerned, will begin to be felt in Third World countries as well. These are countries wherein, up until recent times, work has not been a dominant cultural value. Whether work will have the same significance in the twenty-first century that it acquired by way of the Protestant Reformation in the sixteenth century remains to be seen.

Alba, R. D., & Chamblin, M. B. (1983). A preliminary examination of ethnic identification among whites. *American Sociological Review*, 48(2), 240–247.

Amato, J. A. (1980). Social class discrimination in the schooling process: Myth and reality. *The Urban Review*, 12(3), 121–130.

Arbona, C. (1989). Hispanic employment and the Holland typology of work. *The Career Development Quarterly*, 37(3), 257–268.

Austin, H. S. (1984). The meaning of work in women's lives: A sociological model of career choice and work behavior. *Counseling Psychologist*, 12(4), 117–126.

Ballesteros, E. (1986). Do Hispanics receive an equal opportunity? The relationship of school outcomes, family background, and high school curriculum. In M. Olivas (Ed.), *Latino college students* (pp. 47–70). New York: Teachers College Press.

Baltes, P. B., Reese, H. W., & Lipsitt, L. P. (1980). Life development psychology. *Annual Review of Psychology*, 31, 65–110.

Best jobs for the future. (1989, September 25). *U.S. News and World Report*, pp. 60–72.

Blumberg, P., & Murtha, J. (1977). College graduates and the American dream. *Dissent*, 24, 45–53.

Brazelton, T. B. (1989). Interview. In B. Moyers (Ed.), *A World of Ideas* (pp. 140–155). New York: Doubleday.

Brenner, M. H. (1976). *Estimating the social costs of national economic policy: A study prepared for the Joint Economic Committee, U.S. Congress.*

Burtless, G. (1984). Manpower policies for disadvantaged: What works? *Brookings Review*, 3(1), 18–22.

Cahill, M., & Salomone, P. R. (1987). Career counseling for work life extension: Integrating the older worker into the labor force. *The Career Development Quarterly*, 35(3), 188–196.

Cain, G. G. (1984). The economics of discrimination: Part I. *Focus* (University of Wisconsin Institute for Research on Poverty) 7 (Summer), 1–11.

Cetron, M., & Davies, O. (1989). *American Renaissance.* New York: St. Martin's Press.

Coolidge, C. (1925, January 17). Address, Society of American Newspaper Editors.

Cyert, R. M., & Mowery, D. C. (1989). Technology, employment and US competitiveness. *Scientific American*, 260(5), 54–62.

DeChick, J. (1988, July 19). Most mothers want a job too. *USA Today*, p. D1.

Dement, E. F. (1982). *Results-oriented work experience programming.* Salt Lake City: Olympus Publishing.

Despite Bush, parental-leave policies are here to stay. (1990, July 2). *U.S. News and World Report*, p. 19.

Dresch, D. P. (1975). Demography, technology, and higher education: Towards a formal model of educational adaptation. *Journal of Political Economy*, 83(3), 535–569.

Droughton, M. (1975). Relationship between economic decline and mental hospital admissions continues to be significant. *Psychological Reports*, 36, 882.

Education Commission of the States. (1985). *Reconnecting youth: The next stage of reform.* Denver: Author.

Emery, F. (1985). Public policies for healthy workplaces. *Human Relations*, 38(11), 1013–1022.

Erikson, E. H. (1963). *Childhood and society* (2nd ed.). New York: Norton.

Fitzgerald, L. R., & Betz, N. E. (1983). Issues in the vocational psychology of women. In W. B. Walsh & S. H. Osipow (Eds.), *Handbook of vocational psychology* (Vol. I, pp. 83–159). Hillsdale, NJ: Erlbaum.

Fligstein, N., & Fernandez, R. M. (1985). Educational, transitions of Whites and Mexican-Americans. In G. J. Borjas & M. Tienda (Eds.), *Hispanics in the U.S. economy* (pp. 161–192). Orlando, FL: Academic Press.

Foner, N., & Napolic, R. (1978). Jamaican and black-American migrant farm workers: A comparative analysis. *Social Problems*, 25(5), 491–503.

Fox, A (1976). *Work status and income change, 1968–1972: Retirement history study preview.* Report no. 10, DHEW Publication No. (SSA) 76–11700.

Fox, M. F., & Hesse-Biber, S. (1984). *Women at work.* Palo Alto, CA: Mayfield.

Freeman, R. (1975). Overinvestment in college training. *Journal of Human Resources*, 10(3), 287–311.

Freeman, R. (1976). *The overeducated American.* New York: Academic Press.

Freeman, R. (1977). The decline in economic rewards to college education. *Review of Economics and Statistics*, 59(1), 18–29.

Freeman, R. (1980). The facts about the declining economic value of college. *Journal of Human Resources*, 15(1), 124–142.

Galper, H., & Dunn, R. H. (1969). A short-run demand function for higher education in the U.S. *Journal of Political Economy*, 77(5), 765–777.

Ginzberg, E. (1981). *The school/work nexus: Transition of youth from school to work.* New York: Phi Delta Kappa Educational Foundation.

Glenn, N., & Weaver, C. (1982a). Enjoyment of work by full-time workers in the United States, 1955 and 1980. *Public Opinion Quarterly, 46,* 459–470.

Glenn, N., & Weaver, C. (1982b). Further evidence on education and job satisfaction. *Social Forces, 61*(1), 46–55.

Goddard, R. W. (1987). The crisis in workplace literacy. *Personnel Journal, 66*(12), 72–81.

Gottfredson, L. S. (1978). An analytical description of employment according to race, sex, prestige, and Holland type of work. *Journal of Vocational Behavior, 13*(2), 210–221.

Gottfredson, G. D., & Gaiger, D. C. (1977). Using a classification of occupations to describe age, sex, and time differences in employment patterns. *Journal of Vocational Behavior, 10*(2), 121–138.

Green, G. P., & Epstein, R. K. (Eds.). (1988). *Employment and earnings* (Vol. 35(2)). Washington, DC: U.S. Department of Labor, Bureau of Labor Statistics.

Greenberger, E., & Steinberg, L. D. (1986). *When teenagers work.* New York: Basic Books.

Grossman, F. K., Pollack, W. S., & Golding, E. (1988). Fathers and children: Predicting the quality and quantity of fathering. *Developmental Psychology, 24*(1), 82–91.

Gruneberg, M. (1980). The happy worker: An analysis of educational and occupational differences in determinants of job satisfaction. *American Journal of Sociology, 86*(2), 247–271.

Gurney, R. (1980). Does unemployment affect the self-esteem of school leavers? *Australian Journal of Psychology, 32,* 175–182.

Hall, R. H. (1986). *Dimensions of work.* Beverly Hills, CA: Sage Publications.

Harpaz, I. (1985). Meaning of working profiles of various occupational groups. *Journal of Vocational Behavior, 26*(1), 25–40.

Harris, L. (1979). *1979 study of American attitudes towards pension and retirement.* New York: Johnson and Higgins.

Hauser, R. M., & Featherman, D. L. (1977). *The process of stratification: Trends and analyses.* New York: Academic Press.

Hofstede, G. (1980). *Culture's consequences: International differences in work-related values.* Beverly Hill, CA and London: Sage Publications.

Hofstede, G. (1984). The cultural relativity of the quality of life concept. *Academy of Management Review, 9*(3), 389–398.

Holland, J. L. (1985). *Making vocational choices: A theory of vocational personalities and work environments.* Englewood Cliffs, NJ: Prentice-Hall.

Hsia, J. (1980, September). *Cognitive assessment of Asian Americans.* Paper presented at the National Institute of Education—National Center for Bilingual Research Symposium on Bilingual Research at Los Alamitos, CA.

Jacobson, B. (1980). *Younger programs for older workers: Case studies in personnel policies.* New York: Van Nostrand Reinhold.

Janson, P., & Martin, J. K. (1982). Job satisfaction and age: A test of two views. *Social Forces, 60*(4), 1089–1102.

Jones, R. C. (1984). Changing patterns of undocumented Mexican migration to south Texas. *Social Science Quarterly, 65*(2), 465–481.

Kalleberg, A. L. (1977). Work values and job rewards: A theory of job satisfaction. *American Sociological Review, 42*(1), 124–143.

Kalleberg, A. L., & Loscocco, K. A. (1983). Aging, values, and rewards: Explaining age differences in job satisfaction. *American Sociolgical Review, 48*(1), 78–90.

Kaufman, R. L. (1983). A structural decomposition of black-white earnings differential. *American Journal of Sociology, 89*(3), 585–611.

King, M., Murry, M., & Atkinson, T. (1982). Background, personality, job characteristics, and satisfaction with work in a national sample. *Human Relations, 35*(2), 119–133.

Kolodny, H., & Stjernberg, T. (1986). The change process of innovative work designs: New design and redesign in Sweden, Canada, and the US. *Journal of Applied Behavioral Science, 22*(3), 287–301.

Lefkowitz, B. (1979). *Breaktime: Living without work in a nine to five world.* New York: Hawthorne Books.

Leigh, D. E. (1978). Racial discrimination and labor unions: Evidence from the NLS sample of middle-aged men. *Journal of Human Resources, 13*(4), 568–577.

Leong, T. L. (1985). Career development of Asian Americans. *Journal of College Student Personnel, 26*(6), 539–546.

Lieberson, S. (1980). *A piece of the pie: Black and white immigrants since 1880.* Berkeley: University of California Press.

Maccoby, M. (1988). *Why work: Leading the new generation*. New York: Simon & Schuster.

Manpower Demonstration Research Corporation Summary and Findings of the National Supported Work Demonstration. (1980). Cambridge: MA: Ballinger.

Maslow, A. H. (1954). *Motivation and personality*. New York: Harper & Row.

Matthews, K. A., & Rodin, J. (1989). Women's changing work roles. *American Psychologist*, 44(11), 1389–1393.

McClelland, D. C. (1961). *The achieving society*. New York: Van Nostrand Reinhold.

Merton, R. K. (1957). The role-set: Problems in sociological theory. *British Journal of Sociology*, 8, 106–120.

Miller, D. C., & Form, W. (1964). *Industrial sociology*. New York: Harper & Row.

Minatoya, L. Y., & Sedlacek, W. E. (1981). Another look at the melting pot: Perceptions of Asian American undergraduates. *Journal of College Student Personnel*, 22(4), 328–336.

Mohran, S. A., & Mitroff, I. A. (1987, June). Business not as usual. *Training and Development Journal*, pp. 37–43.

Moore, W. E. (1969). Occupational socialization. In D. A. Goslin (Ed.), *Handbook of socialization theory and research* (pp. 861–883). Chicago: Rand McNally.

Morrison, M. H. (1979). International development in retirement flexibility. *Aging and Work*, II(Fall), 221–233.

Morrison, M. H. (1986). Work and retirement in an aging society. *Daedalus*, 115(1), 269–293.

Mottaz, C. J. (1984). Education and work satisfaction. *Human Relations*, 37(11), 985–1004.

Mottaz, C. (1985). The relative importance of intrinsic and extrinsic rewards as determinants of work satisfaction. *The Sociological Quarterly*, 26(3), 365–385.

Mottaz, C. J. (1986). An analysis of the relationship between education and organizational commitment in a variety of occupational groups. *Journal of Vocational Behavior*, 28(3), 214–228.

Mottaz, C. J. (1988). Determinants of organizational commitment. *Human Relations*, 41(6), 467–482.

MOW International Research Team. (1981). The meaning of working. In G. Dlugos & K. Weiermair (Eds.), *Management under different value systems: Political, social and economical perspectives in a changing world* (pp. 565–630). Berlin/New York: de Gruyter.

National Academy of Sciences, Panel on Secondary School Education for the Changing Workplace. (1984). *High school and the changing workplace, the employers' view*. Washington, DC: National Academy Press.

Ogbu, J. U. (1974). *The next generation: An ethnography of education in an urban neighborhood*. New York: Academic Press.

Ogbu, J. U. (1989). Cultural boundaries and minority youth orientation. In D. Stern & D. Eichorn (Eds.), *Adolescence and work: Influences of social structure, labor markets, and culture* (pp. 101–136). Hillsdale, NJ: Erlbaum.

O'Reilly, C. A., III, & Caldwell, D. F. (1980). Job choice: The impact of intrinsic and extrinsic factors on subsequent satisfaction and commitment. *Journal of Applied Psychology*, 65(5), 559–565.

Orum, L. S. (1986). *The education of Hispanics: Status and implications*. Washington, DC: National Council of La Raza.

Osterman, P. (1989). The job market for adolescents. In D. Stein & E. Eichorn (Eds.), *Adolescence and work: Influences of social structure, labor markets, and culture* (pp. 235–256). Hillsdale, NJ: Erlbaum.

O'Toole, J. (1977). *Working, learning, and the American future*. San Francisco: Jossey-Bass.

Palmore, E. B., & Stone, V. (1973). Predictors of longevity: A follow-up of the aged in Chapel Hill. *The Gerontologist*, 13(1), 88–90.

Person, R. (1988). Female workers in the First and Third Worlds: The Greenery of Women's Labor. In R. E. Pahl (Ed.), *On Work: Historical, Comparative, and Theoretical Approaches* (pp. 449–466). New York: Basil Blackwell.

Peters, T. (1987). *Thriving on chaos*. New York: Knopf.

Pine, G. J., & Innis, G. (1987). Cultural and individual work values. *The Career Development Quarterly*, 35(4), 279–285.

Pineda-Ofreneo, R. (1984). Subcontracting in export-oriented industries: Impact on Filipino working women. In I. Nortrund, P. Wad, & V. Bruin, *Industrialisation and the Labour Process in Southeast Asia*. Papers from the 1983 Copenhagen Conference, Repro Serie no. 6, Institute of Cultural Sociology, University of Copenhagen.

Porter, L. W., Crampom, W. J., & Smith, F. J. (1976). Organizational commitment and managerial turnover: A longitudinal study. *Organizational Behavior and Human Performance*, 15(1), 87–98.

Portes, A. (1984). The rise of ethnicity: Determinants of ethnic perceptions among Cuban exiles in Miami. *American Sociological Review*, 49(June), 383–397.

Priorities. (1990, April 5). *Newsweek*, p. 5.

Quinn, R. P., & Cobb, W. (1971). *What workers want: Factor analysis of importance ratings of job facets*. Ann Arbor: University of Michigan, Survey Research Center.

Quinn, R., & Mandilovitch, M. (1975). *Education and job satisfaction: A questionable payoff*. Ann Arbor: Survey Research Center University of Michigan.

Quinn, R. P., Staines, G. L., & McCullough, M. R. (1974). *Job satisfaction: Is there a trend?* Washington, DC: U.S. Department of Labor.

Rabinowitz, S., & Hall, D. T. (1977). Organizational research on job involvement. *Psychological Bulletin, 84*(2), 265–288.

Rettig, J. L. (1982, June). On the meaning of work. *NSPI Journal, 22*–23.

Robertson, J. (1985). *Future work*. London: Gower Publishing.

Rokeach, M. (1968). A theory of organization and change within value-attitude systems. *Journal of Social Issues, 24*(1), 13–33.

Rosenberg, M. (1987). *Occupations and values*. Glencoe, IL: Free Press.

Rosenblum, M., & Sheppard, H. L. (1977). *Jobs for older workers in U.S. industry: Possibilities and prospects*. Washington, DC: American Institute for Research.

Rumberger, R. W. (1980). The economic decline in college graduates: Fact or fallacy? *Journal of Human Resources, 15*(1), 99–112.

Sayers, S. (1988). The need to work: A perspective from philosophy. In R. E. Pahl (Ed.), *On work: Historical, comparative, and theoretical approaches* (pp. 722–752). Cambridge, MA: Basil Blackwell.

Scarr, S. (1984). Mother care/other care. New York: Basic Books.

Scarr, S., Phillips, D., & McCartney, K. (1989). Working mothers and their families. *American Psychologist, 44*(11), 1402–1409.

Schaie, K. W. (1974). Transitions in gerontology: From lab to life. *American Psychologist, 29*, 802–807.

Schnall, M. (1981). *Limits: A search for new values*. New York: Clarkson N. Potter.

Scott, J. W. (1987). 'L'ouvriere! Mot impie, sordide. . .': women workers in the discourse of French political economy, 1840–1860. In P. Joyce (Ed.), *The historical meaning of work* (pp. 119–142). Cambridge: Cambridge University Press.

Sheldon, A., McEwan, P. J., & Ryser, C. P. (1975). *Retirement: Patterns and predictions*. National Institute of Mental Health, DHEW Publication No. (ADM) 74–149.

Sheppard, H. L. (1977). *Research and development strategy on employment related problems of older workers*. Washington, DC: American Institute for Research.

Sherman, B. (1986). *Working at leisure*. London: Methuen.

Shkop, Y. M. (1982). The impact of job modification options on retirement plans. *Industrial Relations, 21*(2), 261–267.

Silvestri, G. T., & Lukasiewicz, J. M. (1985). Occupational employment projections: The 1984–95 outlook. *Monthly Labor Review, 108* (11), 42–57.

Smith, H. L. (1986). Overeducation and underemployment: An agnostic review. *Sociology of Education, 59*(2), 85–99.

Soumerai, S. B., & Avorn, J. (1983). Perceived health, life satisfaction, and activity in urban elderly: A controlled study of the impact of part-time work. *Journal of Gerontology, 38*(3), 356–362.

Stein, D., & Nakata, Y. (1989). Characteristics of high school students' paid jobs, and employment experience after graduation. In D. Stern & D. Eichorn (Eds.), *Adolescence and work: Influences of social structure, labor markets, and culture* (pp. 189–211). Hillsdale, NJ: Erlbaum.

Stern, D., & Eichorn, D. (1989). Overview. In D. Stern & D. Eichorn (Eds.), *Adolescence and work: Influences of social structure, labor markets, and culture* (pp. 1–12). Hillsdale, NJ: Erlbaum.

Suddenly, high tech is a three-way race. (1990, June 15). *Business Week*, pp. 118–123.

Sue, D. W., & Sue, S. (1972). Ethnic minorities: Resistance to being researched. *Professional Psychology, 3*(1), 11–17.

Sue, S., Sue, D. W., & Sue, D. (1975). Asian Americans as a minority group. *American Psychologist, 30*(Sept), 906–910.

Sue, S., & Wagner, N. (Eds.). (1973). *Asian Americans: Psychological perspectives*. Palo Alto, CA: Science and Behavior Books.

Sum, A. (1983, December). *Educational attainment, academic ability, and the employability and earnings of young persons*. Northeastern University.

Super, D. E. (1984). Leisure: What it is and might be. *Journal of Career Development, 11*(2), 71–80.

Taggart, R. (1981). *A fisherman's guide, an assessment of training and remediation strategies*. Kalamazoo, MI: Upjohn Institute.

Tausky, C. (1960). Meaning of work among blue collar men. *Pacific Sociological Review, 12*(1), 49–55.

Terman, L. M., & Oden, M. H. (1959). *Genetic studies of genius: V. The gifted group at midlife.* Stanford, CA: Stanford University Press.

The Face of Change (1989). An Environment Scan for the United Ways of Southwestern Pennsylvania. Pittsburgh: United Way.

Thompson, G. B. (1973). Work versus leisure roles: An investigation of morale among employed and retired men. *Journal of Gerontology, 28*(3), 339–344.

Thurow, L. C. (1974). Measuring the economic benefits of education. In M. S. Gordon (Ed.), *Higher education and the labor market* (pp. 373–418). New York: McGraw-Hill.

U.S. Bureau of the Census. (1981). *Statistical abstract.* Washington, DC: GPO.

U.S. Department of Labor (1990, January 29). Jobs for the year 2000. *U.S. News and World Report,* p. 62.

Vroom, V. H. (1962). Ego involvement, job satisfaction, and job performance. *Personnel Psychology, 15*(2), 159–177.

Walker, J. W., & Lazer, H. (1978). *The end of mandatory retirement: Implications for management.* New York: Wiley.

Westley, W., & Westley, M. (1971). *The emerging worker: Equality and conflict in the mass consumption society.* Montreal: McGill-Queen's University Press.

Wilson, K., & Porters, A. (1980). Immigration enclaves: An analysis of the labor market experiences of Cubans in Miami. *American Journal of Sociology, 86*(2), 295–313.

Wilson, W. J. (1978). *The declining significance of race.* Chicago: University of Chicago Press.

Winefield, A. H. (1989). Job loss vs. failure to find work as psychological stressors in the young unemployed. *Journal of Occupational Psychology, 62*(1), 79–85.

Winefield, A. H., & Tiggermann, M. (1985). Psychological correlates of employment and unemployment: Effects, predisposing factors and sex differences. *Journal of Occupational Psychology, 58*(3), 229–242.

Work in America Institute. (1980). *The future of older workers in America: New options for an extended work life.* Scarsdale, NY: Author.

Wright, J. D., & Hamilton, R. F. (1978). Work satisfaction and age: Some evidence for the 'job change' hypothesis. *Social Forces, 56*(4), 1140–1158.

Yankelovich, D. (1979). Work, values, and the new breed. In C. Kerr & J. M. Rosow (Eds.), *Work in America, the decade ahead* (pp. 3–26). New York: Van Nostrand.

Zemke, R., & Schaaf, D. (1989). *The service edge.* New York: New American Library.

18

Masculine Gender Role and Midlife Transition in Men

RICHARD M. EISLER AND KIM RAGSDALE

INTRODUCTION

Most studies of the human lifespan have focused on infancy, childhood, adolescence, and old age. The potential for developmental changes in adulthood has remained relatively uncharted. An exception to the relative absence of developmental perspective on adulthood has been the attention given to the midlife period. The object of study during midadulthood has typically been American men. From various theoretical perspectives, the middle adult years for men have been described as a time of reappraisal and inevitable turmoil, which has sometimes been called the midlife crisis. Whether the midlife period for men typically results in problems of sufficient intensity to label them a *crisis* has been difficult to document empirically.

For the present chapter, we plan to view middle adulthood as a developmental transition phase associated with certain age- and gender-related problems and stresses. Certainly, the biological changes associated with aging, increasing awareness of one's own mortality, the gap between early aspirations and present accomplishments, as well as important role changes powerfully impact both sexes during middle adulthood. The appraisal of these events and the evaluation of oneself in relation to these events is probably gender specific and quite different for men and women. Rather than attempt to look at these events for both men and women, the present chapter will focus primarily on the midlife transition in men.

RICHARD M. EISLER AND KIM RAGSDALE • Department of Psychology, Virginia Polytechnic Institute and State University, Blacksburg, Virginia 24061-0436.

Handbook of Social Development: A Lifespan Perspective, edited by Vincent B. Van Hasselt and Michel Hersen. Plenum Press, New York, 1992.

RICHARD M.
EISLER and KIM
RAGSDALE

In this chapter we seek to develop a theoretical perspective on the adult developmental midlife transition in men that focuses on the problems and tasks of midlife as they interact with masculine gender roles. In the first part of the chapter, we will review various theories of adult development that have something to contribute to our understanding of the period of middle adulthood. Additionally, we will review some of the major life events issues that have a high probability of being associated with this period. In the next section of the chapter, we wish to focus on male gender-role development and describe our conceptualization of masculine gender-role stress that we believe, in part, determines the difficulties that men will face as they age and the ways in which they will cope with these problems. Finally, we focus on how the issues of work and family relationships may be affected by masculine gender-role commitment during the midlife transition.

THEORETICAL MODELS OF MIDLIFE

When considering theories that address midlife one is confronted with great diversity. Each perspective offers unique explanations and salient issues that usher in this era of life. However, most theories of adult development share certain structural assumptions that make it possible to classify them. Most of these probably can be classified as either developmental "stage" theories (Lerner, 1986) or "life event" theories (George, 1982). Stage theories, reflecting their dynamic roots, propose qualitative or structural changes that occur in an invariant sequence or succession with cultural factors enhancing, or arresting, development, but not altering the sequence (Kohlberg), 1973). Some stage theorists, such as Levinson (1977) stress the link between specific chronological ages and the emergence of developmental periods, whereas others deny the importance of age in prompting developmental tasks. On the other hand, theories that emphasize the critical role of environmental events may be classified as "life event" theories (George, 1982). Life event theories do not necessarily deny the existence of stages but consider the nature and timing of "environmental" events to be most critical to development. Life event theories vary in the degree to which they emphasize an individual's subjective interpretation of an event. Stage versus life event theories are not conceptualized as pure types but are felt to reflect different degrees of focus on either intrapsychic factors or social and environmental factors in producing developmental changes.

Stage Theories

Stage theories of midlife have historically tended to focus on intrapsychic development reflecting the Freudian or neo-analytic derivations of many of their proponents. Although the environment is often acknowledged to play some role in development, primary focus centers on distinct intraindividual changes over time (Lerner, 1986). The stages are generally considered to be associated with age-linked social roles or maturational cycles that are to a large extent fixed by chronological age. Although stage theorists believe that environmental events may alter the stages, normal development inevitably involves certain experiences during specific periods of the lifespan.

We now turn to a more specific discussion of the proposals of four of the most well-known stage theorists: Erik Erikson, George Vaillant, Daniel Levinson, and Roger Gould. Erikson and Erikson (1981) proposed that "generativity" versus "stagnation" was the crucial developmental task that arose at midlife. During this period of adulthood, it was expected that a person would examine his accomplishments and then would wish to develop a major role in providing guidance to the younger generation. Thus a "normal" outcome of midlife reappraisal would be an increased interest in the larger community, with a corresponding decrease in self-absorption. Gould (1972, 1978), reflecting a Jungian perspective, proposed that people carry "childhood demons" of fear, anger, hatred, and "false assumptions" into adulthood. Developmental stages provide the opportunity to resolve the influence of these demons and false assumptions at a particular life stage. Thus at midlife one would have to challenge the false assumption of one's invincibility and ultimately face the reality of one's own mortality. This position is akin to that of Jacques (1965), who writes that at the prime period of life, a person's confrontation with the inevitably of death becomes a highly salient and very personal matter. This realization of the finiteness of one's life according to Jacques, results in major psychological disruption during midlife.

Vaillant (1977), in a longitudinal study of male Harvard University graduates, determined that there was a shift of emphasis from career to forming intimate relationships. Thus a conflict between work and intimacy would arise at this stage that could reactivate earlier adolescent conflicts over intimacy. Levinson, Darrow, Klein, Levinson, and McKee (1978), in their classic study of 40 midlife men, also placed heavy emphasis on the concept of universal age-determined life stages during which some variations may occur. Presumably these stages cycle alternatively between periods of relative calm and stability to periods of major upheaval and stress. Levinson (1977) has proposed that the midlife transitional period that ordinarily starts at about age 40, give or take 2 years, lasts about 4 to 6 years. During this period men must deal with various "polarities" described as young/old, destructive/creative, masculine/feminine, and attachment/separateness dichotomies. In addition, the degree of psychological upheaval during the midlife reappraisal depends on the man's perception of the adequacy of his previous vocational, family, and value commitments for the second half of his life.

Life Event Theories

Life event theories consider development to be a product of interaction between the person and environment, with emphasis placed on the role of the environment in fostering development. The quality of development is considered to be plastic, rather than on a relatively fixed maturational timetable. The theories of Neugarten (1976) and Lowenthal, Thurnher, and Chiriboga (1975) focus on changes in social status and role during the midlife transition.

Neugarten (1976) studied adults 40 to 70 years of age and found that this period was characterized by the restructuring of time left to live rather than time since birth. Also, she found a heightened sense of stock taking and reappraisal of one's accomplishments. Women's cues about middle age were defined in terms of events within the family cycle (e.g., the launching of children). On the other hand, men's cues were largely outside the family, including changes in work status. Men were also far more sensitive to changes in their biological functioning and health than women. In terms of gender-role changes, men seemed to become more receptive to affiliation and nurturance, whereas women became more able to express aggression and self-centeredness. Neugarten also noted that "social clocks" operate with respect to major life events, such as marriage, having children, and retirement. That is, most adults become aware of whether they are "late," "early," or "on time" with respect to familial or occupational events. Relatively greater disruption is caused should these events happen "off time" or be unanticipated. For example, the midlife baby is rarely received with the fondest anticipation. Finally, Neugarten discussed the social and class context in which events are perceived. For instance, an upper-middle-class man may not see himself as middle aged until age 50, whereas a working-class man may perceive himself to be middle aged at 40. The upper-middle-class man may see middle age as the most powerful productive period in his life, whereas the working class man may see middle age as marking a major decline in his life.

Placing more emphasis on the role of environmental events in development, Lowenthal *et al.* (1975) focused on the predictable sequence of changes in status and roles that occur during adult transitions. In a study of adults aged 20 through 70, he found that as men approached postparenthood they seemed absorbed in work-related problems, although some were remorseful that they had not achieved greater ties with their children or wives. During the next 5 years, however, they seemed to develop greater comfort and ease with themselves. Similar to the findings of Neugarten (1976), Lowenthal (1977) found as men moved through the midlife transition they tended to decrease their aggressive coping styles and move toward more nurturant, sensual, and affiliative coping styles.

Is There a Midlife Crisis?

Defining the midlife period and the problems associated with it elicits little agreement about precisely when it is, or how severe the problems associated with it are from those who have written most extensively about middle age. Levinson (1977) gives us the most narrow time frame for this stage, including ages 40 through 43, give or take a few years. McGill (1980) has proposed a 40 to 60 agespan, Neugarten (1976), designates 35 to 45, and Brim (1976) uses 40 to 50, just to name a few possibilities. Whether midlife is a time of crisis, maladaptive coping reactions, healthy changes, or really any different than any other time of life also appears controversial. Evidence bearing on these issues come from a variety of sources, including clinical case studies, field studies, and longitudinal research.

There is a fair amount of evidence to support the view that entrance into middle age is often associated with certain kinds of stresses and maladaptive coping patterns. In a review of studies on the incidence and prevalence of psychological problems in middle-aged men, Rosenberg and Farrell (1976) found evidence for decreased marital satisfaction, increased psychosis and adjustment reactions, as well as more hospital admissions for alcoholism as well as other psychiatric problems. Their review also noted increases in the incidence of psychosomatic illnesses, including peptic ulcers, hypertension, and heart disease relative to younger age groups. Levinson *et al.* (1978), who defined midlife transition as a period when the meaning, value, and direction of one's life is called into question, noted that about 80% of his male subjects from different occupational classes experienced "tumultuous struggles within the self and with the external world." The men were described as "full of recriminations against themselves and others," suggesting dissatisfaction with their lives.

Gould (1975) studied 524 male and female subjects ranging in age from 19 to 60. He characterized the ages from 40 to 43 as "acutely unstable," with many from 35 to 43 questioning whether they had made the right choices in life. Those in their late 40s and older typically showed greater acceptance of their life situation. Henry (1961) found that male executives in their 40s were more likely to question their choice of career than those in their 30s.

Although the aforementioned investigators have found evidence of psychological disruption during midlife, others have reported evidence of relative stability and satisfaction. Clausen (1976), in examining 135 female and 112 male middle-class participants in the Berkeley Institute of Human Development Project, found that few gave any indication of midlife crisis or crisis of middle age, though their lives were certainly not free of tension. Neugarten (1968), who examined 100 middle-aged men and women who were successful in their vocations, found relatively little evidence for midlife crisis. Lowenthal and Chiriboga (1972) did not find that the "empty nest syndrome" associated with middle age to be a crisis-precipitating event, although males did seem to be reluctant to admit to difficulties associated with middle age.

To resolve these apparently contradictory findings about whether middle adulthood, however defined, is a time of increased personal disorganization, or a period of new growth and development, suggests the need for a more adequate conceptualization of the relationships among biological, psychological, social, and gender-role issues. Based on our review, we may conclude that not every man approaching middle age inevitably experiences sufficient turmoil that could be labeled a *crisis*. However, some men do experience significant increases in stress associated with the universally experienced era of middle age. Perhaps like the "adolescent," the middle-aged male must confront biological changes and social-role changes that may precipitate a reappraisal of how he has lived his life thus far.

Based on a review of the literature, Collin (1979) has discussed some relatively widespread issues that nearly all men must cope with during midlife. All men must confront the physical effects of aging, including changes in appearance and declines in physical endurance. There are also changes in the perception of time left to live associated with an increased awareness of mortality. Most writers have agreed that nearly all men reappraise their work or career objectives in light of their previous achievements sometime during the midlife period. It is also generally agreed that men reevaluate their participation and satisfaction with their family lives. During the midlife period there is the inevitability of family events that force changes in a man's social roles and commitments at home. One's parents are aging and will in the foreseeable future pass from the scene. In the meantime they may become more dependent upon him. If he is married and has children, the children are becoming more independent, requiring a readjustment to them and a changed relationship with his spouse.

It is our view that how each man evaluates the inevitable changes in his life associated with middle adulthood, combined with his ability to cope with these changes, are the factors that determine the intensity of the difficulties he experiences in navigating the midlife transition. We further propose that masculine gender-role socialization and ideology also affect the ability of men to cope with midlife changes and stress. As Levinson (1977) has pointed out, men at midlife are inclined to reevaluate their "sense of masculinity." Therefore, we next turn our attention to a discussion of masculine sex typing and masculine gender-role behavior. We believe that rigid adherence to traditional masculine values may limit a man's adaptive flexibility during the midlife transition.

MASCULINE GENDER ROLE AND THE MIDLIFE TRANSITION

Theories of psychosocial development have previously postulated that strong gender-role identification is necessary for healthy adjustment. According to this perspective, "normal" adaptive coping patterns develop, in part, through the incorporation of sex-typed attitudes and behaviors associated with one's biological sex. For males, commitment to traditional masculine values, such as self-reliance, competitiveness, and assertiveness, are presumed essential adaptive skills in many cultures. Increasingly, however, it has been shown that rigid adherence to masculine sex-typed values and male gender-role behavior may produce stress. For example, Eisler and Skidmore (1987) and Eisler, Skidmore, and Ward (1988) found that some men experience stress when they judge themselves unable to cope with the demands of the male role or must confront issues requiring sex-typed "feminine" behavior such as the expression of tender emotions. Additionally, studies by Skidmore, Eisler, Blalock, and Sikkema (1988) and Lash, Eisler, and Shulman (1990) have shown that men who are highly dedicated to the imperatives of the male gender role show greater cardiovascular reactivity to social and physical stressors than men who are less committed to male gender-role behavior.

In this next section, we will elaborate on a number of masculine gender-role imperative areas that may predispose men to conflict and stress as they approach middle age. We believe that the ways in which men deal with these masculine scripts are related to some of the disruptions that they may experience during the midlife transition. The following four behavior patterns appear to be strongly influenced by masculine gender-role socialization: (1) emotional expressiveness and intimacy; (2) socialized control, power, and competition; (3) obsession with achievement and success; and (4) body focus and health care.

Emotional Expressiveness and Intimacy

Researchers in gender role-development believe that men in most cultures tend to be more instrumental and goal oriented than women in their approach to life. On the other hand, women tend to be more affiliative and motivated by emotional connectedness in their view of life. Developmentally, it is speculated that a diffusion of gender roles occurs as people age, with the sexes becoming more alike in middle age. Men tend to become more emotionally reactive and sensual, whereas women become more aggressive and less sentimental. Levinson *et al.* (1978) described midlife as the time for men to integrate their masculine and feminine feelings. Lowenthal and Weiss (1976) described "intimacy" as the major challenge. Vaillant (1977) contends that for men, issues of intimacy collide with those involving career aspirations during middle adulthood.

Historically, male socialization has devalued emotional expressiveness, which has proven to be a barrier to intimate or supportive relationships with spouse, children, or even other men. As men approach middle age, their lack of ability to develop intimate connections with others may have greater untoward consequences than in earlier years. For example, Lowenthal (1967) found that widowerhood was far more traumatic for men than widowhood for women. Women tend to have a larger circle of individuals whom they describe as close friends and to have more confidants than men (Antonucci & Akiyama, 1987). Husbands, in contrast, tend to name their spouses as confidants more often than do wives. In fact, wives typically express dissatisfaction regarding their husband's inability to be intimate or emotionally supportive (Balswick & Peek, 1971). Women have been shown to develop larger, more multifaceted social support networks than men (Campbell, 1980). Comparing middle-aged males and females, Lewis (1978) and Lowenthal and Weiss (1976) showed that women had the greater capacity for mutuality and were more willing to self-disclose (Jourard, 1971). Within the group of middle-aged males examined by Lowenthal and Weiss (1976), those males with the greatest capacity for intimacy had the fewest psychological and health problems.

In reviewing these findings, then, it would appear that masculine inexpressiveness is a threat to husband and wife bonds as women are likely to become less satisfied with their marriages especially as women become more independent during midlife. Additionally, if close bonds with children are not made by fathers during their early years, the potentially supportive relationships with one's children may be less likely in middle age. It also appears that men with diminished capacity for significant relationships are at greater risk for cardiovascular disease, suicide, alcoholism, and mental health problems than those who have emotional ties with family.

Socialized Control, Power, Competition

O'Neill (1982) has pointed out that males are socialized to exercise power and authority as evidence of one's masculinity. In their classic review of gender differences, Maccoby and Jacklin (1974) found that young boys appear more biologically aggressive than girls and are reinforced to be active, dominant, and in control of situations. Also, young boys learn the value of power by modeling their behavior after adult men in their families or from media heros. Sports has always been highly competitive for boys from elementary school through college. Unfortunately, the often quoted statement by football coach Vince Lombardi, "Winning is not everything, it's the only thing," typifies the traditional males' view of competition, that competing without winning is not worth very much, and neither is the man who loses.

Masculine socialization for power and control is most evident in "climbing up the ladder" at the workplace. Here satisfaction with work is replaced with the importance of ever-increasing earnings, prestige, and control over others at the workplace. Sometimes the competition for less room at the top can produce a high level of work stress and dysfunctional relationships both at work and at home. Because very few men reach it to the most powerful positions at the top, by middle age, most men have to deal with the fact of not being as successful as they had hoped when they were young.

Although masculine attitudes toward exhibiting power and control may serve useful instrumental purposes when males are younger, it would appear that there are increasing drawbacks to this gender-role commitment in later adulthood. With children growing more independent and leaving home, and wives becoming more autonomous, male insistence on authority and control at home is simply less viable. Lowenthal and Weiss (1976) have noted middle-aged couples whose children have left home were on a "collision" course, as men hoped to receive increased attention from their wives, whereas women hoped to become increasingly involved in activities away from the home. Meanwhile at work, middle-aged men are beginning to worry about losing status and power to younger men. During this period, men should be reevaluating the value and meaning of their work apart from its financial aspects. The masculine gender-role mandate for power and control may have to be relinquished and replaced by greater concern for developing the abilities of the next generation.

Obsession with Achievement and Success

Related to male preoccupation with power and control is his socialized obsession with achievement and success. O'Neil (1982) has theorized that "fear of femininity" shapes much of a man's obsessive work behavior in his early adult years. In fact, a major element of the masculine gender role has been characterized by David and Brannon (1976) to be "the big wheel," achieving a respectable measure of fame and fortune in his vocational pursuits. It is during the midlife period that masculine sex-typed attitudes and gender-role behavior intersect with a reevaluation of a man's commitments to work.

Erikson (1959) viewed the developmental task of men in relation to work one of "generativity versus stagnation." Levinson *et al.* (1978) noted the reemergence of "the dream," which involved a new appraisal of how one has measured up to one's earlier anticipations of success. Brim has (1976) noted that workers at midlife had developed an awareness of the gap between "career dreams" and actual attainments. Clausen (1976), examining longitudinal data from the Berkeley Growth Studies, found that between ages 30 to 40 approximately one-fourth of the men became dissatisfied with their careers.

Masculine imperatives to be successful are well documented in what has been described by Friedman and Rosenman (1974) as the Type A behavior pattern. The Type A behavior pattern, a major risk factor for coronary artery disease primarily in men, is summarized as an unrelenting, aggressive, hard-driving struggle for achievement and success (Price, 1982). The cost of excessive achievement striving may be high. Goldberg (1977) has written that the masculine ingredients for success may twist men's lives into combative competitive struggles that leave little time for relaxation, pleasure, or a healthy life outside of work.

Given the importance of the role of achievement in how men define themselves, it seems likely that a fair amount of stress may be generated in middle adulthood, especially in those men who have not created alternative self-defining roles outside of the work setting. Negative changes in work status or loss of job in middle age may precipitate major psychological problems. On the other hand, reappraisal of the dedication to work versus other pursuits at midlife may lead a man to conclude that he is not defined by work success alone and that other roles and values are more important to his sense of well-being.

From a historical perspective, physical strength, vigor, and sexual potency have been defining aspects of masculine self-concept. Whether a warrior on the battlefield, a mountain climber scaling Everest, or a little leaguer on the soccer field, males have been expected to demonstrate physical strength and endurance. Eisler and Skidmore (1987) recently developed a measure of masculine gender-role stress (MGRS) to determine what internal and external events men appraise as stressful compared to women. The largest factor to emerge from the factor analysis of the MGRS was physical inadequacy, a major concern about "maintaining masculine standards of physical fitness, sexual prowess, and manly appearances" (p. 130). Some of the major stresses men felt they might encounter were feeling that they were not in good physical condition, being perceived as a poor lover, or losing in a sports competition.

Somewhat paradoxically, masculine gender-role training leads men to neglect their bodies in order to portray themselves as tireless machines (Fasteau, 1974), who must ignore pain and illness in the service of maintaining an aura of physical invincibility. As Goldberg (1977) has pointed out, the masculine stance of ignoring the body's warning signals of impending damage does little to preserve the health of many men. Admission of pain or illness is associated with femininity, helplessness, and weakness. This sex-typed attitude probably accounts for the fact that men are less likely than women to visit health professionals for physical and mental health problems (Cleary, 1987). Cleary also cites statistics that show that men are much more likely than women to abuse alcohol or illegal drugs to reduce stress. It would appear that although men, more than women, have their self-concept invested in physical strength and fitness, masculine values paradoxically limit men from engaging in self-care behaviors to preserve their health.

The evidence does indeed indicate that there are significant declines in physical functioning during middle adulthood. While some major sports athletes are pushing their careers into their late 30s and early 40s, most like the tennis star Jimmy Connors are beginning to succumb to younger rivals. Schultz and Ewen (1988) reports that as males approach middle age, decreased efficiency is evidenced in the lungs, heart, kidneys, reflexes, and sense organs. Although many of these bodily changes are gradual, they do provide cues that a man is indeed losing some of his physical powers. Masters and Johnson (1970) have noted that although male sexual capacity remains well into the 70s, there is a slowing of sexual responsiveness, with longer refractory periods following orgasm, and greater stimulation is required for erection and ejaculation.

Many of the adult developmental theorists agree that men are especially sensitive to the perception of physical decline that is inevitable during the midlife transition. Gould (1978) has written that the primary issue precipitating midlife disruption was the development of an acute awareness of one's own mortality. Jacques (1965) proposed that the reality and inevitability of one's own eventual death was "the central and crucial" feature of the midlife phase. Neugarten (1976) has considered the reorientation in time perspective from time since birth until time until death as a major perceptual change in evaluating one's life during middle age.

As men approach middle age, it would appear that the masculine investment in physical power and invincibility must confront the biological facts of aging, however gradual their onset. For men who are highly committed to a youthful physical strength and endurance definition of their masculinity, middle age could signal a significant threat to their sense of well-being.

CHANGES IN WORK AND FAMILY RELATIONSHIPS AT MIDLIFE

The old masters Freud, Adler, and Erikson all emphasized the universal components of work and love in influencing the development of mens' lives. As we have previously noted, entrance into middle age brings about a reappraisal of accomplishments and satisfactions in both of these arenas for most men. The purpose of this section is to review developments and events in the areas of work, family, and social life that are salient during midlife. Further, it is our intention to show how these areas of life are affected by masculine gender-role scripts. It is felt that men who reduce some of their commitments to traditional masculine gender-role values are more likely to make a successful transition through the difficulties of midlife.

Masculine Gender Role and Work

As men move into the second half of life, the nature and extent of their investment in careers or vocations are often reevaluated. Typically reexamined are the extent to which a man has fulfilled his early aspirations, the costs involved in his successes and failures, as well as the relative importance of work when compared to other aspects of his life. A man's appraisal of the meaning and importance of his work during midlife can sometimes be emotionally charged, leading to major career changes in some cases. On the other hand, Neugarten (1968) who examined 100 successful middle-aged males, found relatively little evidence for a midlife crisis during this period.

Murphy and Burck (1976) have proposed that a separate stage of career development occurs for men at midlife. In reviewing the literature on career development, they noted that as men approach 40, the period is characterized by decreased self-esteem, questioning of the meaning of life, examination of personal values, and stock taking of one's personal attainments. These deliberations are usually resolved by the late 40s. Henry (1961) found that among a group of 45 male executives, those in their 40s were more prone to question their career choice and wish they had devoted more time to personal relationships than those in their 30s. Clausen (1976), in examining over 240 male and female participants in the Berkeley Institute of Human Development studies, found that men between the ages of 30 and 40 changed jobs because of major dissatisfactions. He noted that by the age of 50, "most men have seemed to come to terms with the job that they have." Those men who were rated as most markedly disturbed, as indicated by being anxious, self-defeating, given to psychosomatic ailments, and concerned with their own adequacy, had been downwardly mobile in their occupational class. Sofer (1970), in a study of the career attitudes of 81 British scientists, found that many felt that they had not done as well in their careers as they had hoped. Their perceived lack of success resulted in lowered self-esteem and career disappointment.

It appears, then, that the vast majority of men have had significant psychological investments in their work and careers. As middle age approaches, most men reassess their vocational choices, aspirations, and dreams as well as the priority that they have assigned to work in their lives. The outcomes associated with this reappraisal are complex, requiring examination of each individual's characteristics, his level of attainment in relationship to his aspirations, and the various work and other life circumstances that may affect his satisfaction with work. However, nearly all men must come to terms with the masculine gender-role script that places a relatively high value on achievement in the workplace.

Males in American society tend to identify and define themselves in terms of their career success (Levinson *et al.*, 1978). Clausen (1976) noted that three-fourths of middle-aged men defined themselves as "heavily invested" in their career roles as compared to a small minority of the working women examined. O'Neil (1982) noted that early male gender-role socialization determines each man's "persistent and disturbing preoccupation with work, accomplishments, and eminence as a means of substantiating and demonstrating his masculinity." Men learn that their definition of what it means to be masculine is inextricably intertwined with their career success, the breadwinner role, being competitive, and in control of their work role.

This heavy emphasis on the importance of work in defining one's self-worth may create difficulties in the midlife adjustment of males who ascribe strongly to the masculine prototype of what David and Brannon (1976) have called "the big wheel." Sherman (1987) found that a common problem for middle-aged men was that they spent a disproportionate amount of time, effort, and self in work related endeavors rather than in family relationships. Difficulty in achieving one's career goals has been found to be related to poorer psychological adjustment (Clausen, 1976).

Men who are socialized to be successful at work may develop the overly competitive, hard-driving, aggressive behavior patterns that have been identified by Solomon (1982) as the Type A personality pattern. Type A behavior, which reflects many traditional masculine values, is associated with greater risk of coronary artery disease. It is masculine for men to endure pain and not ask for help when under stress. Therefore, it is not surprising to find that men are more likely to relieve stress through alcohol abuse and heavy smoking than women. They are also less likely to seek medical advice or perform preventative health care behaviors than women (Nathanson, 1977).

Loss of the work role through illness or forced early retirement often has especially detrimental consequences to men during middle age. Most men derive a sense of self-worth from their abilities to be providers to their families through work. Being forced to give up the work role deprives men of a major defining aspect to their lives associated with a loss of masculinity. "Off-time" retirement due to physical problems has been related to significant dissatisfaction with retirement (Harris, 1976). Not only has a man's sense of invulnerability been threatened by illness, but his sense of potency has been threatened by loss of the work role. For those men who have not developed sources of satisfaction and self-esteem outside of work, readjusting career aspirations during the midlife period because of perceived lack of success or health problems may be vulnerable to increased adjustment difficulties during the midlife transition.

There is little doubt that men associate their work roles with their sense of masculinity. Eisler and Skidmore (1987) showed that being unemployed, not making enough money, lacking occupational skills, and failure to get promoted at work comprised a major factor in masculine gender-role stress.

During the midlife period, when most men reevaluate their work roles, changes in both their attitudes toward work as well as changes in their actual work situation may present a challenge to their sense of masculine self-worth. The resolution of this challenge is important to successful adjustment during the midlife transition.

Masculine Gender Role and Family Life

Entrance into the era of midlife frequently ushers in family developmental events that must be successfully navigated. The family is typically in the "launching" stage, with adolescent and young adult children preparing to leave home to live independently (Kelley, 1981). The strain on many families of coping with adolescent children has been the impetus for countless books on parenting. Many fathers have devoted relatively small increments of time to their growing children, having placed primary responsibility for child care on the mother. As children become more difficult to manage during adolescence, mothers will place more demands on their husbands to play a larger role in the parenting chores. The stresses that fathers may experience in fulfilling a more active parenting role during this period may be heightened by fathers' perception of the adolescent's behavior as a challenge to his authority. Men tend to resort to the expression of angry feelings more readily than women when their authority is challenged. Additionally, fathers are likely to have more difficulty than their wives in being nurturant or supportive, particularly toward male adolescents (Balswick, 1982). Men who are heavily invested in the traditional male role may have difficulty in openly expressing feelings with their teenager in other than an authoritarian style. Typically "masculine" methods of solving family problems may serve to increase family upheaval during this period.

During middle age, the emptying of the "nest" may reduce some family problems, and yet create new ones. Indeed, the "empty nest" period has not necessarily been found to be the traumatic event it was once believed to be, with approximately three-fourths of parents maintaining weekly face-to-face contact with their children (Cicirelli, 1981). Also, the children leaving home is typically perceived as an "on-time" event (Lowenthal et al., 1975), permitting years of family preparation.

For many couples, there is some difficulty in making this transition to the absence of the children as they are forced to deal with one another without the buffer or diversion of additional family members. Relatively little investigative attention has been given to ascertaining the effects of the children's leaving on fathers due to the stereotypical views that this event primarily impacts on mothers. Yet recent evidence has suggested that fathers are more emotionally affected by this event than previously realized (Lewis, Freneau, & Roberts, 1979).

Occurring with increasing prevalence, midlife parents are experiencing the return of adult offspring to the home for financial and emotional support (Mancini & Blieszner, 1985). Such an unanticipated event is likely to create additional strain and conflict within the marital or family unit (Kelley, 1981). Also occurring with greater frequency, due to increasing lifespan, is the dependence of aging parents on their middle-aged children (Cicirelli, 1981). Evidence has dispelled the myth of the family rejecting the elderly or ill parent, elucidating the critical role that middle-aged children play in the caring of chronically ill or poorly functioning parents

(Atchley, 1980; Cicirelli, 1981; Shanas, 1980). Although these midlife adults assume tremendous responsibilities in this area, the result can be a major intergenerational conflict, greatly increasing stresses of the midlife transition. Although women play a major role in the caretaking duties, men must assume greater financial responsibilities (Troll, 1971). In addition, the wives' preoccupation with aging parents reduces husbands' access to their spouses.

As children depart from the home, middle-aged women in ever increasing numbers are going back to school or entering the work force. Husbands who have been socialized to see themselves as the "breadwinner" may feel threatened by their wive's newfound economic independence (Goldberg, 1977). Engaging in activity outside of the home is an increasing source of satisfaction for women, who have spent nearly half their adult lives as homemakers (Lowenthal, 1977). Men who rigidly cling to stereotyped masculine roles may create significant marital discord. This problem has been noted with increasing regularity in a clinical settings, where the women decided to divorce their husbands whom they perceived as holding them back (Moulton, 1980).

The physical effects of aging during midlife may potentially impact on the marital relationship in adverse ways. Changes in the youthful appearance of both partners and the onset of menopause in the wife signaling the end of fertility as a couple may be difficult for either or both spouses. For those men who are exceptionally sensitive for the need to maintain youthful masculine appearances, aging may be perceived as a threatening process involving loss of self-esteem. Griffitt (1981) noted that declines in sexual activity from middle age onward in previously sexually active couples may be ascribed to the societal belief that attractiveness and youth are equated. For some married males, denial that they are aging may occur in the form of extramarital affairs, often with much younger women (Moulton, 1980). At a time of decreasing sexual activity with the spouse of many years, the extramarital relationship may symbolize a man's ability to recapture the youth and vitality of his earlier years.

Many writers in the field of adult development (Golan, 1986; Gutman, 1976; Levinson *et al.*, 1978; Nadelson, Polonsky, & Mathews, 1978) discuss decreased sex-typed behavior in both genders as men and women enter midlife. Gutman (1976) feels that each sex becomes more androgynous with age. Males may become more nurturant and affiliative, whereas women assume more instrumental roles and interests. Although these gender-role changes may enhance each person's satisfaction with midlife, they may also produce problems that require adjustment efforts by the spouse. Nadelson, Polonsky, and Mathews (1978) found role changes in couples in which the previously passive partner in the relationship becomes increasingly assertive, which then threatens the identified dominant partner. Men who are strongly invested in masculine roles would therefore have problems with wives who become more self-sufficient and independent.

During the midlife period, men seem to be struggling with the need to find meaning in life beyond traditional masculine roles. A frequently neglected area of a man's life has been closeness and intimacy in his social and sexual relationships. There is typically very little in male socialization that prepares men to give or receive emotional closeness. Lowenthal and Weiss (1976) believe that men have been socialized to avoid intimacy. Men have greater difficulty than women in exchanging personal expressions of warmth and caring as a result of masculine gender-role conditioning (Balswick, 1982). The midlife period presents men with an opportunity to develop increased closeness with their spouses and families that might have been previously neglected due to an unbalanced preoccupation with work. Whether or not a man becomes increasingly connected with his family or in some instances entirely separated from them depends on many factors. What is certain, however, is that relationships between a man and his family will be undergoing important changes during the midlife period.

Summary

In this chapter we have endeavored to develop a theoretical perspective on midlife developmental issues in men. Theories of adult development addressing midlife transitions have primarily focused on either maturational-induced stages or on the influence of environmental challenges that presumably precipitate adjustment difficulties during middle age. The effect of socially prescribed gender roles that impact on coping with such transitions as parenthood, work status changes, aging parents, or the "empty nest," and the like have largely been neglected by the previous literature. Therefore, our purpose was to integrate theories that addressed the effects of maturational induced stages, and life event challenges, with our notions of socially learned masculine roles. We believe that assessment of the influence of the masculine gender role on developmental issues at midlife provides a more useful explanatory framework when integrated with developmental stage and contextual life event models.

We have seen that middle age introduces a number of developmental issues, such as the biological effects of aging and an inevitable "psychological" confrontation with one's mortality. Additionally, there may be a variety of "normal" life events issues to cope with, including growing children, aging parents, and a loss or change of job. Additionally, the biological changes of aging are being felt by most men. Although these problems may be particularly salient for many men during midlife, no evidence was found that would support the idea of midlife crisis universally experienced by all men. Nor was there any evidence that these life events inevitably unfold within a specified time period. Instead, we have concluded that as a man ages, maturational changes and exposure to common life events during this period will require coping and adaptation.

We have hypothesized that some of the ways men cope with midlife transitions are based on learned gender-role attitudes and behavior. A review of the literature in this area shows that American males are socialized to associate masculinity with: (a) decreased expression of intimacy; (b) strong requirements for power and control; (c) high needs for achievement and success in work roles; and (d) maintenance of physical strength and sexual potency. We have proposed that successful navigation of the demands of midlife for men may depend on the degree to which they reduce their adherence on the aforementioned imperatives of the masculine role. In part, this is necessary because we believe that the process of coping with aging, from both biological and social-role perspectives, requires a greater flexibility of coping skills than the masculine role typically allows.

During the midlife transition it is not unusual for men to reevaluate their previous achievements and future priorities. These may include youthful ideas of career success and status within their own families. Structural changes in families occur with adult children leaving home, wives returning to work, and aging parents becoming increasingly dependent. The quality of the relationship between the man and his spouse may also need to change in light of these events. Men who have had difficulty in forming intimate or supportive relationships would appear to be at greater risk for midlife adjustment difficulties than those who can ask for and receive help from others close to them. Those men who define themselves and their accomplishments solely in terms of their work achievements may find their lives empty lacking in richness and fulfillment during the midlife transition.

Thus we conclude that consideration of midlife developmental changes is best viewed from the perspectives of biological and maturational changes, typical midlife events, and gender-role ideology. Men typically rely on masculine gender-role socialization to cope with these transition tasks. We have pointed out how excessive reliance on masculine gender-role coping styles may hinder adjustment to the transitions experienced during the midlife period.

REFERENCES

Antonucci, T. C., & Akiyama, H. (1987). An examination of sex differences in social support among older men and women. *Sex Roles, 17,* 737–749.

Atchley, R. C. (1980). *The social forces in later life.* Belmont, CA: Wadsworth.

Balswick, J. O. (1982). Male inexpressiveness: Psychological and social aspects. In K. Solomon & N. B. Levy (Eds.), *Men in transition: Theory and therapy* (pp. 131–150). New York: Plenum Press.

Balswick, J., & Peek C. (1971). The inexpressive male: A tragedy of American society. *Family Coordinator, 20,* 363–368.

Brim, O. (1976). Theories of the male mid-life crisis. *The Counseling Psychologist, 6,* 2–9.

Campbell, A. (1980). *A sense of well-being in America.* New York: McGraw-Hill.

Cicirelli, V. G. (1981). *Helping elderly parents: The role of adult children.* Boston: Auburn House.

Clausen, J. A. (1976). Glimpses into the social world of middle age. *International Journal of Aging and Human Development, 7,* 99–106.

Cleary, P. D. (1987). Gender differences in stress-related disorders. In L. Biener & G. K. Baruch (Eds.), *Gender and stress* (pp. 39–74). New York: Free Press.

Collin, A. (1979). Mid-life crisis and its implications in counseling. *British Journal of Guidance and Counseling, 7,* 144–152.

David, D. S., & Brannon, R. (1976). *The forty-nine percent majority: The male sex role.* Reading, MA: Addison-Wesley.

Eisler, R. M., & Skidmore, J. R. (1987). Masculine gender role stress: Scale development and component factors in the appraisal of stressful situations. *Behavior Modification, 22,* 123–136.

Eisler, R. M., Skidmore, J. R., & Ward, C. H. (1988). Masculine gender-role stress: Predictor of anger, anxiety and health-risk behaviors. *Journal of Personality Assessment, 52,* 133–141.

Erikson, E. H. (1959). Identity and the life cycle: Selected papers. *Psychological Issues Monograph No. 1.* New York: International Universities Press.

Erikson, E. H., & Erikson, J. M. (1981). On generativity and identity. *Harvard Education Review, 51,* 240–278.

Fasteau, M. F. (1974). *The male machine.* New York: McGraw-Hill.

Friedman, M., & Rosenman, R. (1974). *Type A behavior and your heart.* Greenwich, CT: Fawcett.

George, L. (1982). Models of transitions in middle and later life. *Annals of the American Academy of Political and Social Science, 464,* 22–37.

Golan, N. (1986). *The perilous bridge: Helping clients through mid-life transitions.* New York: Free Press.

Goldberg, H. (1977). *The hazards of being male.* New York: New American Library.

Gould, R. L. (1972). The phases of adult life: A study in development psychology. *American Journal of Psychiatry, 129,* 33–43.

Gould, R. (1975). Living through the mid-life crisis. *Psychology Today, 8,* 39–57.

Gould, R. (1978). *Transformations.* New York: Simon & Schuster.

Griffitt, W. (1981). Sexual intimacy in aging marital partners. In R. Fogel, E. Hatfield, S. Kiesler, & E. Shanas (Eds.), *Aging: Stability and change in the family* (pp. 301–315). New York: Academic Press.

Gutman, D. (1976). Individual adaptation in the middle years: Developmental issues in the masculine mid-life crisis. *Journal of Geriatric Psychiatry, 9,* 41–59.

Harris, L. (1976). *The myth and reality of again in America.* Washington: National Council on Aging.

Henry, W. E. (1961). Conflict, age, and the executive. *Business Topics, 9,* 15–25.

Jacques, E. (1965). Death and the mid-life crisis. *International Journal of Psychoanalysis, 46,* 502–514.

Jourard, S. (1971). *The transparent self.* New York: Van Nostrand Reinhold.

Kelley, H. H. (1981). Marriage relationships and aging. In R. Fogel, E. Hatfield, S. Kiesler, & E. Shanas (Eds.), *Aging: Stability and change in the family* (pp. 275–300). New York: Academic Press.

Kohlberg, L. (1973). Stages and aging in moral development: Some speculations. *Gerontologist, 13,* 497–502.

Lash, S. J., Eisler, R. M., & Shulman, R. S. (1990). Cardiovascular reactivity to stress in men: Effects of masculine gender role stress appraisal and masculine performance challenge. *Behavior Modification, 14,* 3–20.

Lerner, R. M. (1986). *Concepts and theories of human development.* New York: Random House.

Levinson, D. J. (1977). The mid-life transition: A period in adult psychosocial development. *Psychiatry, 40,* 99–112.

Levinson, D. J., Darrow, C. M., Klein, E. B., Levinson, M. H., & McKee, B. (1978). *The seasons of a man's life.* New York: Knopf.

Lewis, R. A. (1978). Emotional intimacy among men. *Journal of Social Issues, 34,* 108–121.

Lewis, R. A., Freneau, P. J., & Roberts, C. L. (1979). Fathers and the postparental transition. *Family Coordinator, 28,* 514–520.

Lowenthal, M. F. (1967). *Aging and mental disorder in San Francisco.* San Francisco: Jossey-Bass.

Lowenthal, M. F. (1977). Toward a sociological theory of change in adulthood and old age. In J. E. Biven & K. W. Schaie (Eds.), *Handbook of the psychology of aging* (pp. 116–127). New York: Van Nostrand.

Lowenthal, M. F., & Chiriboga, D. (1972). Transition to the empty nest: Crisis, challenge, or relief? *Archives of General Psychiatry, 26,* 3–14.

Lowenthal, M. F., Thurnher, M., & Chiriboga, D. (1975). *Four stages of life: A comparative study of men and women facing transitions.* San Francisco: Jossey-Bass.

Lowenthal, M. F., & Weiss, L. (1976). Intimacy and crises in adulthood. *The Counseling Psychologist, 6,* 10–15.

Maccoby, E., & Jacklin, C. (1974). *The psychology of sex differences.* Palo Alto, CA: Stanford University Press.

Mancini, J. A., & Blieszner, R. (1985). Return of middle-aged children to the parental home. *Medical Aspects of Human Sexuality, 19,* 192–194.

Masters, W. H., & Johnson, V. E. (1970). *Human sexual inadequacy.* Boston: Little, Brown.

McGill, M. E. (1980). *The 40 to 60 year old male.* New York: Simon & Schuster.

Moulton, R. (1980). Divorce in the middle years: The lonely woman and the reluctant man. *Journal of The American Academy of Psychoanalysis, 8,* 235–250.

Murphy, P. P., & Burck, H. D. (1976). Career development of men at mid-life. *Journal of Vocational Behavior, 9,* 337–343.

Nadelson, C. C., Polonsky, D. C., & Mathews, M. A. (1978). Marital stress and symptom formation in mid-life. *Psychiatric Opinion, 15,* 29–33.

Nathanson, C. A. (1977). *Sex roles as variables in preventive health behavior. Journal of Community Health, 3,* 142–155.

Neugarten, B. L. (1968). *Middle age and aging: A reader in social psychology.* Chicago: University of Chicago Press.

Neugarten, B. L. (1976). Adaptations and the life cycle. *The Counseling Psychologist, 6,* 16–20.

O'Neil, J. M. (1982). Gender-role conflict and strain in men's lives: Implications for psychiatrists, psychologists, and other human-service providers. In K. Solomon & N. B. Levy (Eds.), *Men in transition: Theory and therapy* (pp. 5–44). New York: Plenum Press.

Price, V. A. (1982). *Type A behavior pattern: A model for practice.* New York: Academic Press.

Rosenberg, S. D., & Farrell, M. P. (1976). Identity and crisis in middle aged men. *International Journal of Aging and Human Development, 7,* 153–170.

Schultz, R., & Ewen, R. B. (1988). Physiological aspects of aging. In R. Schultz & R. B. Ewen (Eds.), *Adult development and aging: Myths and emerging realities* (pp. 51–83). New York: Macmillan.

Shanas, E. (1980). Older people and their families. The new pioneers. *Journal of Marriage and the Family, 42,* 9–15.

Sherman, E. (1987). *Meaning in mid-life transitions.* Albany: State University of New York Press.

Skidmore, J. R., Eisler, R. M., Blalock, J. A., & Sikkema, K. J. (1988, March). *Cardiovascular reactivity in men as a function of masculine gender-role stress*. Paper presented at the 19th annual meeting of the Biofeedback Society of America, Colorado Springs.

Sofer, C. (1970). *Men in mid-career: A study of British managers and technical specialists*. Cambridge: Cambridge University Press.

Solomon, K. (1982). The masculine gender role: Description. In K. Solomon, & N. B. Levy (Eds.), *Men in transition: Theory and therapy* (pp. 45–76). New York: Plenum Press.

Troll, L. E. (1971). The family of later life: A decade review. *Journal of Marriage and the Family, 33*, 163–290.

Vaillant, G. E. (1977). *Adaptation to life*. New York: Little, Brown.

V

The Elderly

One of the inevitable consequences of the scientific advances in medical care is the increased longevity that we experience. However, along with such increased longevity are the problems of aging, such as how to spend time in the retirement years, whether to move to a retirement village or center, how to deal with diminished physical ability and illness, and how to deal with the eventualities of widowhood and bereavement. It is very clear from the chapters in Part V that social development does not end in adulthood but is a major factor for the elderly as well. The life events in one's elderly years require marked adjustments in social interaction and flexibility heretofore not associated with the latter portion of one's life.

Lawrence W. Smith, Thomas L. Patterson, and Igor Grant (Chapter 19) examine in great detail the issues of work, retirement, and activity in the elderly. These issues are conceptualized as coping problems for the aging population. The primary thesis of the chapter is that the elderly must remain active and must continue to develop in the social sphere. The elderly must be stimulated, and this includes maintaining physical activity, socializing, learning new skills, and even returning to work or school. All of the aforementioned are geared toward enhanced self-esteem and counter the possibilities of depression. Robert B. Fields (Chapter 20) details the psychosocial response to environment change in the elderly. In so doing he reviews representative theoretical models, examines the physical and social environments of the elderly (including migration and reverse migration), outlines the psychosocial response to reactive environmental change, discusses psychosocial response to nonreactive environmental change, as well as to natural disasters. Finally, Richard K. Morycz presents a comprehensive evaluation of the issues of widowhood and bereavement in late life. Many aspects of this problem are discussed, including the issue of marital relationship experienced before bereavement, mode of death and timing issues, other losses, stresses, life events experienced, coping styles and strengths, acute or initial response to loss, personality and self-esteem, history of medical or psychiatric problems, social support, financial status, and gender and age. Widowhood is presented from a developmental perspective, which is seen as involving both change and possible growth.

473

19

Work, Retirement, and Activity

Coping Challenges for the Elderly

Lawrence W. Smith, Thomas L. Patterson, and Igor Grant

Introduction

To consider the social development of elderly individuals might seem odd to some, given the more common and stereotypic concern with the deterioration of physical and mental capacities in this group. But, in order to interact effectively within a social environment, one must continue to obtain information, acquire skills, and cultivate dispositions conducive to one's own well-being and to the well-being of those with whom one interacts. Thus, despite the greater visibility of social development during the first few decades of life, individuals of all ages continue to develop.

In addition to providing information about the functioning of older people in their work, retirement, and activities, in this chapter we will comment on myths about growing older, examine hypotheses about retirement and adjustment, and discuss a life events and coping perspective on optimizing adjustment during the later years.

Lawrence W. Smith • Management Psychologists, 411 University Street, Seattle, Washington 98101. Thomas L. Patterson and Igor Grant • Psychiatry and Research Services, Veterans Affairs Medical Center, San Diego, California 92161; Department of Psychiatry, University of California, San Diego, California 92093; and Department of Psychology, San Diego State University, San Diego, California 92182.

Handbook of Social Development: A Lifespan Perspective, edited by Vincent B. Van Hasselt and Michel Hersen. Plenum Press, New York, 1992.

LAWRENCE W.
SMITH *et al.*

The importance of a discussion on the social development of the elderly is a function of the familiar demographics: the group of individuals aged 65 and older is the most rapidly growing segment of the population in the United States. Such profound growth will affect the functioning of government, industry, medical and educational institutions, and families. Virtually every dimension of society will feel the effects of increased numbers of elderly individuals, many of whom will function relatively well as they reach their 80s, 90s, and 100s. Perhaps the most dramatic shift will be experienced by the aging individuals themselves. Although the elderly are not a homogeneous group—due, in part, to the wide diversity among older cohorts—they will probably continue to experience expanding political power and have a greater impact on society. Their perceived influence will no doubt shape their own attitudes, and those of younger individuals, about the possibilities for participation in society's roles and activities.

DISENGAGEMENT VERSUS PARTICIPATION

In 1961, researchers reporting findings from a Kansas City study of adult life developed an influential theory of aging (Cumming & Henry, 1961). Their "disengagement theory" described normal aging as an inevitable withdrawal from many of one's social systems. The theory, described as "provisional," held that as individuals age, their participation with others diminishes. Such disengagement supposedly leads to a new equilibrium characterized by a social network with fewer connections to others. Relinquishment of some of one's roles might be initiated by the individual, by members of groups to which one belongs, or by both. The theory allows, however, that a person may remain relatively close to individuals in some groups while withdrawing more completely from others. The originators of the theory also stated that increased preoccupation with oneself often accompanies disengagement.

A theory, *per se*, implies an accumulation of a set of cohesive findings or facts that explain some phenomenon. The phenomenon addressed in the disengagement theory was the apparently (in the sample studied) universal social withdrawal of aging individuals—disengagement. This was the behavior that was to be explained. The theoretical portion of the disengagement theory can be summarized as an explanation: Aging individuals disengage because this is the normal, gradual progression that eventually ends in death. In other words, disengagement as one ages is appropriate for the human species (i.e., it is biologically determined). Increased self-preoccupation could simply indicate that one is attempting to make peace with oneself or to derive meaning from one's life. According to this theory (that disengagement characterizes normal, healthy aging), successful aging would be distinguished by sufficient disengagement, and, excessive reluctance or failure to disengage would lead to decreased morale, and, presumably, to maladjustment or illness.

The disengagement theory was criticized after publication of *Growing Old: The Process of Disengagement* (Cumming & Henry, 1961) as untestable (Hochschild, 1975). It also seemed to run counter to theories of psychological adjustment and evidence suggesting that ample social support and participation with others are hallmarks of mental health. Moreover, Neugarten (1973), relying on the same database used in the development of the disengagement theory, found an inverse, linear relationship between disengagement and life satisfaction. The more disengaged one was, the less one was satisfied with life. Thus, much environmental contact through a wide range of activities is probably more characteristic of high-functioning persons.

This chapter addresses social development in the elderly—not social disengagement. Not being as interested in one's usual activities as one was previously, or withdrawing from friends, family, and avocations that were previously pleasurable can describe common symptoms of depression—not normal aging. Moreover, the essential features of depression do not differ across the various ages of adulthood. Increasing age, nevertheless, presents challenges not faced at younger ages. Optimally, though, these must be faced and dealt with as appropriately and courageously as were the events of previous decades. Thus, the premise of this chapter on work, retirement, and activity in the elderly may be stated in the following way: The essential features of a satisfying and healthy life do not differ across an adult's life span.

AGEISM

The social development of older adults is sometimes hampered by society's views of their capacities. As with younger people, if opportunities for growth are not openly extended to the elderly, their progress may be impeded. In current discussions of work, retirement, and activity in the elderly, the topic of prejudice and discrimination against them must be addressed. A belief that age is an important determinant of one's traits and capacities and that individuals older than a particular age are inherently inferior to younger persons is an example of *ageism*, a term first coined by Robert Butler in 1969. Perhaps the most common institutionalized form of ageism was mandatory retirement. However, in 1986 Congress enacted a law no longer permitting employers to require workers to retire when they reach age 70 (exceptions were temporarily made for certain occupations, e.g., police officers and college professors). Nevertheless, prejudice and discrimination against the elderly continue to limit the opportunities of older individuals and of businesses and institutions that might benefit from the expertise of older workers. If disengagement were a biologically determined pattern of behavior in aging individuals, perhaps this would provide evidence to support discrimination against older people for some purposes. But, there are compelling arguments and evidence against not only the paradigm of disengagement (Hochschild, 1975) but also against the usefulness of age as a meaningful predictor of performance on the majority of tasks (Cerella, Poon, & Williams, 1980). Nevertheless, there are a few general differences between adults of different ages. For example, a slowing of reactions to various stimuli is common among older persons, though the magnitude of this effect is inconsequential for the performance of most tasks (Salthouse, 1987; Schaie, 1988).

Ageism has been a rather pervasive problem. In fact, sometimes, gerontological researchers themselves hold stereotypes of the elderly, which makes them more likely to accept findings of poorer performance among older individuals or to subtly reflect ageism in their conclusions. For example, studying types of work, health, work ability, functional capacity, and symptoms of strain in older workers (mean age = 54.7) as part of a study on the criteria for retirement age at the Institute of Occupational Health in Helsinki, Finland, Ilmarinen (1988) concluded that despite much individual variation, the capabilities for physical work are distinctly impaired after the age of 50 years. The authors stated that this "disability" is chiefly due to declining cardiorespiratory capacity among women and to reduced muscular trunk strength among men. The author concludes by making the following three recommendations: (1) women over the age of 50 who are involved in prolonged physical work should perform tasks that require less than an oxygen consumption of $1.01 \cdot min^{-1}$; (2) an intensive occupational health care system should be available; or (3) early retirement should be available.

Surprisingly, these recommendations follow the author's acknowledgment that there is great variability among older workers. To generally recommend that women over the age of 50 be given light work appears to incriminate the author for discriminating inadvisably on two counts: The first is to generalize across all individuals over the age of 50, despite the considerable variation among persons in this category, and the second is to discriminate against women. It is unclear why the author did not make similar recommendations about light work for "disabled" men over the age of 50.

Moreover, it seems an overstatement to label individuals as *disabled* when they are simply not currently physically fit. The expression "disabled person" usually implies the presence of an illness or injury, and it is objectionable as a label because it implies that a person as a whole is disabled (Wright, 1989). It would seem more prudent to refrain from using labels and to closely examine the differences in lifestyle and health practices between those older workers who function at a higher capacity and those who function at lower levels. It is likely that, in general, those who function better get more exercise and practice other healthful behaviors more often than do those who are less physically fit. Nevertheless, certain physiological changes generally occur as individuals age. For example, decreased speed of information processing, decreased muscular strength and vital capacity, and increased numbers of illnesses (especially chronic illnesses) represent some of the widespread changes that accompany aging. But great individual variation in these changes will be observed across sizable groups of older individuals. Moreover, some changes that were customarily thought to be correlates of aging—for example, "senility"—are now known to be secondary to disease and not normal aging.

We must, however, be careful to admit our ignorance of causation with regard to many health practices and avoid making sweeping generalizations that create guilt and anxiety among the elderly. There are a number of spheres in which the distinct advantages of particular behavioral interventions have not been scientifically substantiated (Brody & Brock, 1985). For example, in a report stemming from a workshop held at the Brookings Institution in 1986 to evaluate the potential of preventive interventions to improve the health of older people, Louise Russell (1987) drew a contrast between the clear impact of exercise on heart disease and the only suggestive effects of exercise on improving bone strength in the elderly. Even less well established are the potential benefits of taking dietary calcium supplements to strengthen bones and prevent fractures in old age; much uncertainty remains regarding how and when calcium strengthens bone structure. Moreover, analyzing the costs and benefits of interventions is sometimes complex, requiring one to weigh direct benefits from an intervention against the costs, considering economics and the potential impact of side effects on the quality of life (Kaplan & Anderson, 1990).

Nevertheless, to coddle older workers—simply because they have reached some age—by generally limiting the strenuousness of tasks, making available extraordinary health care, or encouraging early retirement is as insulting and potentially damaging to them as it would be to younger workers. Efforts to encourage better health and functional capacity would be more helpful to older individuals—employed or retired.

Certainly, regardless of one's age, individuals who are truly limited in their functional capacity due to illness or a debilitating condition should be excused from performing tasks too strenuous or demanding for them. This is only reasonable. But because of the tremendous power of expectations to shape one's destiny, care must be taken not to discriminate against individuals on the basis of any demographic variable that provides little or no information about an individual. Examples of such variables that are nearly useless in most cases are race, gender, sexual orientation, and age.

In order to improve gerontological research and to prevent the promulgation of unfavorable and inaccurate descriptions of the elderly, Schaie (1988) recommends that researchers and consumers of research carefully evaluate findings of performance differences among individuals of different ages. Interpretation of research findings within the context of the aging literature is perhaps the best safeguard against erroneous interpretations.

The truth is that there is considerable variation in personalities, intellectual abilities, skills, functional capacities, and personal resources among the elderly. Stereotypes of 75-year-olds are no more accurate than are standardized mental pictures of 45-year-olds. Addressing some severe forms of stereotyping, Maas and Kuypers (1974) argue that:

> So long as old age is ultimately coupled with criminality, mental illness, and other kinds of "social deviance," and "treated" by institutional means which remove the afflicting persons from the mainstream of life, homogenizing conceptions of "the aged" will persist—conceptions which disregard the great differences among aging persons, as among all human beings. (p. 202)

Birth Cohorts

Social development in the elderly differs from development in infants. The development of a newborn is preceded only by its genetic predisposition and the quality of the prenatal environment. The development of elderly individuals on the other hand is preceded by respective genetic dispositions but also by a fantastic variety of environmental experiences during the preceding decades. Part of this variety stems from one's particular birth cohort. Thus, it becomes difficult to discuss social development in the elderly, *per se*, without first accounting for cohort differences (see Schaie & Schooler, 1989). Willis (1989), for example, discusses evidence indicating that individuals of different birth cohorts, when assessed at the same chronological age, differ in performance on various psychometric ability measures. She indicates that some social environments primarily affect the acquisition of cognitive abilities, whereas others influence the maintenance of cognitive skills as we age.

LAWRENCE W.
SMITH *et al.*

There are numerous anecdotes in the news and popular press about older people who have made significant changes in their lives. Occasionally, an elderly person will obtain a high-school diploma or college degree after spending 50 or 60 years out of school. But many older people make meaningful changes in their lives that are equally personally significant, albeit they are not newsworthy. Maas and Kuypers (1974), for example, examined data spanning approximately 40 years on 142 parents through the Institute of Human Development at the University of California, Berkeley. After analyzing their longitudinal data they addressed the opportunities that old age brings, concluding that

> finally, even when young adulthood is too narrowly lived or painfully overburdened, the later years may offer new opportunities. Different ways of living may be developed as our social environments change with time—and as we change them. In this study we have found repeated evidence that old age can provide a second and better chance at life. (p. 215)

Development and "Aging"

Featherman (1989) describes development as "additions to reserve or adaptive capacity in mind and behavior across the lifespan" (p. 43). Careful attention to this definition reveals that development (and also reductions of developmental reserve or adaptive capacity) is not, as Featherman describes it, an "age-graded process." Aging, according to Featherman, is a reduction in adaptive resources. Thus, one may experience "aging" as a child, as an adolescent, or as an adult. One may also reverse aging processes—that is, replenish adaptive resources—at any age throughout the lifespan. To provide a simple physical example, one may show cardiovascular development after consistent aerobic exercise, then aging, due to failing to exercise for an extended period, then redevelopment, after resuming a steady exercise program. Similar processes apply to other domains, such as social skills, musical abilities, formal intellectual capacities, and so forth. Figure 1 shows this alternative view of development as compared to a popular, stereotypic view of development and decline across the lifespan.

Aging and Intellectual Functioning

Shneidman (1989) added to the overwhelming evidence that as we age our general intellectual powers do not usually decline significantly, if at all. Studying septuagenarians, he found that for relatively bright individuals who had remained intellectually active throughout their lives, there was virtually no decline in general intellectual functioning or working vocabulary. The author speculated that perhaps these individuals in their 70s were able to maintain their high level of intellectual performance because they expected that habitual intellectual work would keep them in shape mentally. It is unclear whether this expectation is responsible for maintaining performance (as if it were a self-fulfilling prophesy), whether scholarly practice itself should be credited, or whether genetic predisposition, alone, or combined with other factors, accounts for the sustained intellectual power. Certainly, presence of a dementia or other pathological condition would influence one's

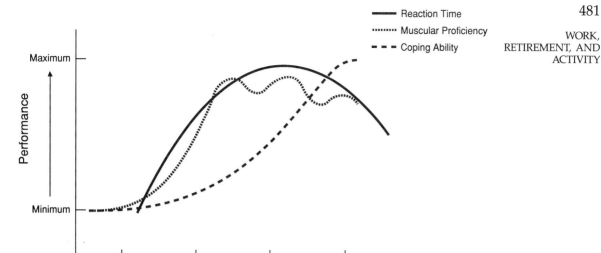

FIGURE 1. Alternative view of development and "aging" exemplified as hypothetical levels of performance for reaction time, muscular proficiency, and ability to cope with threatening life events.

intellectual functioning. Septuagenarians who had remained intellectually active until the onset of Alzheimer's disease, for example, would clearly show impairment upon neuropsychological evaluation due to the new presence of brain pathology. Although Shneidman may have studied a group of unusually fortunate intellectuals, it is possible for healthy elderly *individuals* to exhibit little decline in cognitive functioning (Heaton, Grant, & Matthews, 1986). Some neuropsychological impairment, however, has been detected through the Halstead-Reitan Battery (Reitan & Davidson, 1974) in most normal elderly subjects (Heaton *et al.*, 1986). Determining the extent to which such "normal" impairment is due to an accumulation of insults or to cognitive experience might be a suitable goal of future research.

There is reasonably strong evidence that new experience or training enhances cognitive performance and lasting ability in the elderly (Salthouse, 1989; Willis, 1989). Providing the older individuals are reasonably healthy, these training effects do not seem to be restricted to certain groups of individuals. Nevertheless, it is unclear whether improvement in performance due to training operates by changing the mechanisms responsible for age-related decline (Salthouse, 1989).

Cognitive flexibility in the elderly also seems to be a function of experience. Schooler (1984) reviews extensive evidence that "doing self-directed, substantively complex work leads to increased intellectual flexibility" (Schooler, 1989, p. 130).

A Brief History of Retirement

At the turn of the century retirement was unknown. The worklife of men (women were rare in the work force) was roughly equivalent to life after the age of 16 (Stub, 1982). As human life expectancy increased, the glut of older workers who were limiting the opportunities of younger workers was gradually alleviated by mandating retirement and providing the new Social Security (Minkler, 1981).

The elderly of ancient times might not have been placed in a separate category from the other younger adults. In ancient Greece and Rome, for example, only the wealthy could consider living without working during their later years. Most people, according to Kebric (1988), worked until they could physically no longer do so. Perhaps the most striking difference between our present society's view and that of ancient Rome and Greece about the abilities of the elderly comes from the nonageist expectation that everyone in ancient Greece and Rome, regardless of age, would serve in the military to defend their homeland. Few job requirements today compare with the rigors of serving in an ancient army. The elderly were expected to function even as combat soldiers if they were able (Kebric, 1988). Thus it must be emphasized that in speaking of retirement—especially stereotypic retirement in which individuals participate in progressively fewer enjoyable activities—we are discussing a cultural phenomenon. Currently, in primitive societies, and to a lesser extent in nonindustrialized societies, retirement does not appear to exist.

The demographic factors that created a perceived need to replace older with younger workers during the early twentieth century are now demanding that we rethink retirement. The aging of the baby-boom generation is leading the way to an older America. In 1930, 5.4% of the population was over age 65; today about 12% are over 65, and by 2010 approximately 20% of the population will be older than 65. It will become increasingly more difficult for the smaller number of younger workers to adequately support many members of this retired population. The ratio of workers to retired persons dependent upon Social Security benefits is often referred to as the *dependency ratio*. New laws are already being devised to encourage workers to continue in the work force beyond the age of 65. For example, as mentioned previously, Congress eliminated mandatory retirement for most occupations in 1986. Also, the minimum age to begin collecting Social Security has been raised for future workers (effective in 2010), and income tax laws have changed so that the Social Security benefits of upper-income individuals will be taxed. These changes occur as more employment opportunities are becoming available for older workers in both the public and private sectors.

From this brief account of the history of retirement it should be clear that retirement is an artifact, stemming, in part, from a need to manipulate the number of workers competing for jobs. As the demand for more workers increases, especially in the many service industries, strong incentives will be developed to persuade older workers to continue or return to work.

Stereotyping Wealth

The stereotype that the elderly are generally in financial need might lead some to conclude that it should be relatively easy to persuade them to return or continue to work. Stephen Crystal (1982, 1986), however, provided data that demonstrate the inappropriateness of treating the elderly as an "undifferentiated mass" with regard to their financial resources. Although such stereotypes were understandable in the 1950s when more than a third of the elderly had incomes that fell below the poverty line, a standardized mental picture of the elderly as poor was 87.6% *incorrect* in 1984, when only 12.4% of the elderly had incomes considered below the poverty level (Crystal, 1986). Although it is incorrect to generally characterize the elderly as poor, too many elderly women, members of minorities, and the very old continue to have serious financial needs. It is also true that a substantial cluster of older individuals had 1984 incomes that were between 100% and 125% of poverty-line income.

Although Crystal points out that an effective "scorekeeping" system is needed in order to accurately assess the financial status of elderly individuals (a considerable amount of underreporting and underestimating occurs), clearly the average income of the elderly has improved dramatically relative to that of the nonelderly.

Addressing the potential shift into poverty after retirement, Burkhauser, Holden, and Feaster (1988), relying on longitudinal data covering the time just prior to retirement through up to 10 years after retirement, followed the economic status of couples who were solvent prior to retirement. They found that a sizeable majority of these couples did not become impoverished during their earliest years of retirement, regardless of whether or not they received a pension income. Their findings demonstrated, however, that death of a husband can profoundly modify the risk and pattern of poverty in retirement. Nevertheless, there seems to be reliable evidence to suggest that the risk of becoming poor is no greater for the elderly than it is for younger individuals (Crystal, 1982, 1986; Danziger, van der Gaag, Smolensky, & Taussig, 1984).

THEORIES OF ADJUSTMENT TO RETIREMENT

Substitution or Activity Theory

Friedmann and Havighurst (1954) formulated what Shanas (1972) termed *substitution theory* and Atchley (1976) referred to as *activity theory*. The theory postulates that giving up work creates a void in people's lives, regardless of the fact that work has diverse meanings associated with it for different people. There are four features of the theory: (1) Retirement from work results in an individual experiencing a *sense of loss*; (2) the focus of this sense of loss *will differ between individuals;* (3) individuals must substitute something for that loss or they will not make a satisfactory adjustment to retirement; and (4) this substitution involves replacing one set of activities by another.

Support for one aspect of this theory stems from the fact that the meaning of work differs between members of distinct occupational groups (cf. Powers & Goudy, 1971; Streib & Schneider, 1971). In general, blue-collar workers (i.e., individuals with relatively lower paying jobs), who retire earlier than white-collar workers (Mitchell, Levine, & Pozzebon, 1988), report *a source of income* as the primary meaning of work. White-collar workers, on the other hand, report *satisfaction derived from work* as the primary meaning of work, and they tend to work to more advanced ages. A positive relationship between social activities, in the postretirement period, and adjustment has been found repeatedly (e.g., Havighurst, Munnicks, Neugarten, & Thomas, 1969; Maddox, 1963).

Critics have complained that substitution theory reflects only middle-class values (e.g., Shanas, 1972; Streib & Schneider, 1971). Many blue-collar workers do not find their work interesting or stimulating, have little control over their work, and are dissatisfied with their jobs. For them, leaving a job may be experienced as a relief.

Shanas (1972) posed a more dynamic model that involved a new distribution of energies into other roles and behaviors. According to this theory, the retirement period is a time during which an individual's needs change due to retirement itself, aging, and changes in social circumstances. Some individuals may seek new social roles, whereas others might reduce their social involvement. Thus, retirement is viewed as a rather individual process that requires personalized adjustments rather than simple substitutions. For each individual this process is related to a number of factors, including social-psychological (e.g., perceived health), and social-structural (e.g., income) phenomena, which may or may not constrain a person. Unlike substitution theory, accommodation theory suggests that changes in behavior may occur because of changes in personality. These accumulating changes may reflect one's currently perceived needs or self-concept.

Unfortunately, the accommodation theory is weakened by its limited specificity. As Shanas (1972) herself pointed out, unless new propositions are derived from accommodation theory, empirically differentiating it from substitution theory will be impossible.

Disengagement Theory

As mentioned in the introduction to this chapter, disengagement theory proposes to characterize the later years of life by progressive and mutual withdrawal between individuals and society (Cumming, 1964; Cumming & Henry, 1961; Henry, 1964). This theory's suggestion that a decrease in social activities will be associated with better morale and greater satisfaction in life has failed repeatedly to garner empirical support (e.g., Neugarten, 1973; Schonfield, 1977).

Continuity Theory

Rosow (1963) proposed that adjustment in old age may be evaluated by referring to an individual's adjustment in the early or middle 50s. He views this period as representing the peak years, largely because occupational advancement has usually peaked and responsibilities for rearing children have greatly diminished or ceased. For Rosow, the best life is the one that changes the least, and the measure of an individual's adjustment should be made in reference to his or her own behavior before retirement. Changes, however, that eliminate negative aspects of life (e.g., frustrations, burdens, etc.) or add new positive features (e.g., satisfactions) represent net gains for a person. Conversely, the maintenance of negative patterns contributes to poor adjustment.

Atchley (1972, 1976, 1989a), presenting a similar continuity theory, maintains that habits, preferences, and goals that develop during adulthood generally persist into old age. Subjective, internal compromises are made in order to change or develop the hierarchy of one's personal goals.

Continuity theory, like others discussed previously, seems to lack specificity. It is unclear what stable behaviors constitute *poor* adjustment and what changes in behavior contribute to *good* adjustment. A true test of the theory is impossible due to circular reasoning inherent in continuity hypotheses. For example, it is hypothesized that an individual's adjustment will depend upon the extent to which (a) continuity is maintained, (b) positive changes are made, and (c) negative patterns are abandoned. Unfortunately, because the predictors (continuity/change) are not easily classified independently from the criterion variable (adjustment), they are evaluated after adjustment has been assessed. Thus, instead of predicting adjustment by analyzing one's continuity over a number of years, "postdiction" occurs: that is, if one demonstrates good adjustment, one would reason that the topography of one's life course must exemplify a coherent continuity reflecting favorable preretirement behaviors. Moreover, continuity theory suggests that if one has not demonstrated suitable adjustment during the working years (i.e., one has demonstrated some enduring pathology), pathological adjustment will likely continue in retirement. This probability, in a shorter time frame, has been demonstrated in the general life events and illness literature (e.g., see the Grant, Patterson, Yager and Olshen, 1987, discussion of symptoms as predictors of symptoms).

A Stress and Coping Model

In the stress model, an individual's reaction to retirement depends on the degree to which retirement is perceived as stressful or threatening (see the Lazarus & Folkman, 1984, discussion of primary vs. secondary appraisal, pp. 315–316). A number of variables, including the effectiveness of one's coping responses and the abundance and quality of social support available, may mediate the relationship between retirement and adjustment. George (1980) differentiates between coping responses, which consist of behavioral and intrapsychic reactions, and other moderating and mediating variables, including demographics, situational factors, or personality characteristics. George measures adjustment in terms of life satisfaction and identity (e.g., self-esteem). The model, as it was posited by George, is primarily descriptive and does not make specific hypotheses.

The present authors also view retirement as a life event occurring within a unique context for each individual. One's appraisal of the event (Lazarus & Folkman, 1984), that is, the event's meaning and perceived threat to one's integration and well-being, and the specific context in which the event occurs (Grant *et al.*, 1989), are viewed as relevant to one's postretirement adjustment. Appraisal and context also have implications for coping responses. Optimally, one's coping responses—the more or less strategic cognitive and behavioral reactions to threatening life events—will be appropriate to the specific event or difficulty. Smith, Patterson, McNaughton, Smith, and Grant (1990) developed a method by which the appropriateness of one's coping responses may be evaluated, independent of any type of symptom or functional outcome. Coping Appropriateness Rating (CAR) scores have been found to be associated with fewer physical and psychological symptoms in elderly individuals. Figure 2 diagrams a coping model of adjustment to retirement.

Are Theories of Retirement Really Necessary?

Given the attention that various authors have devoted to describing and explaining adjustment in retirement, one might think that retirement represents a sacred initiation into the final chapter of one's life—that it is a biological birthright or unique phase that all members of the human species undergo, usually between the ages of 58 and 68. Often, one hears the response, "I'm retired," to the question,

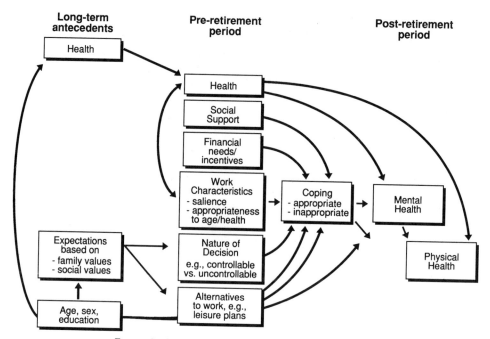

FIGURE 2. A coping model of adjustment to retirement.

"What do you do?" This response (which does not answer the question) accompanies an assumption that almost everyone knows what it means to be retired. But this is not the case. Knowing that someone is retired tells nothing about what a person does. And, the question, "What do you do?", is actually quite important.

Retiring from one's job is an event. It may be viewed as a threat to some and not to others. It will allow (and usually will require) one to make new choices about what to do with one's time.

Available theories of retirement might be viewed as less than adequate because the behavior or state categorized as retirement is *not* a mystery to be solved. Retirement is generally possible because people can afford it through Social Security benefits, pensions, and personal investment income. It has its roots in a social bargain with older workers who make room for younger workers. Likely, the needs of society will also be responsible for making other "deals" with the elderly to get them back into the work force in greater numbers than have been seen in decades.

Retirement as a Life Event

Because retirement is no enigma, future discussions should simply consider it a life event and apply to it the findings of the research on life events, coping, and health status in the elderly (e.g., Folkman, Lazarus, Pimley & Novacek, 1987; Patterson *et al.*, 1990; Smith, Patterson, & Grant, 1990). Because mandatory retirement is no longer a *problem* for most U.S. citizens, older individuals have more choices about how they spend their time. Their involvement with life, whether employed or not, will certainly impact on their mental and physical health.

Clearly there is a significant, positive correlation between involvement in activities and life satisfaction. In fact, satisfaction and participation in life are nearly synonymous. Contrary to the disengagement hypothesis, evidence suggests that one should maintain roles in life (Lemon, Bengtson, & Peterson, 1972). No doubt these roles will change over the life course, but successful or optimal aging has been characterized by continued meaningful involvement in a variety of activities and resistance to preventable, functional decline (Bell, 1978). The maintenance of balanced activity levels is one means of maintaining adaptive capacities, inhibiting deteriorative trends or "aging," and boosting satisfaction in life.

Statistical Retirement Data

Between 1974 and 1981 the percentage of individuals in the 55- to 64-year-old group who reported being employed either full or part time (formally retired or not) grew from 48 to 55% and from 18 to 21% among 65- to 69-year-olds (Harris, 1981). During this same period no changes in the percentage employed were observed among 70- to 79-year-olds (11%), or 80-year-olds (4%).

Fewer older women reported being housewives during this same period. Approximately 24% of women over the age of 65 reported being housewives in 1981, compared to 30% of women in 1974.

Finally, during this same time period, 1974 to 1981, the unemployment level declined in each elderly age segment, while the number of individuals who considered themselves to be retired showed a corresponding rise. For example, as can be seen from Figure 3, among the 65- to 69-year-old age group in 1974, 4% were unemployed and 61% were retired. In 1981, 1% were unemployed and 67% were retired. Harris (1981) also found that elderly African-Americans 65 and older showed an even greater rise in employment between the years 1974 and 1981, a smaller rise in retirement, and an even more dramatic decline in the number of housewives, compared to Caucasians. It appears that as our population ages and economic pressures dictate the necessity to remain employed, more elderly people are employed; at the same time, more are retired, while fewer individuals report being unemployed, being employed part time or being in charge of a household as a housewife.

Actual retirement age increased slightly between 1974 and 1981, 62.9 to 63.5 years old, respectively. The number of people who stated they had been forced to retire remained constant, 37% between 1974 and 1981. Among those who had reported that they had been forced to retire, 67% (27% of all retirees) reported it was because of "disability or poor health," whereas only 20% (8% of all retirees) reported that they had been forced to retire because their "company had fixed retirement age."

Describing the subjective predictability of retirement, Ekerdt, Vinick, and Bosse (1989) found that over a 2-year period (i.e., 2 years after obtaining worker's predictions) 66% of workers were able to predict their ultimate retirement date within 1 year. Forty percent, however, were precise to within 3 months. The workers who best predicted their retirement date were pleased with their current salary, expected to obtain a good pension, maintained positive thoughts about retirement, participated in retirement preparation (either formally or informally), and planned to retire at older ages.

Morrow-Howell and Leon (1988) found that workers participating in the labor

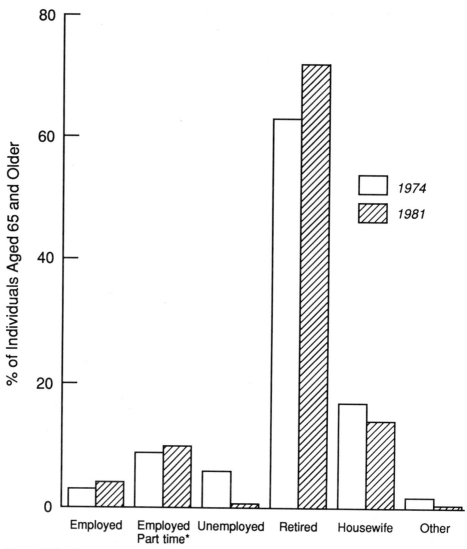

FIGURE 3. Employment status of individuals aged 65 and older during the years 1974 and 1981 in the U.S. *1981 includes "employed part time" 3%, and "retired, but working part time" 7%.

force after retirement (during the first 3 years) had more successful employment histories prior to retirement. Conversely, people with more marginal work histories were not as likely to seek work after retirement, despite their lower income.

At the same time the attitudes of Americans became even stronger in response to the question of mandatory retirement. In 1981, 90% of those polled agreed with the statement that "nobody should be forced to retire because of age" compared to 86% in 1974. In addition, most of the public still believed that "most employers discriminate against older people and make it difficult for them to find work" (p. 18) (in 1981, 79%, compared to 80% in 1974).

Many workers reported that they did not look forward to retiring, about 45% in 1981, and as one ages this negative attitude strengthens. Among those individuals aged 65 to 69, 81% said that they do not look forward to retirement compared to 49% among individuals aged 18 to 64. These attitudes are modified by individual income. The higher the annual income, the more positive the attitude about retirement. Fifty-four percent of individuals with incomes over $20,000 looked forward to work, whereas 34% of individuals with incomes under $5,000 looked forward to retirement.

Satisfaction in Retirement

Schnore (1985) reported on a study of 750 male and female workers and retirees in Ontario, Canada. The focus of this research was to predict adjustment to retirement, examine the relationship between work attitudes and retirement, and sex differences in retirement. He found that a high level of well-being was associated with modest expectations, positive evaluation of one's life situation, and a high level of perceived self-competence. Those workers who indicated a high level of work *saliency* endorsed more negative attitudes toward retirement. *Satisfaction* with one's job, however, was not related to retirement attitudes. Thus, being satisfied with one's job is differentiated from perceiving one's job as significant. Workers whose jobs are regarded as of great importance to their lives will tend to view retirement more negatively. This study found that women viewed their work as less salient and preferred to retire earlier than did men.

Schnore's work supports the hypothesis that when work holds a central position in the meaning of one's life, attitudes toward retirement tend to be more negative. Interestingly, a number of previous studies did not support this hypothesis (e.g., Glamser, 1976; Grubbs & Powers, 1980). In those studies, however, work saliency was inferred from assessed attitudes toward one's job. When a distinction is made between work saliency and degree of satisfaction with one's work, saliency, but not satisfaction, predicts attitudes toward retirement (Schnore, 1985).

Perhaps most interestingly, it was the individual's perceived evaluations of health, wealth, and education, for example, and not objective measures of these factors that predict satisfaction with life. This conclusion has also been supported by other investigators (e.g., Fengler & Jensen, 1981; Liang, Drorkin, Kahana, & Mazian, 1980). Steitz and McClary (1988) found that subjective age was determined by age, education, health, self-esteem, financial satisfaction, and job satisfaction. Positive self-esteem and financial satisfaction were important mediators between chronological age and subjective age. It would be interesting to examine whether these findings would hold among the lower one-third of the distributions of each of these domains. In any case, it is clear that personal expectations and perceptions provide significant contributions to our understanding of attitudes toward retirement. Figure 4 diagrams the factors that influence the decision whether to retire or continue working.

The results of the Schnore study indicate that relinquishing the work role does not necessarily have negative consequences, such as an identity crisis. In fact, retirees were found to be happier and more satisfied with their lives than were middle-aged workers. In addition, no evidence was found that retirement has a deleterious effect on health. Actually, 43% of retirees reported that their health had *improved* since their retirement. This is true, despite the fact that aging is usually associated with a decline in heath and that poor health is a familiar reason for retirement.

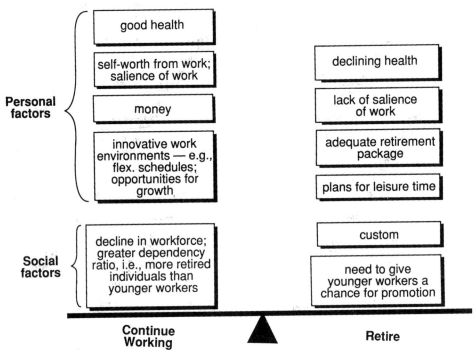

FIGURE 4. Personal and social factors that influence one's decision to retire or to continue working.

What Is Missed after Retirement?

After retiring, the aspects of employment most missed did not change between 1974 and 1981. Money (71% in 1981) and people (70% in 1981) were the two factors missed most. Other factors also reported as being important to many retirees included "the work itself" (57%), "the feeling of being useful" (55%), "things happening around me" (51%), "the respect of others" (48%), and "having a fixed schedule every day" (44%). Thus, it is clear that many important benefits, including financial, social and psychological benefits, are derived from the workplace.

THE MEANING OF RETIREMENT

The importance of work and retirement continue to be central in theories concerning aging (Atchley, 1982). Theorists emphasize either the negative aspects of retirement—loss of income, for example—or its positive aspects, such as increased leisure time. In fact, not surprisingly, there are considerable individual differences in the changes associated with this life stage, and most individuals experience both positive and negative features of retirement, to some degree. In this section we will discuss some of the changes that individuals undergo when they retire.

The most obvious change that occurs for most retiring individuals is a reduction in income. The U.S. Senate Special Committee on Aging (1982) found that the average income was reduced by 50% to 67%. Some changes in the distribution of spending mitigate, to a small degree at least, this reduction in income. For example, costs of transportation may be reduced; the proportion of income allocated for leisure-time activities, however, may increase, offsetting any gains. In fact, most retired individuals appear to be relatively satisfied with their financial situations. The 1981 Harris Poll for the National Council on Aging found that more individuals under age 65 reported financial problems than did individuals over the age of 65 (see previous discussion of stereotyping wealth in the elderly). Having adequate funds, consequently, entices many individuals to retire. This finding confutes the popular misconception that retired persons are generally poor.

Psychological Adjustment

There is a relatively large literature on the impact of retirement on psychological adjustment. The loss of social status and occupational identity has often been addressed by researchers (e.g., Miller, 1965), as has retirement as a role change (e.g., Bengtson, 1973), change in associates (Lowenthal & Robinson, 1976), and shifts in time utilization (e.g., Blau, 1973). These studies emphasize the problems of change associated with retirement. Comparisons of retirees with comparable nonretired men, however, have found high levels of satisfaction among the retired. If one does not remove those individuals who have retired because of poor health from the comparison, this bias will tend to make retirees appear less satisfied. In addition to health, other variables that must be examined for their effects on reported satisfaction in retirement are gender, income, type of occupation, preretirement well-being, age, achieving style, social participation, and attitudes toward retirement (e.g., Die, Sealbach, & Sherman, 1987; Schaie & Geiwitz, 1982).

Health Problems

It is commonly reported by both the popular press and professionals that the event of retirement contributes to health problems and the probability of premature death (e.g., Bernard, 1982; Minkler, 1981). This notion is sometimes based on anecdotes in which retirement was involuntary. Generalizations are then made about the deleterious effects of retirement, *per se*. For example, football coach Paul "Bear" Bryant of the University of Alabama died of a heart attack 37 days after his retirement. To the casual observer, the retirement might be viewed as having "caused" his death. For example, one can imagine hearing such statements as "Sports meant everything to him—he shouldn't have retired," and so forth. The truth is that Bear Bryant had been ill for 3 years and retired *because* of his ill health. A review of the literature indicates that retirement does not increase the risk of either death or a deterioration in health (e.g., Ekerdt, Baden, Bosse, & Dibbs, 1983; Palmore, Burchett, Fillenbaum, George, & Wallman, 1985). In fact, it has been suggested that retirement may have beneficial effects on some existing medical conditions (cf. Ekerdt, Bosse, & LoCastro, 1983).

The picture is not rosy for all retirees, however. Schnore found that at least

10% of workers became maladjusted after retiring. For them, work held a central position in their lives. It would seem a worthy challenge to attempt to identify these individuals and offer assistance to them in preparing for the changes ushered in by retirement. Assisting them in making a suitable vocational change that allows them to achieve new goals, perhaps with a flexible work/leisure schedule, might be helpful to some.

Why does the idea persist that retirement causes illness and death? Ekerdt (1987), providing a many-sided answer to this question, pointed out that provocative anecdotes about retirement, based on both popular and clinical observations, reach an enormous audience through mass media. Consequently, Ekerdt's first point is that an event will seem to occur more frequently or appear plausible to the extent that people can easily imagine it (Tversky & Kahneman, 1982). Because anecdotes such as that about Bear Bryant are mentioned in headlines, whereas happy stories of individuals experiencing a healthy retirement are not considered newsworthy (precisely because they are too common), we sometimes form the erroneous conclusion that retirement is often associated with premature death. Second, people tend to seek order and understanding in their lives. Because retirement is frequently considered a milestone, individuals will often consider its connections with other dimensions of life. For example, when asked about any life events that might have preceded illness, people often attribute causality to a single, important, vivid, and recent event (Brim & Ryff, 1980), such as retirement. In prospective studies that obviate such a bias, however, retirement, *per se*, does not appear to predict ill health. Third, some individuals have a prejudice against retirement, which stems from our culture's celebration of work as the major source of self-worth, self-esteem, identity, and personal fulfillment. Those having this bent might find it difficult to imagine living a truly healthy life without being employed. Fourth, there sometimes exists an *a priori* assumption that retirement must have some effect because it is of such great importance that it is anticipated by many individuals for decades. Any event as significant as that might be thought to have astounding effects. As the reader will surmise from this chapter, we propose that retirement is not necessarily a momentous event. Certainly, however, if one maintains a disliked or unfulfilling job for 30 or 40 years while imagining beginning to truly live after retirement, this expectation will probably have noticeable effects on one's lifestyle, and perhaps, health. Under the present senario, however, one might expect retirement to be, in fact, a glorious introduction into a fresh existence, that is, providing the worker who long delayed "truly living" still possesses the requisite skills. Therefore, researchers and readers should not necessarily expect that there will exist a relationship between retirement and ill health. One should, however, keep in mind the context in which the retirement occurs. For some individuals, retirement might in fact provide the provocation for ill health. This may, however, be due to a number of factors including the reason for retirement (e.g., forced vs. voluntary), coping mechanisms utilized (appropriate vs. inappropriate), social support (satisfactory vs. unsatisfactory), and preexisting health conditions, among others. These are but a few reasons for the persistence of the unsupported generalization that retirement is harmful to health.

Active Life Expectancy

The meaning of retirement will be colored by one's health and quality of well-being or functional capacity (Kaplan & Anderson, 1990, discuss the qualitative dimension of functioning vs. "health outcomes"). Katz *et al.* (1983) suggested a measure of functional health in the elderly, which is used to calculate one's "active life expectancy" or the expected duration of one's functional well-being. An elderly person's active life expectancy is assessed based on his or her ability to perform functions essential to independence (i.e., bathing, dressing, transfer, and eating). With regard to independence/dependence, elderly women tend to have longer periods of remaining dependent years than do men, possibly because of their longer life expectancy and tendency to have chronic as opposed to acute disease.

Maladaptive Behavior Patterns in Retirement

Alcohol Abuse

At least one study has found that 71% of the late-onset alcohol abusers began drinking heavily when they retired (Carstensen, Rychtarik, & Prue, 1985). This study provides support for the hypothesis that retirement can occasion maladaptive behavior patterns. It should be noted that alcohol abuse is a problem for elderly individuals, although there are fewer elderly alcohol abusers than middle-aged abusers (Drew, 1968). This difference may, in part, be due to selective attrition—younger alcohol abusers tend to die or remit their drinking as they age. It has been estimated that 2 to 10% of the elderly actively abuse alcohol (National Institute on Alcohol Abuse and Alcoholism, 1971). This is particularly meaningful because, in the elderly, alcohol remains in the body longer, and, thus, has a more toxic effect (Zimberg, 1978). The elderly also tend to take more medications, especially for insomnia, that may further potentiate the sedative effects of alcohol (Forni, 1978).

It has been estimated that about 70% of older alcohol abusers are young alcoholics grown old, and 30% are individuals for whom the abuse began late in life (Dunham, 1981). The latter group is potentially relevant to discussions of retirement because onset of alcohol abuse could be theoretically attributed to stresses of aging and retirement. Aside from the Carstensen *et al.* study, however, little empirical evidence for this hypothesis can be found (cf. Schuckit, Atkinson, Miller, & Berman, 1980).

Self-Esteem

The potential threat to one's self-image due to retirement was addressed by Young (1989), who found no differences in subjective perception of social standing, contentment, self-reliance, outlook, and dependence between retired and working individuals. This supports the view that, generally, retirement is not so unsettling that it damages one's self-image. To the extent that retirement is a major change for someone, it will require adaptation, as do most major life events. But it appears that the self-image generally endures, whereas one's experience expands through retirement.

Retirement Preparation

How do most workers prepare for retirement? Harris (1981) reported that in 1981 fewer individuals reported preretirement preparation than did those in 1974. For example, in 1981, 64% reported planning for retirement by "building up your own savings" (73% in 1974), learning "about pensions and social security benefits" (73% in 1981 vs. 87% in 1974), or deciding "whether you want to move or continue to live where you are" (56% in 1981 vs. 72% in 1974). Among those 55 to 64 years of age, about half (51%) reported having taken five or more steps toward retirement. This trend is particularly acute among minorities; African-Americans and Hispanics, about 20%; the poor, 33% with incomes under $10,000; and the less educated, 31% with less than high-school education. Thus, it would appear that more focus needs to be placed on modifying the public's perception of the need to prepare for retirement, with a particular emphasis on the poor, minorities, and those with limited education.

The construct of "locus of control" (see later discussion) might play a role in one's participation in preretirement programs and in one's expectations of well-being in retirement. Aging is sometimes associated with a decrease in the perception of control over the events of one's life, and one's responses to them (Reid, Haas, & Hawkings, 1977). Conversely, positive retirement attitudes may lead one to participate in preretirement planning (Glamser, 1981). Abel and Hayslip (1987) found that participation in a preparation program was related to more desirable attitudes about retirement, and an expectancy of internal control was related to more positive psychological functioning. Their program did not, however, increase internal control. In any case, it appears that locus of control may perform as an important moderating factor between retirement preparation and attitudes toward retirement.

More effort needs to be placed on developing comprehensive preretirement programs for all segments of the population. The proportion of potential retirees currently participating in these types of programs is small (cf. Phoon, 1985). This is especially true among those with limited education and among manual workers. These individuals would potentially benefit most from a preretirement program because their postretirement outcomes are least favorable. We might choose to institute incentive programs to enroll these workers or enlist the support of organizations involved with them, such as trade unions. Abel and Hayslip (1987) lament the fact that individuals most in need of preretirement counseling are least likely to obtain it. Those with lower income or poorer health should be urged to participate in programs that will help them to secure a more satisfying lifestyle after retirement.

Leisure in Retirement

The retirement years represent the phase of the life cycle during which, for many, leisure activities become central. Best (1980) describes the "linear life plan" that is predominant in our culture, in which whole blocks of our lives are first devoted to education, next to work or child rearing, or both, and finally to leisure. He argues that individuals would function better if life cycles were more flexible, so that education would occur throughout the lifespan and work would not necessarily fill so much of any single period in one's life.

In fact, it is already true to some extent that retirement is not a unitary concept. Work and leisure are mixed in many cases (Atchley, 1980), and retirement can take on aspects of employment. For example, many "retired" individuals earn money through their "hobbies" (Shanas *et al.*, 1968). Thus, as Robinson (1985) points out, the line between leisure and work is blurring.

Not only is it difficult to categorize work and leisure, it is difficult to define leisure itself (e.g., Gordon, Gaitz, & Scott, 1976; Robinson, Coberly, & Paul, 1985). It has been variously defined as "valuable" (DeGrazia, 1962), a value-laden definition; work versus nonwork (e.g., Kreps, 1972), which means retirement is synonymous with leisure; unobligated discretionary time (e.g., Kabanoff, 1980); or as unplanned actions that are being pursued as ends in themselves (Atchley, 1971). Given the complexities of defining leisure, it is not surprising that it is difficult to operationalize that activity. The challenge is to define components of leisure in a measurable fashion. We may then determine if the quality/quantity of leisure is important.

Optimal Adjustment

Theoretically, there are multiple components that lead to optimal adjustment in persons of any age—the aggregate of these could be considered the minimum requirements for a person's sense of well-being. The premise, stated in the introduction of this chapter, that the essential features of a satisfying and healthy life do not differ across an adult's lifespan, is analogous to the relatively stable dietary needs of the human organism across the lifespan. Of course, minor modifications of diet are necessary for those undergoing unusually strenuous periods, such as pregnancy or athletic performance, or for those recuperating from disease or injury. Many elderly individuals faced with making decisions about work and retirement and attempting to achieve an adequately balanced life during their later years might benefit by paying attention to particular psychosocial factors that appear to be associated with optimal functioning, better morale, and perhaps a decreased mortality rate. For example, coping well with life events and maintaining a sense of control or self-efficacy seem to be crucial to well-being at any age, but perhaps these factors are especially important for the elderly.

Appropriately coping with life events (both major and minor) will have a positive influence on well-being and health. A number of significant events, which threaten well-being, occur in the lives of older individuals. Deaths of loved ones, losses of status, roles, or financial wealth, and decreases in social support (such as seeing family members less often) are commonly experienced by older persons. Certainly, the less severe problems of daily living, impairment of the senses (especially vision and hearing), and chronic pain also need to be dealt with adequately. Although there is much to be learned about the process of coping, the present authors consider *appropriate* coping (Smith *et al.*, 1990) to consist minimally of the following basic dimensions: (a) *ratio of problem-focused to emotion-focused responses* (see Lazarus & Folkman, 1984): suitable to the situation; (b) *activation*: adequate to deal with the situation; (c) *coherence*: the responses should form a reasonably consistent set or an integrated whole; and (d) *self-nurturance*: the responses should be self-enhancing, not self-destructive.

Coping with pain can be a major challenge for some elderly individuals. In fact, in the United States there is more disability stemming from chronic pain than from any other cause (Slater & Good, 1991). There has been some progress in the treatment of those who suffer from chronic pain (i.e., pain that was originally caused by tissue damage but in which healing has occurred). Psychologists and other practitioners working in behavioral medicine have developed cognitive and behavioral strategies to assist elderly individuals in coping with chronic pain. For example, Slater and Kodiath (1991) describe a comprehensive treatment regimen that has proven to be effective in significantly improving the objective functioning and subjective well-being of patients with chronic pain. Their treatment includes education, physical reconditioning, behavior management to increase the frequency of healthy behaviors, cognitive-behavioral and marital therapies, and vocational counseling. Enhancing the quality of life and increasing the use of the body often helps to limit the influence of the pain. According to Fordyce (1988) "patients must be helped to understand the dictum, 'To make it better, use it'" (p. 282). Fordyce (1988) also asserted a law that is relevant to the topic of activity in the elderly, especially those with chronic pain. The following is Fordyce's law: "People who have something better to do don't suffer as much" (p. 282).

There is evidence that a sense of personal-environmental control enhances the well-being of elderly individuals (Langer & Rodin, 1976; Rodin & Langer, 1977). Slivinske and Fitch (1987) found that wellness, muscular strength, and flexibility were associated with increases in perceived control in an elderly group. In their study, individuals who participated in a control-enhancing intervention sought medical care and reported illness less often, and consequently spent less money for medical care than did control group members.

Self-efficacy, a construct related to an internal locus of control, has to do with individuals' beliefs about their ability to exert control over events affecting their lives. Bandura (1989), discussing the importance of people's self-efficacy beliefs, suggests that individuals with a strong sense of self-efficacy will tend to set higher goals and maintain firmer commitments to them. Elderly individuals who successfully return to work or obtain employment in an entirely new type of job, will tend to visualize themselves skillfully performing during an interview or while learning new occupational tasks. Efficacious older people will also prepare themselves educationally for different occupational or leisure pursuits. There are multiple avenues by which older individuals may attend college and obtain degrees or participate in a variety of learning experiences regardless of their educational history (e.g., see Thornton, 1987).

Summary

In order to function well throughout life, elderly individuals must remain active regardless of their employment status and must continue to develop within their social groups. There is, however, great diversity among older cohorts and among individuals within those cohorts. These differences preclude the making of specific recommendations for all, but it seems that self-esteem and a sense of well-being are contingent, at least to some degree, upon adequate participation with others, the maintenance of fulfilling roles, and a belief in one's self-efficacy. The view of aging as a reduction in adaptive resources carries a promise of "reversing" aspects of the aging process by changing one's behavior. Although decline is inevitably related to growing older, viewing aging as a *reduction* of adaptive resources implies that *increasing* the frequency of behaviors that have adaptive value might be quite beneficial to many older persons for some functions. For example, physically exercising, practicing various interpersonal skills, learning about interesting topics, or even returning to work or school will provide stimulation, increase one's sense of self-efficacy, and act against depression. New experience or training can even enhance cognitive performance and development in the elderly. Thus, it is a pessimistic and erroneous notion that a significant loss of adaptive capacities and an inability to learn are inevitable concomitants of growing older.

It seems clear that theories of retirement, *per se*, are of limited usefulness. Retirement is probably best viewed as another of many transitions in life that require appropriate coping. A fruitful area for research might be the enhancement of performance in the elderly, whether in work or in other pursuits.

As more people retire, the need increases to develop programs for the elderly directed toward the needs of both the active retired and the frail elderly. One such program has been outlined by Habib and Gutwill (1985), who utilized the workers' union as a means of disseminating the program. This retiree reach-out program through the union has four major components: (1) individual home visits to retired members; (2) retiree activity groups in each county; (3) a statewide retiree executive board; and (4) outreach to the homebound retired. This type of program is probably not needed by many if not the majority of retirees. Some retirees, however, may be isolated, unaware of community resources or afraid or unable to venture out to use them. Habib and Gutwill reported that their union-based program was successful because it provided a familiar base for former workers to identify with, whereas programs with other sponsors might be suspect. The success of this program points to the need to tailor reach-out programs to the special needs of individual groups.

The vast majority of research on retirement focuses on men. Minimal attention has been devoted to retirement among women. In part, this may be due to our history of relatively fewer formally employed women. This, of course, is no longer the case, as has been discussed by Richardson (1985). Research indicates that employment is generally becoming increasingly central to the lives of most women (e.g., Baruch & Barnett, 1983; Pepitone-Rockwell, 1980). Commitment to work has, in fact, increased among women recently, whereas it has remained relatively stable among men (Veroff, Douvan, & Kulka, 1981). With more women currently in the work force, data on women and retirement will become more readily available.

The change in demographics will, no doubt, lead to more research on improving the functioning of the elderly. As industrial needs increase, the potential profits from utilizing trained older workers will motivate industry and government to support interventions to enhance the functioning of older people. As a result of the small birth cohorts entering the labor force, older workers will be needed to fill jobs to meet the demands of industry. Employees of retirement age will be asked to delay retirement, an action they will not easily agree to, given the strong evidence suggesting that most older workers prefer retirement to continuing to work (Atchley, 1989b). Also, some retired persons will no doubt be asked to reenter the work force, possibly after reviewing responsibilities previously performed or receiving training for new tasks. Employers, however, will need to develop innovative inducements to successfully attract older workers.

Before acceptable solutions may be found to problems associated with a shortage of younger workers, institutional and business leaders must become cognizant of the needs and desires of older potential workers. From a behavioral perspective, the stimuli that are reinforcing to the potential elderly employee must be determined.

To a person who has been delaying gratifications for perhaps 50 years or longer in order to earn a living, time off to pursue avocations, and freedom from having to complete unpleasant, delegated assignments might be powerful reinforcers. Thus, one key to recruiting such older individuals who have adequate financial resources might be to offer them, wherever possible, the opportunity to obtain satisfactions or pleasures that they have been postponing. Certainly, for a smaller group of elderly workers, the opportunity to obtain even the minimum wage working at McDonald's would be viewed favorably. Working in such an environment may be regarded positively or negatively, depending upon the appeal of that particular work environment to the abilities, goals, and needs of individuals. It cannot be emphasized enough that diversity characterizes the elderly.

Evidence suggests that generous salaries might be relatively weak reinforcers for some individuals (Atchley, 1989a) compared to opportunities that cannot be easily obtained with monetary funds. The success of educational programs for the elderly indicates that a sizable number of older learners seek out opportunities for growth (Thornton, 1987). Industrial leaders might benefit by applying the law of supply and demand at the personal level. To entice older workers who have adequate pensions and sufficient other financial resources, industrial leaders will begin to focus more on experiential opportunities, customized work schedules, and the personal growth of their older employees.

REFERENCES

Abel, B. J., & Hayslip, B. (1987). Locus of control and retirement preparation. *Journal of Gerontology, 42*, 165–167.

Atchley, R. C. (1971). Retirement and leisure participation: Continuity or crisis? *The Gerontologist, 2*, 13–17.

Atchley, R. C. (1972). *The social forces in later life: An introduction to social gerontology* (1st ed.). Belmont, CA: Wadsworth.

Atchley, R. C. (1976). *The sociology of retirement.* Cambridge, MA: Schenkman Publishing Company.

Atchley, R. C. (1980). *The social forces of later life: An introduction to social gerontology* (3rd ed.). Belmont, CA: Wadsworth.

Atchley, R. C. (1982). Retirement as a social institution. *Annual Review of Sociology, 8*, 263–287.

Atchley, R. C. (1989a). A continuity theory of normal aging. *The Gerontologist, 29*, 183–190.

Atchley, R. C. (1989b). Demographic factors and adult psychological development. In K. W. Schaie, & C. Schooler (Eds.), *Social structure and aging: Psychological processes* (pp. 29–30). Hillsdale, NJ: Erlbaum.

Bandura, A. (1989). Human agency in social cognitive theory. *American Psychologist, 44*, 1175–1184.

Baruch, G., & Barnett, R. (1983). *Lifeprints: New patterns of love and work for today's women.* New York: McGraw-Hill.

Bell, J. Z. (1978). Disengagement versus engagement—a need for greater expectation. *Journal of the American Geriatric Society, 26*(2), 89–95.

Bengtson, V. L. (1973). *The social psychology of aging.* Indianapolis: Bobbs-Merrill.

Bernard, K. (1982). The first step to the cemetery. *Newsweek*, February 22, p. 15.

Best, F. (1980). *Flexible life scheduling.* New York: Praeger.

Blau, Z. S. (1973). *Old age in a changing society.* New York: New Viewpoints.

Brim, O. G., & Ryff, C. D. (1980). On the properties of life events. In P. B. Baltes & O. G. Brim (Eds.), *Life-span development and behavior* (Vol. 3, pp. 368–388) New York: Academic Press.

Brody, J. A., & Brock, D. B. (1985). Epidemiologic and statistical characteristics of the United States elderly population. In C. E. Finch & E. L. Schneider (Eds.), *Handbook of the biology of aging* (2nd ed., pp. 3–26). New York: Van Nostrand Reinhold.

Burkhauser, R. V., Holden, K. C., & Feaster, D. (1988). Incidence, timing, and events associated with poverty: A dynamic view of poverty in retirement. *Journal of Gerontology: Social Sciences, 43*(2), S46–52.

Butler, R. N. (1969). Age-ism: Another form of bigotry. *The Gerontologist, 9*, 243–246.

Carstenson, L. L., Rychtarik, R. G., & Prue, P. M. (1985). Behavioral treatment of the geriatric alcohol abuser: A long term follow-up study. *Addictive Behaviors, 10*, 307–311.

Cerella, J., Poon, L. W., & Williams, D. M. (1980). Age and the complexity hypothesis. In L. W. Poon (Ed.), *Aging in the 1980s* (pp. 332–340). Washington, DC: American Psychological Association.

Crystal, S. (1982). *America's old age crisis: Public policy and two worlds of aging.* New York: Basic Books.

Crystal, S. (1986). Measuring income and inequality among the elderly. *The Gerontologist, 26*, 56–59.

Cumming, E. (1964). New thoughts on the theory of disengagement. In R. Kastenbaum (Ed.), *New thoughts on old age* (pp. 3–18). New York: Springer.

Cumming, E., & Henry, W. E. (1961). *Growing old: The process of disengagement.* New York: Basic Books.

Danziger, S., van der Gaag, J., Smolensky, E., & Taussig, M. (1984). Implications for the relative economic status of the elderly for transfer policy. In H. Aaron & G. Burtless (Eds.), *Retirement and economic behavior* (pp. 175–196). Washington, DC: Brookings Institution.

DeGrazia, S. (1962). *Of time, work, and leisure.* Garden City, NY: Archer Books.

Die, A. H., Sealbach, W. C., & Sherman, G. D. (1987). Achievement motivation, achieving styles, and morale in the elderly. *Psychology and Aging, 2*(4), 407–408.

Drew, L. R. H. (1968). Alcoholism as a self-limiting disease. *Quarterly Journal of Studies of Alcohol, 29*, 956–967.

Dunham, R. G. (1981). Aging and changing patterns of alcohol use. *Journal of Psychoactive Drugs, 13*, 143–151.

Ekerdt, D. J. (1987). Why the notion persists that retirement harms health. *The Forum, 27*, 454–457.

Ekerdt, D. J., Baden, L., Bosse, R., & Dibbs, E. (1983). The effect of retirement on physical health. *American Journal of Public Health, 73*, 779–783.

Ekerdt, D. J., Bosse, R., & LoCastro, J. S. (1983). Claims that retirement improves health. *Journal of Gerontology, 38*, 231–236.

Ekerdt, D. J., Vinick, B. J., & Bosse, R. (1989). Orderly endings: Do men know when they will retire? *Journal of Gerontology: Social Sciences, 44*(1), S28–35.

Featherman, D. L. (1989). "What develops in adulthood?": A developmentalist's response to Atchley's demographic view. In K. W. Schaie & C. Schooler (Eds.), *Social structure and aging: Psychological processes* (pp. 41–56). Hillsdale, NJ: Erlbaum.

Fengler, A. P., & Jenson, L. (1981). Perceived and objective conditions as predictors of the life satisfaction of urban and non-urban elderly. *Journal of Gerontology, 36*, 750–52.

Folkman, S., Lazarus, R. S., Pimley, S., Novacek, J. (1987). Age differences in stress and coping processes. *Psychology and Aging, 2*, 171–184.

Fordyce, W. E. (1988). Pain and suffering: A reappraisal. *American Psychologist, 43*, 276–283.

Forni, P. J. (1978). Alcohol and the elderly. In R. C. Kayne (Ed.), *Drugs and the elderly* (pp. 75–83). Los Angeles: University of California Press.

Friedman, E., & Havighurst, R. J. (1954). *The meaning of work and retirement.* Chicago: University of California Press.

Genevay, B. (1986). Intimacy as we age. *Generations*, Summer, 12–14.

George, L. K. (1980). *Role transition in later life.* Monterey, CA: Brooks/Cole.

Glamser, F. D. (1976). Determinants of a positive attitude toward retirement. *Journal of Gerontology, 31*, 104–107.

Glamser, F. D. (1981). Predictors of retirement attitudes. *Aging and Work, 4*, 23–29.

Gordon, C., Gaitz, C. M., & Scott, J. (1976). Leisure and lives: Personal expressively across the life span. In R. H. Binstock & E. Shanas (Eds.), *Handbook of aging and the social sciences* (1st ed., pp. 310–341). New York: Van Nostrand Reinhold.

Grant, I., Brown, G. W., Harris, T., McDonald, W. I., Patterson, T. L., & Trimble, M. R. (1989). Severely threatening events and marked life difficulties preceding onset or exacerbation of multiple sclerosis. *Journal of Neurology, Neurosurgery, and Psychiatry, 52*, 8–13.

Grant, I., Patterson, T. L., Yager, J., & Olshen, R. (1987). Life events do not predict symptoms: Symptoms predict symptoms. *Journal of Behavioral Medicine, 10*, 231–240.

Grubbs, M. J., & Powers, E. A. (1980). *A multiplemeasure approach to the relationship between work and retirement attitudes.* Paper presented at the Annual Meeting of the Gerontological Society of America, San Diego, November.

Habib, M., & Gutwill, S. (1985). The union setting: Working with retirees. In E. Schwartzman (Ed.), *Gerontological social work practice in the community* (pp. 247–255). New York: Haworth Press.

Harris, L., & Associates, Inc. (1981). *Aging in the eighties: America in transition.* A survey conducted for the National Council on Aging, November.

Havighurst, R. J., Munnicks, J. M., Neugarten, B. L. & Thomas, H. (1969). *Adjustment to retirement: A cross-sectional study.* New York: Humanities Press.

Heaton, R. K., Grant, I., & Matthews, C. G. (1986). Differences in neuropsychological test performance associated with age, education, and sex. In I. Grant & K. M. Adams (Eds.), *Neuropsychological assessment of neuropsychiatric disorders* (pp. 100–120). New York: Oxford University Press.

Henry, W. E. (1964). The theory of intrinsic disengagement. In P. F. Hausen (Ed.), *Age with a future* (pp. 415–418). Copenhagen: Munksgaard.

Hochschild, A. (1975). Disengagement theory: A critique and a proposal. *American Sociological Review, 40,* 553–569.

Ilmarinen, J. (1988). Physiological criteria for retirement age. *Scandinavian Journal of Work and Environmental Health, 14,* Suppl. 1, 88–89.

Kabanoff, B. (1980). Work and nonwork: A review of models. *Psychological Bulletin, 88,* 60–77.

Katz, S., Branch, L. G., Branson, M. H., Papsidero, J. A., Beck, J. C., and Greer, D. S. (1983). Active live expectancy. *New England Journal of Medicine, 309,* 1218–1224.

Kaplan, R. M., & Anderson, J. P. (1990). The general health policy model: An integrated approach. In B. Spilker (Ed.), *Quality of life assessments in clinical trials* (pp. 131–149). New York: Raven Press.

Kebric, R. B. (1988). Old age, the ancient military, and Alexander's army: Positive examples for a graying America. *The Gerontologist, 28,* 298–302.

Kreps, J. M. (1972). Lifetime tradeoffs between work and play. In G. M. Shatto (Ed.), *Employment of the middle-aged* (pp. 31–41). Springfield, IL: C. C. Thomas.

Langer, E. J., & Rodin, J. (1976). The effects of choice and enhanced personal responsibility for the aged: A field experiment in institutional setting. *Journal of Personality and Social Psychology, 34,* 191–198.

Lazarus, R. S., & Folkman, S. (1984). *Stress, appraisal, and coping.* New York: Springer.

Lemon, W. B., Bengtson, V. L., & Peterson, J. A. (1972). An exploration of the activity theory of aging: Activity types and life satisfaction among inmovers to a retirement community. *Journal of Gerontology, 27,* 511–523.

Liang, J., Drorkin, L., Kahana, E., & Mazian, F. (1980). Social integration and morale: A re-examination. *Journal of Gerontology, 35,* 746–57.

Lowenthal, M. F. & Robinson, B. (1976). Social networks and isolation. In R. H. Binstock & E. Shanas (Eds.), *Handbook of aging and the social sciences* (1st ed., pp. 432–456). New York: Van Nostrand Reinhold.

Maas, H. S., & Kuypers, J. A. (1974). *From thirty to seventy: A forty-year longitudinal study of adult lifestyles and personality.* San Francisco: Jossey-Bass.

Maddox, G. L. (1963). Activity and morale: A longitudinal study of selected elderly subjects. *Social Forces, 42,* 195–204.

Miller, S. J. (1965). The social dilemma of the aging leisure participant. In A. M. Rose & W. E. Peterson (Eds.), *Older people and their social world* (pp. 77–92). Philadelphia: F.A. Davis.

Minkler, M. (1981). Research on the health effects of retirement: An uncertain legacy. *Journal of Health & Social Behavior, 22,* 117–130.

Mitchell, O. S., Levine, P. B., & Pozzebon, S. (1988). Retirement differences by industry and occupation. *Gerontologist, 28*(4), 545–551.

Morrow-Howell, N., & Leon, J. (1988). Life-span determinants of work in retirement years. *International Journal of Aging and Human Development, 27*(2), 125–140.

Neugarten, B. L. (1973). Personality changes in later life: A developmental perspective. In C. Eisdorfer and M. P. Lawton (Eds.), *The psychology of adult development and aging* (pp. 311–335). Washington, DC: American Psychological Association.

NIAA (1971). U.S. Department of Health, Education and Welfare. *First special report to congress on alcohol and health* (pp. 23–26). National Institute of Alcohol Abuse and Alcoholism, Rockville, MD.

Palmore, E. B., Burchett, B. M., Fillenbaum, G. G., George, L. K., & Wallman, L. M. (1985). *Retirement: Causes and consequences.* New York: Springer.

Patterson, T. L., Smith, L. W., Grant, Clopton, P., Josepho, S., & Yager, J. (1990). Internal vs. external determinants of coping responses to stressful life-events in the elderly. *British Journal of Medical Psychology, 63,* 149–160.

Pepitone-Rockwell, F. (1980). *Dual career couples.* Beverly Hills, CA: Sage Publications.

Phoon, F. N. (1985). *Adding more life to years.* Paper presented at the SMA Jubilee National Medical Convention. Department of Social Medicine and Public Health, National University of Singapore, Outram Hill: Singapore.

Powers, E. A., & Goudy, W. H. (1971). Examination of the meaning of work to older workers. *Aging and Human Development, 2*, 38–45.

Reid, D. W., Haas, G., & Hawkings, D. (1977). Locus of desired control and positive self-concept of the elderly. *Journal of Gerontology, 32*, 441–450.

Reitan, R. M., & Davidson, L. A. (Eds.). (1974). *Clinical neuropsychology: Current status and applications*. New York: Wiley.

Richardson, V. (1985). Projective measurement of adult peer relations as a function of chronological age. *International Journal of Aging and Human Development, 19*, 11–23.

Richardson, V. (1985). Status concerns among retired women: Implications for social work practice. *The Journal of Applied Social Sciences, 9*, No. 2, 177–186.

Robinson, P. K., Coberly, S., & Paul, C. E. (1985). Work and retirement. In R. H. Binstock & E. Shanas (Eds.), *Handbook of aging and social sciences* (2nd ed.; pp. 503–527). New York: Van Nostrand Reinhold.

Rodin, J., & Langer, E. J. (1977). Long term effects of a control-relevant intervention with the institutionalized aged. *Journal of Personality and Social Psychology, 35*, 897–902.

Rosow, I. (1963). Adjustment of the normal aged. In R. H. Williams, C. Tibbitts, & W. Donahue (Eds.), *Processes of aging* (Vol. 2, pp. 195–223). New York: Atherton Press.

Russell, L. B. (1987). *Evaluating preventive care: Report on a workshop*. Washington, DC: Brookings.

Salthouse, T. A. (1987). Age, experience, and compensation. In C. Schooler & K. W. Schaie (Eds.), *Cognitive functioning and social structure over the life course* (pp. 142–150). New York: Ablex.

Salthouse, T. A. (1989). Training-controlled social structure? In K. W. Schaie, & C. Schooler (Eds.), *Social structure and aging: Psychological processes* (p. 123). Hillsdale, NJ: Erlbaum.

Schaie, K. W. (1988). Ageism in psychological research. *American Psychologist, 43*, 179–183.

Schaie, K. W., & Geiwitz, J. (1982). *Adult development and aging*. Boston: Little, Brown.

Schaie, K. W., & Schooler, C. (Eds.). (1989). *Social structure and aging: Psychological processes*. Hillsdale, NJ: Erlbaum.

Schnore, M. (1985). *Retirement: Bane or blessing?* Waterloo, Ontario, Canada: Wilfrid Laurier University Press.

Schonfield, D. (1977). Retirement and the commitment to activity. In B. T. Wigdor (Ed.), *Canadian Gerontological Collection I: Selected papers*. Canadian Association of Gerontology.

Schooler, C. (1984). Psychological effects of complex environments during the lifespan: A review and theory. *Intelligence, 8*, 259–281.

Schooler, C. (1989). Social structure effects and experimental situations: Mutual lessons of cognitive and social science. In K. W. Schaie & C. Schooler (Eds.), *Social structure and aging: Psychological processes* (p. 130). Hillsdale, NJ: Erlbaum.

Schuckit, M. A., Atkinson, J. H., Miller, P. L., & Berman, J. (1980). A three year follow-up of elderly alcoholics. *Journal of Clinical Psychiatry, 41*, 412–416.

Seeman, J. (1989). Toward a model of positive health. *American Psychologist, 44*, 1099–1109.

Shanas, E. (1972). Adjustment to retirement: Substitution or accomodation? In F. M. Carp (Ed.), *Retirement* (pp. 219–243). New York: Behavioral Publications.

Shanas, E., Townsend, P., Wedderburn, D., Friis, H., Milhoj, P., & Stehouwer, E. (1968). *Old people in three industrial societies*. New York: Atherton Press.

Shneidman, E. (1989). The Indian summer of life: A preliminary study of septuagenarians. *American Psychologist, 44*, 684–694.

Slater, M. A., & Good, A. B. (1991). Behavioral management of chronic pain. *Holistic Nursing Practice, 6*, 66–75.

Slater, M. A., & Kodiath, M. (1991). Comprehensive management of the chronic pain patient: A case study. *Holistic Nursing Practice, 6*, 1–8.

Slivinske, L. R., & Fitch, V. L. (1987). The effect of control enhancing interventions on the well-being of elderly individuals living in retirement communities. *The Gerontologist, 27*, 176–181.

Smith, L. W., Patterson, T. L., & Grant, I. (1990). Avoidant coping predicts psychological disturbance in the elderly. *Journal of Nervous and Mental Disease, 178*, 525–530.

Smith, L. W., Patterson, T. L., McNaughton, M. E., Smith, K. S., & Grant, I. (1990). *Coping appropriateness ratings are associated with physical and psychological symptoms in the elderly*. Paper presented at the annual meeting of the Society of Behavioral Medicine, April 18–21.

Steitz, J. A., & McClary, A. M. (1988). Subjective age, age identity, and middle-age adults. *Experimental Aging Research, 14*(2), 83–88.

Streib, G. F., & Schneider, C. J. (1971). *Retirement in American society: Impact and process*. Ithaca, NY: Cornell University Press.

Stub, H. R. (1982). *The social consequences of long life*. Springfield, IL: C. C. Thomas.

Thornton, J. E. (1987). Third-age colleges. *Generations*, Winter, 1987.

Tversky, A., & Kahneman, D. (1982). Judgement under uncertainty: Heuristics and biases. In D. Kahneman, P. Slovic, & A. Tversky (Eds.), *Judgement under uncertainty: Heuristics and biases*. Cambridge: Cambridge University Press.

U.S. Senate Special Committee on Aging. (1982). *Toward a national older worker policy*. Washington, DC: U.S. Government Printing Office.

Veroff, J., Douvan, E., & Kulka, R. (1981). *The inner American*. New York: Basic Books.

Willis, S. L. (1989). Cohort differences in cognitive aging: A sample case. In K. W. Schaie, & C. Schooler (Eds.), *Social structure and aging: Psychological processes* (pp. 95–112). Hillsdale, NJ: Erlbaum.

Wright, B. A. (1989). Extension of Heider's ideas to rehabilitation psychology. *American Psychologist, 44*, 525–528.

Young, J. B. (1989). Effects on retirement on aspects of self-perception. *Archives of Gerontological Geriatrics, 9*, 67–76.

Zimberg, S. (1978). Treatment of the elderly alcoholic in the community and an institutional setting. *Addictive Disease: An International Journal, 3*, 417–427.

20

Psychosocial Response to Environment Change

Robert B. Fields

Introduction

The inclusion of a chapter on psychosocial response to environment change among the elderly in this volume is a tribute to three decades of theoretical and applied research contributions in the areas of environmental psychology and social gerontology. Although initially challenged to provide explanations for eye opening, but somewhat misleading, early findings such as those suggesting that placement of elderly in institutions could dramatically shorten their lifespan (Carmargo & Preston, 1945; Josephy, 1949; Lieberman, 1961), the field has subsequently been marked by the development of theoretical models and methodological strategies to account for the impact of a variety of environmental changes on the physical and emotional well-being of the elderly.

The contributions of Robert Kleemeier are often cited as central to the development at this field. In his chapter of the first handbook on aging, Kleemeier (1959) stressed the importance of taking into account age-related changes in sensory-perceptual functioning (e.g., vision, hearing) and physical status (e.g., size, body fat, tolerance of extreme temperatures) when evaluating and planning environments for the elderly. The work of Kleemeier as well as individuals such as Lawton, Kahana and Kahana, Carp and Carp, Moos and Lemke, their colleagues, and many others has led to significant changes in the way in which environments for

Robert B. Fields • Allegheny Neuropsychiatric Institute, Oakdale, Pennsylvania 15071 and Department of Psychiatry, Medical College of Pennsylvania, Allegheny Campus, Pittsburgh, Pennsylvania 15212.

Handbook of Social Development: A Lifespan Perspective, edited by Vincent B. Van Hasselt and Michel Hersen. Plenum Press, New York, 1992.

healthy and impaired elderly are designed (Moos & Lemke, 1985; Parmelee & Lawton, 1990) and to our understanding of the response of elderly to their naturally occurring environments (Lawton, 1980; Scheidt & Windley, 1985).

One outcome of this research has been an increased appreciation for the heterogeneity of the elderly population as well as the enormous complexity of person–environment interactions within this population. Thus, the elderly are no longer conceptualized simply as passive responders to their environment but rather as individuals with varying capacities to shape it as well. Similarly, there are now studies exploring the adjustment of healthy, and even "adventurous" (Kahana & Kahana, 1983), elderly who choose to make major environmental changes upon retirement, as well as the adjustment of impaired elderly who are relocated to old age or nursing homes out of necessity. Outcome measures now focus less on gross measures, such as survival following environment change, and more on the specific component parts of physical and emotional well-being following environment change, such as perceived autonomy and control, perceived safety, social contacts, congruence between personal needs and environmental resources, and the dynamics of interactions with caregivers. Unfortunately, the research productivity in this area has slowed in the past decade, prompting some (Parmelee & Lawton, 1990) to suggest that it is at a crossroad. Thus, in addition to serving as a tribute to the area's rich past, it is hoped that this chapter may be an impetus for new research as well.

Implicit in the study of the topic of aging and environment are at least two assumptions or hypotheses about the elderly. The first is that certain environmental changes are not only more prevalent among the elderly than nonelderly but are relatively common occurrences among the over-65 population as a whole. The second is that older adults may be more vulnerable than younger adults to changes in the environment. Although it is clear that certain environmental changes and vulnerabilities are more common among the elderly, it is also clear from the literature of the past three decades that the description of an impaired individual struggling to adjust to nursing home relocation does not capture the modal interaction between elderly individuals and their environments.

What also seems clear is that although the variable of age plays a very important role in explaining why certain environmental changes occur, it may play a less important role as one of several variables in the hypothetical regression equation that determines psychosocial response to those changes. The potential "benefit" of considering non-age-related variables when evaluating psychosocial response is that it opens the door for the application of findings from other areas of environmental, social, developmental, and clinical psychology to our understanding of, and intervention with, the elderly. The potential "cost," which is an extreme one, is that the unique portion of the variance that is accounted for by the variable of age might be overlooked, which could result in decreased attention to the elderly and a reduction of sorely needed services and interventions.

With this cost/benefit ratio in mind, this chapter will attempt to provide a broad context for understanding the person–environment interactions among the elderly by reviewing three representative theoretical models, as well as the environmental demographics of the elderly, and by applying this information to three areas of person–environment interaction. The first is the well-researched area of relocation as a reaction to impairments in functioning, referred to here as "reactive environment change." The second is an area that has received increased interest over the past decade and takes into account the proactive efforts of elderly to change their environments, permanently or temporarily, referred to here as "non-reactive environment change." The third is a relatively understudied area that directly addresses the issue of differential vulnerability of the elderly to environment change; that is, the comparative response of elderly and nonelderly to natural disasters.

REPRESENTATIVE THEORETICAL MODELS

Interest in examining how elderly individuals respond to changes in their environment comes from several sources. These include (a) the importance of environmental factors in influencing human behavior in general, (b) the expectation that elderly individuals will be more vulnerable to environmental stress due to their increased physical and cognitive limitations, (c) the aforementioned evidence from early studies that dramatically changing the environment of already impaired elderly can significantly shorten their lives, and (d) studies demonstrating that environmental interventions can enhance those lives.

Attempts to provide conceptual models to explain available data and to make predictions for the millions of elderly who will at some point undergo an environment change have focused on understanding the competencies and vulnerabilities of elderly individuals and the demands and resources of their environments. Central to the major theoretical models in this areas has been the notion that positive response to environment change is most likely when there is congruence between individual abilities and needs and environmental demands and resources.

Not surprisingly, these models were derived from more broad-based theories of environmental impact on behavior. Lewin's (1951) field theory, for example, which applied topological terms from mathematics to psychology, is a typical starting place. According to this model, behavior can be conceptualized as a function of person and environment: that is, $B = F(P,E)$. Murray's (1938) needs–press theory also has been applied to this age group. This theory suggested that well-being depends, in part, on the appropriate satisfaction of needs by the environment and that environmental forces (i.e., press) activate interpersonal needs.

Applying such broad theories to specific populations, specific environments, or specific person–environment interactions is not accomplished easily. As Lawton (1989b) suggests, accounting for the variance in the P and E terms in Lewin's equation is essentially the task of understanding all of personality and environmental psychology. Another difficulty has been a stumbling block for much of gerontology (i.e., the use of an impaired subgroup as a basis for making generalizations about the elderly population as a whole). Thus, although the literature on psychosocial response to relocation to a nursing home is relevant (and potentially life prolonging) to impaired elderly who need nursing homes, it is less relevant, and possibly misleading, to our understanding of the majority of elderly who do not require nursing home care. It has, in fact, been the desire to account for healthy as well as impaired elderly and to understand the enormously complex and dynamic nature of person–environment interactions that has characterized theoretical formulations and reformulations in this area over the past decade.

ROBERT B. FIELDS

As much, or perhaps, more than anyone else, M. Powell Lawton and his colleagues have contributed to our theoretical and practical understanding of the intricate interactions between the elderly and their environments. Lawton and Nahemow's (1973) ecological model of adaptation and aging, in fact, emphasizes the importance of these interactions by adding an interaction term to Lewin's field theory equation. They propose that behavior, in this case adaptive behavior and affective response among the elderly, is a function of person factors, environment factors, and person by environment interaction factors; that is, $B = f(P, E, P \times E)$.

Person (P) factors are described primarily as an individual's overall level of competence (in Lawton's terms, the "theoretical upper limits of capacity"). Measuring the competence of elderly individuals involves assessing their functional capacity along dimensions such as physical health, sensation–perception, motor behavior, and cognitive abilities. Initially, the model focused on the reactions of individuals to their environments and proposed that greater competence led to more adaptive responses. As the model developed, Lawton gave increased emphasis to the proactive behavior of individuals to shape or exert control over their environment as well; that is, personal competence as a determinant of the environment as well as a predictor of successful adaptation to it.

Environment (E) factors or "press" are the demands of a particular environment that have the potential for activating behavior or challenging an individual's competencies. Lawton and Nahemow (1973) discussed press in terms of the normative influence that environmental factors have on behavior. Thus, response to the press of lack of food, cold weather, and crime requires the activation of some behavior whether it is shopping and cooking versus obtaining "meals on wheels," purchasing warm clothing and shoveling snow versus moving to a warm climate, or adding locks to doors and windows versus moving to a safer location.

The interaction term in the equation ($P \times E$) allows for the inclusion of the transactional nature of person–environment overlap and acknowledges that some portion of the variance in the $B = f(P, E)$ equation cannot be explained solely on the basis of P and E factors. The model assumes that maintaining a relatively stable balance between environmental demands and personal competencies is desirable. The adaptation level (AL) (from Helson, 1964) represents the rarely achievable and affectively neutral condition when there is a perfect balance between personal competencies and environmental demands. Because these demands and competencies are constantly changing, stable adaptation is short lived. Consistent with Wohlwill's (1966) work on environmental stimulation, the model assumes that minor deviations from the adaptation level (AL) are not problematic and in fact may be experienced as pleasurable. However major departures from this equilibrium are experienced negatively. Thus mild discrepancies between competence level and environmental press are perceived as either stimulating (i.e., when demand is increased) or supportive (i.e., when demand is decreased). Excessive demands, however, lead to increased stress, whereas stimulus deprivation leads to boredom and atrophy of skills. Although some elderly may periodically create press, there exists for everyone a level of press strength beyond which no degree of competence can produce a positive outcome.

Although this general principle applies to all levels of competence, the model assumes that the likelihood of positive outcome is greatest when competence is high. Thus more competent individuals can, according to the theory, adapt to a wider range of environmental press and have a greater likelihood of experiencing positive affect and of displaying successful adaptation. Conversely, as competence declines, individuals become more vulnerable to the effects of their environment and have a greater likelihood of experiencing environmental press in negative terms and exhibiting a narrower range of adaptive behavior.

Lawton and Simon (1968) referred to the notion that lowered competence results in greater vulnerability to environmental press as the "environmental docility" hypothesis. Since then, Lawton (1989b,c) has suggested an "environmental proactivity" hypothesis as well, which proposes that more competent individuals are better able to make use of environmental resources. Inclusion of this hypothesis is a noteworthy step in that it stimulates greater exploration of the effects of personal competencies, as well as environmental stressors, on psychosocial outcome.

Discussions of proactive behavior include, but are not limited to, elderly of high competence. Healthy elderly who use their retirement years to travel, move, do volunteer work, enroll in college, and generally search for novelty and stimulation are probably better understood by exploring their efforts to address needs for fulfillment and self-actualization (which may increase press) rather than by examining their reactions to the day-to-day demands of their environment. Impaired elderly, however, also engage in proactive behavior to cope with increased press or decreased competence. Rowles (1983) has described the efforts of homebound rural elderly in Appalachia to maximize their participation in their environment by positioning themselves by strategic windows to increase their "surveillance zone." This zone, which consists of the area that can be visualized from home serves two purposes; increased participation in the environment and a means of sending signals to neighbors (i.e., via drawing shades or turning on lights) about their condition. Lawton (1985a) has described the use of a "control center" by homebound elderly to increase their control over their environment, thereby increasing autonomy and affective stimulation. Typically, the control center involves use of a well-placed chair that provides visual and manual access to the door, window, television, and telephone, as well as valued personal possessions.

In addition to a greater emphasis on the bidirectional quality of person–environment interactions, Lawton (1985a, 1989b; Parmelee & Lawton, 1990) has recently stressed their dynamic nature as well proposing that old age is characterized by a dialectic between autonomy and security needs. Although the needs for physical security, feelings of safety, and social and community support among the elderly are fairly obvious, Lawton concludes that there are many empirical data to suggest, that at virtually all levels of competence, maintenance of personal autonomy and a sense of self-efficacy is also extremely important (Kahana, Kahana, & Riley, 1989; Parmelee & Lawton, 1990; Schulz & Brenner, 1977). Lawton and his colleagues (Lawton, 1989b,c; Parmelee & Lawton, 1990) have suggested that security and autonomy are the "primary environmental motives" among the elderly and that there is a constant pull to have both of these sets of needs met. They suggest further that these needs can be seen as contributing to a "life plan" that is continuously modified as the balance between autonomy and security changes with personal development and changes in the environment. The notion of an autonomy–security dialectic fits well into Lawton's extension of his theoretical framework, which takes into account both reactive and proactive behavior as contributing to psychosocial outcome. It conceptualizes an elderly individual not simply as a passive reactor to an environmental stimulus but rather someone who is actively assessing his or her own inventory of needs and attempting to influence the environment to get those needs met.

The theoretical and empirical contributions of Lawton and his colleagues have had a tremendous impact on the field of gerontology, as well as public policy. His earlier work has been particularly instrumental in increasing our understanding of the effects of various environmental variables (e.g., the physical and social attributes of buildings, neighborhoods, and communities) on the well-being and housing satisfaction of the elderly (Lawton, 1980, 1981b, 1989a; Lawton & Hoffman, 1984; Lawton & Nahemow, 1979; Lawton, Nahemow, & Yeh, 1980; Lawton & Yaffee, 1980), whereas his later work has drawn more attention to the importance of personal variables (i.e., proactivity, needs, emotional factors) in this process (Lawton, 1989b,c; Parmelee & Lawton, 1990). This work has also been helpful in providing strategies for the development of improved environments for elderly with varying needs and competencies. Finally, this work has helped us recognize both the importance and the limitations of considering the $P-E$ interaction when assessing overall well-being in the elderly (Lawton, 1983). Lawton's model emphasizes the complexity and bidirectional quality of $P-E$ interactions and implies that from a $P-E$ interaction perspective, an optimal environment is one in which the environmental demands and resources are consonant, or congruent, with the competencies and needs of the individual. This implication is central to the theoretical models of Kahana and Carp.

Kahana's Congruence Theory

The congruence theory of Eva Kahana (1975; 1982) also derived from Lewin's field theory and Murray's needs–press theory and their applications to environmental psychology and social ecology (i.e., French, Rogers, & Cobb, 1974). In Kahana's model, the person–environment interaction is probably best represented by the term "PcE" rather than "$P \times E$" where PcE reflects the congruence between personal needs and the properties of the environment (Carp & Carp, 1984). The model assumes that individuals are motivated to find environments that are congruent with their needs. In keeping with Murray's model, Kahana suggested that environmental press provides a "situational counterpart" to internalized needs that may either facilitate or hinder the gratification of those needs.

In broad terms, the model assumes that a positive outcome will result when specific personal needs or preferences are congruent with environmental demands and resources or when an individual's behavior results in the removal of an incongruous situation. Therefore, when dissonance between press and needs exists, an individual must utilize his or her adaptive coping strategies to modify the press, alter his or her hierarchy of needs, or remove himself or herself from the field. When these three options are not possible, stress and discomfort result.

In addition to her emphasis on person-specific $P-E$ congruence, Kahana stressed the importance of exploring the various dimensions of person–environment interactions and of testing the different forms of the congruence mode. Following Lewin (1951) and French *et al.* (1974), Kahana proposed that a test of person–environment congruence requires the assessment of commensurate dimensions of person and environment variables using common and quantifiable measures. Three dimensions of primarily environmental factors and four dimensions of primarily person factors were identified for inclusion in the evaluation of environments and individuals in studies of P–E congruence.

The environmental variables (from Kleemeier, 1961) included the segregate dimension (i.e., factors such as the homogeneity, stability, continuity, and similarity of an environment), the congregate dimension (i.e., whether treatment is collective or individualized and whether privacy is available), and the institutional control dimension (i.e., whether control over decisions/resources is institutionally or individually based). The person variables included structure (i.e., tolerance of ambiguity, need for structure), stimulation-engagement (i.e., preference/tolerance for stimulation and activity), affect (i.e., need for emotional expression), and impulse control (i.e., ability to delay gratification).

Kahana also described three forms of the general congruence model that could be empirically investigated. The nondirectional model predicts that the absolute size of the deviation from congruence predicts outcome rather than the direction. Thus, according to this model, excessive resources and excessive demands relative to individual needs have a similarly deleterious effect on well-being. The one-directional model predicts that only an undersupply of resources produces a negative outcome and that an oversupply has the same effect as congruence. Finally, the two-directional model predicts that behavioral outcome is different, depending upon whether the departure from congruence is in the positive direction (i.e., oversupply) or the negative direction (i.e., undersupply).

In a test of various aspects of this model, Kahana, Liang, and Felton (1980) interviewed 124 elderly individuals at three homes for the aged. Using resident preferences as person variables, staff ratings as environment variables, and morale as the outcome measure, several important results were found. First, the importance of including congruence in the assessment of person–environment interaction was supported. Person–environment fit (or congruence) was found to be most important in the areas of congregation, impulse control, and segregation. Person and/or environment factors, rather than fit, were more important along the dimensions of affective expression and institutional control. Second, the importance of examining multiple aspects of congruence was supported. Five of the seven dimensions assessed contributed significantly to the determination of morale, suggesting the methodologies targeting fewer dimensions of P–E fit may omit important sources of variance. Third, the importance of exploring the direction of the incongruence was supported. Although the amount of variance explained by the nondirectional model approached that explained by the two-directional model, the latter provided more information regarding the relationship of fit to positive outcome. Thus, depending on the dimension assessed, either oversupply or undersupply of environmental features was related to higher morale. This point also underscores the importance of examining multiple dimensions as conclusions about directionality based on one dimension could not be generalized to another.

Although presumably applicable to all elderly, the initial work with the congruence model focused on relatively impaired elderly (i.e., those living in old age or nursing homes). Paralleling the development of Lawton's model to include the proactive behavior of elderly and the dynamic nature of person–environment interactions, Kahana and her colleagues attempted to include in her model their observation that elderly at various levels of competence (but in particular, healthy elderly) demonstrated tremendous individual differences in coping strategies and environmental preferences.

In addition to the application of the congruence model to institutional populations (Kahana *et al.*, 1989), Kahana and her colleagues have been interested in healthy elderly as well. They have found, for example, that some elderly seem to break the rules of the congruence model as well as accepted gerontological theory (e.g., the desire for continuity as a means of congruence and the lack of future orientation). Kahana and Kahana (1983; Harris, Kahana, & Kahana, 1989) have followed groups of elderly who changed their environment because of a lifelong plan, or because it was "too" continuous and stable. Their samples of "adventurous aged" who voluntarily relocated to Israel or Florida demonstrated attributes such as future orientation. These individuals often chose discontinuity over stability, ostensibly because their needs for adventure, stimulation, self-growth, generativity, and the like were not being met by their environments.

The successful outcomes for many of these elderly supported Kahana's emphasis on the individual differences in coping strategies among elderly and prompted a reassessment of the static nature of the initial congruence model. Kahana and her colleagues suggested that an appreciation of adaptation over time requires a more dynamic interpretation of person–environment fit. They proposed that

> self-initiated environment change may provide a possible and meaningful avenue to the elderly to extend themselves in to the future, to find meaningful new stimulation and roles, and to enhance their satisfaction during later life. (Kahana & Kahana, 1983, p. 213)

Carp's Complementary/Congruence Model

The development of the models of Lawton and Kahana has included attempts to account for individuals of greater competence with a model first tested among individuals of lower competence and to define the relevant main and moderator variables for the modified Lewinian equation. Thus the proactivity hypothesis followed the docility hypothesis, and studies of adventurous aged followed studies of person–environment fit among residents of old age homes. One of the questions about these models has been how well do the original "rules" apply as the models expand to include individuals of increased competence and attempt to become more well defined. Another has been what are the relevant person, environment, and person by environment variables that affect or modify the $B = f(P,E,P \times E)$ equation.

Carp and Carp (1984) have suggested a complex two-part model of person and environment predictors and modifiers of behavioral outcome in the elderly to address these issues. This model is based on the underlying rationale of Lawton's and Kahana's models (and, therefore, Lewin's and Murray's as well) and attempts to define many of the terms of these models in more detail. The model is based on Murray's notion that the appropriate satisfaction of needs by the environment leads to well-being and emphasizes Kahana's notion of congruence as the critical aspect of person–environment interaction. Thus, in this model, $B = f(P,E,PcE)$. The model addresses the issue of applicability to the range of elderly by proposing that needs are organized according to Maslow's hierarchy and that the relative importance of the terms of the Lewinian equation differ based on where in the hierarchy the need is. Carp and Carp also depart from Lawton and Kahana by using a dichotomous classification system to differentiate elderly individuals based on their level of need and propose that the congruence term has a different meaning at each of these levels.

Part 1 of the model focuses on elderly whose needs are lower on Maslow's hierarchy. The task for these relatively impaired elderly is to satisfy their lower order, or life maintenance (LM), needs such as the acquisition of food and shelter independently by successful completion of their activities of daily living (ADLs). The relevant person (P) and environment (E) variables in this part of the model are the individual's competencies and the environment's resources/barriers that facilitate or inhibit the satisfaction of those needs. The congruence term in Part 1 of the model refers to the complementarity with, or compensation for, P competencies by the environment. Thus if an elderly individual has deficits in areas such as mobility, vision, and numerical reasoning skills, a complementary environment would provide specially equipped rooms (e.g., bathrooms with handrails, increased lighting) and assistance with finances. Failure to provide such resources would lead to an inability to perform some categories of ADL's which might be critical for continued independent existence. At this level, successful adaptation depends on P factors, E factors, and P–E complementarity.

Part 2 of the model focuses on elderly whose needs are higher on Maslow's hierarchy. Thus it is assumed that lower order needs are met without difficulty and are less important to the determination of well-being and positive affect. Instead, the focus is on higher order (HO) needs, such as affiliation, similarity, and privacy. In Part 2 of the model, P factors and E factors are seen as neither positive or negative and are less important than P–E congruence in determining successful adaptation to the environment. However, unlike Part 1 of the model, congruence at this level refers to similarity between personal needs and preferences and environmental resources, rather than complementarity of the environment with personal competencies and deficits. The congruence term is a reflection of the similarity between the strength of a need or personality trait (e.g., need for similarity) and the amount of environmental supply (e.g., availability of age or ethnically segregated housing). Thus the presence or absence of a specific need or preference is less important than the environment's ability to meet that need.

A valuable contribution of Carp and Carp's model is the detailed description of the specific variables involved (e.g., ADL categories of nutrition, sleep/rest, medication, medical care, hygiene, phoning, handling money, housecleaning, shopping, banking, and the like in Part 1 and higher order needs such as harm, avoidance, order, affiliation, similarity, privacy, and esthetic experience in Part 2) and the assignment of different levels of importance to variables at different places in the model. They also point out the need to take into account the effects of moderating variables such as intrapersonal characteristics (e.g., sense of personal competence, coping style, and attitude toward health), extrinsic situations that reflect the results of previous P–E transactions, and life events when determining outcome.

As with most broad theories, those of Lawton, the Kahanas and the Carps raise many issues that remain open to theoretical debate and empirical investigation. For example, the relative detrimental effects of excessive demand versus understimulation, the identification and relative weighting of critical variables for determining successful adaptation in specific situations, the ability of one model to account most parsimoniously for elderly individuals at differing levels of competence, and the relative efficacy of "person" (e.g., psychotherapy) versus "environment" (e.g., structural/caregiver environment change) based interventions for different problems under different conditions require further study.

The contributions of other theorists have also been helpful in providing explanations for the process by which elderly individuals interact with, make judgments about, and attempt to shape their environments (Scheidt & Windley, 1985). Schooler (1976), for example, has applied the stress-theoretical formulation of Lazarus (1966) to the environmental appraisal process. He proposed that elderly continuously evaluate their environments and the degree of potential threat that exists therein. When situations are perceived as harmful (vs. beneficial or irrelevant), a range of direct and intrapsychic coping responses are reviewed and applied to remove harmful stimuli or to adapt to them. Moos and Lemke have explored the relationships between a variety of physical, architectural, social, administrative, and caregiver features and the behavior of elderly in sheltered settings (see Moos, Lemke, & David, 1987, for a review). Others have focused on issues such as the cognitive maps used to perceive the environment (Regnier, 1981), the ecological and architectural attributes of environments (Scheidt & Windley, 1985), the decrease in life space (or age-loss continuum) that occurs with age (Pastalan, 1975), and what appears to be a gradual transition with age from physical participation in the environment to vicarious environmental experience via observation and fantasy (Rowles, 1981).

Like most broad theories, those reviewed here are in need of additional empirical support. They do, however, provide a valuable framework for interpreting existing data as well as generating research hypotheses and intervention strategies at both the individual and environmental levels. With regard to the topic of environment change, the three theoretical models discussed predict that (1) environment changes are likely to occur in situations when P–E incongruence is increasing, 2) environment changes that result in a more congruent fit between personal needs/desires and environmental resources/demands are likely to produce positive outcomes, and (3) the variance associated with general psychosocial well-being following an environment change will be due to person factors, environment factors, complex person–environment interaction factors, as well as other factors not accounted for in the $B = f(P,E,P \times E)$ equation. Before turning to the literature on three types of environment change, it may be helpful to obtain a broad perspective of P–E interactions by reviewing demographic data on the environments and environmental changes of the elderly.

ENVIRONMENTS AND ENVIRONMENTAL CHANGE AMONG THE ELDERLY

Physical and Social Environments of the Elderly

Where, and with whom, do the elderly live? Five percent of those above age 65 in this country reside in nursing homes or other institutions (Parmelee & Lawton, 1990; U.S. National Center for Health Statistics, 1987). Among this population, women outnumber men by approximately 3 to 1. The proportion of elderly who cannot successfully manage in the community by themselves, or with the help of others, increases with age. Thus, over 20% of those who are 85 or older reside in nursing homes (Parmelee & Lawton, 1990; U.S. National Center for Health Statistics, 1987).

In addition to age, several other factors contribute to the risk of becoming and remaining institutionalized, including absence of a spouse, absence of children, presence of cognitive and physical dysfunction, and length of previous institutionalization (Bear, 1990; Dolinsky & Rosenwaike, 1988; Litwak, 1985; Retsinas & Garrity, 1986). The availability of a family support network is particularly relevant in preventing or delaying institutionalization. Marital status is of greater relative importance for elderly males than females (Dolinsky & Rosenwaike, 1988) but is an important variable for both. Lawton (1981b) reported, for example, that only 12% of nursing home residents were married, compared to a rate of 54% among community elderly. For elderly women, risk of institutionalization depends, in part, on the number of availability of offspring. Above age 75, for example, rate of institutionalization is almost 70% higher for women with no children compared to those with three or more children (Dolinsky & Rosenwaike, 1988). Given that the actual numbers of elderly continue to increase, that the "old-old" are the fastest growing segment of the population, and that the American family is becoming smaller and more geographically spread out, our ability to understand the unique needs of elderly who require institutionalization remains a clinical imperative and an important research challenge. An overview of the psychosocial response to this type of environment change is presented later.

The overwhelming majority of the 95% of elderly who are not institutionalized live in their own homes in the community (Chevan, 1987; Lawton, 1990; Struyk & Soldo, 1980). Studies of these elderly have focused on factors such as location of residence (e.g., urban vs. suburban vs. rural) and degree of age concentration in the area. Historically, greater concentrations of elderly have been found in central cities and small rural areas than in suburbs; however, this trend has recently been changing (Golant, 1990; Rogers, 1989). Due in part to changes in the definition of metropolitan and nonmetropolitan areas, the nonmetropolitan elderly population has declined from 35.8% in 1970 to 26% in 1988 (Golant, 1990). Over the same time period, the suburban (vs. central city) portion of the metropolitan elderly population rose from 46.2% to 57.4% (Golant, 1990). The rate of "suburbanization" is now higher for both young-old and old-old than the general population (Golant, 1990). This trend has resulted in additional service needs in suburban areas and has contributed to a decrease in age segregation among the elderly.

Living in an age-segregated area has traditionally been somewhat of a mixed blessing (Jirovec, Jirovec, & Bosse, 1984; Usui & Keil, 1987). Although accessibility to same-age peers and needed services are often seen as desirable features of age-concentrated environments (Adams, 1985–86; Kendig, 1976; Lawton & Nahemow, 1979; Rosow, 1967; Ward, 1979), the increased level of poverty and crime in many of these settings, as well as the preference of some for a wider social age mix obviously are not desirable (Kendig, 1976; Lawton, 1985b; Rogers, 1989). In a study of elderly residential data through 1980, Tierney (1987) found that age segregation was on the decline among the young-old but was still increasing among those above age 75. Golant (1990), however, found that from 1980 through 1988, age segregation declined for both the young-old and the old-old.

The majority of community-dwelling elderly own their own home, with a trend over the past five decades toward increased home ownership (Chevan, 1987; Struyk & Soldo, 1980). In 1940, the proportion of elderly who owned their homes was less than 50%, whereas in 1980 it was 70.1% (Chevan, 1987). This rate of increase was higher for the elderly than the general population (Chevan, 1987). Home ownership peaks among the young-old, with a change from owner to renter status thereafter (Newman, Zais & Struyk, 1984; Struyk, 1980). For example, rate of home ownership above age 85 is approximately 35% (Chevan, 1987). Thus factors such as the rapidly increasing population of old-old, as well as housing market changes may affect the elderly owner–renter ratio over time (Newman et al., 1984).

Once in their homes, elderly are the least likely segment of the population to move (Struyk & Soldo, 1980). In fact, examining data from the late 1970s, Newman et al., (1984) found the elderly to be four times less likely than nonelderly to change residences. Elderly renters are also much less likely to relocate than nonelderly renters but more likely than elderly homeowners. This reluctance to move occurs even when the need for service increases faster than the environment can provide such services (Lawton, Moss, & Grimes, 1985). Among those who do change residences, 40% move from their own homes to rental units, whereas the reverse is true only 15% of the time (Newman et al., 1984).

Of those who continue to maintain their own residence, Lawton (1985b) estimates that up to 10% have made structural changes (e.g., the addition of handrails) to compensate for physical deficits, or in Carp and Carp's model to assist in the successful completion of life maintenance ADLs. Approximately 5% to 10% of elderly live in specialized age-segregated residential settings that range from the provision of virtually no supervision to almost complete supervision (Lawton, 1985b; Marans, Hunt, & Valkalo, 1984; Moos & Lemke, 1985). Such settings include foster families, boarding care homes, residential care facilities (Mor, Sherwood, & Gutkin, 1986), congregate apartments (Erlich, Erlich, & Woehlke, 1982; Muller, 1987), single-room-occupancy hotels, planned housing developments, homesharing (Danigeles & Fengler, 1990; Jaffe & Howe, 1988; Schreter & Turner, 1986), retirement communities (Cohen, Tell, Batten, & Larsen, 1988; Marans et al., 1984), and so forth. Reviews of the literature on the design of specialized facilities for the elderly and the variety of types of alternative community housing are available (Eckert & Murrey, 1984; Lawton, 1985b; Moos & Lemke, 1984; 1985).

The social environments of the elderly vary as a function of several factors, including age, sex, cultural norms, and family size. Because of sex differences in lifespan, the sex-by-age interaction is particularly relevant. For example, above age 65, the percentage of men who are widowed is 13.7%, whereas the percentage of widowed women is 50.5% (U.S. National Center for Health Statistics, 1987). Thus, among the elderly, 75% of men live with their spouse (vs. 38% of women), 15% live alone (vs. 41% of women), and 9% live with someone else (vs. 20% of women). For both men and women, the likelihood of living alone increases with age (25% for those between 65 and 74, 43% for those between 75 and 84, and over 70% for those over 85) (Muller, 1987). This likelihood also increases with decline in personal income and functional capacity (Soldo, Sharma, & Campbell, 1984), life-cycle-related events (Fillenbaum & Wallman, 1984) as well as the passage of time in this culture. In 1900, 60% of elderly resided with their children, whereas in 1984, 18% of older persons coresided with children (Aizenberg & Texas, 1985; Crimmins & Ingegneri, 1990). By comparison, approximately 70% of the Japanese elderly population in 1980 resided with their adult children (Kamo, 1988). Increased mobility, higher rates of divorce, and smaller family size, as well as other demographic, economic, and social support variables have been cited as reasons for the increase in those living along in this county (Crimmins & Ingegneri, 1990; Krivo & Mutchler, 1989; Newman *et al.*, 1984).

Soldo (1978, cited in Lawton, 1981) found a relationship between the residences of elderly widows and their family size. In her study of widowed women, 9% of those with no children lived with relatives, 17% of those with one child lived with a relative, whereas 38% of those with four or more children lived with a relative. Living with others has also been related to health status. But, as Magaziner, Cadigan, Hebel, and Parry (1988) noted, poor health does not result from living alone or with others. Rather, the choice of live with others is made because poor health limits the individual's capacity to live independently. When given a choice, the elderly strongly prefer to live independently (Dolinsky & Rosenwaike, 1988; Marans *et al.*, 1984).

Emphasizing only health of the elderly and child availability may, however, be a somewhat age-biased view of living arrangements that leaves out an important source of variance; that is, the needs of the child (Crimmins & Ingegneri, 1990; Wolf & Soldo, 1988). In their study of coresidence between elderly parents and their adult children, Crimmins and Ingegneri (1990) found that 56% of the children who coresided with elderly parents had done so for their entire lives, indicating that age of parent was not the primary reason for the living arrangement. In addition, of those who made a decision to coreside after living independently, approximately half cited reasons that were of primary benefit to the child (e.g., death of child's spouse, etc.). In a separate sample, only 36% of the older sample living with their children cited their own health or the need to share living expenses as the reason for the coresidence.

The data of Crimmins and Ingegneri (1990) underscore the need to test, rather than assume an assigned role for age when assessing the environmental behavior of the elderly. In general, the question of where and with whom the elderly live is probably best answered by considering personal competencies (e.g., physical and mental health, cognitive integrity, financial resources), family and other environmental resources (e.g., availability of spouse, children, friends), and cohort effects (e.g., recent trends toward increased suburbanization and decreased age segregation), as well as at least two age-related conclusions regarding the environments of the elderly. First, with advancing age, elderly in this country are more likely than the general population to face the psychosocial stressors of living alone or placement in a nursing home. Second, the elderly appear to be more strongly attached to their home environments than the nonelderly. Reasons for the first conclusion are relatively straightforward, in particular with regard to the need for nursing home placement. Consistent with Lawton's environmental docility hypothesis, as personal competencies decline, an elderly individual is more vulnerable to the press of the environment and more likely to require a new or adapted environment that is more congruent (Kahana, 1975) with his or her life maintenance (Carp & Carp, 1984) needs. The lack of environmental supports caused by the death of a spouse or the absence of children contributes to such vulnerability.

The second conclusion is less easily understood. Several explanations have been proposed for the phenomenon of increased attachment to home among the elderly. These include (a) reluctance to give up a home environment that has become associated with personal achievement, personal meaning, affectively positive memories, and strong neighborhood and social attachments, (b) reluctance to give up a major financial asset, (c) deficient knowledge of alternative housing possibilities, (d) absence of suitable housing, (e) increased reluctance to experience the stress of moving, and (f) perceived loss of decisional control (Golant, 1984; Lawton, 1985b; Newman et al., 1984; Rowles, 1980; Rubinstein, 1989). As Newman et al. (1984) point out, many of these explanations require additional empirical support. Attachment to home may be best understood as one important variable in the ongoing decision-making process of assessing congruence between personal needs/desires and the resources/opportunities offered by the home environment. Factors, such as psychological attachment, financial situation, and family life cycle stage, as well as the influence of personal, environmental, and life event variables of this decision process are discussed in Wiseman's (1980) model of residential behavior. For many elderly, the desire to change residence is outweighed by the lack of financial resources to do so. For others, a desire to live in a warmer climate or in closer proximity to relatives because of declining health outweighs attachment to home. However, as the aforementioned data suggest, for many elderly, attachment to home and neighborhood remains an important aspect of the unique person environment interaction among the elderly.

Types and Patterns of Environmental Change in the Elderly

As noted, the frequency of environmental change declines with age. Reviewing U.S. Census data, Golant (1984) noted that for the 5 years prior to 1980, 21% of the elderly population of the United States changed residence compared to 45% of the total population. The data on moves across county (Bohland & Rowles, 1988) and state (Rogers & Watkins, 1988) lines by elderly and nonelderly are similarly discrepant. For example, 4.6% of the elderly population moved to different states between 1975 and 1980 compared to an interstate migration rate of 9.9% for the general population (Rogers & Watkins, 1988). From their review of the elderly migration data across three census periods, Rogers and Watkins (1988) observed that although the volume of elderly moves has continued to increase, an increase in the rate of interstate migration is a relatively recent phenomenon and has corresponded in time with a decline in the rate of local moves.

Patterns of movement among the elderly, such as those noted have been of particular interest to those attempting to plan for the tremendous potential impact of a substantial change in the elderly population on the economies and service needs of local communities (Longino & Biggar, 1982; Monahan & Greene, 1982). As a result, comprehensive studies in this area have been conducted (e.g., the Retirement Migration Study of Flynn, Longino, Wiseman, & Biggar, 1985). Types of moves have been discussed from geographic and demographic (Biggar, 1980; Carter, 1988; Flynn et al., 1985; Krout, 1983; Rogers & Watkins, 1988; Serow, 1987a), as well as psychosocial (Litwak & Longino, 1987; Speare & Meyer, 1988; Wiseman, 1980) perspectives. Thus interstate moves have been characterized by migration to the sunbelt and return migration to place a birth (or former residence) and differentiated from local moves. From a demographic standpoint, those moving across state lines tend to be married, white, younger, of higher education, and more financially secure than other movers or nonmovers. Those who return from the sunbelt to northern states tend to be older and more socially and economically dependent, whereas local movers are more economically dependent and in poorer health than elderly nonmovers or long distance movers.

From a psychosocial perspective, moves by elderly in search of improved climate and/or quality of life, increased proximity to family, and/or increased assistance following gradual functional decline or major disability have been studied (Litwak & Longino, 1987; Oldakowski & Roseman, 1986; Serow, 1987a; Wiseman, 1980). As several reviewers of this literature have suggested (Gober & Zonn, 1983; Lawton, 1985a,b; Watkins, 1989; Wiseman, 1980) these moves represent a dynamic P–E interaction process that is influenced by changing personal situations, environmental resources, and cultural perception about what constitutes a desirable environment. Wiseman's (1980) typology of moving has been particularly helpful in understanding the many variables involved in the decision to move or remain in place. Consistent with the environmental docility and proactivity hypotheses, as well as with P–E congruence models, Wiseman suggests that the decision to move results from a process of continuous evaluation of residential satisfaction. This process take into account "push" factors (e.g., environmental stress, loss of a spouse), "pull" factors (e.g. retirement amenities, family/friends), and "triggering mechanisms" (e.g., change in preferred lifestyle, critical life events, change in social support network, P–E incongruence) and weighs them against personal needs/desires, available personal and environmental resources, and perceived postrelocation outcome. Wiseman's typology specifies three types of long-distance moves (i.e., amenity, assistance, and return migration) and allows for predictions about psychosocial outcome for elderly whose decision to move or stay is made voluntarily or involuntarily.

More recently, Litwak and Longino (1987) have suggested a developmental perspective for understanding the migration patterns of the elderly. They propose that three types of moves characterize the elderly and support their model with census data on migration, return migration, and institutionalization. The first move described in the model occurs soon after retirement and is made primarily for amenity reasons. Relocation to a retirement community in the sunbelt is an example. In Carp and Carp's model, this is clearly a decision based on higher order, rather than life maintenance, needs and is more common among the young-old who are healthy, have intact marriages, and can afford it. Interstate migration data are consistent with the notion of increased amenity moves following retirement. In 1980, for example, 8.9% of those who changed states of residence in the general population moved to the most frequent destination (Florida). Among the elderly, 25.9% of those who moved across state lines, chose Florida as a destination with California (8.8%), Arizona (5.7%), New Jersey (4.5%), and Texas (3.1%) next in line (Rogers & Watkins, 1988).

The second move is proposed to occur when the need to focus on life maintenance needs takes center stage. Thus moves to obtain assistance, rather than for amenity reasons, are prompted by widowhood or the development of chronic disabilities that make tasks such as cooking, cleaning, and shopping, as well as access to medical services, more difficult. These moves are presumed to be more common in the old-old and typically are designed to increase proximity to children or to return to a former residence where necessary resources are available. Data on return migration reviewed by Litwak and Longino (1987) and Watkins (1988) supported the contention that migration to sunbelt states is more frequent among those below age 75, whereas return migration is more common among those over 75. Serow and Charity (1988) did not find that return to state of birth was more common among the old-old, but they did find that return migration accounted for more than one-fourth of all interstate moves among the elderly and that it was more common among females and elderly who were not married.

Speare and Meyer (1988) suggested that this second stage actually consists of two types of moves. The first is a move designed to increase proximity to family in anticipation of future needs, and the second, a true assistance move, occurs following a change in health or functional status. The third type of move proposed by Litwak and Longino (1987) is typically a local one: that is, relocation to an institution when there either are no caretakers available, or the caretaker can no longer provide the necessary care.

The notion of a unique developmental sequence for the elderly is consistent with studies of elderly and nonelderly movers from the 1970s (Long & Hansen, 1979) and 1980s (Speare & Meyer, 1988), which found that although employment is the most commonly cited reason for moving below age 55, amenity, kinship/family, retirement, and widowhood are the most common reasons cited by movers over age 55. This perspective is also consistent with Serow's (1987b) review of elderly migration patterns across nine countries. He found evidence for two main types of elderly migration; one by younger, relatively more affluent elderly seeking improvements in their quality of life, and a second by older, more dependent elderly seeking additional care and support. Lawton's (1985b) review of this literature underscores the relationship between health and type of residential relocation. He points out that good health facilitates moves for amenity reasons, whereas poor health leads the elderly to make moves for assistance. He also points out that some return migration and local moves are clearly amenity moves as well. Thus evaluating psychosocial response following a move requires a consideration of personal competencies, as well as environmental and cultural/cohort-specific contextual factors.

A final type of modified residential change has also received increased attention (Happel, Hogan, Pflanz, 1988; Hogan, 1987; Krout, 1983; Monahan & Greene, 1982). Elderly who choose to migrate on a seasonal basis (the so-called "snowbirds") seem to have the best of both worlds. By retaining residences in their home states, they are able to maintain social and emotinoal attachments to home and neighborhood. By changing residences during the winter they are able to reap the benefits of an amenity move without experiencing the loss of previous ties. For many, returning to the same location each year allows for the development of new social and environmental attachments. This process is made easier if members from social networks in the states of origin actively attempt to keep in contact with friends or acquaintances who seek the same winter destination.

Because of the nature of seasonal migration, estimates of its prevalence have been difficult to obtain. However, it seems clear that his phenomenon is increasing and will have a very significant impact on specific communities. Happel *et al.* (1988) estimate that approximately 200,000 elderly spent part or all of the 1986–1987 winter season in the Phoenix area. Compared with a total permanent immigration estimate of 95,000 between 1975 and 1980, this number is quite significant. Happel *et al.* (1988) found that the most frequent residence type was mobile homes (47%), followed by apartments (23%), single-family homes/condos (15%), motels (8%), and friends/relatives (7%). The geographic pattern of seasonal migration is similar to permanent sunbelt migration with Florida the most frequent destination, followed by Arizona, California, and Texas (Hogan, 1987). Demographically, elderly seasonal migrants are similar to permanent migrants with the exception that they are more likely to be married and less likely to be widowed (Hogan, 1987; Krout, 1983; Martin, Hoppe, Larson, & Leon, 1987). In general, seasonal migrants are more likely than nonmigrants to be white, married, retired, in good health, to own a car, have more education, and have a higher income (Hogan, 1987; Krout, 1983).

These data, like the data on elderly who age in place, point out that there are age-related differences in the mobility patterns of the elderly compared to the nonelderly. Because of the increases in permanent and seasonal migration, considerable interest will be generated by the migration pattern results of the 1990 census. Whatever the results, it is safe to assume that aging in place will remain the modal choice for the elderly (Lawton, 1985b).

Although the focus of this chapter is on psychosocial response to significant environmental changes, it is important to emphasize that aging in place does not mean the absence of significant environmental change. Alterations in social and physical aspects of "stable" environments of the elderly have very significant psychosocial implications. It has been well documented, for example, that the death or prolonged illness of a spouse can exact a tremendous psychological toll on widows and caregivers (Pruchno & Resch, 1989). Decreases in an elderly individual's ability to perceive his or her environment accurately (e.g., due to hearing loss, vision loss, or misperception or visual/spatial deficits following a stroke) also can, but do not always, produce a "changed" environment with psychosocial or behavioral consequences.

In a similar vein, a variety of physical and social environmental factors have been shown to contribute significantly to the psychological well-being and environmental satisfaction of the elderly. This literature has obvious implications for our understanding of the decisions behind, and the adaptation process following, an environment change. Thus, for example, factors such as the physical and architectural features of a new setting (Moos & Lemke, 1985), whether those features are congruent with resident preferences (Brennan, Moos, & Lemke, 1988), and the composition, quality, and safety of the new neighborhood (Chapman & Beaudet, 1983; Jirovec et al., 1984; LaGrange & Ferraro, 1987; Lawton, 1980; Lawton & Yaffee, 1980; Normoyle & Foley, 1988) are all likely to influence postrelocation outcome.

PSYCHOSOCIAL RESPONSE TO REACTIVE ENVIRONMENTAL CHANGE

The reactions of the elderly when environments do change have been discussed from a variety of perspectives. As a result, attention has been focused on Person factors, such as desire or willingness to move, Environment factors, such as type and quality of relocation setting, and Person × Environment interaction factors, such as relocation preparation programs. For understandable reasons, greater emphasis has been placed on assessing the effects of relocation of relatively impaired elderly who were presumed to be more vulnerable to this type of life event. Use of the terms *reactive* and *nonreactive* environment change is designed to include healthy, as well as impaired, elderly in this discussion.

Reactive environmental changes are operationalized here as those that are

(a) triggered (Wiseman, 1980) by life or environmental events (e.g., chronic illness, functional decline, widowhood, condominium conversion), (b) designed to provide greater access to needed or anticipated services, and (c) more common among the elderly than the nonelderly. Relocation to nursing homes or senior citizen apartments are examples. Nonreactive environmental changes are operationalized as those moves made by the elderly who are searching not for additional assistance but rather an environment that can provide resources that will presumably lead to an improved quality of life. Amenity moves to the sunbelt are examples. In general terms, this distinction is consistent with the distinction between lower order and higher order needs in Carp and Carp's complementary-congruence model of Person × Environment interaction among the elderly as well as Lawton's environmental docility and proactivity hypotheses. Admittedly, use of this terminology produces a significant amount of gray area. For example, whether a move made by a healthy elderly widow from a sunbelt state to her place of former residence in order to be closer to friends and family is reactive, nonreactive, or both, is open to debate. The point of making this distinction is to question whether findings based on relatively impaired elderly apply to healthy elderly as well or whether different explanatory models are needed.

The literature covered by the general topic of reactive relocation ranges from healthy elderly who move to new residences in the community to those elderly making inter- or intrainstitutional moves. Relocation to age-segregated facilities and institutional settings has received the most attention. In fact, few topics in gerontology have been as widely studied or as heatedly debated as the issue of survival following relocation of the elderly. Despite their methodological weaknesses, early studies that reported strikingly increased mortality rates among the elderly admitted or transferred to institutional settings (e.g., Carmago & Preston, 1945; Whittier & Williams, 1956) raised sufficient concern to prompt a series of relocation, or "transplantation shock," studies. The results of these follow-up studies were contradictory. Some (e.g., Aldrich & Mendkoff, 1963; Killian, 1970; Markus, Blenker, Bloom, & Downs, 1972; Pablo, 1977) found evidence for negative effects of relocation such as increased rates of stress, depression, and mortality. Others (e.g., Borup, Gallego, & Heffernan, 1979; Carp, 1967; Lawton & Yaffee, 1970; Wittels & Botwinick, 1974) found that relocation had no negative effects and in some cases positive effects on well-being, longevity, and survival (Newman & Owen, 1982; Pastalan, 1983).

Reviews of this literature have also been contradictory. One group of researchers (Borup, 1981, 1982, 1983; Borup & Gallego, 1981) concluded that relocation does not lead to increased mortality or other adverse consequences for the elderly. As a result, they also concluded that relocation preparation programs are valuable only as a means of general stress reduction and that fear of relocation effects might unfairly prevent elderly from moving to improved environments. Coffman (1981, 1983) also concluded that there was not evidence for a generalized relocation effect on postmove mortality. He suggested that relocation *per se* is not inherently harmful or beneficial to survival among the institutionalized elderly and also cautioned that under certain conditions not moving someone may be more dangerous than moving them. Coffman (1983) proposed further that postrelocation mortality effects may have more to do with caretaking and social support system changes than with physical environment changes.

On the other side of the controversy, strong objections were raised to the conclusion that relocation does not produce negative effects (Bourestom & Pastalan, 1981; Horowitz & Schulz, 1983). It was suggested that although many environmental changes are not harmful, those that are would place the elderly at even greater risk if the vulnerabilities of this group were not recognized. It was also suggested that some of the studies upon which the conclusions of no-relocation effect were based were biased in that direction on methodological grounds (Schulz & Horowitz, 1983). This group of researchers (Bourestom & Pastalan, 1981; Horowitz & Schulz, 1983; Pastalan, 1983; Schulz & Brenner, 1977; Schulz & Horowitz, 1983) concluded that relocation outcome is affected by several variables including whether the move was voluntary, prepared for, to a similar or improved environment, and made by an individual in good or failing health.

It is likely that generalized conclusions about the negative versus neutral/ positive effects of relocation based primarily on mortality data have been misleading. Numerous methodological criticisms of these studies provide support for this contention. One area of criticism has been the lack of comparability between the health and cognitive status of the samples of the elderly studied and the quality of pre- and postrelocation and environments (Lieberman & Tobin, 1983; Moos & Lemke, 1985; Tobin & Lieberman, 1976). A second area has been the emphasis on the variable of mortality to the relative exclusion of variables that might be more likely to change prior to and/or following a significant stressor (Coffman, 1983; Elwell, 1986; Horowitz & Schulz, 1983; Lieberman, 1974; Schulz & Horowitz, 1983). A third area has been the failure to isolate the impact of factors, such as demographic variables (e.g., age, sex), health and functional capacity, self-selection, anticipation of moving, exposure to noxious aspects of institutional life, and pre- and postrelocation differences in social support and quality of care when assessing relocation effects (Coffman, 1981, 1983; Elwell, 1986; Horowitz & Schulz, 1983; Moos & Lemke, 1985; Tobin & Leiberman, 1976). A final area has been the relative lack of emphasis on differences in the extent of environmental change that occurs following relocation (Elwell, 1986; Moos & Lemke, 1985).

From the perspective of individual elderly, even if eventual adaptation takes place, the global life changes associated with the experience of becoming institutionalized are likely to have significant psychosocial consequences (Baltes & Reisenzein, 1986; Piper & Langer, 1986). It is not surprising, therefore, that increased symptoms of depression have been reported among elderly nursing home residents (Parmelee, Katz, & Lawton, 1989), as well as among the family members who care for them (Brody, Dempsey, & Pruchno, 1990). On the other hand, for some, institutionalization or change in institutional setting may provide a level of care that has been long overdue. Thus literature reviews and new research that emphasize the need to consider the effects of the event of relocation within a broader context may provide the most helpful recommendations. Given that the elderly are reluctant to move, that these moves often follow a very significant life event such as disability or widowhood, and that the postrelocation environment may differ dramatically from their previous environment, the effects of "pure relocation" are often difficult to discern and may be less meaningful than the entire sequence of events within which an environment change is embedded (Coffman, 1983; Moos & Lemke, 1985; Stokols & Shumaker, 1982).

The issue of control, or perceived control, has been central to this sequence of events. In general, it has been well established that loss of control leads to feelings of helplessness that have been associated with decreased physical and mental health, decreased general well-being, and increased mortality (Kahana *et al.*, 1989; Maiden, 1987; Schulz & Brenner, 1977). Schulz and Brenner (1977) applied models derived from human and animal studies of control to the relocation literature. They hypothesized that the potential negative effects of relocation would be reduced if an individual had more control over the move and if it was more predictable. They also suggested that aspects of personality and previous experience (e.g., locus of control and type of relocation setting) would contribute to psychosocial response. Reviews of the relocation literature have generally supported these hypotheses (Moos & Lemke, 1985; Pastalan, 1983; Parmelee & Lawton, 1990; Schulz & Brenner, 1977).

Two, now-classic field studies have also lent support. Schulz (1976) found that the ability to control or predict the occurrence of a positive event (i.e., a visit from an undergraduate) led to increases in physical and psychological well-being among nursing home residents compared to residents who received random or no visits. These increases, however, stopped when the experimental intervention stopped (Schulz & Hanusa, 1978). Along similar lines, Langer and Rodin (1976) found that communications to nursing home residents emphasizing their opportunities for choice and their responsibility for themselves and the care of a plant led to improvements in alertness, active participation, and a general sense of well-being. In this project, the intervention was continued, and the initial improvements were maintained at an 18-month follow-up (Rodin & Langer, 1977). The impact of these and similar control-enhancing strategies has been reviewed by Rodin, Timko, and Harris (1985). More recent programs designed to enhance control and self-help activities have also been associated with positive effects on perceived level of control and overall functioning for the elderly living in nursing home (Rodin, 1983) and other settings such as retirement communities (Berkowitz, Waxman, & Yaffe, 1988; Slivinske & Fitch, 1987).

In addition to control, the contention that increased predictability of post-relocation environment due to preparation programs can reduce the negative effects of relocation has also received attention (Kowalski, 1981; Pastalan, 1983; Schulz & Brenner, 1977; Zweig & Csank, 1975). Although the impact of preparation programs on mortality remains in question (Borup, 1982; Pastalan, 1983), most researchers agree that these programs can reduce prerelocation anxiety and/or facilitate postrelocation adjustment. In his review of this literature, Pastalan (1983) concluded that the most effective programs tailored the use of site visits, group discussions, and individual counseling to the specific competencies of the individual. The importance of specific components of these programs has also been suggested, including targeting the most vulnerable subpopulations for increased assistance (Kowalski, 1981; Mirotznik & Ruskin, 1985), recognizing the importance of preserving relationships with staff, family, and personal possessions in the new setting (Kowalski, 1981; Mirotznik & Ruskin, 1985; Tesch, Nehrke, & Whitbourne, 1989; Wells & Macdonald, 1981), involving residents and staff (whenever possible) in the process of relocation planning (Kowalski, 1981; Mirotznik & Ruskin, 1985; Tesch *et al.*, 1989), and assessing the utility of specific behavioral skills and coping styles to deal with postrelocation changes (Kahana, Kahana, & Young, 1987; Nirenberg, 1983).

Thus, although somewhat less heated, the relocation controversy has not disappeared. Recent work has attempted to refine methodological strategies in order to explore the multiple possible predictors of a variety of outcome variables in a more systematic manner. Although Coffman (1981) did not find evidence for a systematic effect of any specific variable on mortality, the majority of the studies that he reviewed did not attempt to factor out the effects of other possible predictor variables or to address a representative sample of the range of possible outcome variables. The slow process of understanding this complex multiple predictor–multiple outcome matrix has focused on the effect of variables such as control, predictability, social network, and person–environment congruence on psychosocial outcome following three types of environmental change (home to home, home to institution, and institution to institution).

Home to Home

Moves from one home to another occur for a variety of reasons. As operationalized here, the term *reactive* relocation fits this type of move least well in that many elderly change residences for nonreactive reasons, whereas others are forced to move for reasons that are not age related. Ferraro (1982) pointed out the differences between voluntary and involuntary moves as well as between moves to senior citizen residences and those to non-age-segregated dwellings in the community. He proposed that voluntary moves to senior citizen facilities are likely to have neutral or positive effects because of the physical and social support resources available in them, whereas involuntary moves in the community are likely to have detrimental effects on health especially if they disrupt social networks and do not result in an improved environment.

The literature generally supports the first contention. The great majority of studies of elderly making voluntary moves to senior citizen residences found no significant ill effects on variables such as mortality or overall well-being (Carp, 1967; Lawton & Yaffee, 1970; Sherwood, Greer, Morris, & Mor, 1981; Wittels & Botwinick, 1974). For example, Carp's (1967) study of the elderly who relocated to the Victoria Plaza apartment complex in San Antonio found positive changes in satisfaction, need for services, and social functioning. When reassessed 8 years later (Carp, 1977), evidence for improved health and declining death rates was found and related to increased life satisfaction and reduced stress associated with the new environment. The finding that positive outcome follows moves to improved environments (Carp, 1967, 1977) that offer a sense of long-term security and, in cases, opportunities to enhance personal control and increased social involvement (Berkowitz *et al.*, 1988; Slivinske & Fitch, 1987) are in keeping with Lawton's proposed dialectic between security and autonomy needs (Parmelee & Lawton, 1990).

Ferraro's conclusion that postrelocation outcome is not as favorable for the elderly who are forced to move to community settings without physical and social resources has received mixed support. Increased health problems have been reported following involuntary moves by the elderly prompted by highway construction and urban renewal (Brand & Smith, 1974; Ferraro, 1982; Kasteler, Gray, & Carruth, 1968). However, recent studies of forced relocation of urban elderly single-room occupancy (Eckert & Haug, 1984) and Manhattan hotel (Cohen, Teresi, & Holmes, 1985) residents did not report negative outcome. In these studies, the importance of social networks, congruence between old and new neighborhoods, and satisfaction with the new environment were cited as mediating variables.

To summarize, the literature on moves from one residence to another is most conclusive under extreme conditions. Voluntary relocations by the elderly to settings designed to meet their needs do not produce ill effects and can, in fact, be beneficial whereas involuntary relocations within the community may place the elderly at increased risk for health and adjustment problems. Although there do appear to be risks associated with involuntary relocations to senior citizen residences and semivoluntary relocations within the community, especially among those in poorer health (Pastalan, 1983; Schulz & Brenner, 1977), these risks can apparently be modified by factors such as quality of and satisfaction with postrelocation environment as well as social support.

Home to Institution

Moves from home to an institution were hypothesized by Schulz and Brenner (1977) to be the most disruptive because of the significant dissimilarity between environments. That institutionalization in general has been associated with iatrogenic effects, such as increased dependency, helplessness (Avorn & Langer, 1982; Baltes, Kinderman, Reisenzien, & Schmid, 1987; Baltes & Reisenzien, 1986), and depression (Parmelee et al., 1989) as well as reduced perceived control, in particular for those with less education and more functional impairments (Arling, Harkins, & Capitman, 1986), supports this hypothesis. That problems such as inappropriate placement (Knight & Walker, 1985), lack of staff training (Heumann, 1988), and inadequate use of the literature on architectural design for the impaired elderly (e.g. Calkins, 1988) have also been reported in institutional settings also lend support. Furthermore, as Kahana et al. (1989) point out, the typical elderly individual making this type of move is a widowed female in her 80s whose self-care skills are declining, who is reliant on the assistance of others for decision making, and who fears being institutionalized.

It is not surprising, therefore, that early studies also supported Schulz and Brenner's hypothesis. Ferrari (1963), for example, reported that 16 of 17 patients relocated involuntarily died within 10 weeks of admission, whereas only 1 of 38 patients relocated voluntarily died in the same timespan. Schulz and Alderman (1973) found that cancer patients transferred from home survived on average 1 month less than cancer patients transferred from a similar inpatient setting. More recently, Stein, Linn, and Stein (1989) also found increased mortality rates in cancer patients who had increased feelings of hopelessness and helplessness following relocation to a nursing home.

In their reviews of this literature, both Schulz and Brenner (1977) and Pastalan (1983) stressed the importance of the variable of control. They concluded that involuntary relocation, in particular to an environment that is dissimilar to the prerelocation environment, places the elderly at increased risk for death, whereas voluntary relocation reduces this risk. Adjustment, they contend, appears to be affected by the nature of the prerelocation environment, the degree of change in control over the environment, the response style of the individual (i.e., active vs. passive), as well as the congruence between personality attributes and environmental demands. More recent studies continue to support the importance of predictability and control prior to, and following, moves to institutional settings. Rodin (1983) for example, found that programs designed to enhance coping skills by focusing on self-regulatory behavior (e.g., positive and negative self-statements) in helplessness-provoking situations had positive effects on the behavior and well-being of nursing home residents. In addition, Hunt and Roll (1987) found that elderly volunteers who were prepared to enter an unknown building via simulation training or a site visit displayed better and more confident "way-finding" behavior than controls. They suggest that similar simulation programs could be used prior to institutional moves.

Other studies (Kahana *et al.*, 1987; Turner, Tobin, & Lieberman, 1972) have also documented the importance of aspects of postrelocation environment as well as an individual's coping style in moderating postrelocation effects and have suggested that positive outcome following institutional relocation is not an impossibility (Kahana *et al.*, 1989). From a family/social network perspective, it seems likely that for many elderly, nursing home relocation represents the best possible psychosocial decision. That this decision is often made when the social support system has been exhausted (Bear, 1990) and allows families some relief from physical caretaking and the opportunity for social and emotional caretaking as well as other social outlets (Aizenberg & Treas, 1985) supports this contention.

Thus the event of nursing home placement among the elderly represents a complex interaction between a number of demographic, (e.g., age, number of offspring, marital status), health (e.g., physical and mental competence), and psychosocial (e.g., availability and type of social support system, degree of personal control) variables. Future studies of response to home to institution relocation will be most helpful if they take into account preexisting differences in these variables as well as differences in quality of setting, social support system, perceived control, and degree of person–environment congruence in the postrelocation environment.

Intra- and Interinstitutional Moves

For reasons that are primarily practical, research on inter- and intrainstitutional moves has been the most abundant. By definition, these moves typically involve impaired elderly who are relocated for administrative rather than personal choice reasons. Although it is possible to line up these studies solely on the basis of negative (Aldrich & Mendkoff, 1963; Csank & Zweig, 1980; Killian, 1970; Markus *et al.*, 1972; Pablo, 1977) versus neutral or positive (Bonardi, Pencer, & Tourigny-Rivard, 1989; Borup, 1982; Borup & Gallego, 1981; Elwell, 1986; Haddad, 1981; Mirotznik & Ruskin, 1985) outcome, the aforementioned methodological criticisms of this area clearly suggest a more fine-grained analysis. As with other types of relocation, variables of premove health status, degree of environmental change, perceived control over the move, degree of preparedness, impact on social support network, and effect on available services have been postulated as predictors of postrelocation outcome on a variety of outcome variables (Bonardi *et al.*, 1989; Elwell, 1986; Mirotznik & Ruskin, 1985; Pastalan, 1983; Schulz & Brenner, 1977).

As with other types of relocation, methodological approaches have become more focused for this type of move as well. In the area of personal competence, for example, whereas early studies suggested increased mortality among elderly who were classified in general terms as helpless, psychotic, or demented (Aldrich & Mendkoff, 1963; Csank & Zweig, 1980), more recent work (Pruchno & Resch, 1988) has attempted to specify the levels of personal competence (i.e., moderate vs. high or very low) and environmental dependence (i.e., high vs. low) that predict increased risk of mortality following this type of relocation. Regarding the impact of severity of environmental change, the debate continues about the possible negative effects of radical (e.g., individual transfers to a new setting with new caretakers) versus moderate or slight (mass moves with the same staff to similar or improved settings) change. Elwell (1986) did not find an increase in institutional dependence in his sample of elderly who underwent individual patient transfers to institutional settings. Likewise, Mirotznik and Ruskin (1985) failed to find negative effects following an interinstitutional move. In fact, they reported decreases in depression, alienation, and distress for many of their elderly sample following a moderate environment change. Overall improvement in morale and self-concept was found for those who were willing to move and for those experiencing fewer disturbances, and no change in morale was found for those who experienced significant relocation related disturbances.

Although helpful, these studies point out the complex nature of P–E interactions in institutional settings. It is possible, for example, that changes in aspects of physical and emotional health other than those measured by Elwell (1986) do occur, following single-patient transfers. In addition, the sample of Mirotznik and Ruskin's (1985) study was unique, in that they moved to a new facility that was specifically designed for them, and into which a panel of residents had active input. Work in the areas of enhancing perceived control, maintaining social support and increasing preparedness and available services (Bonardi et al., 1989; Haddad, 1981; Mirotznik & Ruskin, 1985; Shamain, Clarfield, & Maclean, 1984; Tesch et al., 1989; Wells & Macdonald, 1981) as well as specific skills training programs (Nirenberg, 1983) continue to suggest that, as with other types of relocation, a number of variables contribute to the prediction of positive or negative psychosocial outcome following intra- or interinstitutional moves.

From a research perspective, the literature reviewed provides a rationale for continuing to draw distinctions between the types of reactive environmental changes made by the elderly. As several reviewers have pointed out, comparing voluntary moves by relatively healthy married elderly to service-rich senior citizen complexes with involuntary moves by widows to nursing homes to explore a "relocation effect" is not methodologically sound. An understanding of the effects of relocation requires an appreciation of the context in which it occurs and the relative importance, based on that context, of a number of variables. From a theoretical perspective, the issue of control, predictability, social support, and quality of environment, as well as postrelocation adjustment, can be seen as a function of the congruence between the pre- and postrelocation environment and the needs and desires of the individual. An environment change can, therefore, be conceptualized as a landmark event in the ongoing dynamic process of person–environment interactions. Faced with relocation, elderly individuals become keenly aware of their own and their environment's ability to meet their needs. From the perspective of Lawton's model, involuntary moves clearly threaten an individual's desire for autonomy and, as a result, may lead to negative consequences. On the other hand, voluntary moves to settings where autonomy and security (Parmelee & Lawton, 1990) as well as health and socialization (Namazi, Eckert, Kahana, & Lyon, 1989) needs are addressed may lead to positive outcomes. Congruence between individual needs and environmental resources has in fact been found in the selection of sheltered care settings by the elderly (Lemke & Moos, 1981). From this perspective, relocation to a service-rich setting may be particularly helpful for those elderly who become lonely and fearful living alone but are reluctant to express their desire to move, particularly if accomplished voluntarily.

Long-term adjustment following reactive relocation has also been viewed from a congruence perspective (Kahana *et al.*, 1980; Kahana *et al.*, 1989). Kahana *et al.* (1989) propose that positive outcome (e.g., well-being) in institutional settings is likely to result if congruence between resident needs for perceived control and environmental responsiveness exists or can be achieved via coping efforts by residents and/or the actions of staff. Reduced symptoms of depression and increased levels of satisfaction with care have, in fact, been reported in nursing homes where staff were given specific training programs (Linn, Linn, Stein, & Stein, 1989). Negative outcome (e.g., learned helplessness, depression) is likely when coping efforts are unsuccessful at reducing incongruence and when residents learn that staff responses are not contingent on their behavior (Kahana *et al.*, 1989). Inherent in this model is the assumption that institutions do not exert one set of influences and that residents do not have one set of needs. Thus positive outcome may depend on the congruence between the specific needs of the resident and the specific behavior of their caregiver staff. From this perspective, interventions, such as those designed to increase perceived control, reduce learned helplessness, and/or modify the contingencies of staff behavior, will optimally include programs at the institutional (Langer & Rodin, 1976; Linn *et al.*, 1989; Rodin *et al.*, 1985; Rodin & Langer, 1977; Schulz, 1976; Schulz & Hanusa, 1978; Slivinske & Fitch, 1987) as well as individualized levels (Kahana *et al.*, 1989; Lawton, 1989c).

Psychosocial Response to Nonreactive Environmental Change

Turning to the elderly whose environmental changes are made for reasons other than the immediate or anticipated need for assistance, the question posed is whether the theoretical models and specific predictors of psychosocial outcome based on elderly reactive relocation apply? From several perspectives, elderly nonreactive relocators are quite different from elderly reactive relocators. Demographically, those making long-distance moves for amenity or personal growth reasons are younger, healthier, more financially secure, more often married, and typically more willing to take risks than reactive relocators and elderly in general (Harris *et al.*, 1989; Hogan, 1987; Kahana & Kahana, 1983; Litwak & Longino, 1987; Serow, 1987b; Wiseman, 1980).

From a psychosocial perspective, these moves are not only nonreactive in the sense that they are not triggered by a stressful or negative life event, they are in fact typically proactive in that they represent the culmination of a process of assessing prerelocation person–environment fit and investigating possible alternatives (Gober & Zonn, 1983; Kahana & Kahana, 1983; Marans *et al.*, 1984). Whereas reactive relocators are more often "pushed" from environments where their capacities to meet basic needs and to function independently are challenged, nonreactive relocators are "pulled" to new environments where they believe their higher order needs will be met (Carp & Carp, 1984; Kahana & Kahana, 1983; Wiseman, 1980). As a result, expectations for positive outcome are likely to be much greater among nonreactive relocators. Thus, when predicting postrelocation adjustment for these two groups, the enormous differences in prelocation competence (i.e., vulnerable vs. competent), impetus for the move (i.e., following negative life event vs. years of planning), and attitude about the new environment (i.e., fear of institutionalization vs. enthusiasm and high expectations) must be taken into account.

Despite these very significant *a priori* differences in prerelocation status, as noted, not all reactive relocators do poorly, and not all nonreactive relocators do well. Although the research on nonreactive relocators has primarily focused on demographic variables and their socioeconomic implications, the limited psychosocial data on seasonal, permanent, and cross-national movers provides an initial look at the factors relating to their postrelocation adjustment.

Permanent and Seasonal Long-Distance Movers

Not surprisingly, the majority of elderly who move on a temporary or permanent basis to settings such as retirement communities in sunbelt states adjust quite well. Self-reports indicate that physical and mental health are maintained and in some cases improved, following relocations of this type (Harris *et al.*, 1989; Marans *et al.*, 1984; Mullins, Tucker, Longino, & Marshall, 1989; Sullivan & Stevens, 1982). Indirect indexes of satisfaction among seasonal relocators are reports of "instant comradeship" (Sullivan & Stevens, 1982), the tendency to return to the same locale each year, and the stated preference to make an eventual permanent move to that locale (Martin *et al.*, 1987). In addition to better climate (Krout, 1983), residents of retirement communities in the sunbelt express high levels of satisfaction with the age concentration of the area, opportunities for recreational and social pursuits, and the mutual assistance in time of illness that is available to them in these settings (Kahana & Kahana, 1983; Marans *et al.*, 1984).

Most assuredly, nonreactive relocations are not without stressful components. Increased distress among subgroups of elderly following desired relocations has been associated with the actual move as well as postrelocation adaptation difficulties (Golant, 1984; Harris *et al.*, 1989). Lack of social support and greater discrepancies between pre- and postrelocation environments have been linked to some of these increased adjustment problems (Harris *et al.*, 1989; Mullins *et al.*, 1989; Prager, 1986). However, similar postrelocation adjustment problems have been documented among subgroups of nonelderly movers as well (Stokols & Shumaker, 1982).

For the elderly in relatively supportive and familiar settings, such as planned retirement communities, unexpected adjustment problems may also arise relating to issues of self-government (for residence owners) and the possibility of forced relocation due to new ownership (for renters) (LaGreca, Streib, & Folts, 1985). Declining competence and diminished resources are also potential stressors for the elderly in retirement communities. Some communities prepare for this eventuality by including a range of services that do not require an individual to leave when increased assistance is needed, whereas others do not (Marans *et al.*, 1984). Marans *et al.* (1984) point out that well-being becomes threatened in retirement communities when incongruence between personal needs and environmental resources increases. Analogously, Mullins *et al.* (1989) found that even among a generally very healthy and satisfied group of Canadian seasonal residents in Florida, some adjustment difficulties related to issues of personal competence and social integration into the new environment occurred. For example, those who acknowledged feelings of loneliness tended to be younger, female, less educated, not married, in poorer physical health, and were found to have smaller social networks available to them in Florida (compared to Canada) than their nonlonely counterparts.

It seems plausible to argue that nonreactive relocators report well-being and life satisfaction because it is too cognitively dissonant (Festinger, 1957) to voluntarily change one's entire environment and then dislike it. Although this may be the case for some elderly, for the majority, well-being and satisfaction seem to relate to personal attributes, environmental resources, and the process by which the decision to change environments was made.

Regarding Person variables, success following relocation has been linked to factors such as future (vs. past/present) orientation, risk-taking attitude, and desire for new opportunities/challenges for some, and positive identification with same-age peers and desire for a child-free quiet lifestyle for others (Kahana & Kahana, 1983; Marans et al., 1984; Martin et al., 1987). Differential coping styles have also been linked to successful adaptation to relocation stressors (Harris et al., 1989). Consistent with the theoretical formulations of Carp and Carp, as well as those of Kahana and Kahana, Environment factors seem to be most important to the extent that they are congruent with prerelocation expectations. Kahana and Kahana (1983) noted that successful long-distance relocators expressed enthusiasm about the move prior to its occurrence and had a positive view of the postrelocation environment following the move. In contrast, they found that those seeking to move primarily on the basis of reducing discomfort or inconvenience of the prerelocation environment were less satisfied and more disappointed following the move.

That the majority of these elderly end up in settings that are, at least initially, congruent with their needs is not accidental. The available literature points out that these moves are not the result of impulsive postretirement decisions (Gober & Zonn, 1983; Kahana & Kahana, 1983; Marans et al., 1984; Wiseman, 1980). Rather, the norm seems to be that permanent moves follow years of planning and information gathering, often via Person × Environment interaction efforts such as visits to potential retirement locations (Gober & Zonn, 1983; Kahaha & Kahana, 1983). Kahana and Kahana (1983) found that one aspect of this investigation process (i.e., the feeling of lack of relocation permanence among seasonal migrants to Florida) correlated positively with self-report of health. Gober and Zonn (1983) found that over 70% of a cohort of new residents to Sun City, Arizona, had friends or family in that community or the surrounding area and that the average number of visits made prior to moving was 2.5. These authors suggest that this process allows for the establishment of social networks that are already in place when an elderly individual faces the stress of relocation.

Cross-National Movers

The extreme case of nonreactive relocation is the cross-national mover. These so called "adventurous" elderly (Kahana & Kahana, 1983), such as those moving from the United States to Israel, seem to be responding to lifelong dreams or religious and family commitments when deciding to relocate to different countries. Consistent with the literature on permanent and seasonal nonreactive relocators, it has been found that successful cross-national relocators have satisfactory levels of personal competence and coping skills, an even greater risk-taking perspective, and positive premove expectations (Harris *et al.*, 1989; Kahana & Kahana, 1983; Prager, 1986). These individuals, however, are reported to be more driven by altruism and needs for personal fulfillment than those elderly making pure amenity moves, and as a result, may be more tolerant of the taxing conditions they find in their new environments (Kahana & Kahana, 1983; Prager, 1986).

The limited data on elderly relocators to Israel suggest that the majority eventually adapt well to their new environments (Kahana & Kahana, 1983; Prager, 1986) and report maintained or improved levels of health, activity, and volunteerism. They also report, however, that the physical move and postrelocation adjustment process are often difficult. Relatively smaller differences between pre- and postrelocation environments, individual coping styles (instrumental and avoidant vs. affective) and premove attitudes (e.g., risk-taking perspective) have been associated with reduced adjustment problems (Harris *et al.*, 1989; Kahana & Kahana, 1983; Praeger, 1986).

The issues of social integration, continuity, and person–environment congruence are of particular interest among this group given that their actions are so discrepant from most elderly. Kahana and Kahana (1983) imply that long-distance relocation may be the most congruent choice for elderly whose needs for adventure, new opportunities, and/or religious/personal fulfillment are primary. They found that those seeking discontinuity and challenge were more satisfied with their choices and more able to tolerate difficult environmental conditions. On the other hand, dissatisfaction resulted for those who did not find what they were seeking or experienced more change than their need for continuity would comfortably allow. Prager (1986) also characterizes this subgroup as unique in their search for novelty, adventure, and new problems to solve as well as their willingness to disrupt the continuity of their lives but argues that both congruence and continuity are critical for successful postrelocation adjustment. From his study of elderly relocators to Israel, Prager (1986) proposed six components of successful adjustment that relate to the dimensions of congruence with the new environment (i.e., establishment of a physical/geographic niche, feeling of psychosocial and cultural belonging, maintaining and maximizing control and independence in interactions with the new environment) and continuity with the past (i.e., perceived fulfillment through satisfaction of spiritual, ideological, or cultural needs, attainment of goals in accordance with prerelocation expectations, subjective sense of well-being). Prager (1986) contends that establishment of $P–E$ congruence and maintenance of continuity with one's cognitive and affective past are preconditions for successful adjustment and preservation of mental health.

Kahana and Kahana (1983) have suggested a typology of successful relocators (explorers, helpers, fun seekers, and comfort seekers) that also underscores the notion that positive outcome will occur if the type of relocation setting is congruent with the reasons and expectations for the move by acknowledging the individual differences in motivations/expectations among nonreactive relocators. A possible addition to the Kahana's typology is the freedom seeker. No less adventuresome, but perhaps more at risk, are elderly relocators to the United States from other countries. These individuals often cannot return to their countries of origin if they do not adapt well, have not had the preparation or resources that U.S. relocators have, and report relatively greater levels of poor health and adjustment problems than U.S. relocators (Gelfand, 1986; Kiefer *et al.*, 1985; Tran, 1990). Although significant intra- and intersample as well as cross-cultural differences exist in areas such as reasons for moving (dissident status vs. desire to be with family), coping styles (reliance on government agencies vs. reliance on friends/family) and family structure, the limited data suggest that Person (e.g., level of education), Environment (e.g., availability of family), and Person × Environment factors (e.g., length of time in United States, degree of acculturation) also relate to adjustment.

Thus in reviewing what we know about elderly nonreactive relocators as a whole, it appears that they tend to adapt well in their new settings because they approach the stress of an environment change well armed with personal competencies that seem to both select, and prepare, them for the move. Their ability to apply their personal resources, coping strategies, and adventurous attitudes as well as to develop and implement concrete plans for location selection and initial adaptation lead to positive outcome. Although more work in this area is needed, the available data suggest that when expectations are not congruent with the realities of the postrelocation environment, when social integration does not take place, and when a social support network is not established or is significantly discrepant from previous networks, a negative outcome may result. In addition, when personal competencies change, the likelihood of incongruence increases and elderly individuals become more inclined toward return migration (Wiseman, 1980) and a qualitatively and, perhaps, developmentally (Litwak & Longino, 1987) different type of environment change.

These conclusions suggest that the use of explanatory models of relocation that focus on issues of voluntary–involuntary status of the move and predictability/responsiveness of postrelocation environment as well as outcome variables such as mortality rates do not adequately capture the experiences of nonreactive relocations. However, these variables are not irrelevant. The fact that elderly nonreactive relocators report high levels of well-being and life satisfaction may be due to the fact that they exercise control over their environment by preparing for and then changing it to one that is responsive to their needs. Where reactive relocation models fall short is in their emphasis on lower order needs that are taken for granted by this population.

Thus, a nonlinear congruence model (Carp & Carp, 1984; Kahana & Kahana, 1983) that stresses the fundamental differences between elderly at different levels of competence and emphasizes the need for individual P–E congruence based on level of competence may be best suited as a general model for studies of response to environment change. For both reactive and nonreactive relocators, P–E incongruence may be a precondition for an environment change. The fundamental differences are in the reason for the change (i.e., declining competence and need for increased assistance/resources vs. preserved competence and desire for more desirable or challenging environment) and the degree of proactivity (Lawton, 1989c) involved in making it. Although the potential impact of this change remains uncertain, the current evidence suggests that high degrees of congruence between postrelocation environment and individual needs buffers, and often supersedes, this impact. This evidence is, however, clearly preliminary, and more work is needed.

PSYCHOSOCIAL RESPONSE TO NATURAL DISASTERS

The final question to be addressed in this chapter is whether the elderly are particularly vulnerable to changes in the environment that are not unique to their age group. Perhaps the best place to explore this differential vulnerability hypothesis is the literature on psychosocial response to natural disasters. The need to change environments due to a disaster is clearly reactive; however, such moves do not fit the criteria for reactive and nonreactive environment changes as operationalized here. From a theoretical perspective, a traumatic event, such as a natural disaster, is likely to result in significant psychological and perhaps physical consequences (Selye, 1956). The more traumatic the event, the more significant and long-lasting the consequences (Rosen & Fields, 1988). If the differential vulnerability hypothesis is true, it would be expected that elderly individuals would have more postdisaster physical and adjustment problems than their nonelderly counterparts.

The stage for exploring age differences in response to natural disasters was set in the late 1950s and early 1960s (Friedsam, 1962; Moore, 1958). Friedsam (1961, 1962), for example, reviewed the literature on casualties during World War II and following natural disasters, and concluded that in such circumstances the elderly are a "special risk" casualty population in that they are overrepresented among fatalities in the affected populations. He also suggested that they were at greater risk for psychosocial consequences.

Over the past two decades, several aspects of potential vulnerability following disasters have been explored, some of which have conflicting results. The following is a summary of the literature in these areas.

Increased Risk of Death

In studies of natural disasters that assessed this variable, the literature is generally consistent in suggesting that there is an increased risk of death and injury with age. Friedsam (1961) found evidence of this following Hurricane Audrey. Likewise, Hutton (1976) reported increased casualty rates among the elderly following the 1972 Rapid City Flood and Bolin and Klenow (1982–83) following tornadoes in Texas. Several factors have been postulated for these findings. These include factors presumably related to age, such as decreased physical capacity, increased likelihood of being at home, and greater reluctance to heed warnings to evacuate (Friedsam, 1962). Other factors that may be as much related to socioeconomic status as age include lack of available resources in times of crisis and the greater likelihood that they will live in floodplains and/or in less sturdy houses (Kilijanek & Drabek, 1979).

Distorted Perception of Circumstances

Friedsam (1961) suggested that in addition to an increased risk of harm during a disaster, the tendency of the elderly to perceive their losses as relatively greater than the losses of their neighbors contributes to psychosocial their vulnerability. Tests of this "relative deprivation" hypothesis have provided conflicting results. Some studies have concluded that the elderly do in fact suffer greater economic and physical losses following disasters and have greater unmet needs for postdisaster services (Friedsam, 1961; Kilijanek & Drabek, 1979; Moore, 1958). Such findings would suggest that statements by elderly that their losses are greater than their neighbors might not represent exaggerations.

In a direct test of the relative deprivation hypothesis, Bolin and Klenow (1982–83) found "support" for the hypothesis when they discovered that although the elderly did not suffer greater material losses following a disaster, their self-perception of losses was higher than the nonelderly. Use of the criterion of "material" losses may have been misleading, however, because they also reported that the elderly in their sample were significantly more likely to have experienced a death or injury to a household member. In a separate test of this hypothesis, Huerta and Horton (1978) report no evidence to support relative deprivation among survivors of the Teton Dam Collapse in Idaho. In their sample, perceived loss correlated highly with actual loss and was not exaggerated in their elderly group. They, however, included "injuries or disablement" as well as legal problems in addition to material loses in their assessment of actual losses, whereas Bolin and Klenow (1982–83) used damage to the house (in percentage destroyed and dollar amount) only. Thus, at this point it is difficult to conclude that the elderly are likely to exaggerate their losses following a disaster. The literature suggests that in some disasters, the elderly may experience more physical losses and may report more material losses, but the discrepancy between actual and perceived loss appears to be primarily methodological. The fact that elderly and nonelderly attach different significance to different types of possessions may also contribute to the inconsistent findings in this area (Kilijanek & Drabek, 1979). Future studies of this issue will need to include questions that assess actual and perceived losses as well as personal significance of the loss across several dimensions.

Use of Available Resources

Most studies have documented the tendency among elderly victims of natural disasters to seek and to receive less aid than nonelderly victims (Bolin & Klenow, 1982–83; Kilijanek & Drabek, 1979; Poulshock & Cohen, 1975). Kilijanek and Drabek (1979) found what they termed a *dramatic pattern of neglect* among the elderly who received less aid from community resources than other age groups. They also found that the elderly were less likely to use insurance and other economic sources with the exception of home insurance. Other studies have also noted the general underutilization of resources as well as a differential pattern of use. Typically, the elderly seem to be willing to use aid sources such as home insurance and assistance from the Red Cross and Salvation Army but are less likely to seek out or receive assistance from federal agencies such as FEMA and the SBA. It has been suggested that there may be a stigma attached to accepting "government handouts" that contributes to this underutilization (Huerta & Horton, 1978; Kilijanek & Drabek, 1979). It has also been reported that the elderly tend to report a higher level of satisfaction with services even if those services were not adequate (Poulshock & Cohen, 1975). Thus a pattern emerges of a population subgroup who ask less, complain less, and apparently receive less resources than other age ranges of the population. Their reliance on social support networks, which may provide informal aid, however, is very important following a natural disaster (Bell, 1978; Bolin & Klenow, 1988; Hutchins & Norris, 1989). Thus, like other segments of the population, availability of a social support network for the elderly is a significant source of financial and emotional aid in the aftermath of a disaster. Although the elderly who are better off financially prior to a disaster tend to recover more effectively following one (Bolin & Klenow, 1988), the underutilization of aid among the elderly in general suggests the need for greater diligence on the part of disaster-related agencies (e.g., FEMA) as well as community and elderly advocacy groups (e.g., Area Agencies on Aging) to insure that the physical and financial needs of this population get addressed.

Psychosocial Consequences

Early studies in this area predicted an increased vulnerability to long-term emotional problems for the elderly following natural disasters (Lifton & Olson, 1976; Moore & Friedsam, 1959). The findings of increased vulnerability to injury and underutilization of aid would tend to strengthen this prediction. However, the majority of the research over the past two decades suggests that although there are emotional consequences for the elderly following natural disasters, these consequences do not appear to be significantly greater than those for the nonelderly.

Comparing studies in this area is somewhat problematic because of large differences in variables such as the severity of the disaster and the instruments used to obtain the data. In most studies, disasters are presumed to be relatively equivalent (Phifer, Kanasky, & Norris, 1988), whereas the trauma literature indicates that the severity and duration of a traumatic experience are important factors in predicting its effects (Phifer & Norris, 1989; Rosen & Fields, 1988). In addition, only a minority of studies have specifically or adequately assessed the symptoms of posttraumatic stress disorder (Shore, Tatum, & Vollmer, 1986), whereas most have instead focused on a wide range of general indicators of perception of health and well-being. Therefore, the presence/absence of some postdisaster problems (e.g., nightmares, startle response, anniversary reactions, etc.) may have gone undetected.

Despite these methodological shortcomings, there appears to be evidence that most natural disasters are events of sufficient significance to produce at least short-term emotional consequences in the elderly as well as the nonelderly victims (Phifer & Norris, 1989; Shore et al., 1986; Shore, Vollmer, & Tatum, 1989). The duration of these effects, however, remains somewhat unclear. Therefore, for example, in two posttornado studies, Bolin and Klenow (1982–83, 1988) report that one- to two-thirds of their elderly and nonelderly samples acknowledged continuing problems 8 to 12 months following the disaster. Poulshouk and Cohen (1975) found that 25% of their sample of elderly victims of Hurricane Agnes cited emotional factors as the most significant consequence of the flood even though over 80% of their sample had not returned to their preflood housing 1 year later. The symptoms reported by this sample included nightmares, fear, nervousness, depression, isolation, and loneliness. Other studies, however, have concluded that the long-term (i.e., 1 to 3 year) physical and psychological effects of disasters on the elderly are minimal (Cohen & Poulshock, 1977; Huerta & Horton, 1978; Kilijanek & Drabek, 1979).

In the most comprehensive study of physical and psychological sequelae following natural disasters among this population to date, Phifer et al. (1988; Phifer & Norris, 1989) evaluated a sample of 200 older residents (i.e., 55 and above) of Kentucky prior to and four times following a flood of moderate severity in 1981, and then 18 months following a severe flood in 1984. Both short- and long-term physical and emotional health consequences were observed. Regarding physical health, the effects of the flood of moderate severity were relatively weak and limited to the first year. Although an increase in functional impairment was noted immediately after the flood and although fatigue persisted as a complaint, all problems assessed improved over time. The health effects of the more severe flood that were more persistent than the flood of moderate severity were correlated with the degree of personal loss and community destruction and were not limited to season or "anniversary" effects (Phifer *et al.*, 1988).

The psychological consequences of these floods also correlated with the severity of disaster (Phifer & Norris, 1989). In general, individuals who experienced both extensive personal losses and high levels of community destruction were at greatest risk for psychological symptoms (e.g., anxiety, depression). Specifically, although personal loss was strongly associated with the experience of negative affect (e.g., dysphoric mood, anxiety, discouragement, worry) and seen as a prerequisite of psychological distress, the level of community destruction predicted the longevity of the symptoms. Thus the psychological effects of personal loss alone were limited to the first postflood year, whereas the combination of personal loss and high community destruction predicted the continuation of negative affect 2 years later. Exposure to community destruction alone predicted declines in positive affect (i.e., happy, pleasant, satisfied, hopeful feelings) but not negative affect. Finally, seasonal variations (anniversary reactions) were also noted in psychological symptoms.

The question posed in this chapter is whether the elderly have more postdisaster adjustment problems than the nonelderly, and the general conclusion from studies over the past two decades is that they do not. Several studies have suggested that the elderly are no more affected than younger victims following disasters (Cohen & Poulshouk, 1977; Kilijanek & Drabek, 1979), and some have suggested that they are in fact less vulnerable (Bell, 1978; Bolin & Klenow, 1982–83; Huerta & Horton, 1978). Bell (1978) found that the younger victims (18 to 59) in his sample reported more physical and emotional indicators of stress following a tornado than older victims and that the elderly did not seem to require more time to recover from disaster-related anxieties. Bolin and Klenow (1982–83) found that their elderly reported similar frequencies of family disruption and nervousness in bad weather as younger victims but that they scored consistently lower on all other measures (e.g., anxiety about future disasters). They concluded that the storms were apparently less traumatic or disruptive to them than the general population.

Although it has been suggested that the elderly may have less adaptational requirements than the nonelderly following some disasters (Hutchins & Norris, 1989), it has also been suggested that factors such as greater experience with life events (including previous disasters) as well as the opportunity for an increase in social/community activity might contribute to their relatively low levels of anxiety and depression. Phifer and Norris (1989) found that experience with a prior disaster promoted, rather than inhibited, adaptation to a subsequent one. As Bell (1978) and Melick and Logue (1985–86) have suggested, the healthy elderly may actually find more productive roles within their families and communities following disasters that might improve their overall adjustment.

Finally, the issue of differential vulnerability due to age may be best understood when placed in a broader context. Although age differences in psychosocial response have important theoretical and practical implications, it is possible that focusing on the variable of age skews its importance. It may be helpful, therefore, to explore the question of what percentage of the total variance in psychosocial response is accounted for by age compared to other factors. A partial answer to this question comes from a study by Bolin and Klenow (1988) that found that SES, marital status, availability of family and friends, and social support all correlated with emotional recovery for both elderly and nonelderly whites, although these and other variables were differentially important within age and racial groups. Although the variable of age was not specifically addressed in the studies of Phifer and his colleagues, their research attempted to explore the relative contribution of predisaster variables to postdisaster outcome. For example, it was found that 50% to 70% of the variance in postdisaster physical health status was determined by predisaster health status, whereas flood status variables accounted for approximately 2% to 12% of the change in physical status across the follow-up interval (Phifer *et al.*, 1988). Preflood symptom index was also the strongest predictor of postfloor psychological status, although the pre-post correlations were lower for psychological status than for physical health. Presumably, age correlates with predisaster health status, however, whether the change following the flood was mediated by age remains unknown. These findings, as well as those reviewed, led Phifer and Norris (1989) to conclude that observance of physical and/or psychological effects among older adults following a disaster depends on the severity of the disaster as well as the methodological strategies utilized (e.g., the length of the follow-up interval, the relation in time of the interview to specific external trigger events or seasons, and the type of assessment measure used).

The studies reviewed have added considerably to our understanding of the potential vulnerability of the elderly following natural disasters. The literature suggests that the overall health status of elderly can be affected by natural disasters particularly severe ones. Although the elderly may be at greater risk for injury during a disaster and for underutilization of aid following it, they do not appear to be significantly more vulnerable than the nonelderly for psychosocial adjustment problems. In fact, there is evidence that in some cases, the elderly may be less prone to psychosocial problems than younger victims. What is needed in this area is a more rigorous examination of factors, such as premorbid psychosocial functioning, the severity of the stressor experienced, the prevalence and course of PTSD symptoms following the disaster, and the interaction between age and change in psychological status following a disaster. Along with the already established findings of the importance of financial and social support resources following a disaster, this information will help us determine the relative importance of a larger subset of the relevant variables, including age, that predict psychosocial adjustment following disasters among older adults. What is also needed is additional work in the application of models of person–environment congruence, social role, posttraumatic stress disorder, and social support to the exposure of elderly following disasters.

SUMMARY

In this chapter, an attempt has been made to review the literature on three types of environment change from the perspective of current theoretical models and the demographic characteristics of person–environment interactions among the elderly. Although the majority of the elderly "age in place," for a number of reasons the likelihood of some type of environment change for older Americans is increasing. The literature reviewed indicates that the search for a specific effect of an environment change on the elderly is misleading because of the enormous differences in the populations studied and the types of environment changes made. Rather than looking for a unitary influence, environment change is perhaps best seen as a significant life event that has the potential for positive or negative consequences. Environment changes take place within a broad content that includes personal history, competence, needs, and desires, as well as environmental stressors and resources.

From a broad theoretical perspective, it appears that environment changes that lead to increased person–environment congruence will be most successful. At this level of explanation, for the majority of the elderly the issues of congruence, autonomy/control, security, and social support are important variables. It may be helpful to point out, however, that none of these is necessary or sufficient to guarantee psychosocial well-being. At the next level of explanation, the theoretical models and literature reviewed suggest that subgroups of elderly exist for whom different environmental issues are relevant. Carp and Carp discussed two levels of $P–E$ congruence; however, it is likely that more could be specified.

Finally, at the level of the individual, it seems clear that optimizing $P–E$ congruence requires an assessment of specific personal needs and competencies as well as specific environmental demands and resources. From a research perspective, numerous questions remain unanswered regarding specific P, E, and $P \times E$ variables that produce congruence and incongruence for various groups of elderly in different environmental situations.

The role of age in this equation also remains in need of further exploration. For all three types of environmental change, some of the elderly were clearly more at risk for negative outcome because of age-related impairments, whereas others seemed no worse off than the nonelderly, and still others appeared to adjust better than the general population. For many reactive environmental changes, age seems to be an affectively negative variable in that age-related changes in functioning required environmental changes that underscore declining competencies and need for assistance. On the other hand, age may be an affectively positive variable for many nonreactive relocators who, because of their age, have the opportunity for increased enjoyment of life. Following natural disasters, age may place some elderly at greater risk for physical, psychosocial, and financial consequences while providing others with an opportunity for increased participation in activities that increase role satisfaction. The present challenge, it seems, is to continue to develop theoretical models and research strategies of $P–E$ interactions among the elderly that allow for the inclusion of all relevant variables, including age, in predicting, measuring, and intervening with the elderly before and following environmental changes.

References

Adams, R. G. (1985–86). Emotional closeness and physical distance between friends: Implications for elderly women living in age-segregated and age-integrated settings. *International Journal of Aging and Human Development, 22*, 55–76.

Aizenberg, R., & Treas, J. (1985). The family in late life: Psychosocial and demographic considerations. In J. E. Birren & K. W. Schaie (Eds.), *Handbook of the psychology of aging* (pp. 169–189). New York: Van Nostrand Reinhold.

Aldrich, C. K., & Mendkoff, E. (1963). Relocation of the aged and disabled: A mortality study. *Journal of the American Geriatrics Society, 11*, 185–194.

Arling, G., Harkins, E. B., & Capitman, G. A. (1986). Institutionalization and personal control: A panel study of impaired older people. *Research on Aging, 8,* 38–56.

Avorn, J., & Langer, E. (1982). Induced disability in nursing home patients: A controlled trial. *Journal of the American Geriatrics Society, 31,* 137–143.

Baltes, M. M., Kindermann, T., Reisenzein, R., & Schmid, U. (1987). Further observational data on the behavioral and social world of institutions for the aged. *Psychology and Aging, 2,* 390–403.

Baltes, M. M., & Reisenzein, R. (1986). The social world in long-term care institutions: Psychosocial control toward dependency? In M. M. Baltes & P. B. Baltes (Eds.), *The psychology of control and aging* (pp. 315–343). Hillsdale, NJ: Erlbaum.

Bear, M. (1990). Social networks and health: Impact on returning home after entry into residential care homes. *The Gerontologist, 30,* 30–34.

Bell, B. D. (1978). Disaster impact and response: Overcoming the thousand natural shocks. *The Gerontologist, 18,* 531–539.

Berkowitz, M. W., Waxman, R., & Yaffe, L. (1988). The effects of a resident self-help model on control, social involvement and self-esteem among the elderly. *The Gerontologist, 28,* 620–624.

Biggar, J. C. (1980). Who moved among the elderly, 1965–70. *Research on Aging, 2,* 73–91.

Bohland, J. R., & Rowles, G. D. (1988). The significance of elderly migration to changes in elderly population concentration in the United States: 1960–1980. *Journal of Gerontology, 43,* S145–S152.

Bolin, R., & Klenow, D. J. (1982–1983). Response of the elderly to disaster: An age-stratified analysis. *International Journal of Aging and Human Development, 16,* 283–296.

Bolin, R., & Klenow, D. J. (1988). Older people in disaster: A comparison of black and white victims. *International Journal of Aging and Human Development, 26,* 29–43.

Bonardi, E., Pencer, I., & Tourigny-Rivard, M. F. (1989). Observed changes in the functioning of nursing home residents after relocation. *International Journal of Aging and Human Development, 28,* 295–304.

Borup, J. H. (1981). Relocation: Attitudes, information network and problems encounterd. *The Gerontologist, 21,* 501–511.

Borup, J. H. (1982). The effects of varying degrees of interinstitutional environmental change on long-term care patients. *The Gerontologist, 22,* 409–417.

Borup, J. H. (1983). Relocation mortality research: Assessment, reply, and the need to refocus on the issues. *The Gerontologist, 23,* 235–242.

Borup, J. H., & Gallego, D. T. (1981). Mortality as affected by interinstitutional relocation: Update and assessment. *The Gerontologist, 21,* 8–16.

Borup, J. H., Gallego, D., & Heffernan, P. (1979). Relocation and its effect on mortality. *The Gerontologist, 19,* 135–140.

Bourestom, N., & Pastalan, L. (1981). The effects of relocation on the elderly: A reply to Borup, Gallego and Hefferman. *The Gerontologist, 2,* 4–7.

Brand, F., & Smith, R. (1974). Life adjustment and relocation of the elderly. *Journal of Gerontology, 29,* 336–340.

Brennan, P. L., Moos, R. H., & Lemke, S. (1988). Preferences of older adults and experts for physical and architectural features of group living facilities. *The Gerontologist, 28,* 84–90.

Brody, E. M., Dempsey, N. P., & Pruchno, R. A. (1990). Mental health of sons and daughters of the institutionalized aged. *The Gerontologist, 30,* 212–219.

Calkins, M. (1988). *Design for dementia.* Owings Mills, MD: National Health Publishing.

Carmago, O., & Preston, G. H. (1945). What happens to patients who are hospitalized for the first time when over sixty-five? *American Journal of Psychiatry, 102,* 168–173.

Carp, F. M. (1967). The impact of environment on old people. *The Gerontologist, 7,* 106–108.

Carp, F. M. (1977). Impact of improved living environment on health and life expectancy. *The Gerontologist, 17,* 242–249.

Carp, F., & Carp, A. (1984). A complimentary/congruence model of well-being on mental health for the community elderly. In I. Altman & M. P. Lawton (Eds.), *Elderly people and their environment* (pp. 279–336). New York: Plenum Press.

Carter, J. (1988). Elderly local mobility. *Research on Aging, 10,* 399–419.

Chapman, N. J., & Beaudet, M. (1983). Environmental predictors of well-being for at-risk older adults in a mid-sized city. *Journal of Gerontology, 38,* 237–244.

Chevan, A. (1987). Home-ownership in the older population. *Research on Aging, 9,* 226–255.

Coffman, T. L. (1981). Relocation and survival of institutionalized aged: A re-examination of the evidence. *The Gerontologist, 21,* 483–500.

Coffman, T. L. (1983). Toward an understanding of geriatric relocation. *The Gerontologist, 23,* 453–459.

Cohen, E. S., & Poulshock, S. W. (1977). Societal response to mass relocation of the elderly. *The Gerontologist, 17,* 262–268.

Cohen, M. A., Tell, E. J., Batten, H. L., & Larson, M. J. (1988). Attitudes toward joining continuing care retirement communities. *The Gerontologist, 28,* 637–643.

Cohen, C. I., Teresi, J., & Holmes, D. (1985). Social networks and adaptation. *The Gerontologist, 25,* 297–304.

Crimmins, E. M., & Ingegneri, D. G. (1990). Interaction and living arrangements of older parents and their children. *Research on Aging, 12,* 3–35.

Csank, J. Z., & Zweig, J. P. (1980). Relative mortality of chronically ill geriatric patients with organic brain damage, before and after relocation. *Journal of the American Geriatrics Society, 28,* 76–83.

Danigelis, N. L., & Fengler, A. P. (1990). Homesharing: How social exchange helps elders live at home. *The Gerontologist, 30,* 162–170.

Dolinsky, A. L., & Rosenwaike, I. (1988). The role of demographic factors in the institutionalization of the elderly. *Research on Aging, 10,* 235–257.

Eckert, J. K., & Haug, M. (1984). The impact of forced residential relocation on the health of the elderly hotel dweller. *Journal of Gerontology, 39,* 735–755.

Eckert, J. K., & Murrey, M. (1984). Alternative modes of living for the elderly. In I. Altman, M. P. Lawton, & J. Wohlwill (Eds.), *Human behavior and the environment: The elderly and the physical environment* (pp. 95–128). New York: Plenum Press.

Elwell, F. (1986). The effect of single-patient transfers on institutional dependency. *The Gerontologist, 26,* 83–90.

Erlich, P., Erlich, I., & Woehlke, P. (1982). Congregate housing for the elderly: Thirteen years later. *The Gerontologist, 22,* 399–403.

Ferrari, N. (1963). Freedom of choice. *Social Work, 8* 104–106.

Ferraro, K. F. (1982). The health consequences of relocation among the aged in the community. *Journal of Gerontology, 38,* 90–96.

Festinger, L. (1957). *A theory of cognitive dissonance.* Stanford: Stanford University Press.

Fillenbaum, G. G., & Wallman, L. M. (1984). Change in household composition of the elderly: A preliminary investigation. *Journal of Gerontology, 39,* 342–349.

Flynn, C. G., Longino, C. F., Wiseman, R. F., & Biggar, J. C. (1985). The redistribution of America's older population: Major national migration patterns for three census decades, 1960–1980. *The Gerontologist, 25,* 292–296.

French, J. P. R., Rodgers, W., & Cobbs, S. (1974). Adjustment as person-environment fit. In G. V. Coelho, D. A. Hamburg, & J. E. Adams (Eds.), *Coping and adaptation* (pp. 316–333). New York: Basic Books.

Friedsam, H. J. (1960). Older persons as disaster casualties. *Journal of Health and Human Behavior, 1,* 269–273.

Friedsam, H. (1961). Reactions of older persons to disaster caused losses: An hypothesis of relative deprivation. *The Gerontologist, 1,* 34–37.

Friedsam, H. J. (1962). Older persons in disaster. In G. W. Baker & D. W. Chapman (Eds.), *Man and society in disaster* (pp. 151–182). New York: Basic Books.

Gelfand, D. E. (1986). Assistance to the new Russian elderly. *The Gerontologist, 26,* 444–448.

Gober, P., & Zonn, L. E. (1983). Kin and elderly amenity migration. *The Gerontologist, 23,* 288–294.

Golant, S. M. (1984). The effects of residential and activity behaviors on old people's environmental experiences. In I. Altman, M. P. Lawton, & J. E. Wohlwill (Eds.), *Elderly people and the environment* (pp. 239–278). New York: Plenum Press.

Golant, S. M. (1990). The metropolitanization and suburbanization of the U. S. elderly population: 1970–1988. *The Gerontologist, 30,* 80–85.

Haddad, L. B. (1981). Intra-institutional relocation: Measured impact upon geriatric patients. *Journal of the American Geriatrics Society, 29,* 86–88.

Happel, S. K., Hogan, T. D., & Pflanz, E. (1988). The economic impact of elderly winter residents in the Phoenix area. *Research on Aging, 10,* 119–133.

Harris, P. B., Kahana, E., & Kahana, B. (1989). *Risk taking and coping effects as buffers of stress for newly arrived relocators.* Paper presented at the annual meeting of the Gerontological Society of America, Minneapolis.

Helson, H. (1964). *Adaptation level theory.* New York: Harper & Row.

Heumann, L. F. (1988). Assisting the frail elderly living in subsidized housing for the independent elderly: A profile of the management of its support priorities. *The Gerontologist, 28,* 625–631.

Hogan, T. D. (1987). Determinants of the seasonal migration of the elderly to sunbelt states. *Research on Aging, 9,* 115–133.

Horowitz, M. J., & Schulz, R. (1983). The relocation controversy: Criticism and commentary on five recent studies. *The Gerontologist, 23,* 229–233.

Huerta, F., & Horton, R. (1978). Coping behavior of elderly flood victims. *The Gerontologist, 18,* 541–546.

Hunt, M. D., & Roll, M. K. (1987). Simulation in familiarizing older people with an unknown building. *The Gerontologist, 27,* 169–175.

Hutchins, G. L., & Norris, F. H. (1989). Life change in the disaster recovery period. *Environment and Behavior, 21,* 33–56.

Hutton, J. (1976). The differential distribution of death in disaster: A test of theoretical propositions. *Mass Emergencies, 1,* 254–261.

Jaffe, D. J., & Howe, E. (1988). Agency-assisted shared housing: The nature of programs and matches. *The Gerontologist, 28,* 318–324.

Jirovec, R. L., Jirovec, M. M., & Bosse, R. (1984). Environmental determinants of neighborhood satisfaction among urban elderly men. *The Gerontologist, 24,* 261–265.

Josephy, H. (1949). Analysis of mortality and causes of death in a mental hospital. *American Journal of Psychiatry, 106,* 185–189.

Kahana, E. (1975). A congruence model of person-environment interaction. In P. Windley & G. Ernst (Eds.), *Theory development in environment and aging* (pp. 181–214). Washington, DC: The Gerontological Society of America.

Kahana, E. (1982). A congruence model of person-environment interaction. In M. P. Lawton, B. G. Windley, & T. O. Byerts (Eds.), *Aging and the environment: Theoretical approaches* (pp. 97–120). New York: Garland Publishing.

Kahana, E., & Kahana, B. (1983). Environmental continuity, futurity, and adaptation of the aged. In G. D. Rowles & R. J. Ohta (Eds.), *Aging and milieu: Environmental perspectives on growing old* (pp. 205–228). New York: Academic Press.

Kahana, E., Kahana, B., & Riley, K. (1989). Person-environment transactions relevant to control and helplessness in institutional settings. In P. S. Fry (Ed.), *Psychological perspectives of helplessness and control in the elderly* (pp. 121–153). North-Holland: Elsevier.

Kahana, E. F., Kahana, B., & Young, R. (1987). Strategies of coping and post institutional outcomes. *Research on Aging, 9,* 182–199.

Kahana, E., Liang, J., & Felton, B. (1980). Alternative models of person-environment fit: Prediction of morale in three homes for the aged. *Journal of Gerontology, 35,* 584–595.

Kamo, Y. (1988). A note on elderly living arrangements in Japan and the United States. *Research on Aging, 10,* 297–305.

Kasteler, J., Gray, R., & Carruth, M. (1968). Involuntary relocation of the elderly. *The Gerontologist, 8,* 276–279.

Kendig, H. (1976). Neighborhood conditions of the aged and local government. *The Gerontologist, 1976,* 148–156.

Kiefer, C. W., Kim, S., Choi, K., Kim, L. Kim, B-L., Shon, S., & Kim, T. (1985). Adjustment problems of Korean American elderly. *The Gerontologist, 25,* 477–482.

Kilijanek, T. S., & Drabek, T. E. (1979). Assessing long term impacts of a natural disaster: A focus on the elderly. *The Gerontologist, 19,* 555–566.

Killian, E. C. (1970). Effects of geriatric transfer on mortality rates. *Social Work, 15,* 19–26.

Kleemeier, R. W. (1959). Behavior and the organization of the bodily and the external environment. In J. E. Birren (Ed.), *Handbook of aging and the individual* (pp. 400–451). Chicago: University of Chicago Press.

Kleemeier, R. W. (Ed.). (1961). *Aging and leisure.* New York: Oxford University Press.

Knight, B., & Walker, D. L. (1985). Toward a definition of alternatives to institutionalization for the frail elderly. *The Gerontologist, 25,* 358–363.

Kowalski, N. C. (1981). Institutional relocation: Current programs and applied approaches. *The Gerontologist, 21,* 512–519.

Krivo, L. J., & Mutchler, J. E. (1989). Elderly persons living alone: The effect of community context on living arrangements. *Journal of Gerontology, 44,* S54–S62.

Krout, J. A. (1983). Seasonal migration of the elderly. *The Gerontologist, 23,* 295–299.

LaGrange, R. L., & Ferraro, K. F. (1987). The elderly's fear of crime. *Research on Aging, 9,* 372–391.

LaGreca, A. J., Streib, G. F., & Folts, W. E. (1985). Retirement stages and their life communities. *Journal of Gerontology, 40,* 211–218.

Langer, E. J., & Rodin, J. (1976). The effects of choice and enhanced personal responsibility for the aged: A field experiment in an institutional setting. *Journal of Personality and Social Psychology, 34,* 191–198.

Lawton, M. P. (1980). *Environment and aging.* Monterey, CA: Brooks-Cole.

Lawton, M. P. (1981a). An ecological view of living arrangements. *The Gerontologist, 21*, 59–66.

Lawton, M. P. (1981b). Community supports for the aged. *Journal of Social Issues, 37*, 102–115.

Lawton, M. P. (1983). Environment and other determinants of well-being in older people. *The Gerontologist, 23*, 349–357.

Lawton, M. P. (1985a). The elderly in context: Perspectives from environmental psychology and gerontology. *Environment and Behavior, 17*, 501–519.

Lawton, M. P. (1985b). Housing and living environments of older people. In R. H. Binstock & E. Shanas (Eds.), *Handbook of aging and the social sciences* (pp. 450–478). New York: Van Nostrand Reinhold.

Lawton, M. P. (1989a). Knowledge resources and gaps in housing for the aged. In D. Tillson (Ed.), *Aging in place* (pp. 287–309). Glenview, IL: Scott Foresman.

Lawton, M. P. (1989b). Environmental proactivity and affect in older people. In S. Spacapan & S. Oskamp (Eds.), *Social psychology and aging* (pp. 135–164). Beverly Hills, CA: Sage.

Lawton, M. P. (1989c). Behavior-relevant ecological factors. In K. W. Schaie & C. Schooler (Eds.), *Social structure and the psychological aging process* (pp. 57–78). Hillsdale, NJ: Erlbaum.

Lawton, M. P. (1990). Residential environment and self-directedness among older people. *American Psychologist, 45*, 638–640.

Lawton, M. P., & Cohen, J. (1974). The generality of housing impact on the well-being of older people. *Journal of Gerontology, 28*, 194–204.

Lawton, M. P., & Hoffman, L. (1984). Neighborhood reactions to elderly housing. *Journal of Housing for the Elderly, 2*, 41–53.

Lawton, M. P., Moss, M., & Grimes, M. (1985). The changing service needs of older tenants in planned housing. *The Gerontologist, 25*, 258–264.

Lawton, M. P., & Nahemow, L. (1973). Ecology and adaptation in the aging process. In C. Eisdorfer & M. P. Lawton (Eds.), *Psychology of the aging process* (pp. 619–674). Washington, DC: American Psychological Association.

Lawton, M. P. & Nahemow, L. (1979). Social areas and well-being of tenants in planned housing for the elderly. *Multivariate Behavioral Research, 14*, 463–484.

Lawton, M. P., Nahemow, L., & Yeh, T. (1980). Neighborhood environment and the well-being of older tenants in planned housing. *International Journal of Aging and Human Development, 11*, 211–227.

Lawton, M. P., & Simon, B. (1968). The ecology of social relationships in housing for the elderly. *The Gerontologist, 8*, 108–115.

Lawton, M. P., & Yaffe, S. (1970). Mortality, morbidity, and voluntary change of residence by older people. *Journal of the American Geriatrics Society, 18*, 823–831.

Lawton, M. P., & Yaffe, S. (1980). Victimization and fear of crime in elderly public housing tenants. *Journal of Gerontology, 35*, 768–779.

Lazarus, R. (1966). *Psychological stress and the coping process.* New York: McGraw-Hill.

Lemke, S., & Moos, R. H. (1981). The suprapersonal environments of sheltered care settings. *Journal of Gerontology, 36*, 233–243.

Lewin, K. (1951). *Field theory in social science.* New York: Harper & Row.

Lieberman, M. A. (1961). The relationship of mortality rates to entrance to a home for the aged. *Geriatrics, 16*, 515–519.

Lieberman, M. A. (1974). Relocation research and social policy. *The Gerontologist, 14*, 494–501.

Lieberman, M. A., & Tobin, S. S. (1983). *The experience of old age.* New York: Basic Books.

Lifton, R. J., & Olson, E. (1976). The human meaning of total disaster. *Psychiatry, 39*, 1–18.

Linn, M. W., Linn, B. S., Stein, S., & Stein, E. M. (1989). Effect of nursing home staff training on quality of patient survival. *International Journal of Aging and Human Development, 28*, 305–315.

Litwak, E. (1985). *Helping the elderly: The complementary roles of informal networks and formal systems.* New York: Guilford Press.

Litwak, E., & Longino, C. F. (1987). Migration patterns among the elderly: A developmental perspective. *The Gerontologist, 27*, 266–272.

Long, L., & Hanson, K. (1979). *Reasons for interstate migration: Jobs, retirement, climate and other infuences.* Washington, DC: U.S. Bureau of the Census.

Longino, C. F., & Biggar, J. C. (1982). The impact of population redistribution on service delivery. *The Gerontologist, 22*, 153–159.

Longino, C. F., Wiseman, R. F., Biggar, J. C., & Flynn, C. B. (1984). Aged metropolitan-non-metropolitan migration streams over three census decades. *Journal of Gerontology, 39*, 721–729.

Magaziner, J., Cadigan, D. A., Hebel, J. R., & Parry, R. E. (1988). Health and living arrangements among older women: Does living alone increase the risk of illness? *Journal of Gerontology, 43*, M127–M133.

Maiden, R. J. (1987). Learned helplessness and depression: A test of the reformulated model. *Journal of Gerontology, 42,* 60–64.

Marans, R. W., Hunt, M. E., & Vakalo, K. W. (1984). Retirement communities. In I. Altman, J. Wohlwill, & M. P. Lawton (Eds.), *Human behavior and the environment: The elderly and the physical environment* (pp. 57–93). New York: Plenum Press.

Markus, E., Blenker, M., Bloom, M., & Downs, T. (1972). Some factors and their association with post-relocation mortality among institutionalized aged persons. *Journal of Gerontology, 27,* 376–382.

Martin, H. W., Hoppe, S. K., Larson, C. L., & Leon, R. L. (1987). Texas snowbirds. *Research on Aging, 9,* 134–147.

Melick, M. E., & Logue, J. N. (1985–86). The effect of disaster on health and well-being of older women. *International Journal of Aging and Human Development, 21,* 27–38.

Mirotznik, J., & Ruskin, A. P. (1985). Inter-institutional relocation and its effects on psychosocial status. *The Gerontologist, 25,* 265–270.

Monahan, D. J., & Greene, V. L. (1982). The impact of seasonal population fluctuations on service delivery. *The Gerontologist, 22,* 160–163.

Moore, H. (1958). *Tornadoes over Texas.* Austin: University of Texas Press.

Moore, H., & Friedsam, H. (1959). Reported emotional stress following a disaster. *Social Forces, 38,* 135–139.

Moos, R., & Lemke, W. (1980). Assessing the physical and architectural features of sheltered care settings. *Journal of Gerontology, 35,* 571–583.

Moos, R. H., & Lemke, S. (1984). Supportive residential settings for older people. In I. Altman, M. P. Lawton, & J. Wohlwill (Eds.), *Human behavior and the environment: The elderly and the physical environment* (pp. 159–190). New York: Plenum Press.

Moos, R. H., & Lemke, S. (1985). Specialized living environments for people. In J. E. Birren & K. W. Schaie (Eds.), *Handbook of the psychology of aging* (pp. 864–889). New York: Van Nostrand Reinhold.

Moos, R. H., Lemke, S., & David, T. G. (1987). Priorities for design and management in residential settings for the elderly. In V. Regnier & J. Pyroos (Eds.), *Housing the aged: Design directives and policy considerations* (pp. 179–205). New York: Elsevier.

Mor, V., Sherwood, S., & Gutkin, C. (1986). A national study of residential care for the aged. *The Gerontologist, 26,* 405–417.

Muller, C. (1987). Homesharing and congregate housing. *Research on Aging, 9,* 163–181.

Mullins, L. C., Tucker, R., Longino, C. F., & Marshall, V. (1989). An examination of loneliness among elderly Canadian seasonal residents in Florida. *Journal of Gerontology, 44,* S80–S86.

Murray, H. A. (1938). *Explorations in personality.* New York: Oxford University Press.

Namazi, K. H., Eckert, J. K., Kahana, E., & Lyon, S. M. (1989). Psychological well-being of elderly board and care home residents. *The Gerontologist, 29,* 511–516.

Newman, S. J., & Owen, M. S. (1982). Residential displacement: Extent, nature, and effects. *Journal of Social Issues, 38,* 135–148.

Newman, S. J., Zais, J., & Struyk, R. (1984). Housing older America. In I. Altman, M. P. Lawton, & J. F. Wohlwill (Eds.), *Human behavior and the environment: Elderly people and the environment* (pp. 17–55). New York: Plenum Press.

Nirenberg, T. D. (1983). Relocation of institutionalized elderly. *Journal of Consulting and Clinical Psychology, 51,* 693–701.

Normoyle, J. B., & Foley, J. M. (1988). The defensible space model of fear and elderly public housing residents. *Environment and Behavior, 20,* 50–74.

Oldakowski, R. K., & Roseman, C. C. (1986). The development of migration expectations: Changes throughout the life course. *Journal of Gerontology, 41,* 290–295.

Pablo, R. (1977). Intra-institutional relocation: Its impact on long-term patients. *The Gerontologist, 17,* 426–435.

Parmelee, P. A., Katz, I. R., & Lawton, M. P. (1989). Depression among institutionalized aged: Assessment and prevalence estimation. *Journal of Gerontology, 44,* M22–M29.

Parmelee, P. A., & Lawton, M. P. (1990). The design of special environments for the aged. In J. E. Birren & K. W. Schaie (Eds.), *Handbook of psychology and aging* (3rd ed., pp. 464–487). New York: Academic Press.

Pastalan, L. A. (1975). Research in environment and aging: An alternative to theory. In P. G. Windley, T. O. Byerts, & F. G. Ernst (Eds.), *Theory development in environment and aging.* Washington, DC: Gerontological Society.

Pastalan, L. A. (1983). Environmental displacement: A literature reflecting old person-environment transactions. In G. D. Rowles, & R. J. Ohta (Eds.), *Aging and milieu: Environmental perspectives on growing old* (pp. 189–203). New York: Academic Press.

Phifer, J. F., Kaniasty, K. Z., & Norris, F. H. (1988). The impact of natural disaster on the health of older adults: A multiwave prospective study. *Journal of Health and Social Behavior, 29,* 65–78.

Phifer, J. F., & Norris, F. H. (1988). Psychological symptoms in older adults following natural disaster: Nature, timing, duration, and course. *Journal of Gerontology, 44,* S207–S217.

Piper, A. I., & Langer, E. J. (1986). Aging and mindful control. In M. M. Baltes & P. B. Baltes (Eds.), *The Psychology of control and aging* (pp. 71–89). Hillsdale, NJ: Erlbaum.

Poulshock, S. W., & Cohen, E. S. (1975). The elderly in the aftermath of a disaster. *The Gerontologist, 15,* 357–361.

Prager, E. (1986). Components of personal adjustment of long distance elderly movers. *The Gerontologist, 26,* 676–680.

Pruchno, R. A., & Resch, N. L. (1988). Intrainstitutional relocation: Mortality effects. *The Gerontologist, 28,* 311–317.

Pruchno, R. A., & Resch, N. L. (1989). Aberrant behaviors and Alzheimer's disease: Mental health effects on spouse caregivers. *Journal of Gerontology, 44,* S177–S182.

Regnier, V. (1981). Neighborhood images and use: A case study. In M. P. Lawton, & S. Hoover (Eds.), *Community housing choices for older Americans* (pp. 180–197). New York: Springer.

Retsinas, J., & Garrity, P. (1986). Going home: Analysis of nursing home discharges. *The Gerontologist, 26,* 431–436.

Rodin, J. (1983). Behavioral medicine: Beneficial effects of self-control training in aging. *International Review of Applied Psychology, 32,* 153–181.

Rodin, J., & Langer, E. J. (1977). Long-term effects of a control-relevant intervention with the institutionalized aged. *Journal of Personality and Social Psychology, 35,* 897–902.

Rodin, J., Timko, C., & Harris, S. (1985). The construct of control: Biological and psychological correlates. In M. P. Lawton & G. L. Madox (Eds.), *Annual review of gerontology and geriatrics* (pp. 3–55). New York: Springer.

Rogers, A. (1989). The elderly mobility transition. *Research on Aging, 11,* 3–32.

Rogers, A., & Watkins, J. (1988). General versus elderly interstate migration and population reidstribution in the United States. *Research on Aging, 9,* 483–529.

Rosen, J., & Fields, R. B. (1988). The longterm effects of extraordinary trauma: A look beyond PTSD. *Journal of Anxiety Disorders, 2,* 179–191.

Rosow, I. (1967). *Social integration of the aged.* New York: Free Press.

Rowles, G. D. (1980). Growing old "inside": Aging and attachment to place in an Appalachian community. In N. Datan & N. Lohmann (Eds.), *Transitions of aging* (pp. 153–170). New York: Academic Press.

Rowles, G. D. (1981). Geographical perspectives on human development. *Human Development, 24,* 67–76.

Rowles, G. D. (1983). Geographical dimensions of social support in rural Appalachia. In G. D. Rowles & R. J. Ohta (Eds.), *Aging and milieu: Environmental perspectives on growing old* (pp. 111–130). New York: Academic Press.

Rubinstein, R. L. (1989). The home environments of older people: Psychosocial processes relating person to place. *Journal of Gerontology, 44,* S45–S53.

Scheidt, R. J., Windley, P. G. (1985). The ecology of aging. In J. E. Birren & K. W. Schaie (Eds.), *Handbook of the psychology of aging* (pp. 245–258). New York: Van Nostrand Reinhold.

Schooler, K. K. (1976). Environmental change and the elderly. In I. Altman, & J. F. Wohlwill (Eds.), *Human behavior and environment* (pp. 265–298). New York: Plenum Press.

Schreter, C. A., & Turner, L. A. (1986). Sharing and subdividing private market housing. *The Gerontologist, 26,* 181–186.

Schulz, R. (1976). Effects of control and predictability on the physical and psychological well-being of the institutionalized aged. *Journal of Personality and Social Psychology, 33,* 563–573.

Schulz, R., & Alderman, D. (1973). Effect of residential change on the temporal distance of terminal cancer patients. *Omega: Journal of Death and Dying, 4,* 157–162.

Schulz, R., & Brenner, G. (1977). Relocation of the aged: A review and theoretical analysis. *Journal of Gerontology, 32,* 323–333.

Schulz, R., & Hanusa, B. H. (1978). Long-term effects of control and predictability-enhancing interventions: Findings and ethical issues. *Journal of Personality and Social Psychology, 36,* 1194–1201.

Schulz, R., & Horowitz, M. (1983). Meta-analytic biases and problems of validity in the relocation literature: Final comments. *The Gerontologist, 23,* 460–461.

Selye, H. (1956). *The stress of life*. New York: McGraw-Hill.

Serow, W. J. (1987a). Determinants of interstate migration: Differences between elderly movers and nonelderly movers. *Journal of Gerontology, 42*, 95–100.

Serow, W. J. (1987b). Why the elderly move: Cross-national comparisons. *Research on Aging, 9*, 582–597.

Serow, W. J., & Charity, D. A. (1988). Return migration of the elderly in the United States. *Research on Aging, 10*, 155–168.

Shamain, J., Clarfield, A. M., & Maclean, J. (1984). A randomized trial of intra-hospital relocation of geriatric patients in a tertiary-care teaching hospital. *Journal of the American Geriatrics Society, 32*, 794–800.

Sherwood, S., Greer, D. S., Morris, J. N., & Mor, V. (1981). *An alternative to institutionalization: The Highland Heights Experiment*. Cambridge, MA: Ballinger.

Shore, J. H., Tatum, E., & Vollmer, W. (1986). Psychiatric reactions to disaster: The Mt. St. Helens experience. *American Journal of Psychiatry, 143*, 590–595.

Shore, J. H., Vollmer, W. M., & Tatum, E. L. (1989). Community patterns of post traumatic stress disorders. *Journal of Nervous and Mental Disease, 177*, 681–685.

Slivinske, L. R., & Fitch, V. L. (1987). The effect of control enhancing interventions on the well-being of elderly individuals living in retirement communities. *The Gerontologist, 27*, 176–181.

Soldo, B. J., Sharma, M., & Campbell, R. T. (1984). Determinants of the community living arrangements of older unmarried women. *Journal of Gerontology, 39*, 492–498.

Speare, A., & Meyer, J. W. (1988). Types of elderly residential mobility and their determinants. *Journal of Gerontology, 43*, S74–S81.

Stein, S., Linn, M. W., & Stein, E. M. (1989). Psychological correlates of survival in nursing home cancer patients. *The Gerontologist, 29*, 224–228.

Stokols, D., & Shumaker, S. A. (1982). The psychological context of residential mobility and well-being. *Journal of Social Issues, 38*, 149–171.

Struyk, R. J. (1980). Housing adjustments of relocating elderly households. *The Gerontologist, 20*, 45–55.

Struyk, R. J., & Soldo, B. J. (1980). *Improving the elderly's housing*. Cambridge, MA: Ballinger.

Sullivan, D. A., & Stevens, S. A. (1982). Snowbirds: Seasonal migrants to the sunbelt. *Research on Aging, 4*, 159–177.

Tesch, S. A., Nehrke, M. F., & Whitbourne, S. K. (1989). Social relationships, psycho-social adaptation, and intrainstitutional relocation of elderly men. *The Gerontologist, 29*, 517–523.

Tierney, J. P. (1987). A comparative examination of the residential segregation of persons 65 to 74 and persons 75 and above in 18 United States Metropolitan Areas for 1970 and 1980. *Journal of Gerontology, 42*, 101–106.

Tobin, S. S., & Lieberman, M. A. (1976). *Last home for the aged*. San Francisco: Jossey-Bass.

Tran, T. V. (1990). Language acculturation among older Vietnamese refugee adults. *The Gerontologist, 30*, 94–99.

Turner, B., Tobin, S., and Liberman, M. (1972). Personality traits as predictive of institutional adaptation among the aged. *Journal of Gerontology, 27*, 61–68.

U.S. National Center for Health Statistics (1987). *Use of nursing homes by the elderly: Preliminary data from the 1985 national nursing home survey, advance data, no. 135*. Washington, DC: U.S. Government Printing Office.

Usui, W. M., & Keil, T. J. (1987). Life satisfaction and age concentration of the local area. *Psychology and Aging, 2*, 30–35.

Ward, R. A. (1979). The implications of neighborhood age structure for older people. *Sociological Symposium, 26*, 42–63.

Watkins, J. F. (1989). Gender and race differentials in elderly migration. *Research on Aging, 11*, 33–52.

Wells, L., & Macdonald, G. (1981). Interpersonal networks and post-relocation adjustment of the institutionalized elderly. *The Gerontologist, 21*, 177–183.

Whittier, J. R., & Williams, D. (1956). The coincidence and constancy of mortality figures for aged psychotic patients admitted to state hospitals. *Journal of Nervous and Mental Disease, 124*, 618–620.

Wiseman, R. F. (1980). Why older people move: Theoretical issues. *Research on Aging, 2*, 141–154.

Wittels, I., & Botwinick, J. (1974). Survival in relocation. *Journal of Gerontology, 29*, 440–443.

Wohlwill, J. F. (1966). The physical environment: A problem for a psychology of stimulation. *Journal of Social Issues, 22*, 29–38.

Wolf, D., & Soldo, B. (1988). Household composition choices of older unmarried women. *Demography, 25*, 387–403.

Zweig, J. P., & Csank, J. Z. (1975). Effects of relocation on chronically ill geriatric patients of a medical unit: Mortality rates. *Journal of the American Geriatric Society, 23*, 132–136.

21

Widowhood and Bereavement in Late Life

Richard K. Morycz

Everyone can master grief but he that has it.
Shakespeare, *Much Ado About Nothing*

Introduction

Loss is a part of life and grief is a universal response to loss. Throughout a person's life, a variety of losses can occur: losses that are a normal part of a particular life stage, losses that are part of a culture or society in which one lives, and losses that are a product of an interaction betweem other losses. For example, one may lose a relationship due to death or disability or a divorce and be relocated because of a job. The result is a loss of social interaction. As one ages, losses occur with more variety, more frequency, and less time between them. Losses can include a change or loss in role, ownership, physical or mental capacity, finances, group or club membership, environment, relationship, neighborhood or community, and social interaction or contact. These major losses are sources of grief and causes of stress; the losses can occur so close to each other in time that another loss happens before the person gets over the previous loss. Life can be a chain of losses, and the most recent loss can resurrect old, seemingly unrelated losses and make a person feel quite inadequate. Time may not necessarily be the great healer.

Although grief is a commonly shared human experience and is not pathological, it can be painful. The popular advice to deal with grief is *not* to push it aside but to encourage emotional catharsis to promote psychological healing. Individ-

Richard K. Morycz • Western Psychiatric Institute and Clinic, Pittsburgh, Pennsylvania 15213.

Handbook of Social Development: A Lifespan Perspective, edited by Vincent B. Van Hasselt and Michel Hersen. Plenum Press, New York, 1992.

uals experience acute grief in a variety of ways, including auditory, visual, and olfactory hallucinations. Faced with a dual problem of managing grief and assuming more responsibilities, the grieving individual is likely to be in continual conflict between the need to withdraw and the need to engage. The death of a spouse is particularly a major stressor, requiring more adaptation and adjustment than other life events (Dohrenwend & Dohrenwend, 1984; Holmes & Rahe, 1967; Windholz, Marmar, & Horowitz, 1985).

The impact of both this role loss of being a spouse and also this role transition from being a married to a widowed person requires a variety of coping responses. The death of a spouse necessitates personal changes because of loss of companionship, loss of a source of caring, a change in a financial situation, assumption of new responsibilities and tasks, decreased opportunity for physical and sexual contacts, and an increase in being alone. For some, the loss may also mean the relief of being free of a poor marriage and of being a blessing after a spouse's long illness (see Kalish, 1987).

For many, when one loses a spouse, one loses the object of one's affection, and the person on whom one has come to depend, the one person in life with whom one expects to share the remainder of a life course. Most people expect a permanence in life with a spouse that does not exist in other relationships. Thus, for most persons, the death of a spouse means the end of a life partner and a deterioration of a resource for social support.

In any case, loss of a spouse does mean role changes for survivors. This is a unique life event and a stressor that reverberates throughout the lives of widows and widowers. The loss is irreversible, breaks long-term bonds, necessitates acquiring new roles, leads to economic hardship, and may have a major impact on the bereaved's support system (Zisook, Schuchter, & Lyons, 1987). Studies of grief and mourning indicate a variety of effects for the survivor. For instance, widowhood has been associated with depression (Clayton, Halikas & Maurice, 1972), suicide (Jacobs & Ostfeld, 1977; Kaprio, Koskenvuo, & Rita, 1987; McMahon & Pugh, 1965), an increase in physician visits (Maddison & Viola, 1968), an increase in alcohol consumption (Parkes & Brown, 1972), an increase in physical illnes (Jacobs & Douglas, 1979), and even in increased mortality (Helsing, Szklo, & Comstock, 1981; Kaprio *et al.*, 1987; Stroebe, Stroebe, Gergen, & Gergen, 1981).

Terminology in this area is not accurate, and meanings of various terms are not discrete. Bereavement can be considered the state in which one is deprived by death, and mourning can include some ritual behaviors through which grief is expressed. Bereavement can be accompanied by mourning, but contemporary society has few mourning customs and ritual behaviors. With exceptance of particular religious or ethnic groups, mourning customs are not codified. The ritual of mourning no longer serves the function of prescribing for the living the exact way to express respect for the dead. The mourners are left to decide the ways that respect will be shown. This potential uncertainty may produce additional hardship in the sufferer by adding the anxiety of vagueness and uncertainty to the pain of the loss. Loss of mourning conventions imposes on the widow the burden of inventing new patterns of behavior at a time of great personal stress.

Grief, bereavement, and mourning are not rigid terms but overlapping ones. However, as Kalish (1987) has indicated, an individual may (a) be formally *bereaved without mourning* (someone has died but the survivor is not behaving in certain accepted ways); (b) be *mourning without being bereaved* (a nonbereaved, nonsurvivor, but still upset because of identification or empathy with someone else who is grieving); and (c) be *mourning without grieving* (attending a funeral or wearing somber clothes in the respect of others). This chapter will focus on the grief process associated with loss of a spouse and explore the impact of widowhood on a person's life. In particular, emphasis will be on grief and widowhood in late life. It should be noted that the literature on bereavement and widowhood is complex, inconsistent, and methodologically weak. In spite of this, the present chapter attempts to explore two major questions: Is the impact of widowhood greater for the young than for the old? And is the effect of widowhood greater for women than for men?

BACKGROUND ON BEREAVEMENT AND WIDOWHOOD IN THE ELDERLY

The death of a spouse is a disruptive and stressful life event (Parkes & Brown, 1972) that places demands on personal, social, and economic resources (Lund, Caserata, Dimond, 1986). The *elderly* bereaved can have an even more difficult time because of the normal losses that occur with age, including reduced resources and limited social support. Old age is a time of multiple losses that are natural to that phase in life (the loss of friends and relatives, physical changes) and societally induced losses (such as retirement, reduced income, increased crime). The interaction of multiple losses can affect bereavement as well and produce reduced opportunities for mourning, delayed grief, or incomplete mourning. Bereavement in the elderly exacerbates already existing symptoms, disabilities, and problems (Sanders, 1988). In old age, losses can produce enormous change in short periods of time. The older person anticipates things to come, rehearses his or her own future, and worries about what is to be. There is loss both in the world and in the environment as well as in personal capacity. One of the most important changes in late life is the death of others, including one's spouse. It is rare that two members of a marital couple encounter death at the same instant. Almost certainly, one partner, probably the woman, will become widowed in late life. Although the elderly probably have the same internal experience of mourning that others' have, the sense of *meaning* of a death may not be the same for persons of various age groups. As Kalish (1987) notes, widowhood

> destroys a relationship of many decades standing, one with an immense network of memories and associations. The death is also a reminder of one's own vulnerability to death. It usually has a tremendous impact on daily living as well as on personal feelings, although both of these sources of impact may diminish as increasing age and worsening health lead to heightened awareness of the likely imminence of death. (Kalish, 1987, p.37)

In old age, a major source of social support is removed by widowhood at just the time when social support is most needed. The elderly are at risk not only because widowhood is more likely to increase with age but also because the aged are more likely to experience anxiety and social isolation from this event (see Sanders, 1980–1981). In late life, loss of a spouse can have physical, psychological, and social effects that can extend for years. This includes not only the feelings and emotional impact related to grief but also adaptations to new role transitions and changes in functions forced by new responsibilities. In late life, it is difficult to find any substitute for losses that occur in widowhood. A variety of changes do occur: the modification or elimination of the social world that existed prior to the death of a spouse; reduced ties with the families and in-laws; changes in instrumental function that occurred over the years through a division of labor with the spouse; and changes in self-identity. In late life, more than at any other time, grief is not for only the loss of the *person* but also for loss of *functions* that the person performed within marriage.

The loss and stress of widowhood is the most common one in late life. The average age of widowhood is 69 years old for men and 66 years old for women (U.S. Bureau of Census, 1984). Widowhood happens more often to older women than to older men. The older population has more women than men due to a higher death rate for the male population and the more rapid improvement in mortality for women. The ratio of males to females declines with increasing age; in 1980, there were 80 males between the ages of 65 to 69 years old for every 100 females, aged 65 to 69; in the 85 and overage group, the ratio of men to women is 44:100. By the year 2020, this ratio will fall even further, to 36:100. As Gilford (1988) notes: "Since the vast majority of the oldest old are female, many of the health, social, and economic problems of this group are those of women" (p. 55). For the over 75 age group, only 22% of males are widowed whereas 65% of females are widowed (see Kovar, 1986). Thus elderly men are much more likely to be married while elderly women are just as likely to be widowed. Among elderly men, more than 74% are married and living with wives, whereas only 36% of women are married and living with husbands. The number of older females living alone has doubled in the last 15 years and will substantially increase by 1995 (Gilford, 1988). Widowhood thus becomes the most common experience for the majority of older women. The life expectancy for an older woman, after being widowed, is an additional 14 years, whereas for men it is only 7 years (U.S. Bureau of Census, 1984).

Although there is much literature on bereavement and widowhood in general, there is much less on bereavement and widowhood in late life. Also, because of a high degree of individual variability in this age group, what is true for some older widowed people is not true for everyone. Little is known of the determinants of the mourning process for the elderly. There is wide variation in the experience of and response to grief.

BEREAVEMENT EXPERIENCE IN LATE LIFE

Little theoretical work has been done in the area of bereavement. There have been a variety of descriptions of stages, syndromes, and symptoms of grief, pathological grief, delayed grief, normal grief, and general bereavement. Most outcome and intervention studies have a variety of methodological shortcomings. There are few controlled studies and many unvalidated hypotheses (see Middleton & Raphael, 1987; Schackleton, 1984). Most studies are inconsistent and lack generalizability (see Stroebe *et al.*, 1981).

Table 1 summarizes various dimensions or stages of grief as depicted in some of the literature. There are similarities in many of these stages or phases of bereavement. Many of these similarities include *shock* or initial numbness, protest or a reliving or pining for the past; *disorganization*, feeling of aloneness and

TABLE 1. Stages and Dimensions of Grief

5 features of grief (Lindemann, 1944)
1. Somatic distress (exhaustion)
2. Preoccupation with image of deceased
3. Guilt/wrongdoing
4. Hostile reactions (anger toward self or others)
5. Loss of normal pattern of conduct/functioning

3 stages of grief (Gorer, 1965)
1. Shock—last few days
2. Intense grief—last 6 to 12 weeks and includes (a) listlessness, (b) disturbed sleep, (d) failure of appetite, and (d) weight loss
3. Gradual reawakening to interest in life

7 phases of grief[a] (Kavanaugh, 1972)
1. Shock and denial—important to have listener, reassurer
2. Disorganization—physical contact important
3. Volatile emotions—reassurance that feelings should be accepted, will pass
4. Guilt—need to listen, accept, allow griever to forgive self
5. Loss and loneliness—need to offer social support
6. Relief
7. Reestablishment

Stages of grief and possible symptomatology (DeVaul & Zisook, 1976), (Zisook & DeVaul, 1985)

Stage	Clinical symptom that can develop if stage unresolved
1. Shock	1. Psychotic denial
2. Acute mourning with 3 substages	2. Acute mourning with 3 substages
3. a. Intense feeling state	a. Agitated depression
b. Social withdrawal	b. Hypochondriasis
c. Identify with deceased	c. Psychosomatic production of persistent physiological symptoms of deceased
	3. Chronic mourning

Phases of grief (Greenblatt, 1978)
1. Shock, numbness, denial, disbelief
2. Pining, yearning, depression, somatic distress
3. Emancipation from loved one and readjustment to new environment
4. Identify reconstruction, new relationships, new roles

Bereavement reaction (Greenblatt, 1978)
1. Denial
2. Searching for lost person
3. Anger, guilt
4. Internal loss
5. Identify; adoption of tracts, symptoms, mannerisms of deceased
6. Excessive, prolonged, inhibited, distorted grief

[a]Not necessarily experienced in same order.

indecision and uncertainty; and *reorganization* or integration in discovering new relationships and new outlets. These various stages or emotions can have clinical utility. These stages are not distinct and do not necessarily go in a particular order but can occur at the same time. Feelings of *shock or denial* can be an adaptive device for coping that assist the surviving spouse in dealing with the death more slowly rather than being completely overwhelmed by the catastrophic fact of this irreversible loss (Zisook & Schuchter, 1985). Denial buys time to build inner strength and to find external support to deal with disruption that this death has produced. The unacceptable will not be accepted until support is found to cope with it. *Guilt* can help the bereaved reevaluate internal beliefs about what is controlled or not controlled and about what the meaning of life is. Older women have been noted to have a relative paucity of overt, conscious feelings of guilt, with more feelings of isolation, identity with the deceased, and hostility toward the living (see Stern & Williams, 1957). Feelings of *depression* may permit the bereaved to reassess personal values and competencies, capacities, and potentials. *Anger* may allow the bereaved person to examine and redefine the internal conception of justice that has been disrupted by the loss. The anger is at the disruption in their own lives. *Anxiety* permits the bereaved person to restructure their lives and attitudes about personal responsibility; what is expected of the survivor, and what is realistic, and what is not.

Many of the stages or phases of grief are parallel and revolve around some experience of the sense of denial of the loss, a recoiling or disorganization as a reaction to the loss, and eventual accommodation (see Silverman, 1981). Katz and Florian (1987) draw on previous literature and propose a three-dimensional theoretical model of psychological reaction to loss that includes a process or stage dimension, subjective reactions, and psychosocial factors. The *process or stage dimension* of loss includes shock (Glick, Weiss, & Parkes, 1974; Rando, 1984), mourning (Marris, 1974; Parkes & Brown, 1972), and adjustment (Bowlby, 1980). Particular responses or *reactions* to loss include feelings of depression or grief (Parkes, 1975; Schoenberg, Carr, Peretz, Kutcher, 1970), somatic production of symptoms (Epstein, Weitz, Roback, & McKee, 1975; Madison, 1968), guilt (Glick *et al.*, 1974; Lindenmann, 1944; Parkes, 1970), denial (Marris, 1974), and reestablishment of the meaning of life (Marris, 1974). Finally, *psychosocial or contextual factors* include individual consideration such as gender, age, religion, mode of death, educational level, and occupational history; family considerations including history of marital relation and perception of the family's role in the mourning process (see Maddison, 1968); and sociocultural environment where society changes toward a person who is widowed (see Charmaz, 1980; Eisenbruch, 1984; Marris, 1974). Here, any religious traditions or cultural customs attached to mourning may provide some structure or expectations for the survivor.

Once again, the expectation is that, whatever the process, there is eventual reestablishment, adjustment, and resolution of grief. However, as Zisook and Schuchter (1985) note: "Anger, guilt, loneliness, withdrawal, depression, and anxiety may become *permanent* affects for a significant minority of widows and widowers" (p. 99, emphasis added). If grief is not resolved, abnormal or pathological grief can occur. Such is the case with enshrinement, a grief reaction in which survivors attempt to keep things as they were before the death of a loved one. Butler and Lewis (1977) thought this is often due to survival guilt and a misplaced fear of infidelity; it especially occurs in spouses whose identity was closely tied to the deceased.

The lack of prescribed behavior associated with grief means that various functioning and behaviors of the widowed are uncertain, ambiguous, and vague. Prescribed mourning rituals with all their restrictions and constrictions served a healing function by emphasizing periods of privacy and aloneness that allowed for reintegration and reflection. It is quite difficult to say what is normal or abnormal grief. Hallucination and delusions of contact with the lost spouse can last for years, especially among happily married couples. These hallucinations, including feeling the spouse's presence, visual and auditory hallucinations, and delusions of touch occur often enough and in a time-limited way to be considered normal (Butler & Lewis, 1977). There has been some attempt to differentiate normal from abnormal, pathological, or neurotic grief (for example, see DeVaul & Zisook, 1976; Stern & Williams, 1957; Wahl, 1970). Grief and mourning has been viewed as an adaptive mechanism that allows the person to accept the reality of a loss and begin to find ways of filling the emptiness caused by the death of a spouse. It is thought that grief helps promote an identification of a new style of life and new interaction with new social contacts. Delayed or suppressed grief has been thought to indicate a poor prognosis for outcome (see Greenblatt, 1978). If grief is not resolved, implication is that it becomes abnormal, pathological, delayed, inhibited, or chronic.

However, in late life, the course of bereavement is characterized by conflicting behaviors and feelings that occur simultaneously. Lund and colleagues (1986) found that when depression scores and emotional impact were highest, coping ability and life satisfaction scores were also relatively high. They note that, "during bereavement, it is possible to experience mild depression, shock, anger, and confusion, while roughly at the same time to feel positive about oneself, confident, and proud of coping abilities" (p. 319). How long grief lasts is also a matter of debate; it is generally noted that bereavement is a longer term experience for older people and does not end even after 24 months after the death of a spouse (see Lund *et al.*, 1986). This is quite different than the 6 to 12 weeks of acute grief associated with Lindemann's early depiction of bereavement. Grief does not end in a circumscribed period of time but rather has a variable life course with many interrelated and partially discreet dimensions (Zisook & Schuchter, 1985).

In late life, grief, in well-defined stages, probably does not exist; there is no documentation of specific times, events, or markers of bereavement in late life. It is clearly a complex and multidimensional experience (Lund *et al.*, 1986) where improvement and recovery are more gradual in late life. Zisook and Schuchter (1985) surveyed 300 widows and widowers with a mean age of 53 years (age range 20 to 76 years). They found that dysphoric feelings, various symptoms, and behaviors occurred more often during the first year of bereavement; however, these *remained 4 more years* after the loss! Anger, guilt, depression, and anxiety diminished over time but not to statistically significant levels. This prolonged time course included an incomplete acceptance of the loss and attachment to the deceased. Self-reports, especially of adjustment, are much poorer (see Zisook & Schuchter, 1986). "Thus, spousal bereavement is often an ongoing life struggle rather than an acute crisis that is simply mastered or resolved over a circumscribed period of time" (Zisook *et al.*, 1987, p. 356).

Wortman and Silver (1989), in a provocative paper, challenged the inevitability of depression and distress following loss and the need for all mourners to "work through" the grief process. Although not focusing on widowhood in the elderly, Wortman and Silver do emphasize that, in the study of widowhood and bereavement, few systematic studies support widely held views about coping successfully with bereavement. From the perspective of the aged, not only is loss more expected, especially for women, but there may be also a period of anticipatory grief where some of the prescribed phases of grief occur prior to the death of a spouse. It is not surprising that elderly widows may not always experience the typical stages of grief following the loss. Indeed, Lund, Caserta, and Dimond (1985), maintain that, for older widows and widowers, difficulties in long-term coping are best predicted by strong emotional responses following the loss, such as suicidal ideation and weeping. Wortman and Silver thus conclude that "the bulk of research provides little support for the widely held view that those who fail to exhibit early distress will show subsequent difficulties" (1989, p.351). Not yearning for or being preoccupied with the deceased does not demonstrate poor adaptation or unsuccessful coping. For older adults, acute grief lasts longer when the death of an adult child is involved, and elderly parents may never be able to resolve their grief. The loss of a spouse through death leaves an indelible mark on the survivors. Eventual acceptance of the loss does not imply forgetfulness of the loss. Various aspects of bereavement can continue as painful reminders of what was and will never be again. Many widowed persons never fully accept the fact of the loss.

If loss is a stress and grief is a normal reaction to the stress, are there other physical or biological responses to the stress of bereavement? Some past studies have found a relationship between alterations in immune functions and bereavement, but it has been difficult to actually correlate lymphocyte response to mitogens and the affective state of widows (see Laudenslager & Reite, 1984; Middleton & Raphael, 1987). Jacobs, Mason et al. (1986) studied bereavement and catecholamines in 59 middle-aged and elderly persons who were acutely bereaved or threatened with the loss of a spouse. They were looking for elevated urinary catecholamine output because of stress and distress. They did not find this relationship and found no difference between those who had experienced actual loss 2 months earlier and those threatened with loss. They also note that, for older subjects in the sample, there were high levels of norepinephrine output due to the stress of loss and an inverse correlation between depression scores and norepinephrine output. They explain this by maintaining that "it is possible that the chronic stress of bereavement for elderly bereaved persons leads to sustained sympathetic-adrenal medullary function at a high level and particularly slow adaptation by comparison with younger bereaved counterparts" (Jacobs, Mason et al., 1986, p. 495). More recently, Pettingale, Watson, Tee, and Inayat (1989) examined the incidence of pathological grief and psychiatric morbidity in 33 bereaved spouses who had suffered a loss the year earlier and their present immunological status. They wanted to test the hypothesis that altered immune function is related to chronically increased psychological morbidity. Results showed the high incidence of psychological morbidity but no significant differences in cellular or humoral immune profile between subjects with high scores and low scores of psychiatric morbidity. Although the responses indicated a high incidence of physical complaints, no significant correlations were found between these complaints and either psychological or immunological variables.

SPECIAL CASES OF GRIEF IN LATE LIFE

Although this chapter deals with bereavement and widowhood in the elderly, it should be noted that older adults can still experience the loss of very old parents and that elderly persons can still suffer the loss of an adult child. The bereaved older adult child may need to mourn the type of death of a parent, experience possible regret at not being present at the parent's death or at the time of the last lucid interval, and grieve any unsatisfying or incomplete aspect of the parent–child relationship. If the period before the death of the parent involved caregiving by the adult child, anticipatory grief may have occurred, and there may have been premature disengagement from parental relationships. If the time before death affirmed a resolved relationship, death could be grieved appropriately. If incapacity, division, discomfort, conflictual relationships, and economic hardship comprised the time before death, then the meaningfulness of the period of dying may be difficult to resolve (Kowalski, 1986). Although the death of a very old parent may represent minimal destructive impact on the surviving elderly adult children, such demise can still be a painful loss of an important and loved family member. Kalish (1987) insightfully notes two other potential effects of this loss: (1) The elderly adult child is now an *orphan* and may experience a sense of meaning that one is really alone now, and (2) the older adult child survivor may now be the elder of the family, and this may mean not only newly perceived responsibilities but also the realization that he or she may be the next to die.

Loss of a child can still be one of the most difficult issues to resolve for an elderly person; it goes against nature, and it is unexpected. Although much has been studied about the stressful loss of the death of a child for younger widows (see Rando, 1983; Sanders, 1980–81), little has been reported on elderly parents losing adult children. On the one hand, the loss of a young child can still haunt parents in their old age. On the other hand, elderly parents who lose an adult child find that loss more difficult than even the expected loss of a spouse. There may be fear by the older adult about who will be caring for him or her now that an adult child is gone.

Grief increases in intensity, and there may be more depression and anger and guilt. Children or grandchildren are not supposed to die before their parents. Older adults do live near their children, and death means the loss of social interaction, family intergenerational relationships, and perhaps the loss of someone who performed essential functions for the older parent. The elderly bereaved feel that the time with their adult child has been robbed; they identify with losses of the adult child and feel those losses acutely (Kalish, 1987). Divorce of children can also be viewed as a loss by the aged parent, with grief for the subsequent loss in time and contact with grandchildren.

DIMENSIONS OF WIDOWHOOD FOR THE AGED

Personality

This section explores issues of personality, timing of death, gender, social support, and finances within the context of widowhood in late life. There is stability of personality throughout adult life; this has been manifested in a variety of longitudinal studies (Eichorn, Clausen, Haan, Honzik, & Mussen, 1981; Leon, Gillum, Gillum, & Gouze, 1979; McCrae & Costa, 1984; Schaie & Parham, 1976; Siegler, George, & Okun, 1979). Individual personality characteristics can be important, not only in adaptation to loss, but also in developing social support networks; an older person with low self-esteem or poor self-image and with a high degree of passivity may be less likely to construct, access, maintain, or utilize a support network in later life. A person who is flexible, sociable, assertive, persevering, or empathic may be much more able to construct an appropriate and effective support network. Insecure, apprehensive, anxious, fearful, and depressed individuals tend to react to the stress of bereavement with excessive grief, depression, and preoccupation with the image of the deceased (Parkes, 1985, Parkes & Weiss, 1983; Sanders, 1980–81). Those with previous dependent or ambivalent marital relationships may cling to the past relationship and chronically grieve (see Parkes & Weiss, 1983; Raphael, 1983). Zisook *et al.* (1987) found that personality characteristics, such as yearning, self-directed anger, and numbness, correlated with poor adjustment. Also, some studies of bereavement have looked at locus of control as an important personality variable. Stroebe and Stroebe (1987) found that individuals with a low internal control and high neuroticism were more depressed after sudden loss.

The Expectedness of Death

Those widows whose spouse died suddenly have a more difficult time in bereavement; this includes prolonged grief, diminished coping capacity, increased somatic complaints, and feelings of helplessness and increased anger (Glick *et al.*, 1974; Parkes & Weiss, 1983; Rando, 1983; Raphael, 1983). Parkes (1975) details an "unexpected loss syndrome" that is marked by withdrawal, bewilderment, and protest. Although this is probably less of an issue for the elderly, one would assume that when no life-threatening or serious chronic illness is present and death is more unexpected, outcome will be worse. Also, the elderly people are a heterogeneous group, with a large number of years of expected life past age 60; the young-old widowed, where the spouse was in relatively good health, probably have a more difficult time with an unexpected death than the older-elderly widowed. The expectation, after retirement, is for there to be a number of years of fairly adequate functioning where one enjoys increased leisure time. Having a death occur in early old age may thus be much more difficult than in late old age, but no definitive research studies have explored this area.

When death is more *expected*, some literature maintains that widowhood can be more *benign*. Rehearsal for widowhood—that is, discussing funeral arrangements, income, feelings of abandonment, what the future will be like, and so on—appears to make adjustment better for younger widows. Hansson and Remondet (1988) note that "there is some evidence that a majority of widows have some warning of the impending death, and that using the subsequent time to prepare or rehearse for widowhood is associated with better long-term adjustment" (p. 65). However, this may not be true for older widows. Hill, Thompson, and Gallagher (1988) followed 95 older widows at 2 months, 6 months, and 1 year following the death of their spouse. They found that rehearsal for widowhood appeared to make no difference related to adjustment and bereavement. This contradicts intuitive issues of anticipatory grief but is probably better explained by the fact that "critical events in life that occur on time are less disruptive than events in life that occur off time or earlier than expected" (Hill *et al.*, 1988, p. 795). Widowhood may thus be perceived as an on-time event whether actual death of a spouse was expected or not. Balkwell (1981) found that elderly persons whose spouses died of chronic illness did worse but maintains that forewarning is more important when the likelihood of being widowed is very small, no matter what the age.

The evidence of the timing or expectedness of death is thus not conclusive. In one study, lonelier older widows were found to be less likely to have engaged in actual rehearsal prior to the husband's death and reported a greater proportion of

their time ruminating about the consequences of the impending death of a spouse
(see Hansson, Jones, Carpenter, & Remondet, 1986). In this study, loneliness in old
age was associated with maladaptive behavior patterns including less rehearsal for
disruptive life events such as widowhood. Here, rehearsal for widowhood is
viewed to be quite important related to adaptation. However, in Hill and colleagues' viewpoint, even when elderly women lose a spouse suddenly and quite
unexpectedly, there may have been some anticipated or spontaneously rehearsed
bereavement for this loss because widowhood is more likely to occur in old age
than earlier. "Thus, these women might exhibit post-bereavement adjustment
similar to those elderly women who expected the death of their spouse as the result
of a known life-threatening illness" (Hill *et al.*, 1988, p. 795). In an earlier study by
Breckenridge, Gallagher, Thompson, and Peterson (1986), 196 bereaved elders were
studied; no differences were found in the Beck Depression Inventory for those
elderly widows or widowers who expected their spouses' death versus those who
did not.

In late life, when anticipatory death does occur, it may be a protective device to
prepare the bereaved for loss. Although it has commonly been viewed as leading to
problems if loved ones disengage themselves prematurely from the dying person
(leaving that person isolated and alone), Rando (1986) believes that this does not
have to result in premature withdrawal but can support continued involvement
with the dying patient. Anticipatory grief is a multidimensional process that occurs
mainly during the terminal illness of a loved one and includes grief over future
losses but also over past and present ones as well. When a family caregiver is a
spouse who is providing day-to-day care for her husband or his wife, she or he may
fall into a social limbo where there is no partner to share. Moreover, there is no
freedom to be single. Spouses have lost a mate but cannot mourn decently. Sexual
and affectional roles are frustrated early. Memories of the elderly person in his or
her prime is in bitter contrast to the present.

Gender and Widowhood

The transformation from a married to a widowed person can create a challenging role change. Adaptation to this life event depends upon many psychosocial
factors. Although popular view holds that widows do better than widowers in
adjusting to the death of a spouse, the research literature on the predictive power of
gender is contradictory and unclear (see Arens, 1983). On one hand, the sex of the
survivor has been found to be the single biggest predictive role in determining how
well the survivor adapts; whether widows or widowers do better depends upon
the research that is reviewed. On the other hand, there is also support for no
difference between males and females in their adjustment to widowhood.

There is some evidence that women have more difficulty in adjustment, have
increased morbidity following conjugal bereavement (Heinemann, 1982), and have
experienced more somatization, depression, and physical symptoms following
loss of a spouse (Cowan & Murphy, 1985). Also, widows have been found to have
more health difficulties than widowers (e.g., Carey, 1979; Lopata, 1973). In some
studies, this particular sex difference continues into later life. Older women have
been found to be more affected by the stress of particular life events and life
transitions than older men (West & Simons, 1983). Older widows have been
reported to be more distressed than older widowers (Gallagher, Breckenridge,

Thompson, & Peterson, 1983). Elkowitz and Virginia (1980) maintain that there are significant relationships between gender and the expression of feelings of distress—mainly that widows showed dejection more freely than widowers, visit the doctor more often, and score higher on the Zung Depression Scale. However, this study looked at only 10 widows and 8 widowers, 69 to 74 years old. Zisook *et al.* (1987) looked at the early stages of widowhood from a panel study of widows and widowers, who were being evaluated at intervals from 2 months to 25 months after death of spouses. This particular sample looked at 89 bereaved persons with a mean age of 60 (age range of 26 to 83 years). Sex, age, and family income were significantly related to outcome variables, such as the Hopkins Symptoms Checklist, Zung Depression Scale, and the Global Adjustment score. Women in lower age and lower income groups had poorer outcomes than men or those at the higher end of the age and income scales. In Gass and Chang's Study (1989), older male widows tended to have higher education and income; this influenced the use of more problem-focused coping and reduced psychosocial health dysfunction.

A more consistent finding is that *widowers* have greater difficulty than widows. Marital roles have been found to be more beneficial to males than females related to survivorship (Balkwell, 1981). Men express grief less openly, lack familiarity with household chores, and do not maintain ties with extended families (Berado, 1970). Widowers do not share feelings because males lack nonspouse confidantes (Elwell & Maltbie-Crannel, 1981). Widowed men tend to exhibit higher rates of mental illness (Balkwell, 1981; Gove, 1972). In general, men have more problems following the death of a spouse (Rees & Lutkins, 1967; Stroebe & Stroebe, 1983) and can be at risk for increased mortality and morbidity (Berado, 1970; Helsing, Szklo, & Comstock, 1981; Parkes, 1970; Parkes, Benjamin, & Fitzgerald, 1969; Parkes & Brown, 1972; Rees & Lutkins, 1967; Stroebe, Stroebe, Gergen, & Gergen, 1981).

Younger male widows have a difficult time working through grief (Glick *et al.*, 1974). Widowers at any age tend to be more socially isolated and have a difficult time in managing the house (Berado, 1970). Traditionally, men have been more likely to depend upon the spouse for social participation, activities, and support. When his wife dies, a man may have less resources available for social interaction and thus become more isolated (Sanders, 1988). Women have tended to utilize social participation for adaptation and this has better long-term effects after acute grief. The implications from this research are that women adjust fairly well to widowhood and thus are able to be independent. In Lopata's studies of widows, those who have had more education and who have created a middle-class lifestyle when the husband was alive do initially have more disorganization in their lifestyles, self-concept, and support system at his death. At the same time, these women have more available resources to assist them in their reorganization (see Lopata, 1986). Indeed, Lopata believes that because there is not a prescribed social role of widow in this country, a woman can become even more individuated when she becomes a widow (Lopata, 1986). Finally, when one compares widowed women to married women, and widowed men to married men, there does appear to be more depressive symptomatology for widowed men than married men, whereas widowed women were no more depressed than married women (Weissman & Klerman, 1977).

Males were found to be at more risk, not only at a younger age (less than 45 years old—see Parkes, 1975), but older males were also more at risk with stressful life events (West & Simons, 1983). Jacobs and Ostfield (1977), in evaluating mortality associated with conjugal bereavement, note that the "risk of mortality is greater for men at all ages" (p. 356). Widowers have consistently been at more risk than widows for health problems in acute bereavement. For young widows, there is some risk, but it lessens with increasing age. This is not true for older widowers (Jacobs & Ostfeld, 1977; Osterweis, Solomon, & Green, 1984). Jacobs, Kasl, Ostfeld, Berkman, and Charpentier (1986) looked at a group of 114 widowed persons, with an average age of 62.5 years (with 60% being over 61 years old). In this study, no significant differences were found between widows and widowers in the experience of grief—that is, in the intensity of separation, anxiety, sadness, and loneliness in the acute stages of grief. Widows did report more numbness, disbelief, and neurovegetative symptoms than widowers. Jacobs and his colleagues believed that this is because women tend to avoid, deny, and defend more than men against the reality of the loss. "It also raises a question if this avoidance is protective of health since women are at lower risk of morbidity from bereavement than men" (Jacobs et al., 1986, p. 309). Younger widowers scored lower on separation anxiety and its components than older men. From this point of view, older men do not suppress their grief. Thus with age, men showed more separation anxiety in widowhood. This change may reflect an age-associated one. Some personality studies have shown that men become more nurturing and emotional with age and that women become more managerial and functional (see Neugarten & Gutmann, 1964). Thus there appears to be an inversion of sex roles in late life. For men, the increase in emotional distress may help explain the poor health consequences for older widowers and some of the pattern of risk (Jacobs, Kasl et al., 1980).

Finally, there is also some evidence that shows *no difference* between males and females in widowhood in general (Clayton, Halikas, & Maurice, 1972; Heyman & Gianturco, 1973), and this lack of difference persists in late life (see Gallagher et al., 1983; Lund, Caserta, & Dimond, 1986).

A variety of studies have found no differences between widows and widowers in adjustment, happiness, depression, or grief resolution (Clayton, 1974; Clayton, Halikas, & Maurice, 1972; Gallagher et al., 1983; Lund, Caserta, & Dimond, 1986). In a 2-year longitudinal study comparing 192 elderly male and female surviving spouses between the ages of 50 and 93, Lund and colleagues (1986) found no statistically significant gender differences at any of the time periods. In a 2-year span, six repeated measures were carried out on five global outcome scales encompassing emotional shock, psychological strength and coping, anger-guilt-confusion, helplessness/avoidance, and grief resolution. There were no significant differences between older widows and widowers on social-psychological bereavement outcomes. Feelings, behaviors, and changes were at similar levels of intensity and frequency. Thus for older males and females, the bereavement process can be more similar than different (Gallagher et al., 1983; Lund, Caserta, & Dimond, 1986). Finally, Gass (1988) looked at 100 elderly widows and 59 older widowers in investigating differences in appraisal, coping, resources, type of death, and health dysfunction. She found no significant differences between gender and physical or psychosocial health dysfunction, appraisal of bereavement, coping strength, and resources. She suggests, once again, that older men and women are more similar than different within 2 years following the loss of a spouse. Gass, however, did find that the *type of death* and *gender* were significant. Widowers whose wife died *suddenly* needed more coping methods to manage bereavement and may have experienced more stress, whereas widowers whose wife died after a *chronic* illness may have had more helpful social supports and opportunities for anticipatory grief.

Thus it is quite difficult to be conclusive about the role of gender as a significant risk factor in bereavement outcome. *The balance of the evidence leans slightly to men, at any age, being more at risk after widowhood.* Part of the difficulty in summarizing this area is in how to interpret findings. For instance, in the West and Simons Study (1983), the contention is that older women are more affected by life events, such as widowhood than older men. However, West and Simons maintain that this is related to "the well recognized tendency for males to be less emotional, to intellectualize and to deny or suppress their feelings more than females" (1983, p. 255). Yet, this contradicts findings that older men experience more separation anxiety in widowhood and that older women suppress this grief more (Jacobs, Kasl *et al.*, 1986). Thomas, DiGiulio, and Sheehan (1988) conclude that evidence from much of the literature manifests that, despite the challenge and discomfort of widowhood, most women at any age survive without psychological damage and view themselves as stronger for having undergone the experience.

Age as a Factor in Widowhood

There is some indication that the young widowed tend to have more acute problems than the old widowed (Parkes & Weiss, 1983) and that the older widowed have shown better adjustment than younger widowed (Ball, 1976–77; Carey, 1979; Morgan, 1976). The likelihood of being widowed at advanced ages may make acceptance of this event easier than earlier in life (Balkwell, 1981). Women, especially, appear to have more support from peers who have had to go through similar life events (Neugarten, 1968). Older people can adapt well in widowhood (Heyman & Gianturco, 1973). Clayton (1975) found that bereavement itself, not the effects of living alone, influences depressive symptoms in widows and widowers 1 month after the death of a spouse. Her study of 109 widowed persons, with an average age of 61, indicated that younger people showed more physical depressive symptomatology and required more hospitalization than matched controls or older widowers at one year.

Gass and Chang (1989) found that older widows and widowers had lower threat appraisal and used fewer coping strategies. This is probably because the elderly tend to lose family and friends more often and have an idea of what to expect. They have also had time to develop more coping skills. Thus loss of a spouse may be perceived as less threatening and reduce the need to cope. In this study, older persons did have more psychosocial dysfunction than younger widowed, but this was probably due to factors independent of grief (preexisting depression, social isolation due to aging, hearing loss, decreased mobility). Walker, MacBride, and Vachon (1977) suggest that younger widows' own networks fail to validate their social and personal identities as single women in need of new contacts and lifestyles. Networks shrink as couples no longer invite them to social occasions. This is in contradistinction to the experience of elderly widows who have social networks with consistently shared experiences that validate the experience of widowhood.

Older widows are actually at less risk, compared to younger widows, for immediate adverse health and psychological outcomes within the first year or two. This may reflect such circumstances as that the death was less unexpected, not considered premature, or a relief from the intense burden of caregiving for an ill spouse. (Hansson & Remondet, 1988, p. 160)

It is actually difficult to evaluate whether age alone is a risk factor, especially in late life when other concurrent life events and losses occur more often. For instance, Sanders (1980–81) found that younger widows showed more acute grief initially than older widows but that, after 18 months, most variables were reduced in intensity. Older widows, after 18 months, show *elevated* scales in the Grief Experience Inventory (Sanders, Mauger, & Strong, 1979) and MMPI personality variables. Loneliness and anxiety were the most common problems for older widows with feelings of helplessness frequently expressed. "The results of the study suggest that being older does not contribute *directly* to grief symptoms, per se, but rather the constellation of debilitating variables that commonly plague the elderly" (Sanders, 1988, p. 98, emphasis added).

Social Support in Widowhood

Social support has been found to be an important factor in adjustment to bereavement: When it is not there, poor adaptation can occur (Lopata, 1973); when it is there, it can act as a prevention for depression (Clayton *et al.*, 1971) and an aid in adjustment (Heyman & Gianturco, 1973). In general, after the death of a spouse, initially there may be an increase in social contacts, interactions, and activities with family members. However, contact eventually decreases, and relations with friends may increase in importance. Loneliness is found to be greater among the younger widowed than the never married (Gubrium, 1974). Many widows refuse to interact in a "society of widows" where same-sex members share stigmatized criteria (Balkwell, 1981).

Widowhood can have disadvantageous outcomes in the social relationship of the elderly (see, for example, Lund, Caserta, Dimond, & Gray, 1986; Pihlblad & Adams, 1972). However, less is known about whether changes in social relationship following widowhood are as true among the elderly as among younger widows. Lopata (1987) has maintained that most older widows can be engaged in a variety of activities and social supports; they have good life satisfaction, self-esteem, morale, and are involved with community, family, neighbors, friends, and organizations. Bereavement for males has been noted to be marked by a poor social network that is not very extensive (see Berado, 1970).

Widowed elderly women reported a greater reliance on extended kin in times of personal crisis than their married counterparts (Anderson, 1984). Older women may also have a better, more extensive nonfamilial social network than younger women or men at any age. Lopata (1975) looked at 301 Chicago women, aged 50 and over, and found that almost half of this group (46%) felt that they themselves and their social life were unaffected by their husbands' death. These widows did not go through the structured sequence of the stages of grief.

Morgan (1989), through the use of focused group discussions, examined older widows ($n = 41$) and positive/negative aspects of social support networks. Family members received more negative assessments. Morgan believes that friends are more useful to older widows in the role transition to widowhood because these relationships are more flexible and accepting; family relationships show more commitment to the basic relationship. During intense grief, widows benefit more from a smaller set of very close relationships with family but later benefit from a broader ranging, flexible network of friends. The ideal social network can provide access to various types of relationships at various points in the role of transition.

> In present terms, the early stages of adaptation require others who are intensely committed, and those with less commitment may present an obstacle, but in the later stages of the transition, the role of resource and obstacle are reversed. Those whose commitments take the form of demands become the hindrance, whereas those who provide flexibility are the crucial resources. (Morgan, 1989, p. 107)

Family relations to the older widow may also be problematic when the aged woman has provided support to other family members. The expectation may be to now resume the role of mother–confidante or sister–confidante. Not only can this produce resentment or withdrawal from these relationships, but a decrease in self-confidence because of the widow's own reluctance to stop grieving. She may not be ready to return to life as usual (see Lopata, 1975). Thus loneliness can occur during widowhood in late life. Elderly widows, even those with frequent contact with families, can still be lonely. Arling (1976), for example, notes that only contact with relatives other than one's children ease the experience of loneliness for elderly widows. Permissive support from others who allow the expression of grief is central to overcoming loneliness (Balkwell, 1981; Maddison, 1968).

Considering social support and gender, male widowers appear to do less well in socialization after death of a spouse. Men may be more likely to depend upon their spouses for social participation, activities, and support. When the wife dies, a man may have less resources available for social interaction and thus become more isolated (Sanders, 1988). Women utilize social participation for adaptation, and this has better long-term effects after acute grief. Thus social support may facilitate the bereavement process over time for widows (Stroebe & Stroebe, 1987). Older widowers may be more hesitant to develop social resources for support, activities, and interaction, not only because there are less men with the experience of widowhood (i.e., it is not the majority experience or way of life for most older men), but they are even more reluctant because they have had more years of emotional and social interdependency on their spouses. One not only loses a loved one, but one also grieves for the functions that that loved one performed; this includes not only instrumental tasks but social ones as well. Older widows, on the other hand, may not know some necessary financial information and may be reluctant to make financial decisions, especially if this is something she has not done before. Older widowers may have depended upon the wife for social contacts and may now have a difficult time not only with household management functions but also with organizing or reorganizing a social network.

However, a study by Wister and Strain (1986) looked at 288 older widows and 66 older widowers and examined social support and well-being. After introducing control variables, there were differences in some components of social support but no gender differences found for measures of well-being. It should also be noted that personality characteristics can be more important than gender in developing social support networks. An older person with low self-esteem or poor self-image, or with a high degree of passivity, may be less likely to construct, access, maintain, or utilize a support network in late life. Someone who is flexible, sociable, assertive, persevering, and empathic may be more likely to organize, maintain, and use social support (see Hansson, Jones, & Carpenter, 1984; Hansson & Remondet, 1988; Hogan, Jones, & Cheek, 1984).

One of the most interesting studies of social support and widowhood in late life was conducted by Dimond and colleagues (1987). They examined 192 bereaved persons between the ages of 50 and 93 years and collected data at six time points (from 3 weeks to 2 years) after the spouses' death. They sought to determine the role of structural and qualitative aspects of social support in outcomes such as depression, coping, health, and life satisfaction. The *qualitative* aspects of social support played a significant role in bereavement outcomes. In terms of the stress of widowhood, then, presence of adequate social support assisted in adaptation. Qualitative aspects of support (i.e., the opportunity to express oneself, levels of interaction, shared confidences, feelings of closeness, mutual helping) were as important as *structural* characteristics (i.e., size, strength of ties, density, homogeneity, extent to which network members maintain contact with each other, dispersion of network membership). The study by Dimond and colleagues (1987) was unique because it focused on *elderly* widows and widowers and social support in a longitudinal design. The mean age of the participants was 67.6 years, with an age range of 50 to 93 years. Although the actual variance explained by social network variables—both structural and qualitative—were still only from 4% to 14%, these variables still explained more of the variation of the dependent variables than either demographic or psychological variables. In summary, social support does play a significant role in coping with widowhood in late life during the first 2 years of bereavement.

Economic Factors in Widowhood

The economic resources of widowhood are not adequate. Deprivation can be caused by lack of income. The economic conditions of widowhood can directly and negatively affect poor adjustment (Glick *et al.*, 1974), self-reported health (Sheldon *et al.*, 1981), and lowered morale (Atchley, 1975; Morgan, 1976).

Lowered income can mean decreased social participation and an increase in social isolation and loneliness. Lopata (1986) has noted that there are isolated widows who can be described by the disengagement theory of Cummings and Henry (1961) because they lack the personal resources to reengage with each break in social relationships. Part of these resources are certainly economic. Besides decreased economic resources, older widowed women, in this generation, still can be financially inept; this makes them easy victims for swindlers who bilk thousands of unfortunate women out of millions of dollars annually.

The Social Security system and private pensions have begun to improve the economic lot of widows; older women are not dependent upon their children for their main economic support. However, results of studies on the economic resources for older widowed persons are inconsistent. Morgan (1986) examined reports from 606 white widows over 50 from the 1975 Longitudinal Retirement History Survey. These widows had experience in handling and managing money; a majority were poor. It was not the lack of experience in managing money or poor advice in managing money matters, either before or after the death of husbands, that contributed to poverty among older widows. For older widowed women in this study, the *reality* was a risk of poverty and limited economical alternatives. Smith and Zick (1986) had similar findings; they looked at data from the 1983 Panel Study of Income at the survey research center at the University of Michigan. This included data collected since 1968 on socioeconomic and demographic characteristics of 5,000 families. Zick and Smith considered the economics of households while both spouses were alive and followed the economic situation of the household after the death of a spouse. This matched-controlled study manifests that the sample of initially nonpoor men and women experienced decline in economic well-being subsequent to the death of a spouse (compared to married couples). Widowers as well as widows suffered economic hardship. After 5 years, almost half of the *initially* nonpoor sample experienced at least 1 year of poverty.

Thus it is now widowhood itself that causes poverty but the way in which the current Social Security system and pensions provide for surviving spouses that produce poor economic situations (Warlick, 1985). The aforementioned studies examined actual income and poverty levels. Additional methods of investigating the economic situation of widowhood are to examine financial strain, the perception of the economic situation in widowhood, or the economic situation as perceived by those widowed. Keith and Lorenz (1989), in a study of 1782 older unmarried persons, found no evidence that widowed or divorced/separated were at any greater risk for financial strain or poor health. Older unmarried females did not express dissatisfaction with finances. Keith and Lorenz concluded this suggested an accommodation to their economical or financial situation. Similarly, O'Bryant and Morgan (1989) analyzed 300 widowed women over age 60 up to 22 months after that death of their spouses. In this sample, 86% of the subjects were white, and 14% were black. The study looked at the financial experience of older widows prior to widowhood, assessed the amount and type of planning taken before the death of their husbands, and analyzed effects on well-being in early widowhood. The results indicate that financial preparation was associated with somewhat better well-being among elderly widows but that experiences with finances prior to widowhood had no effect on well-being. Less than one-half of widows in the sample reported their economic conditions had declined since the death of their husbands; over two-thirds stated their current economic situation was comfortable. However, O'Bryant and Morgan note that

> the fact that current economic status is only moderately related to income levels suggested that the subjected level of economic well-being may depend strongly on the woman's prior economic status and expectations regarding her financial lot of widowhood. (1989, p. 249)

ADAPTING AND ADJUSTING TO WIDOWHOOD

This section briefly reviews the literature on how one adapts to widowhood, resolves grief, maintains well-being and self-esteem, adjusts, and copes with the stress of widowhood.

Stress, Coping, and Resolution of Grief

The stressful life of widowhood can have adverse effects on survivors; this is true not only because of the grief of the loss itself but also because of the need to readjust to new roles and different lifestyles. Subsequently, the brunt of coping with daily living (e.g., "hassles"—cf. Pearlin, Lieberman, Menaghan & Mullen, 1981) may have an effect on morale, well-being, and adjustment. Resolving grief is probably dependent upon a variety of factors: coping strengths, social support networks, the accumulated loss and stresses within a short period of time, and even the mode of death (Ball, 1976–77; Faberow, Gallagher, Gilewski, & Thompson, 1987). Coping strengths may also be related to religious participation, personality factors, and the quality of relationship with the deceased spouse (Gallagher *et al.*, 1981–82). Wortman and Silver (1989) suggest not one but three common patterns of coping with loss: (1) shock, distress, withdrawal, resolution (the bereaved is able to *cope after awhile*); (2) little or no distress, acceptance (survivor is able to cope *immediately* due to belief system or outlook on life); and (3) continued or extended distress (the bereaved is unable to cope).

Coping is also dependent upon resources, marital relationships, and personality characteristics. A hundred older widows and 59 older widowers were assessed by Gass and Chang (1989) within the context of threat appraisal, coping *resources*, and psychosocial health dysfunction. They found the following: (a) Higher threat appraisal caused more stress that manifested itself in poor health functioning; (b) emotion-focused coping strategies prevented the person from confronting the reality of loss by denial, avoidance, or wishing things were different—problem-solving strategies were more adaptive, and emotion-focused strategies were less useful for managing bereavement and were inadequate in reducing threat, thereby contributing to more psychosocial health dysfunction; and (c) threat was less in the presence of resources.

> Widowed persons with more resources were less likely to perceive loss as a threat and were more likely to have better psychosocial health after bereavement. Lower resource strength increased threat appraisal which in turn influenced greater dysfunction. (Gass & Chang, 1989, p. 34)

Poor marital *relationships* (bad, distant, unsupportive, tense, uncomfortable, ambivalent, clinging) have been found to be related to poor adjustment (Parkes & Weiss, 1983; Shanfield, 1983; Zisook *et al.*, 1987). Lopata (1973) noted that increased communication in the marriage and increased joint social and organizational activities in more companionate relationships tended to produce more of a sense of loss of organization in the life of the older female. There may be different resources used for coping with an adaptation to widowhood for older men and older women. The end result of the process of that adaptation to widowhood could be either disengagement (Cummings & Henry, 1961) or the restructuring of one's identity and support system (see Lopata, 1973, 1979). Women tend to utilize social participation for adaptation (Elwell & Maltbie-Crannell, 1981), and this has a long-term effect after acute grief is over. Social support may facilitate the bereavement process for widows and help in the coping with loss, providing relationships and a positive self-concept (see Lopata, 1979; Silverman, 1985; Stroebe & Stroebe, 1987). Indeed, Morgan (1976) found that the life satisfaction of young widows to be poorer than young married women, but older widows reported higher degrees of life satisfaction than elderly married women. Older widowers, as previously noted, may be more hesitant to develop social resources for support, activities, and interaction, not only because there are less men with the experience of widowhood but also because older men had more years of utilizing their wives as confidantes and resources for establishing social networks. Those with previous dependent or ambivalent marital relationships may cling to the partnership and chronically grieve (see Parkes & Weiss, 1983; Raphael, 1983).

Many factors thus effect adaptation in widowhood. This certainly include *personality* factors. Because there is stability of personality throughout the lifespan (Eichorn *et al.*, 1981; Leon *et al.*, 1979; McCrae & Costa, 1984; Schaie & Parham, 1975; Siegler *et al.*, 1979), particular personality characteristics may predict maladaptation. For example, insecure, apprehensive, anxious, fearful, and depressed individuals tend to react to the stress of bereavement and with excessive grief, depression, and preoccupation with the image of the deceased (Parkes, 1985; Parkes & Weiss, 1983; Sanders, 1980–81). Locus of control has also been an important factor in studies of bereavement in general. Stroebe and Stroebe (1987) found that individuals with low internal control and high neuroticism were more depressed after a sudden loss. For older widows and widowers, Gass (1988) has found that belief in control over bereavement was associated with better physical and psychosocial health and encouraged problem-solving coping behaviors.

Self-Concept, Identity, and Self-Esteem

Some reintegration of identity in widowhood is necessary. Each widow or widower must move from a self-concept of being a member of a pair to a self-concept that focuses on the self as an independent and self-sufficient entity. Self-view is influenced by social interaction—who one is depends on how others see one and how one understands such views. After losing a spouse, the source of expectations about who one is and how one behaves may also be lost. Lopata (1973) has noted that this is especially true for companionate marriages. Knowing who one *is* is an integral part of the sense of well-being. Where roles in the marriage are intertwined, new identity formation may be needed, especially when one functions in roles such as homemaker, domestic, confidante, hostess, keeper of social life, mother of children, and in-law. These diverse roles, tied to identity, are now unraveled due to the death of the spouse. One must now gain acceptance with family, friends, and in-laws by oneself, on one's own.

Although the conception of roles and identity as inextricably bound in marriage makes intuitive sense, little real support for this is found in the literature. Thompson *et al.* (1988) looked at 83 widows, age 22 to 74, and found little evidence for the contention that widowhood leads to loss of identity. They maintain that any issues with identity problems occur immediately after the loss of a spouse, but this (if it occurs at all) is quite temporary. Earlier, Lopata (1975) noted that the widowhood phase, where identity reconstruction takes place, is quite transitory. This is probably because the role of the wife is no longer the premier role tied to identity for most women. Women are increasingly in the work force, and economic necessity and fulfillment have developed additional role considerations. The role of mother is another strong role maintained by women who are widowed. The role of the widow, then, especially an older widow, is certainly not a prescribed one tied into an extended period of time. The role of widower is even more vague and uncommon. Older men, however, who are no longer working, may see spouses as a more important part of themselves. Because they are less likely to have confidantes other than their spouses, restructuring of their identities may be more difficult.

On the one hand, a widow or widower's sense of self-esteem may protect the survivor from the stress and threat of the loss of a spouse. For older adults, "self-esteem in and of itself may be a critical variable adjustment to bereavement" (Burks, Lund, Gregg, & Bluhn, 1988, p. 57). Lund *et al.* (1985–86), for example, looked at 138 older persons age 50 and older coping with widowhood 2 years after the death of a spouse. Poor copers did *not* differ from others with respect to any sociodemographic, health, or social support variables. The poor copers had less self-esteem; low self-esteem, even prior to loss, was predictive of coping difficulties 2 years following death. Poor copers expressed confusion and more suicidal ideation, cried more frequently, and were not as busy early in the bereavement.

On the other hand, Arens (1983) looked at national survey data from the 1974 National Council on Aging conducted by Harris & Associates. This analysis looked at 597 men and 952 women 65 years of age and older who were married or widowed. Conclusions of the study were that the *direct effects* of widowhood on well-being were seldom substantial after health, socioeconomic status, and levels of social participation were considered. Even in the 1975 Parkes study detailing differences in self-esteem in those with little warning of impending death, with multiple life crises, and with initial severe reaction to the loss, there was *no* significant differences in self-esteem *2 to 4 years* later. Even if the differences in role transition, identity reconstruction, self-concept, and social support are accepted between widows and widowers, there is no consistent evidence on gender differences for measures of well-being for older widows and widowers (see, for example, Wister & Strain, 1986).

Finally, Johnson, Lund, and Dimond (1986) found that, even though low self-esteem was predictive of coping difficulties 2 years following the death of a spouse (Lund *et al.*, 1985–86), a high sense of self-esteem was not necessarily protective of the stress of widowhood on a long-term basis. Effects of the stressfulness of widowhood in late life later reappear and have negative effects on self-esteem and coping ability a year later. After 6 months, the initial sense of self-esteem was found to no longer protect against stress.

Adjustment through Remarriage

Especially for older men, remarriage can be a response to the adjustment of being widowed. Remarriage is more likely for older widowers than widows (Cleveland & Gianturco, 1976; Northcott, 1984; Spanier & Glick, 1980). Widowers remarry sooner and choose younger women. Remarriage can have an effect on social interaction. Relationships can change after remarriage, with older remarried couples interacting less with children and friends because now they rely on one another for interaction (Vinick, 1979). When one's self-concept and identity was closely tied to the dead spouse, remarriage can still not result in grief resolution (see Moss & Moss, 1980). However, Burks *et al.*, (1988) found that older widows who remarried eventually displayed more positive outcome than their nonmarried counterparts. Gentry and Schulman (1988) also suggested that remarriage can be an effective coping response in widowhood when there is loneliness, undesirable financial problems, or challenges of home maintenance. However, 36% of the study sample of 752 widows across age groups did not wish to remarry because they liked the independence of being single.

RICHARD K.
MORYCZ

So, do most older adults function well after widowhood and eventually cope with and adapt to this life event? McCrae and Costa's (1988) follow-up on a national sample of 14,000 respondents between the ages of 25 and 74 years from the National Health and Nutrition Examination Survey I (NHANES) is an attempt to examine the long-term consequences of widowhood. This important study was a national probability sample and, although not addressing widowhood in the oldest elderly, it was a representative sample. McCrae and Costa conclude that "in the long run, although it effects lifestyle, widowhood does not appear to have any enduring effect on psychosocial functioning in *older* men and women" (1988, p. 37, emphasis added). Neither bereavement nor widowhood had any long-term impact on psychosocial functioning. This follow-up study on the 14,000 respondents included 167 widowed men age 65 to 74 and 791 widowed women age 65 to 74 and did not include institutionalized respondents. Age, education, and sex were significant predictors of survival, *but marital status was not.* Thus, widowhood *per se* did not affect even mortality for older widows or widowers. For the 65 to 74 age group, both widows and widowers *did* have significantly lower income than the married elderly. Finally, when controlling for effects of age and education, none of the variables assessing psychological or social outcomes distinguished widowed from married counterparts. These variables included social network, personality, traits of extraversion/openness, general well-being, activities of daily living, and depression.

These findings are quite important because they emphasize the consistently remarkable ability of the elderly to cope, adapt, and adjust to unfortunate life events. McCrae and Costa (1988) call this "psychological resilience" (p. 138). There is personality stability across the lifespan, and McCrae and Costa correctly point out that older adults can reconstruct disrupted social networks and demonstrate enduring stable personality dispositions in the context of disruptive changes (see Costa, Zonderman, & McCrae, 1985; McCrae & Costa, 1984). Thompson *et al.* (1988) have reviewed this literature and maintain that there is much evidence that women *at any age* survive widowhood without psychological damage and view themselves as stronger. McCrae and Costa, focusing specifically on the *elderly*, emphasize the following:

> Older widowed men and women have as many friends and confidantes, believe themselves to be as healthy, and are as able to perform daily activities as the older married individuals; they do not differ in the personality traits of extraversion or openness to experience, nor in morale or the presence of depressive symptoms. Clearly, the great majority of individuals show considerable ability to adapt to a major life stress and continuing life strains. (McCrae & Costa, 1988, p. 138)

NEGATIVE OUTCOMES OF WIDOWHOOD

Older widowed persons can and do adapt to the life event of widowhood. They undergo the process of bereavement in an extremely heterogeneous manner, with differing experiences, time course, and behaviors. Part of this differentiation may be determined by the age and gender of the widowed individual. A variety of life experiences, individual characteristics, sociodemographic influences, and environmental factors are all inextricably bound to the adjustment of widowhood. Positive outcomes of widowhood could be greater individuation, increased independence, maintenance of well-being and self-esteem, and a new and valuable pattern of social interaction. There may also be negative outcomes or effects of widowhood: impaired economic resources, social isolation and loneliness, loss of identity, lowered morale and self-esteem, and even increased illness and death. Unfortunately, when considering the impact of widowhood on mortality and morbidity, research continues to be discrepant and divergent.

Mortality

Widowed persons have been found to have higher mortality than married persons; this has been a finding both in some prospective studies (Berkson, 1962; Jacobs, 1977; Jacobs & Ostfield, 1977; Susseri, 1981) and in some smaller retrospective ones (Epstein *et al.*, 1975; Parkes *et al.*, 1969; Rees & Lutkins, 1967; Young, Benjamin, & Wallace, 1963). Is this excess mortality true for both widowed men and widowed women? Is the risk greater for widowers than widows? And what happens to the risk of mortality with age?

There is not clear agreement on the answers to these questions (see Middleton & Raphael, 1987). On the one hand, Jacobs and Ostfield (1977) have found widows to be at increased risk of mortality following the death of their husbands. They note that "high risk for women may not continue in old age although it holds for the second year of bereavement" (Jacobs & Ostfield, 1977, p. 356). On the other hand, Helsing and Szklo (1981) have maintained that widows have no increased mortality following the death of a spouse. The risk of mortality is found to be greater for men at any age and especially during the first 6 months after the death of a spouse (Jacobs & Ostfield, 1977). Some prospective studies have shown widowers, especially old widowers, to be more at risk (Cox & Ford, 1964; Helsing & Szklo, 1981; Young *et al.*, 1963).

The risk of mortality after bereavement may not increase with the age of the survivor (cf. Clayton, Halikas, & Maurice, 1972). Mortality and bereavement for the elderly is difficult to evaluate because of additional confounding factors such as prior illness of the widow or widower, income, and length of illness (Gallagher *et al.*, 1981–82). Kaprio, Koskenvou, and Rita (1987) looked at 95,647 widowed persons in Finland during 1971–76. They found that the highest mortality risk was found immediately after bereavement, and this was two times over the expected rate during the first week. There was a larger risk, in all age groups, especially for ischemic heart disease. However, standardized mortality rates decreased after the first week but still remained high for men *under* 65 through the third year. Older widowers, however, had standardized mortality rates that approached expected levels after the first 6 months from the death of a spouse; women's standardized mortality rates approached expected levels after the first month from the death of a spouse. The conclusion is that "while the greatest excess mortality after bereavement seems to be due principally to the acute effects of becoming widowed, there also seems excessive mortality in younger persons widowed for a longer time" (Kaprio *et al.*, 1987, p. 283). McCrae and Costa (1988) found that age, education, and sex were significant predictors of survival but *marital status* was not; widowhood *per se* did not affect mortality for older widows or widowers.

Such lack of relationship with mortality and widowhood has not been a consistent finding, however, especially when considering older widowers. Bowling (1988–89) followed 503 elderly widowed persons for 6 years after bereavement and found that there was excessive mortality for older males over the age of 75 compared with males of the same ages in the general population. The risk of death for elderly males may be highest during the first year of bereavement and then gradually return to normal (see Rowland, 1977). Middleton and Raphael (1987) note that it makes intuitive sense that older widowers would be at more risk for increased mortality compared to younger widowers or widows because the average elderly widower "at the time of bereavement is older in the proportion of his expected life span completed than is the average widow. Hence, he is presumably more vulnerable in terms of general health to adverse health factors" (p. 339).

Finally, does the death of a widowed person mimic the death of his or her spouse? Looking at the causes of death in a sample of 4,032 white widowed and married persons over 18 years old, Helsing, Comstock, and Szklo (1982) found that the similarity and causes of death of the widowed in predeceased spouses was no greater than expected to occur by chance. Furthermore, widowed males or females suffering from the same chronic disease did not die sooner after bereavement than others.

Physical Illness

Although Murrell and colleagues (1988) found no lasting long-term health effects due to bereavement, past reviews of morbidity and mortality of widowhood have demonstrated consistent physical and psychological consequences of conjugal bereavement. Up to one-quarter of those who lose a spouse may suffer from impaired physical and psychological health for a year or more after the loss (see Carey, 1979; Clayton, 1974; Maddison, 1968; Osterweis, Solomon, & Green, 1984; Parkes, 1970; Windholz, Marmar, & Horowitz, 1985). After the death of a spouse, there can be increased use of alcohol, an increase in physician visits, and increased medication and hospital use. Mor, McHorney, and Sherwood (1986) found that the bereaved spouse is at increased risk for this type of secondary morbidity when factors such as age, sex, and health conditions are controlled for.

> This strongly suggests that the affective bond of what is generally a life-long relationship takes it toll with respect to secondary morbidity . . . it is the nature of the conjugal relationship and the reallocation of functional roles and responsibilities resulting from the death of the spouse that affect bereavement adjustment. (Mor *et al.*, 1986, p. 162)

Thompson, Breckenridge, Gallagher, and Peterson (1984) looked at self-perceived physical health for 212 older widows and widowers 2 months after the death of their spouse; the findings were contrasted to responses of 162 controls. They noted that physician visits and hospitalizations were reported to be no more frequent among the bereaved. However, elderly widowed people did report significantly more worsened or recently developed illness, increased use of medications, and poor health ratings in general. Small but significant differences were found for poorer perceived health among older women. The previously mentioned study of Mor, McHorney, and Sherwood (1986) investigated the health consequences of recent bereavement by analzying data from the national Hospice Study (1,447 subjects completed a bereavement interview). Results indicated that the rates of physician visits were higher, but hospitalization rates were actually lower among the recently bereaved. The strongest predictors of morbidity and health care utilization were spousal relationships to the deceased and previous health-care problems. In this study, although older widowed men and older widowed women had more annual physician visits compared to the norm, the rate of hospitalization was actually less than the norm. A disproportionately high rate of physician visits in the oldest age group may be influenced by the bereaved seeking health care for social support. The widowed are expected to get over grief rather quickly; somatization and physical complaints may replace the psychological distress of grief (Mor *et al.*, 1986).

In summary, the relationship between widowhood and onset or exacerbation of physical problems remains unclear. This relationship is probably mediated by many factors including the nature of the marital relationship, available social support, past history of medical problems, personality, and ongoing life experiences (see Zisook, Schuchter, & Lyons 1987). Also, little has been done to determine who stays healthy (see Middleton & Raphael, 1987).

Depression

Mental illness may occur more often to widowed persons than married persons (Balkwell 1981), and this includes depression (Clayton, 1974). Depression and global adjustment scores have been found to be higher for widowed persons, especially when deaths were sudden or unanticipated (see Parkes, 1975; Zisook *et al.*, 1987). There may be some relationship between poor outcome in bereavement and premorbid mental illness (Parkes, 1975; Sanders, 1988). More mental health problems may occur in widowhood, but this has been a more consistent finding for those *under* the age of 65 (Parkes & Brown, 1972). More depression, psychological distress, and psychosomatic complaints have been found in some studies including the elderly but not in others. Gallagher and colleagues (1981–82) note that the findings on the mental health effects of bereavement are inconsistent and fraught with methodological difficulties,

> and it is very difficult to predict exactly what effects could be expected to have on the psychological status of elderly men and women. There appears to be a need for longitudinal studies in this area in order to investigate the full gamut of emotional responses and to trace their change over time. (p. 87).

Spousal bereavement consists of symptoms similar to a major clinical depression (see Clayton & Darvish, 1979). Clayton and colleagues (1972) found that over one-third of the bereaved to be clinically depressed at 1 month after the death of a spouse, 17% at 1 year, and 13% depressed for the whole year. Bereavement itself, not the effects of living alone, may influence depressive symptomatology in widows and widowers in 1 month after the death of a spouse (Clayton, 1975; $n = 109$, average age = 61). In this study, younger people showed more physical depressive symptomatology and required more hospitalizations than matched controls or older widows and widowers at 1 year.

In those who are vulnerable, spousal bereavement can precipitate depression (Lloyd, 1980), with grief eventually resulting in depression for up to one-third of those widowed (see Jacobs *et al.*, 1989). Loss of a spouse is more strongly associated with the development of subsequent depressive symptomatology in older adults than in losses of other kinds (retirement, living arrangements, friends, income)—even when controlling for preevent depression, socioeconomic resources, and other variables (see Murrell & Himmelfarb, 1989).

When one compares widowed women to married women and widowed men to married men, however, there appears to be more depressive symptomatology for widowed men than married men, whereas widowed women were no more depressed than married women (Weissman & Klerman, 1977). Jacobs and colleagues (1989) found that 32% of bereaved spouses were depressed 6 months after the loss; 27% of bereaved spouses were depressed 1 year after the loss. Age, education, living arrangements, previous history of depression, and death of a spouse from acute illness were *not* related to depression. In this study, depressions were more common in women rather than men. Prior history of depression did not seem to enhance the risk of depression. Depression was characterized by anxiety, restlessness, and psychomotor retardation.

Jacobs, Kasl, Ostfeld, Berkman, Charpentier (1986) looked at 114 widowed persons, with the average age of 62.5 years, with 60% being over 61 years old. In this study, there were no significant differences found between widows and widowers in the experience of grief (i.e., in the intensity of separation anxiety and sadness and loneliness in the acute stages of grief). Women scored higher on depressive dimensions of grief than did men. Widows did report more numbness, disbelief, and neurovegatative symptomatology than widowers. Jacobs and colleagues (1986) believe that this is because women tend to avoid, deny, and defend more than men against the reality of loss. But this may not be negative. As Jacobs, Kasl *et al.* (1986) note: "It also raises a question if this avoidance is protective of health since women are at lower risk of morbidity from bereavement than men" (p. 309).

Gallagher, Breckenridge, Thompson, and Peterson (1983) did not find serious psychopathology for bereaved *elderly* widows and widowers compared to the older control group at 2 months following the death of a spouse. There was a significant reduction of psychological distress from the bereaved after 1 year, although they were still more depressed than the nonbereaved (Gallagher *et al.*, 1983). Although a 2-year longitudinal study by Lund, Caserta, and Dimond (1985) did not show differences in health status between bereaved and nonbereaved elders, death of a spouse for an older adult did result in more depression. Although this decreases over time, widowed elders still are more depressed than nonwidowed elders, even after 2 years.

The psychobiology of bereavement has focused on studying the immune system and the hypothalamus–pituitary–adrenal gland function (see Van Eerde-wegh & Clayton, 1988). Only recent work by Reynolds (1989) has looked at sleep and bereavement-related depression, specifically investigating whether depressed bereaved will differ from nondepressed bereaved by having more abnormal REM sleep and be similar to those elderly nonbereaved depressives.

More recent and important work by Murrell and Himmelfarb (1989), however, is not consistent with the findings of increased depressive symptomatology for older widowed persons when they looked at a large sample of older adults over age 55 ($n = 1,411$) prior to and after bereavement, with a 6-month and 1-year follow-up. Controlling for various prebereavement conditions, Murrell *et al.* (1988) found that those who lost a parent, spouse, or child had more depressive symptoms than other types of losses (for example, material) but that these effects are *temporary* and *dissipate within 1 year*. Breckenridge and colleagues (1986) found that depressive features of bereaved elderly to be of a different relative order and of a relative magnitude than nonelderly bereaved. They conclude that "the bereaved elderly may experience less severe distress than middle-aged people" (p. 167). When prospective designs are used, bereavement appears to have little effect; there is more depressive symptomatology within the first year (Clayton, 1979), but this is short-lived (see Norris & Murrell, 1987). Heyman and Gianturco (1973) also found only *temporary* effects on depression from bereavement. There have been findings from the Duke Longitudinal Project that have shown no effects of bereavement on life satisfaction or affect (Palmore, Cleveland, Nowlin, Ramm, & Seigler, 1979). Murrell and Himmelfarb conclude that

> older adults are quite resilient to the stresses of life changes. Thus, bereavement in particular and life events in general would appear to have quite limited etiological importance for depressive symptoms in older adults. (1989, p. 172)

Suicide

Anomie, the absence of social norms that guide behavior as described by Durkheim (1951), has been associated with suicide. Widowhood lacks norms and roles. Suicide rates are found to be higher for widowed than among married counterparts, with a discrepancy especially for men (see Balkwell, 1981). The survivors of suicide have also been found to be more at risk for physical and mental health problems (Weiss, 1984). There are little comprehensive data available on the bereaved after suicide. The stigma of suicide can be quite difficult for family members; those who grieve may be more at risk for poor outcome (Sanders, 1988). Suicide rates for white males continue to climb with age. One would expect the death of a suicide to be quite difficult for the family of an elderly suicide victim. Gallagher and colleagues (1981–82) maintain that inconsistent findings related to suicide demonstrate that the relationship between bereavement and suicide in elderly men and women needs further study. Finally, Faberow, Gallagher, Gilewski, and Thompson (1987) looked at the impact of 108 survivors of suicides of elderly spouses within the first 2 months of the bereavement process and compared them with other elderly survivors of natural deaths and married, nonbereaved older adults. The bereaved groups scored poorer than the nonbereaved controls for virtually all measures except that anxiety was reported more often by suicide survivors than by survivors of natural death. However, Faberow and colleagues (1987) maintain that the differences between the two bereaved groups could have been blurred due to data collection at only 8 weeks after the death of a spouse. Overall findings in this area are, therefore, quite inconclusive.

INTERVENTIONS

Suggestions for assisting widowed persons have typically included sharing the strain with those who have lost a spouse, assessing various needs and discussing the widowed's feelings of this new reality in their lives, and supporting efforts at both remembrance of the spouse and resolution of this life event. If the widowed person is undergoing typical stages of grief, counseling interventions have responded to those phases. For example, the therapist accepts the widowed person and his or her denial and acknowledges that this is a difficult time. The counselor also acknowledges the feeling of guilt because of responsibility for the events leading to the death of a spouse and asks the widowed person to share these feelings. The therapist can also legitimatize depression and talk about how poorly the bereaved person feels. Finally, the therapist can help the widowed person accept anger and focus on what this bereaved person is really angry about, allowing him or her to talk about this with nonjudgmental support. (For a more complete review of interventions in widowhood, see Gallagher, 1986.)

Unfortunately, most of the literature on interventions is vague and unsupported by good methodology. A widely acknowledged intervention for widows of all ages has been widow-to-widow peer counseling that has provided support and role modeling (Silverman, 1980, 1981). This includes telephone hotlines, socialization resources, home visits, and aids in education. Counselors help the widowed by explaining the grief process, by providing an accepting atmosphere for widows to come to terms with their loss and their needs for continued intimacy, and by assisting the widowed with particular skills and activities of daily living (Balkwell, 1981).

There has also been scant literature on assessing problems in widowhood, especially for older persons. Gabriel and Kirschling (1989) reviewed existing instruments in the assessment of grief in the elderly. These instruments are extremely variable in theoretical base, reliability, and validity. A simple 4-point rating scale of overall adjustment to widowhood may be useful. Zisook, Schuchter, and Lyons (1987) found that overall adjustment correlated higher with various standardized psychometric scale scores, including the Zung and the Hopkins Symptom Checklist. Adaptation was also associated with various affects related to grief. "Assessing global adjustment may, therefore, be a single, time-efficient, yet meaningful area of inquiry in clinical situations" (Zisook et al., 1987, p. 366). Essa (1986) treats abnormal or prolonged grief among elderly patients as a crisis and promotes psychotherapeutic intervention as effective and appropriate in dealing with elderly bereavement. Also, support groups for the elderly who are widowed are probably more beneficial if they include both men and women (Lund, Caserta, & Dimond, 1986).

Marmar, Horowitz, Weiss, Wilner, and Kaltreider (1988) compared interventions of brief psychotherapy with mutual help groups for 61 widows with a mean age of 58 years (age range 26–82 years old). Both treatment interventions resulted in reduced symptoms of stress, anxiety, and depression, with brief psychotherapy being better for only 1 out of 11 outcome measures. Group treatment focused more on support, role modeling, and education. Brief psychotherapy focused on recognizing and resolving maladaptations and barriers to the mourning process. Marmar et al., (1988) note that, compared with brief treatments in other stressful life events, interventions for widows resulted in slower change and in more reduction of symptoms than in an improvement of daily functioning.

For the elderly, *timing* of interventions is probably quite important. McCrae and Costa (1988) suggest that interventions in widowhood recognize that bereavement is a major stressor. They maintain that intervention targeted to improving psychological distress or disruptiveness should be timed on *recently* widowed individuals, whereas interventions *extended over time* should aim for the objective issues in quality of life (low income, institutionalization, poor living arrangements) rather than subjective well-being.

In summary, assessment and treatment of problems in widowhood is still, for the most part, supported only by clinical anecdotal information. More research needs to be done on the effectiveness of differential interventions. No controlled studies for intervention effectiveness with older widows or widowers have been done (Gallagher, 1986).

SUMMARY

The previous sections of this chapter have demonstrated that the literature on bereavement in widowhood has been anything but consistent. In reviewing a variety of studies, with differening methodological qualities, it becomes apparent that multifaceted variables both affect how one adapts to the life event of widowhood and also influence a variety of outcomes. The following is a summary of possible risk factors for psychological, physical, and social dysfunction following the death of a spouse; adapting or resolving grief is dependent upon a variety of these factors.

Type of Marital Relationship

Evidence of any preexisting marital difficulty may contribute to poor outcome; this may include an ambivalent marital relationship or relationships that include dependency. (Epstein, Weitz, Roback, & McKee, 1975; Gallagher et al., 1981–82; Lopata, 1975; Parkes & Weiss, 1983; Raphael, 1983; Sanders, 1980, 1988; Shanfield, 1983; Stroebe & Stroebe, 1983; Vachon, 1976; Zisook et al., 1987).

Mode of Death and Timing Issues

Poor bereavement outcome could be due to a protracted death, no opportunities for anticipatory grief, unexpected loss, or particular mode of death (including accidents, suicides, catastrophes, murders) (Ball, 1976–77; Epstein, Weitz, Roback, & McKee, 1975; Faberow et al., 1987; Fulton & Gottesman, 1980; Glick et al., 1974; Neugarten, 1970; Parkes, 1975; Peterson, 1980; Sanders, 1988; Sheldon et al., 1981; Vachon, 1976; Windholz et al., 1985; Zisook et al., 1987).

Other Losses and Stresses, Life Events, Experiences

Possible mediating factors in adapting to widowhood or in the development of illnesses may include the history of loss and stress prior to widowhood, especially when there are additional stresses or crises in close temporal relationships to the bereavement event. A previous experience with loss assumes some prior knowledge was gained; however, the presence of concurrent life events may mean that those suffering from multiple losses have a more difficult time in widowhood (Clayton et al., 1973; Epstein, Weitz, Roback, & McKee, 1975; Lloyd, 1980; Maddison & Walker, 1967; Osterweis, Solomon, & Green, 1984; Parkes, 1975; Sanders, 1988; Windholz et al., 1985).

Coping Styles and Strengths

Past history of coping styles, including a prior history of severe reaction to the death of a family member, may influence poor bereavement outcome. On the other hand, coping strengths, including a belief in interpersonal control over stress, may help adjustment followoing bereavement (Ball, 1976–77; Epstein, Weitz, Roback, & McKee, 1975; Faberow *et al.*, 1987; Horowitz, 1986; Peterson, 1980).

Acute or Initial Response to Loss

The high *initial* symptomatic response to the loss of a spouse may be one predictor for subsequent difficulties. This would include where there is possible minimal funeral ceremony (that feeds into the denial of death), the ability of the widowed person to understand or accept death, and how one grieves. On the one hand, the deliberate avoidance of affective expression in the controlling of hostile and angry feelings may lead to continued reaction formation and denial and thus poor outcome. However, as Wortman and Silver (1989) have pointed out, previous assumptions about the universal *normative* experience of grief through defined stages is presumptuous and not consistently supported by good, sound, research (Epstein *et al.*, 1975; Parkes & Brown, 1972; Windholz *et al.*, 1985).

Personality/Self-Esteem

Particular personality characteristics may influence the adjustment to widowhood. Preexisting self-esteem and prior sense of life satisfaction may also be contributing resources in resolving grief (Bowlby, 1980; Bowling, 1988–89; Heyman & Gianturco, 1973; Parkes, 1985; Sanders, 1980; Stroebe & Stroebe, 1983; Vachon, 1976; Vachon *et al.*, 1982).

History of Medical or Psychiatric Problems

A prior history of medical illness or depression prior to widowhood may affect various outcomes after the widowhood event (Lund *et al.*, 1985; Osterweis *et al.*, 1984; Parkes, 1975; Sanders, 1988; Vachon, 1976).

Social Support

Dissatisfaction with available help during the bereavement crisis may be a predictor of poor bereavement outcome. Quantitative and qualitative factors in the social support network may be one of the most important influences in the adjustment of the survivor to widowhood. For example, poor interpersonal relationships with remaining family members may influence the adaptation process. It is not only whether an extensive social environment exists for the widowed person, it is how this environment is perceived and utilized. Social support networks also provide resources that assist in adjustment; these include opportunities for social participation, meaningful interpersonal relationships that can help restructure or reaffirm one's identity, participation in meaningful religious and leisure time activities (Ball, 1976–77; Epstein *et al.*, 1975; Faberow *et al.*, 1987; Lopata, 1973; Maddison & Walker, 1967; Peterson, 1980; Raphael, 1977; Sanders, 1988; Stroebe & Stroebe, 1987; Vachon *et al.*, 1982; Windholz *et al.*, 1985).

Finances and Income

The elderly can experience poor economic conditions in widowhood that can have a great impact upon eventual adjustment. Many older widowed persons, however, accommodate to their financial situation without perceived strain. (Atchley, 1975; Gallagher *et al.*, 1981–82; Glick *et al.*, 1974; McCrae & Costa, 1988; Morgan, 1976; Sheldon *et al.*, 1981; Smith & Zick, 1986; Zisook *et al.*, 1987).

Gender and Age

Younger age groups may have poorer outcome than older age groups. However, within the elderly widowed, being *very* old may be an influential factor for outcome. It is unclear whether older men or older women have a more difficult time adjusting to widowhood or whether there are any gender differences at all. The literature on gender is thus inconsistent: Women may do worse than men initially but do better over time. Much literature supports poor outcome, especially in mortality, in males. This may be true for older males as well, but findings are not conclusive (Arens, 1983; Ball, 1976–77; Bowling, 1988–89; Lopata, 1973; Neugarten, 1970; O'Bryant & Morgan, 1989; Parkes, 1975; Parkes & Weiss, 1983; Sanders, 1980–81; Stroebe & Stroebe, 1983; Zisook *et al.*, 1987).

CONCLUSION

Widowhood, as viewed from a human developmental perspective, can involve growth and change. The stressful life event of widowhood should not be viewed as pathological but "inducing states of imbalance which can have either positive or negative outcomes" (Thomas, DiGuilio, & Sheehan, 1988, p. 237). A variety of factors can affect the outcome of widowhood in late life. These factors relate to successful adaptation and are determinants of well-being in late life. If one does not do well in adapting to widowhood in late life, it may be more than just not being able to forge a sense of subjective well-being after this life event but in not being able to meet the new demands of the current environment now that one's marital status is changed. (See the definition of maladaptation in late life presented by George, 1980; and also in Lawton's environmental press theory, in Lawton and Nahemow, 1973). Especially in late life, one grieves not only for the spouse who is lost but also for the functions and assistance performed in a state of interdependency. Because one becomes more individuated with age, experience of widowhood in late life is an extremely heterogeneous one. The *interaction* of risk factors is much more important in predicting outcomes. In general, one would have to conclude that widowhood, in and of itself, is a life event that most older people can adapt to without undue difficulty; the eventual impact of widowhood on an elderly person's life may not be as great as other factors such as health, income, personality, and social support. In fact, these factors may do more to directly affect adjustment, self-esteem, morale, and even mortality than the life event of widowhood, *per se*.

ACKNOWLEDGMENT   I thank my colleague, Kathy Reed, for sharing with me her clinical insights in coping with loss.

REFERENCES

Anderson, T. S. (1984). Widowhood as a life transition: Its impact on kinship ties. *Journal of Marriage and the Family, 46,* 105–114.

Arens, D. A. (1983). Widowhood and well-being: An examination of sex differences within a causal model. *International Journal of Aging and Human Development, 15,* 27–40.

Arling, G. (1976). The elderly widow and her family, neighbors, and friends. *Journal of Marriage and the Family, 38,* 757–768.

Atchley, R. C. (1975). Dimensions of widowhood in later life. *The Gerontologist, 15,* 1976–1978.

Balkwell, C. (1981). Transition to widowhood: A review of the literature. *Family Relations, 30,* 117–127.

Ball, J. F. (1976–77). Widow's grief: The impact of age and mode of depth. *Omega, 1,* 307–333.

Baltes, P. B., Reese, H. W., & Lipsitt, L. P. (1980). Life-span developmental psychology. *Annual Review of Psychology, 31,* 65–110.

Berado, F. M. (1970). Survivorship and social isolation: The case of the aged widower. *Family Coordinator, 19,* 11–25.

Berkson, J. (1962). Mortality and marital status. *American Journal of Public Health, 52,* 1318–1329.

Bowlby, J. (1980). *Attachment and loss: Loss, sadness, and depression.* New York: Basic Books.

Bowling, A. (1988–89). Who dies after widow(er)hood? A discriminant analysis. *Omega, 19,* 135–153.

Breckenridge, J. N., Gallagher, D., Thompson, L. W., & Peterson, J. (1986). Characteristic depressive symptoms of bereaved elders. *Journal of Gerontology, 41,* 163–168.

Burks, V. K., Lund, D. A., Gregg, C. H., & Bluhm, H. P. (1988). Bereavement and remarriage for older adults. *Death Studies, 12,* 51–60.

Butler, R. N. & Lewis, M. I. (1977). *Aging and mental health: Positive psychosocial approaches.* St. Louis: C.V. Mosby.

Carey, R. S. (1979). Weathering widowhood: Problems and adjustment of the widowed during the first year. *Omega, 10,* 163–174.

Charmaz, K. (1980). *The social reality of death.* Boston: Addison-Wesley.

Clayton, P. J. (1974). Mortality and morbidity in the first year of bereavement. *Archives of General Psychiatry, 30,* 747–750.

Clayton, P. J. (1975). The effect of living alone on bereavement symptoms. *American Journal of Psychiatry, 132,* 133–137.

Clayton, P. J. (1979). The sequelae and nonsequelae of conjugal bereavement. *American Journal of Psychiatry, 126,* 1530–1534.

Clayton, P. J. & Darvish, H. S. (1979). Course of depressive symptoms following the stress of bereavement. In J. D. Barrett (Ed.), *Stress and mental disorder* (pp. 121–136). New York: Raven Press.

Clayton, P., Halikas, J., & Maurice W. (1971). The bereavement of the widowed. *Diseases of the Nervous System, 32,* 597–604.

Clayton, P. J., Halikas, J. A., & Maurice, W. L. (1972). The depression of widowhood. *British Journal of Psychiatry, 120,* 71–78.

Clayton, P. J., Halikas, J. A., Maurice, W. L., & Robins, E. (1973). Anticipatory grief and widowhood. *British Journal of Psychiatry, 122,* 47–51.

Cleveland, W. P. & Gianturco, D. T. (1976). Remarriage probability after widowhood: A retrospective method. *Journal of Gerontology, 31,* 99–103.

Costa, P. T., Jr., Zonderman, A. B. & McCrae, R. R. (1985). Longitudinal course of social support among men in the Baltimore Longitudinal Study of Aging. In I. Sarason & B. R. Sarason (Eds.), Social support: Theory, research, and applications (pp. 87–154). The Hague, The Netherlands: Nijhoff.

Cowan, M. E., & Murphy, S. A. (1985). Identification of post-disaster bereavement risk predictors. *Nursing Research, 34,* 71–75.

Cox, P. R., & Ford, J. R. (1964). The mortality of widows after widowhood. *Lancet, 1.*

Cummings, E., & Henry, E. W. (1961). *Growing old: The process of disengagement.* New York: Basic Books.

DeVaul, R. A., & Zisook, S. (1976). Unresolved grief: Clinical considerations. *Postgraduate Medicine, 59,* 267–271.

Dimond, M. (1981). Bereavement and the elderly: A critical review with implications for nursing practice and research. *Journal of Advanced Nursing, 6,* 461–470.

Dimond, M., Lund, D. A., & Easerta, M. S. (1987). The role of social support in the first two years of bereavement in an elderly sample. *The Gerontologist, 27,* 599–604.

Dohrenwend, B. S. & Dohrenwend, B. P. (1984). *Stressful life events and their contexts.* New Brunswick, NJ: Rutgers University Press.

Durkheim, E. (1951). *Suicide.* New York: The Free Press.

Eichorn, D., Clausen, J., Haan, N., Honzik, M., & Mussen, P. (1981). *Present and past in middle life.* New York: Academic Press.

Eisenbruch, M. (1984). Cross cultural aspects of bereavement II: Ethnic and cultural variations in the development of bereavement practices. *Culture, Medicine, and Psychiatry, 8*, 315–347.

Elkowitz, E. B., & Virginia, A. T. (1980). Relationship of depression to physical and psychological complaints in the widowed elderly. *Journal of the American Geriatrics Society, 28*(11), 507–510.

Elwell, F., & Maltbie-Crannel, A. D. (1981). The impact of the role loss upon coping resources and life satisfaction of the elderly. *Journal of Gerontology, 26*, 223–232.

Epstein, G., Weitz, L., Roback, H., & McKee, E. (1975). Research on bereavement: A selective and critical review. *Comprehensive Psychiatry, 16*, 537–546.

Essa, M. (1986). Grief as a crisis: Psychotherapeutic interventions with elderly bereaved. *American Journal of Psychotherapy, 40*(2), 243–251.

Faberow, N. L., Gallagher, D. E., Gilewski, M. J., & Thompson, L. W. (1987). An examination of the long impact of bereavement on psychological distress in survivors of suicide. *The Gerontologist, 27*, 592–598.

Ferraro, K. F. (1984). Widowhood and social participation in later life: Isolation or compensation. *Research on Aging, 6*, 451–468.

Fulton, R., & Gottesman, D. J. (1980). Anticipatory grief: A psychosocial concept reconsidered. *British Journal of Psychiatry, 137*, 45.

Gabriel, R. M., & Kirschling, J. M. (1989). Assessing grief among the bereaved elderly: A review of existing measures. *Hospice Journal, 5*, 29–54.

Gallagher, D. (1986). Assessment of depression in elders by interview methods and psychiatric rating scales. In L. Poon, B. Gurland, C. Eisdorfer, T. Crook, L. Thompson, A. Kazniak, & K. Davis (Eds.), *Handbook of clinical memory assessment* (pp. 202–212). Washington, D.C.: American Psychological Association.

Gallagher, D., Breckenridge, J., Thompson, L. W., & Peterson, J. (1982). Effects of bereavement on indicators of mental health in elderly widows and widowers. *Journal of Gerontology, 38*, 565–571.

Gallagher, D., Breckenridge, J., Thompson, L. W., & Peterson, J. (1983). *Change over time and prediction of one-year post-bereavement status: Selected results from the USC longitudinal study of elder's adaptation to spousal bereavement.* Paper presented at the annual meeting of the Gerontological Society of America, San Francisco, November.

Gallagher, D. E., Thompson, L. W., & Peterson, J. A. (1981–82). Psychosocial factors affecting adaptation to bereavement in the elderly. *International Journal of Aging and Human Development, 14*(2), 79–95.

Gass, K. A. (1988). Aged widows and widowers: Similarities and differences in appraisal, coping, resources, type of death, and health dysfunction. *Archives of Psychiatric Nursing, 2*(4), 200–210.

Gass, K., & Chang, A. S. (1989). Appraisals of bereavement, coping, resources, and psychosocial health dysfunction in widows and widowers. *Nursing Research, 38*(1), 31–36.

Gentry, J., & Shulman, A. D. (1988). Remarriage as a coping response for widowhood. *Psychology and Aging, 3*(2), 191–196.

George, L. K. (1980). *Role transitions in later life: A social stress perspective.* Monterey, CA: Brooks/Cole.

Gilford, D. M. (Ed.). (1988). *The aging population in the twenty-first century: Statistics for health policy.* Washington, DC: National Academy Press.

Glick, I. O., Weiss, R. S., & Parkes, C. M. (1974). *The first year of bereavement.* New York: Wiley-Interscience.

Gorer, G. (1965). *Death, grief, and mourning.* New York: Doubleday.

Gove, W. R. (1972). The relationship between sex roles, marital status, and mental illness. *Social Forces, 51*, 34–44.

Greenblatt, M. (1978). The grieving spouse. *American Journal of Psychiatry, 135*, 43–47.

Gubrium, J. F. (1974). Marital desolation and the evaluation of everyday life in old age. *Journal of Marriage and the Family, 36*, 97–106.

Hansson, R. O., Jones, W. J., & Carpenter, B. N. (1984). Relational competence and social support. In P. Shaver (Ed.), *Review of personality and social psychology* (Vol. 5, pp. 265–884). Beverly Hills, CA: Sage.

Hansson, R. O., Jones, W. H., Carpenter, B. N., & Remondet, J. H. (1986). Loneliness and adjustment to old age. *International Journal of Aging and Human Development, 24*(1), 41–53.

Hansson, R. O., & Remondet, J. H. (1988). Old age and widowhood: Issues of personal control and independence. *Journal of Social Issues, 44*, 159–174.

Hartwigsen, G. (1987). Older widows and the transference of home. *International Journal of Aging and Human Development, 25*(3), 195–207.

Heinemann, G. (1982). Why study widowed women: A rationale. *Women and Health, 7*, 17–29.

Helsing, K. J., Comstock, G. W., & Szklo, M. (1982). Causes of death in a widowed population. *American Journal of Epidemiology, 116,* 524–532.

Helsing, K. J., & Szklo, M. (1981). Mortality after bereavement. *American Journal of Epidemiology, 114,* 41–52.

Helsing, K. J., Szklo, M., & Comstock, G. W. (1981). Factors associated with mortality after widowhood. *American Journal of Public Health, 71,* 802–809.

Heyman, D. K., & Gianturco, D. T. (1973). Long-term adaptation by the elderly in bereavement. *Journal of Gerontology, 28,* 359–362.

Hill, C. D., Thompson, L. W., & Gallagher, D. (1988). The role of anticipatory bereavement in older women's adjustment to widowhood. *The Gerontologist, 28*(6), 792–796.

Hogan, R., Jones, W. H., & Cheek, J. M. (1984). Socio-analytic theory: An alternative to armadillo psychology. In B. Schlenker (Ed.), *Self and identity: Presentations of self in social life* (pp. 175–198). New York: McGraw-Hill.

Holmes, T. H., & Rahe, R. H. (1967). The social adjustment rating scale. *Journal of Psychosomatic Research, 11,* 213–218.

Horowitz, J. J. (1986). Stress-response syndromes: A review of post-traumatic and adjustment disorder. *Hospital and Community Psychiatry, 37,* 241–248.

Jacobs, S. (1977). An epidemiological review of the mortality of bereavement. *Psychosomatic Medicine, 39,* 344–357.

Jacobs, S., & Douglas, L. (1979). Grief: A mediating process between loss and illness. *Comprehensive Psychiatry, 20,* 165.

Jacobs, S., Hansen, F., Berkman, L., Kashl, S., & Ostfeld, A. (1989). Depressions of bereavement. *Comprehensive Psychiatry, 30*(3), 218–224.

Jacobs, S., Kasl, S., Ostfeld, A., Berkman, L., & Charpentier, P. (1986). The measurement of grief: Age and sex variation. *British Journal of Medical Psychology, 59,* 305–310.

Jacobs, S. C., Mason, J. W., Kosten, T. R., Wahby, V., Kasl, S. V., & Ostfeld, A. M. (1986). Bereavement and catecholamines. *Journal of Psychosomatic Research, 30*(4), 489–496.

Jacobs, S., & Ostfeld, A. (1977). An epidemiological review of the mortality of bereavement. *Psychosomatic Medicine, 39*(5), 344–357.

Johnson, R. J., Lund, D. A., & Dimond, M. F. (1986). Stress, self-esteem and coping during bereavement among the elderly. *Social Psychology Quarterly, 49*(3), 273–279.

Kalish, R. A. (1987). Older people and grief. *Generations, 11,* 33–38.

Kaprio, J., Koskenvuo, M., & Rita, H. (1987). Mortality after bereavement: A prospective study of 95,647 widowed persons. *American Journal of Public Health, 77,* 283–287.

Katz, S., & Florian, V. (1987). A comprehensive theoretical model of psychological reaction to loss. *International Journal of Psychiatry in Medicine, 16,* 325–345.

Kavanaugh, R. G. (1972). *Facing death.* Baltimore: Penguin Books.

Keith, P. M., & Lorenz, F. O. (1989). Financial strain and health of unmarried older people. *The Gerontologist, 29,* 684–691.

Kobassa, S. C., Maddi, S. R., & Kahn, S. (1982). Hardiness and health: A prospective study. *Journal of Personality and Social Psychology, 42,* 168–177.

Kovar, M. G. (1986). Aging in the eighties: Preliminary data from the supplement on aging to the National Health Interview Survey. *NCHS Advance Data No. 115:3.* Washington, DC.

Kowalski, N. C. (1986). Anticipating the death of an elderly parent. In T. A. Rando (Ed.), *Loss and anticipatory grief* (pp. 187–199). Lexington, KY: Lexington Books.

Lawton, M. P., & Nahemow, L. (1973). Ecotosy and the aging process. In C. Eisdorfer & M. P. Lawton (Eds.), *Psychology of adult development and aging.* Washington, DC: American Psychological Association.

Laudenslager, M. L., & Reite, M. L. (1984). Losses and separations: Immunological consequences and health implications. *Review of Personality and Social Psychology, 5,* 285–312.

Leon, R., Gillum, B., Gillum, R., & Gouze, M. (1979). Personality stability over a thirty-year period— middle age to old age. *Journal of Consulting and Clinical Psychology, 23,* 245–259.

Lindemann, E. (1944). Symptomatology and management of acute grief. *American Journal of Psychiatry, 101,* 141–148.

Lloyd, C. (1980). Life events and depressive disorder reviewed. *Archives of General Psychiatry, 37,* 529.

Lopata, H. Z. (1973). *Widowhood in an American city.* Cambridge, MA: Schenkman.

Lopata, H. Z. (1975). On widowhood: Grief work and identity reconstruction. *Journal of Geriatric Psychiatry, 8*(1), 41–45.

Lopata, H. Z. (1979). *Women as widows: Support systems.* New York: Elsevier.

Lopata, H. Z. (1986) Time in anticipated future and events in memory. *American Behavioral Scientist,* 29(6), 695–709.

Lopata, H. Z. (1987). Widowhood and husband santification. *Journal of Marriage and Family,* 43(2), 432–450.

Lopata, H. Z. (1988). Support systems of American urban widowhood. *Journal of Social Issues,* 44, 113–128.

Lund, D. A., Caserta, M. S., & Dimond, M. F. (1985). *The impact of bereavement on the subjective well-being of older adults.* Paper presented at the annual meeting of the Gerontological Society of America, New Orleans, November.

Lund, D. A., Caserta, M. S., & Dimond, M. F. (1985–86). Identifying elderly with coping difficulties after two years of bereavement. *Omega,* 16, 213–224.

Lund, D. A., Caserta, M. S., & Dimond, M. F. (1986). Gender differences through two years of bereavement among the elderly. *The Gerontologist,* 26, 314–320.

Lund, D. A., Caserata, M. S., Dimond, M. F., & Gray, R. M. (1986). Impact of bereavement on the self-conceptions of older surviving spouses. *Symbolic Interaction,* 9, 235–244.

Lundin, J. (1984). Morbidity following sudden and unexpected bereavement. *British Journal of Psychiatry,* 144, 84–88.

Maddison, D. (1968). The relevance of conjugal bereavement for preventive psychiatry. *British Journal of Medical Psychology,* 41, 223–233.

Maddison, D., & Walker, W. L. (1967). Factors affecting the outcome of conjugal bereavement. *British Journal of Psychiatry,* 113, 1057–1067.

Maddison, D. C., & Viola, A. (1968). The health of widows in the year following bereavement. *Journal of Psychosomatic Research,* 12, 297.

Marmar, C. R., Horowitz, J. J., Weiss, D. S., Wilner, N. R., & Kaltreider, N. B. (1988). A controlled trial of brief psychotherapy and mutual-help group treatment of conjugal bereavement. *American Journal of Psychiatry,* 145(2), 203–209.

Marris, P. (1974). *Loss and change.* New York: Pantheon Books.

McCrae, R. R. (1982). Age differences in the use of coping mechanisms. *Journal of Gerontology,* 37, 454–460.

McCrae, R. R., & Costa, P. T., Jr. (1984). *Emerging lives, enduring dispositions: Personality in adulthood.* Boston: Little, Brown.

McCrae, R. R. & Costa, P. T., Jr. (1988). Psychological resilience among widowed men and women: A 10-year follow-up of a national sample. *Journal of Social Issues,* 44, 129–142.

McMahon, B., & Pugh, T. F. (1965). Suicide in the widowed. *American Journal of Epidemiology,* 81, 23.

Middleton, W., & Raphael, B. (1987). Bereavement: State of the art and state of the science. *Psychiatric Clinics of North America,* 10(3), 329–343.

Mor, V., McHorney, C., & Sherwood, S. (1986). Secondary morbidity among the recently bereaved. *American Journal of Psychiatry,* 143, 158–163.

Morgan, L. A. (1976). A re-examination of widowhood and morale. *Journal of Gerontology,* 31, 687–695.

Morgan, L. (1986). The financial experience of widowed women: Evidence from the LRHS. *The Gerontologist,* 26, 663–668.

Morgan, D. (1989). Adjusting to widowhood: Do social networks really make it easier? *The Gerontologist,* 29, 101–107.

Moss, M. S., & Moss, S. J. (1980). The image of the deceased spouse in remarriage of elderly widow(er)s. *Journal of Gerontological Social Work,* 3, 59–70.

Murrell, S. A., & Himmelfarb, S. (1989). Effects of attachment bereavement and pre-event conditions on subsequent depressive symptoms in older adults. *Psychology and Aging,* 4(2), 166–172.

Murrell, S. A., Himmelfarb, S., & Phifer, J. F. (1988). Effects of bereavement/loss and pre-event status on subsequent physical health in older adults. *International Journal of Aging and Human Development,* 27, 87–107.

Neugarten, B. (1968). Adult personality: Toward a psychology of the life-cycle. In B. Neugarten (Ed.), *Middle age and aging* (pp. 137–147). Chicago: University of Chicago Press.

Neugarten, B. (1970). Dynamics of transitions of middle age to old age: Adaptation and the life cycle. *Journal of Geriatric Psychiatry,* 4, 71–87.

Neugarten, B. L., & Guttman, D. L. (1964). Age-sex roles and personality in middle age: A thematic apperception study. In B. L. Neugarten & Associates (Eds.), *Personality in middle and late life* (pp. 58–71). New York: Atherton.

Norris, F., & Murrell, S. (1987). Transitory impact of life-event stress on psychological symptoms in older adults. *Journal of Health and Social Behavior, 28*, 197–211.

Northcott, H. C. (1984). Widowhood and remarriage trends in Canada 1956–1981. *Canadian Journal on Aging, 3*, 63–78.

O'Bryant, S. L., & Morgan, K. A. (1989). Financial experience and well-being among mature widowed women. *The Gerontologist, 29*, 245–251.

Osterweis, M., Solomon, F., & Green, M. (Eds.). (1984). *Bereavement: Reactions, consequences, and care.* Washington, DC: National Academy Press.

Palmore, E., Cleveland, W. Nowlin, J., Ramm, D., & Siegler, I. (1979). Stress and adaptation in later life. *Journal of Gerontology, 34*, 841–851.

Parkes, C. M. (1970). The first year of bereavement: A longitudinal study of the reaction of London widows to the deaths of their husbands. *Psychiatry, 33*, 44–467.

Parkes, C. M. (1975). Determinants of outcome following bereavement. *Omega, 6*, 303–323.

Parkes, C. M. (1985). Bereavement. *British Journal of Psychiatry, 146*, 11–17.

Parkes, C. M., Benjamin, B., & Fitzgerald, R. G. (1969). Broken heart: A statistical study of increased mortality among widowers. *British Medical Journal, 1*, 740–743.

Parkes, C. M., & Brown, R. (1972). Health after bereavement: a controlled study of young Boston widows and widowers. *Psychosomatic Medicine, 34*, 449–461.

Parkes, C. M., & Weiss, R. S. (1983). *Recovery from bereavement.* New York: Basic Books.

Pearlin, L. I., Lieberman, M. A., Menaghan, E. G., & Mullen, J. T. (1981). The stress process. *Journal of Health and Social Behavior, 22*, 337–356.

Peterson, J. A. (1980). Social-psychological aspects of death and dying and mental health. In J. E. Birren & R. B. Sloane (Eds.), (*Handbook of mental health and aging* (pp. 922–942). Englewood Cliffs, NJ: Prentice-Hall.

Pettingale, K. W., Watson, M., Tee, D. E., & Inayat, Q. (1989). Pathological grief, psychiatric symptoms and immune status following conjugal bereavement. *Stress Medicine, 5*, 77–83.

Pihlblad, C. T., & Adams, D. L. (1972). Widowhood, social participation and life satisfaction. *Aging and Human Development, 3*, 323–330.

Rando, T. A. (1983). An investigation of grief and adaptation in parents whose children have died from cancer. *Journal of Pediatric Psychology, 8*, 3–20.

Rando, T. A. (1984). *Grief, dying, and death: Clinical intervention for caregivers.* Champaign, IL: Research Press Company.

Rando, T. A. (1986). A comprehensive analysis of anticipatory grief: Perspectives, processes, promises, and problems. In T. A. Rando (Ed.), *Loss and anticipatory grief* (pp. 3–37). Lexington, KY: Lexington Books.

Raphael, B. (1977). Preventive intervention with the recently bereaved. *Archives of General Psychiatry, 34*, 1450.

Raphael, B. (1983). *The anatomy of bereavement.* London: Hutchinson.

Raphael, B. (1986). *When disaster strikes.* New York: Basic Books.

Rees, W., & Lutkins, S. G. (1967). Mortality and bereavement. *British Medical Journal, 4*, 13–16.

Rodin, J. (1986). Aging and health: Effects of the sense of control. *Science, 223*, 1271–1276.

Rowland, K. F. (1977). Environmental events predicting death for the elderly. *Psychological Bulletin, 84*, 349–372.

Sanders, C. M. (1980–81). A comparison of younger and older spouses in bereavement outcome. *Omega, 11*, 217–232.

Sanders, C. M. (1988). Risk factors in bereavement outcome. *Journal of Social Issues, 44*, 97–112.

Sanders, C. M., Mauger, P. A., & Strong, P. N. (1979). *A manual for the Grief Experience Inventory.* Palo Alto, CA: Consulting Psychologists Press.

Schackleton, C. H. (1984). The pathology of grief: A review. *Advanced Behavior Research and Therapy, 6*, 153–205.

Schaie, W., & Parham, I. (1976). Stability of adult personality traits: Fact or fable. *Journal of Personality and Social Psychology, 34*, 146–158.

Schanfield, S. (1983). Predicting bereavement outcome: Marital factors. *Family Systems Medicine, 1*, 40–46.

Schoenberg, B., Carr, A. C., Peretz, D., & Kutscher, A. H. (Eds.). (1970). *Loss and grief: Psychological management in medical practice.* New York: Columbia University Press.

Sheldon, A. R., Cochrane, J., Vachon, M. L. S., Lyall, W., Rogers, J., & Freeman, S. (1981). A psychosocial analysis of risk of psychological impairment following bereavement. *Journal of Nervous and Mental Disease, 169*, 253–255.

Siegler, I. C., George, L. K., & Okun, M. (1979). Cross-sequential analysis of adult personality. *Developmental Psychology, 15,* 350–351.

Silverman, D., & Cooperband, A. (1975). On widowhood: Mutual help and early widowhood. *Journal of Geriatric Psychiatry, 8,* 9–27.

Silverman, P. R. (1980). *Mutual help groups: Organization and development.* Beverly Hills, CA: Sage Publications.

Silverman, P. R. (1981). *Helping women cope with grief.* Beverly Hills, CA: Sage Publications.

Silverman, P. R. (1985). *Widow to widow.* New York: Springer.

Smith, K. R., & Zick, C. D. (1986). The incidence of poverty among the recently widowed: Mediating factors in the life course. *Journal of Marriage and the Family, 48,* 619–630.

Spanier, G. B., & Glick, P. C. (1980). Paths to remarriage. *Journal of Divorce, 3,* 283–298.

Stern, K., & Williams, B. M. (1957). Grief reactions in later life. *American Journal of Psychiatry, 108,* 289–294.

Stroebe, M. S., & Stroebe, W. (1983). Who suffers more? Sex differences in health risks of the widowed. *Psychological Bulletin, 93,* 279–301.

Stroebe, W., & Stroebe, M. S. (1987). *Bereavement and health.* New York: Cambridge University Press.

Stroebe, M. S., Stroebe, W., Gergen, K. J., & Gergen, M. (1981). The broken heart: Reality or myth? *Omega, 12,* 87–105.

Susseri, M. (1981). Widowhood: A situational life stress or a stressful life event. *American Journal of Public Health, 71,* 793–795.

Thomas, L. E., DiGiulio, R. C., & Sheehan, N. W. (1988). Identity loss and psychological crisis in widowhood: A reevaluation. *International Journal of Aging and Human Development, 26*(3), 225–239.

Thompson, L. W., Breckenridge, J., Gallagher, D., & Peterson, J. (1984). Effects of bereavement on self-perceptions of physical health in elderly widows and widowers. *Journal of Gerontology, 39,* 309–314.

U.S. Bureau of the Census. (1984). *Current population report: Demographic and socioeconomic aspects of aging in the United States.* Washington, DC: U.S. Government Printing Office.

Vachon, M. L. S. (1976). Grief and bereavement following the death of a spouse. *Journal of the Canadian Psychiatric Association, 21,* 35–44.

Vachon, M. L. S., Sheldon, A. R., Lancee, W. J., Lyall, W. A. L., Rogers, J., and Freeman, S. J. J. (1982). Correlates of enduring distress patterns following bereavement: Social network, life situation, and personality. *Psychological Medicine, 12,* 783–788.

Van Eerdewegh, M., & Clayton, P. J. (1988). Bereavement. In R. Michaels (Ed.), *Psychiatry* (Chapter 62). Philadelphia: J. B. Lippincott.

Vinick, B. H. (1979). Remarriage in old age. In R. H. Jacobs & B. H. Vinick (Eds.). *Re-engagement in later life.* (pp. 141–243). Stamford, CT: Greylock.

Wahl, C. W. (1970). The differential diagnoses of normal and neurotic grief following bereavement. *Psychosomatics, 11,* 104–106.

Walker, K. N., MacBride, A., & Vachon, M. L. S. (1977). Social support networks and the crisis of bereavement. *Social Science and Medicine, 11,* 35–41.

Wan, T., & Odell, B. (1983). Major role losses and social participation of older males. *Research on Aging, 5,* 173–196.

Warlick, J. L. (1985). Why is poverty after 65 a woman's problem? *Journal of Gerontology, 40,* 751–757.

Weiss, R. S. (1984). Reactions to particular types of bereavement. In M. Osterweis, I. Solomon, & M. Owen (Eds.), *Bereavement reactions: Consequences and care.* Washington, DC: National Academy Press.

Weissman, M. M., & Klerman, G. L. (1977). Sex differences and the epidemiology of depression. *Archives of General Psychiatry, 34,* 98–111.

West, G. E., & Simons, R. L. (1983). Sex differences in stress, coping resources, and illness among the elderly. *Research on Aging, 5,* 235–268.

Windholz, J. J., Marmar, C. R., & Horowitz, M. J. (1985). A review of the research on conjugal bereavement: Impact on health and efficacy of intervention. *Comprehensive Psychiatry, 26,* 433–447.

Wister, A. V., & Strain, L. (1986). Social support and well-being: A comparison of older widows and widowers. *Canadian Journal on Aging, 5,* 205–220.

Wortman, C. B., & Silver, R. C. (1987). Coping with irrevocable loss. In G. R. VandenBos and B. X. Bryant (Eds.), *Cataclysms, crises and catastrophes: Psychology in action* (pp. 198–235). Washington, DC: American Psychological Association.

Wortman, C. B., & Silver, R. C. (1989). The myths of coping with loss. *Journal of Consulting and Clinical Psychology, 57,* 349–357.

Yochelson, L. (1969). The emotional problems of men in the mature years and beyond. *Journal of American Geriatrics Society, 17*(9), 855–860.

Young, M., Benjamin, B., & Wallace, C. (1963). The mortality of widowers. *Lancet, I,* 454–456.

Zick, C. D., & Smith, K. R. (1986). Immediate and delayed effects of widowhood on poverty: Patterns from the 1970's. *The Gerontologist, 26,* 669–675.

Zisook, S., & DeVaul, R. A. (1984). Measuring acute grief. *Psychiatric Medicine, 2,* 169–176.

Zisook, S., & DeVaul, R. A. (1985). Unresolved grief. *American Journal of Psychoanalysis, 45,* 370–379.

Zisook, S., & Shuchter, S. R. (1985). Time course of spousal bereavement. *General Hospital Psychiatry, 7,* 95–100.

Zisook, S., & Shuchter, S. R. (1986). First four years of widowhood. *Psychiatric Annals, 16,* 288.

Zisook, S., Shuchter, S. R., & Lyons, L. E. (1987). Predictors of psychological reactions during the early stages of widowhood. *Psychiatric Clinics of North America, 10*(3), 355–369.

Author Index

Subject Index